Bacterial Immunoglobulin-Binding Proteins
Volume 2

VOLUME 2

Bacterial Immunoglobulin-Binding Proteins

Applications in Immunotechnology

Edited by

Michael D. P. Boyle
Department of Microbiology
Medical College of Ohio
Toledo, Ohio

Academic Press, Inc.
Harcourt Brace Jovanovich, Publishers
San Diego   New York   Boston
London   Sydney   Tokyo   Toronto

NOTE: The University of Florida holds patents for the isolation and use of type IIb and type III Fc-binding proteins. These patents have been licensed to Gator Microbiologicals, Inc., a company in which Drs. Boyle and Faulmann have a financial interest. Although we do not believe that this has influenced our interpretation of any of the data presented in this volume, we believe that the reader should be aware of this interest.

This book is printed on acid-free paper.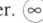

Copyright © 1990 by Academic Press, Inc.
All Rights Reserved.
No part of this publication may be reproduced or transmitted in any form or by any means, electronic or mechanical, including photocopy, recording, or any information storage and retrieval system, without permission in writing from the publisher.

Academic Press, Inc.
San Diego, California 92101

United Kingdom Edition published by
Academic Press Limited
24–28 Oval Road, London NW1 7DX

Library of Congress Cataloging-in-Publication Data

(Revised for vol. 2)

Bacterial immunoglobulin-binding proteins.

   Includes bibliographical references.
   Contents: v. 1. Microbiology, chemistry, and
biology -- v. 2. Applications in immunotechnology.
   1. Bacterial immunoglobulin-binding proteins.
I. Boyle, Michael D. P. [DNLM: 1. Bacterial Proteins.
2. Carrier Proteins. 3. Immunoglobulins. 4. Receptors,
Immunologic.   QW 601 B131]
QR92.I4B33   1990   616'.014   89-6995
ISBN   0-12-123011-2 (v. 1 : alk. paper)
ISBN   0-12-123012-0 (v. 2 : alk. paper)

Printed in the United States of America
90 91 92 93   9 8 7 6 5 4 3 2 1

Contents

Contributors   xv
Preface   xvii

1   Introduction to bacterial immunoglobulin-binding proteins
Michael D. P. Boyle
    I. Introduction   1
    II. The Distribution and Functional Reactivity of Bacterial IgG Fc-Binding Proteins   3
    III. Bacterial IgG-Binding Proteins   4
    IV. Second Generation Immunoglobulin-Binding Proteins   15
    V. Summary   18
    References   18

2   Detection and enhancement of expression of bacterial cell surface immunoglobulin-binding proteins
Kathleen J. Reis and Michael D. P. Boyle
    I. Introduction   23
    II. Preparation of Bacteria   24
    III. Standardization of Bacteria   25
    IV. Assays for the Detection of Immunoglobulin-Binding Proteins   26
    V. Direct Binding of Immunoglobulins to Bacteria   29
    VI. Direct Binding Assay   30
    VII. Absorption of IgG by Bacteria   31
    VIII. Dot Blot Procedure   34
    IX. Methods to Enhance Immunoglobulin-Binding Proteins   37
    X. Mouse Passage   37
    XI. Colony Blot Selection   39
    XII. Storage of Strains   45
    XIII. Conclusions   46
    References   47

3 Extraction and monitoring of soluble immunoglobulin-binding proteins
Michael D. P. Boyle, Kathleen J. Reis, Ronald A. Otten, and Ervin L. Faulmann

  I. Introduction   49
 II. Extraction Procedures   50
III. Secreted IgG-Binding Proteins   55
 IV. Summary   68
    References   69

4 Isolation and functional characterization of bacterial immunoglobulin-binding proteins
Michael D. P. Boyle, Kathleen J. Reis, and Ervin L. Faulmann

   I. Introduction   71
  II. Selection of Immunoglobulin Source to Prepare Affinity Columns   72
 III. Nature of the Sample to Be Purified   73
  IV. Selection of Eluting Agent   74
   V. Affinity Purification of a Type III Fc-Binding Protein Solubilized by Bacteriophage Lysis of the Group C Streptococcus 26RP66   75
  VI. Characterization of Affinity-Purified Immunoglobulin-Binding Proteins   77
 VII. Comparison of Functional Activities of Fc-Binding Proteins   82
VIII. Summary   87
     References   88

5 Determination of protein-binding affinities among bacterial cell surface proteins
Lars Björck and Bo Åkerström

  I. Introduction   91
 II. Binding of Mammalian Proteins to Bacterial Surfaces: Screening Procedures   92
III. Solubilization of Immunoglobulin-Binding Bacterial Surface Proteins   93
 IV. Determination of Immunoglobulin-Binding Protein in Low Concentrations   96
  V. Analysis of the Binding Immunoglobulins and Other Host Proteins to Purified, Bacterial Surface Proteins   97
 VI. Determination of the Affinity Constant for Binding between a Bacterial Cell Wall Protein and Its Ligand   100
    References   104

6 Production of polyclonal antibodies to immunoglobulin-binding proteins
Kathleen J. Reis and Michael D. P. Boyle

    I. Introduction   105
    II. Selection of the Species of Animal to Immunize   105
    III. Preparation of Immunogen and Immunization   107
    IV. Kinetics of Antibody Production   108
    V. Detection of Antibody to Immunoglobulin-Binding Proteins   110
    VI. Conclusion   123
    References   123

7 Use of radiolabeled bacterial Fc-binding proteins as tracers for soluble antigens
Ervin L. Faulmann

    I. Introduction   125
    II. Competitive Inhibition Radioimmunoassay   127
    III. Summary   142
    References   142

8 Application of enzyme-labeled IgG-binding proteins in immunoassay
Kathleen J. Reis and Michael D. P. Boyle

    I. Introduction   145
    II. Types of Assays   147
    III. Preparation of Immunoglobulin Fc-Binding Protein–Enzyme Conjugate Tracers   149
    IV. Development of an ELISA to Quantify Human IgA Using a Type III Fc-Binding Protein–Alkaline Phosphatase Conjugate as Tracer   152
    V. Summary   159
    References   160

9 Use of Fc-binding proteins to identify cell surface and secreted antigens associated with group B streptococci
L. Jeannine Brady, Corey Musselman, Colleen Chun, Elia M. Ayoub, and Michael D. P. Boyle

    I. Introduction   161
    II. Group B Streptococcal Typing Nomenclature   162
    III. Two-Stage Radioimmunoassay for Detection of Group B Streptococcal Type-Specific Antigens   163

IV. Adaptation of the Two-Stage RIA to a Dot Blot Assay 172
V. Adaptation of the Two-Stage RIA to an ELISA Typing Procedure 175
VI. Summary 177
References 177

10 Application of Fc-binding proteins for the detection of specific antibodies
Michael D. P. Boyle, Michael J. P. Lawman, and Adrian P. Gee

I. Introduction 181
II. Development of an Assay for Antibodies to a Soluble Antigen 183
III. Detection of Antibodies to Tumor-Associated Antigens 186
IV. Detection of Rabbit IgM Antibodies to Sheep Erythrocytes 190
V. Summary 194
References 195

11 Use of fluorescent-conjugated bacterial immunoglobulin-binding proteins
Stephen N. Sisson

I. Standard Methods 197
II. Conjugation Method Using GMBS 200
III. Comparison of Recombinant Protein G to Wild Type Protein G Isolated from *Streptococcus* Cell Membranes 201
References 203

12 Biotinylated IgG binding proteins—doubly versatile
Laurence J. McIntyre

I. Introduction 205
II. Biotinylation of IgG-Binding Protein 208
III. Immunohistochemical Staining Using Biotinylated IgG-Binding Proteins 209
References 214

13 Use of IgG-binding proteins in immunoelectronmicroscopy
Sylvia E. Coleman

I. Introduction 217
II. Preparation of Colloidal Gold 217
III. Coupling of Proteins to Colloidal Gold 221

- IV. Use of Gold-Labeling for Localization of Immunoglobulin-Binding Sites and Antigen–Antibody Complexes in Bacteria   225
- V. Double Labeling Techniques with Different Sizes of Colloidal Gold to Localize Two Different Antigens on Thin Sections   231
- VI. Streptavidin/Avidin–Biotin Labeling for Detection of Immunoglobulin-Binding Proteins   236
- VII. Replica Method with Plasma Polymerization Film by Glow Discharge for Three-Dimensional Demonstration of Colloidal Gold Particles   240
- VIII. General Applications of Colloidal Gold Labeling   246
  References   246

14 The use of bacterial Fc-binding proteins as probes for antigen–antibody complexes immobilized on nitrocellulose membranes
Ervin L. Faulmann

- I. Dot Blot Assay   250
- II. Colony and Plaque Blotting of Antigens Expressed by Bacteria   258
- III. Western Blot Analysis   263
- IV. Summary   269
  References   270

15 Application of bacteria expressing immunoglobulin-binding proteins to immunoprecipitation reactions
Michael D. P. Boyle and Ervin L. Faulmann

- I. Introduction   273
- II. General Background   274
- III. Preparation of Bacterial Immunosorbent Reagents   275
- IV. Practical Applications Using Bacterial Immunosorbents   279
- V. Summary   287
  References   287

16 Use of bacteria expressing immunoglobulin-binding proteins in coagglutination assays
Kathleen J. Reis, Michael J. P. Lawman, and Michael D. P. Boyle

- I. Introduction   291
- II. Detection of Cell-Bound Antigens   293

- III. Detection of Specific Antibody 294
- IV. Procedure for Establishing a Coagglutination Assay to Measure a Polyvalent Soluble Antigen 296
- V. Summary 298
  - References 298

17 Utilization of whole bacteria expressing IgG-binding proteins to detect cell surface antigens
Edward J. Siden

- I. Introduction 301
- II. Reagents and Equipment 302
- III. Preparation of Antibodies 304
- IV. Preparation of Anti-Immunoglobulin-Coated Bacteria 304
- V. Preparation of Hybridoma Antibody-Coated Bacteria 305
- VI. Binding Assay 305
- VII. Staining and Quantitation 306
- VIII. Variations on the Theme 307
- IX. Comments 307
  - References 308

18 Use of immobilized protein A to purify immunoglobulins
Larry Schwartz

- I. Introduction 309
- II. Overview of Purification Procedure 313
- III. Choice of Ligand 320
- IV. Choice of Matrix 321
- V. Immobilization Procedure 322
- VI. Available Binding Capacity 323
- VII. Column Preparation 324
- VIII. Sample Preparation 326
- IX. Sample Application 327
- X. Elution Procedures 328
- XI. Collection and Detection Methods 329
- XII. Column Reequilibration, Reuse, and Storage 329
- XIII. Limitations of Method 330
- XIV. General Methods Using Protein A Sepharose CL-4B and Protein A Sepharose 4 Fast Flow for Mouse and Human IgG Purification 332
  - References 337

19 Purification and quantitation of monoclonal antibodies by affinity chromatography with immobilized protein A

Susan M. Scott and Hector Juarez-Salinas

    I. Purification of IgG$_1$ Monoclonal Antibodies   341
   II. Purification of IgM Monoclonal Antibodies   343
  III. Quantitation of Monoclonal Antibodies   345
  IV. Purification of Injectable-Grade Monoclonal Antibodies   346
   V. Conclusions   352
      References   353

20 Use of immobilized protein G to isolate IgG

Barbara Webb Walker

    I. Introduction   355
   II. Determination of Optimal Conditions for Protein G Affinity Chromatography   357
  III. Examples of Affinity Chromatography Using Protein G Agarose   359
  IV. Use of Protein G Agarose to Make an Antigen-Binding Column   363
   V. Summary   366
      References   367

21 Bacterial immunoglobulin-binding proteins and complement

Michael D. P. Boyle

     I. Introduction   369
    II. Measurement of Functional Complement Activity   371
   III. Detection of Classical Pathway Complement Activity   372
   IV. Measurement of the Functional Activity of the Alternate Complement Pathway   378
    V. Application of Functional Complement Titrations to Measurement of Activity of Immunoglobulin-Binding Proteins   379
   VI. Measurement of the Generation of Complement Split Products   380
  VII. Measurement of Complement Split Products Generated as a Consequence of Complement Activation Mediated by Bacterial Immunoglobulin-Binding Proteins   386
 VIII. Studies of Binding of the First Component of Complement   387

  IX. Antigenic Determination of Complement Activation 388
  X. Analysis of Complexes Formed between Bacterial
    Immunoglobulin-Binding Proteins and IgG 388
  XI. Summary 389
    References 390

22 Activation and differentiation of human lymphocytes by bacterial Fc-binding proteins
Douglas J. Barrett

  I. Introduction 393
  II. Lymphocyte Isolation and Purification 394
 III. Assays for Lymphocyte Proliferation 396
 IV. Assays of Lymphocyte Differentiation 398
  V. Conclusion 403
   References 403

23 Measurement of *in vivo* leucocyte chemotaxis mediated by Fc-binding proteins
Michael J. P. Lawman, Adrian P. Gee, Patricia D. Lawman, and Michael D. P. Boyle

  I. Introduction 405
  II. Air Sac Procedure 406
 III. Use of Fc-Binding Proteins in the Air Sac Procedure 410
 IV. Advantages and Limitations of the Air Sac Procedure 413
   References 414

24 The cloning of streptococcal protein G genes
Stephen R. Fahnestock and Patrick Alexander

  I. Colony Immunoassay 417
  II. Streptococcal Clinical Isolates 419
 III. Preparation of Streptococcal DNA 419
 IV. Initial Gene Cloning 420
  V. Cloning of Protein G Genes from Other Isolates 423
   References 424

25 Bacterial immunoglobulin-binding proteins—future trends
Ronald A. Otten and Michael D. P. Boyle

  I. Introduction 425
  II. Role of Bacterial Immunoglobulin-Binding Proteins in Pathogenicity 429

Contents

    III. Structure–Function Relationships of Bacterial
         Fc-Binding Proteins   430
    IV. Applications Involving Immunoglobulin-Binding
         Proteins—Future Trends   442
    V. Summary   447
        References   448

Appendix

    I. General Buffers   453
    II. Iodination Buffers and Related Solutions   455
    III. ELISA Buffers and Related Solutions   456
    IV. Electrophoresis Buffers   456
    V. Buffers for Use in Applications
       Involving Nitrocellulose   458
    VI. General Buffers and Reagents   459

Index   461

Contributors

Numbers in parentheses indicate the pages on which the author's contributions begin.

Bo Åkerström (91), Department of Physiological Chemistry, University of Lund, S-223 62 Lund, Sweden

Patrick Alexander[1] (417), Genex Corporation, Gaithersburg, Maryland 20877

Elia M. Ayoub (161), Department of Pediatrics, University of Florida, College of Medicine, Gainesville, Florida 32610

Douglas J. Barrett (393), Department of Pediatrics, University of Florida, College of Medicine, Gainesville, Florida 32610

Lars Björck (91), Department of Medical Microbiology, University of Lund, S-223 62 Lund, Sweden

Michael D. P. Boyle (1, 23, 49, 71, 105, 145, 161, 181, 273, 291, 369, 405, 425), Department of Microbiology, Medical College of Ohio, Toledo, Ohio 43699

L. Jeannine Brady (161), Department of Oral Biology, University of Florida, College of Dentistry, Gainesville, Florida 32610

Colleen Chun (161), Department of Pediatrics, University of Florida, College of Medicine, Gainesville, Florida 32610

Sylvia E. Coleman (217), Department of Microbiology and Cell Science, University of Florida, Gainesville, Florida 32610

Stephen R. Fahnestock[2] (417), Genex Corporation, Gaithersburg, Maryland 20877

---

[1] Present address: Center for Advanced Research in Biotechnology, Gaithersburg, Maryland 20877.

[2] Present address: National Institute of General Medical Sciences, Bethesda, Maryland.

Ervin L. Faulmann (49, 71, 125, 249, 273), Department of Microbiology, Medical College of Ohio, Toledo, Ohio 43699

Adrian P. Gee (181, 405), Baxter Health Care Corporation, Fenwal Division, Santa Ana, California 92705

Hector Juarez-Salinas (341), Chromatography Business Unit, Bio-Rad Laboratories, Richmond, California 94806

Michael J. P. Lawman (181, 291, 405), Department of Immunology and Medical Microbiology, University of Florida, College of Medicine, Gainesville, Florida 32610

Patricia D. Lawman (405), Department of Oral Biology, College of Medicine, and Department of Immunology/Medical Microbiology, College of Dentistry, University of Florida, Gainesville, Florida 32610

Lawrence J. McIntyre (205), Vector Laboratories, Inc., Burlingame, California 94010

Corey Musselman (161), Department of Immunology and Medical Microbiology, University of Florida, College of Medicine, Gainesville, Florida 32610

Ronald A. Otten (49, 425), Department of Microbiology, Medical College of Ohio, Toledo, Ohio 43699

Kathleen J. Reis[3] (23, 49, 71, 105, 145, 291), Department of Large Animal Clinical Sciences, College of Veterinary Medicine, University of Florida, Gainesville, Florida 32610

Larry Schwartz (309), Technical Service, Pharmacia LKB Biotechnology Inc., Piscataway, New Jersey 08854

Susan M. Scott (341), Chromatography Business Unit, Bio-Rad Laboratories, Richmond, California 94806

Edward J. Siden (301), Division of Clinical Immunology, Department of Medicine, Mount Sinai School of Medicine, New York, New York 10029

Stephen N. Sisson (197), Cascade Immunology Corporation, Springfield, Oregon 97478

Barbara Webb Walker (355), Genex Corporation, Gaithersburg, Maryland 20877

---

[3] Present address: Genex Corporation, 16020 Industrial Drive, Gaithersburg, Maryland 20877.

Preface

Volume 1 brought together in a single book the current state of knowledge of bacterial immunoglobulin-binding proteins. In this volume the focus is on practical approaches to isolation, characterization, and use of these binding proteins. The majority of these studies involve the type I Fc-binding protein (staphylococcal protein A) and the type III Fc-binding protein (streptococcal protein G). These proteins represent the prototypes of a larger family of functionally related bacterial immunoglobulin-binding proteins. The applications described in this volume for the prototype molecules should be adaptable to any new selective binding proteins that become available. An attempt has been made by all the contributors to provide sufficient information to enable any investigator to use bacterial IgG-binding proteins for the specific purpose described without having to consult any secondary references. In addition, the limitations of individual techniques and practical problems experienced by investigators have been stressed. Although it is noted in many of the chapters in this volume, I would like to remind the reader that the species and subclass reactivity of bacterial immunoglobulin-binding proteins is not absolute. In particular, with monoclonal antibodies it is not always possible to predict reactivity just by knowing isotype and subclass.

Finally, I would like to thank the following people: everyone in my laboratory who has contributed to the techniques and methods described; my wife, Carla, and my children, Kieron and Sarah, for their long suffering during the compilation; and my secretary, Shirley Doherty, who battled my handwriting to get this volume to the publisher.

Michael D. P. Boyle

CHAPTER 1

Introduction to bacterial immunoglobulin-binding proteins

Michael D. P. Boyle

I. Introduction

In the early part of the twentieth century, Landsteiner observed that red cells from one individual could be agglutinated by serum from certain other individuals. These findings led to the understanding of blood group antigens and the birth of serological tests for identifying antigens on cells. This hemagglutination assay is still widely used today as the basis for rapid screening and typing assays in blood banks. With the recognition that specific antibodies could neutralize toxins (von Behring and Kitasato, 1890) or cause selective precipitation of soluble antigens (Heidelberger and Kendall, 1932), semiqualitative methods for identifying antigens and antibodies were developed. More recently, the sensitivity of antigen or antibody detection has been increased with the development of radioimmunoassays (RIA) (Yallow and Benson, 1960) and enzyme-linked immunosorbent assays (ELISA) (Engvall and Perlmann, 1971, 1972). These techniques now enable the determination of absolute levels of antigens or antibodies in the nanomolar range or below and have found broad applications for clinical diagnostic procedures and in forensic medicine.

In 1975, Kohler and Milstein described a method for fusing myeloma cells with spleen cells from immunized mice that enabled the selection of a hybrid cell line that produced large quantities of a single antibody. This monoclonal antibody technology has the potential to allow antibodies specific for any desired epitope to be produced. This technology has had a profound impact on immunotechnology and has enabled the development of many new antibody-based detection systems. In particular, the production of monoclonal antibodies to T cell surface markers (Reinherz et al., 1979) coupled with the development of the fluorescence-activated cell sorter has revolutionized many aspects of clinical immunology (for review see Shapiro, 1985; Ault, 1986; Jackson and Warner, 1986). The ability to relate the phenotypes of lymphocytes to their functions, based on their reactivities with specific monoclonal antibodies that recognize surface glycoproteins or cluster determinants, has enabled the clinical immunologist to identify and characterize a variety of acquired and inherited immunodeficiency disorders (for review see Giorgi, 1986). In particular, the inversion of the ratio of CD4 to CD8 T lymphocytes in patients with acquired immunodeficiency syndrome (AIDS) is now characteristic for that disease (Centers for Disease Control (CDC), 1982; Rosenberg and Fauci, 1989).

Over the past decade more sophisticated methods of quantifying and characterizing antigens in complex mixtures and on cell surfaces have been developed. All of these methods require the ability to produce and isolate monospecific antibodies (monoclonal or polyclonal) and to detect these antibodies when complexed with their specific antigens. Proteins can be separated on sodium dodecyl sulfate (SDS)-polyacrylamide gels by virtue of their size. The proteins can then be transferred to nitrocellulose and probed with specific antibody to identify individual antigens, allowing them to be both quantified and characterized for size heterogeneity (Towbin et al., 1979). These Western blotting approaches are now finding wide use both for research applications and for immunodiagnostic purposes. With the increased interest in immunotechnology for analytic methods, quantitative determination of antigens, measurement of antibodies, and monitoring and isolation of specific immunoglobulins, much interest has focused on reagents that facilitate these immunological techniques. Bacterial immunoglobulin-binding proteins represent such a family of valuable immunological reagents (Langone, 1978, 1982b; Langone et al., 1977, 1979; Boyle, 1984; Boyle and Reis, 1987; Forsgren et al., 1983; Richman, 1983; Duboid-Dalcq et al., 1977; Chang et al., 1984; Goding, 1978; Gee and Langone, 1981). The purpose of this volume is to provide a practical guide to the uses of bacterial immunoglobulin-binding proteins, in particular those that bind selectively to constant regions of immunoglobulin molecules, without interfering with the ability of the antibody to bind to its specific antigen. The selection and isolation of these unique groups of bacterial proteins and their application both to the isolation of antibody molecules and to the detection of antigen–antibody complexes will be described in detail. In this chapter, a brief survey of bacterial immunoglobulin-binding proteins and their reactivities is presented. For a more comprehensive treatment, see Volume 1 of this series.

II. The Distribution and Functional Reactivity of Bacterial IgG Fc-Binding Proteins

Bacterial Fc-binding proteins have been found on the surface of a variety of streptococci and staphylococci, and more recently on other organisms (Tables 1 and 2). Bacteria expressing IgG-binding proteins have been detected by a variety of methods, including their ability to agglutinate red cells that have been sensitized with subagglutinating doses of specific antibody and their ability to bind labeled IgG via regions of the immunoglobulin molecule not involved in specific antigen recognition (Chapter 2). Early studies using different species and subclasses of IgG, have demonstrated five distinct patterns of IgG binding to intact bacteria, which led Myhre and Kronvall (1981) to propose a functional classification for bacterial IgG Fc-binding proteins (Figure 1). More recently, we have identified a bacterial isolate that demonstrates a sixth profile of binding to IgG from different mammalian species and we have designated this reactivity as type VI (Figure 1). All of these different functional types of immunoglobulin-binding proteins appear to be mediated by antigenically

TABLE 1
Bacterial IgG Fc-Binding Proteins[a]

Type	Bacterial species	References
Type I	*Staphylococcus aureus* (protein A)	Forsgren and Sjöquist (1966); Sjöquist *et al.* (1972); Langone (1982a)
Type II	Group A streptococci	Havlicek (1978); Grubb *et al.* (1982); Yarnall and Boyle (1986a–c)
Type III	*Streptococcus equisimilus* (group C) *Streptococcus dysgalactiae* (group C) Human group G streptococci Human group G streptococci	Reis *et al.* (1984a,b) Björck and Kronvall (1984)
Type IV	Bovine β-hemolytic group G streptococci	Myhre *et al.* (1979); Reis *et al.* (1990)
Type V	*Streptococcus zooepidemicus* (group C)	Myhre and Kronvall (1980); Yarnall and Widders (1990)
Type VI	*Streptococcus zooepidemicus* (group C) #S212	Reis *et al.* (1988)

[a] Classification originally proposed by Myhre and Kronvall (1981) with the addition of type VI proposed by Reis *et al.* (1988).

TABLE 2
Types of Bacteria that Bind Immunoglobulin in a Nonimmune Fashion

Bacteria	IgG	IgM	IgA	IgD	IgE	References
Streptococcus, Group B			+			Russell-Jones et al. (1984); Brady and Boyle (1989)
	+	+				Jürgens et al. (1987)
Branhamella catarrhalis			+			Forsgren and Grubb (1979)
Clostridium perfringens	+	+	+			Lindahl and Kronvall (1988)
Taylorella equigenitalis	+	+				Widders et al. (1985)
Brucella abortus		(+)[a]				Nielsen et al. (1981)
Coprococcus comes	+					Van der Merwe and Stegeman (1988)
Peptococcus magnus	+	+	+	+	+	Myhre and Erntell (1985) Björck (1988)
Haemophilus somnus	+					Yarnall et al. (1988)

[a] Reactivity limited to a subgroup of bovine IgM antibodies.

distinct proteins (Boyle and Reis, 1990) and are associated with distinct bacterial species (Table 1).

In addition to the six types of bacterial IgG-binding proteins, immunoglobulin-binding proteins for other immunoglobulin isotypes have been identified on other bacteria (Table 2). The properties of these various types of bacterial immunoglobulin-binding proteins are summarized in Section III.

III. Bacterial IgG-Binding Proteins

The chemistry, microbiology, and functional activity of these molecules have been reviewed in a comprehensive manner in Volume 1 of this series. In the next section of this chapter, the properties of certain of these molecules are summarized briefly with respect to their practical values in immunotechnology.

A. Type I

The type I Fc-binding protein is found on the majority of *Staphylococcus aureus* strains and more frequently designated as staphylococcal

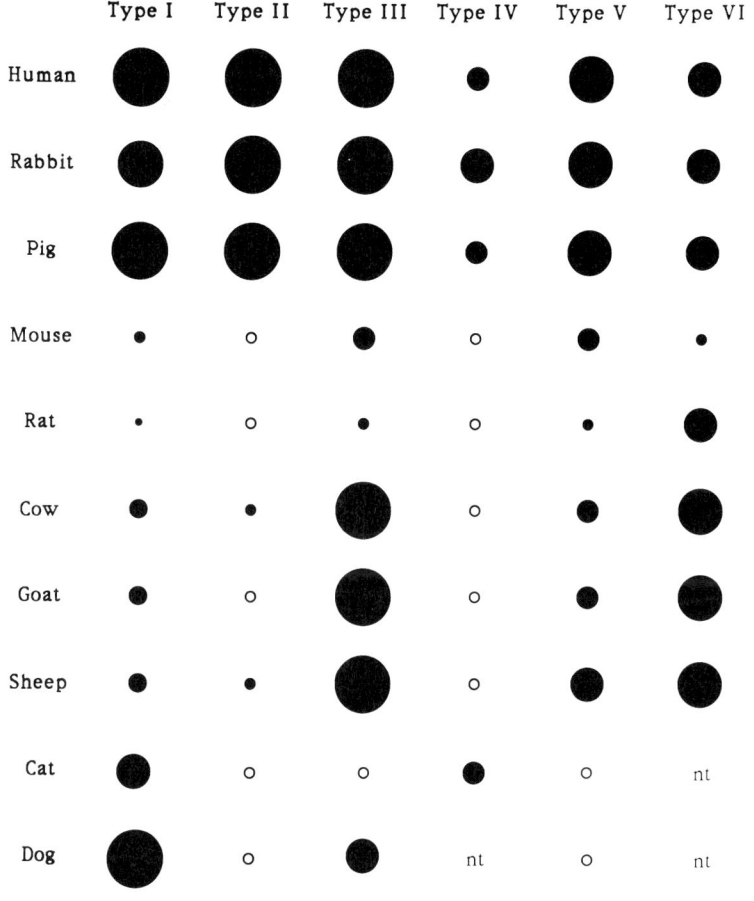

FIGURE 1
Profile of species reactivities of different bacterial IgG-binding protein types. Larger clots represent greater binding activity; o, no reactivity, nt, not tested. Note these reactivities have been determined using polyclonal IgG preparations. Occasional differences have been noted in the reactivity of samples from individual animals. (Reproduced with permission from Boyle and Reis 1990.)

protein A. This protein has been extensively characterized (for review see Langone, 1982a; Boyle, 1990) and the gene coding for it has been cloned and sequenced (Duggleby and Jones, 1983; Uhlén *et al.*, 1984; Löfdahl *et al.*, 1983; Guss *et al.*, 1990). Protein A's binding activity to a variety of different species, classes, and subclasses has been well documented (Tables 3 and 4).

TABLE 3
Comparison of Species Reactivities[a] of the Isolated Type I (Protein A) and Type III (Protein G) Bacterial Fc-Binding Proteins[b]

Species	Type I Fc-Binding Protein (Protein A)	Type III Fc-Binding Protein (Protein G)
Rabbit	+++[c]	+++
Human	++++[d]	++++
Pig	+++	++++
Goat	+[e]	+++
Sheep	+	+++
Cow	+	+++
Dog	+++	+
Rat	0[f]	0
Mouse	++[g]	++
Horse	++	+++

[a] Derived from studies by Langone et al. (1977); Langone (1978); Reis et al. (1984b); and unpublished results from our laboratories. Note that these reactivities have been determined in most cases using polyclonal IgG preparations. However, occasional differences have been noted in the reactivity of samples

[b] The quantity of IgG required to inhibit binding of ^{125}I-labeled Fc-binding proteins by 50% in a competitive binding assay was used.

[c] +++ = > 100 < 1,000 ng
[d] ++++ = < 100 ng
[e] + = > 10,000 < 80,000 ng
[f] 0 = > 50,000 ng
[g] ++ = > 1,000 < 10,000 ng

Protein A was first introduced into the market place as the wild type product by Pharmacia (Piscataway, New Jersey) in 1978. Since that time many commercial sources of the wild type protein have become available. Most commercial protein A preparations contain a single predominant form of the immunoglobulin-binding protein with a molecular weight of approximately 45,000, as well as a number of minor, lower molecular weight breakdown products. Many of these wild type products contain a staphylococcal enterotoxin, which may prove to be a confounding factor in analyzing protein A's reported mitogenic activities for mammalian lymphocytes (Schrezenmeier and Fleischer, 1987; Barrett, 1990). Recombinant forms of protein A are also commercially available and can be obtained from a variety of companies. In addition to the isolated protein, a variety of immobilized and tracer forms of protein A are commercially

TABLE 4
Comparison[a] of Subclass Reactivities of the Type I (Protein A) and Type III (Protein G) Bacterial Fc-Binding Proteins[b]

Species		Type I Receptors (Protein A)	Type III Receptors (Protein G)
Human	IgG_1	+++[c]	+++
	IgG_2	+++	+++
	IgG_3	[d]	+++
	IgG_4	+++	+++
	IgA	[e]	—[f]
	IgM	[e]	—
Mouse	IgG_1	+[g]	+
	IgG_{2a}	++	+++
	IgG_{2b}	++	+++
	IgG_3	++	+++
Cow	IgG_1	—	++
	IgG_2	+	+++
Sheep	IgG_1	—	++
	IgG_2	+	+++
Goat	IgG_1	+/−	++
	IgG_2	+	+++
Horse	IgG(ab)	+	+++
	IgG(c)	+	+++
Dog	IgG	+	not tested
	IgM	+	not tested
	IgA	+	not tested

[a] The majority of these studies have been carried out with myeloma proteins and many instances have been noted in which the expected reactivity with a given mammalian subclass was not observed. This has been particularly evident in studies of mouse monoclonal antibodies (see Chapters 18 and 19). Consequently, this table should only be used as a guide for probable reactivities. Each antibody should be checked directly for reactivity with protein A or protein G prior to its use for any immunochemical procedure (see Chapter 15).
[b] Derived from studies by Reis et al. (1984b); Boyle et al. (1985); Wallner et al. (1987).
[c] +++ = indicates strong reactivity.
[d] Certain IgG_3 allotypes have been reported to react with the type I Fc-binding protein (Haake et al., 1982).
[e] Certain IgM and IgA samples have been reported to react with protein A (Harboe and Fölliny, 1974; Inganäs, 1981).
[f] − = indicates no reactivity.
[g] + = indicates weak reactivity.

available. A representative listing of these products is presented in Table 5. (For a complete listing of commercial sources of protein A and related products, see Linscott, 1989).

Protein A is the prototype IgG-binding protein and has been used extensively for many immunochemical procedures (see reviews by Langone, 1978, 1982b; Goding, 1978). Throughout this volume, many examples of the use of protein A in immunotechnology are presented and the reader should refer to individual chapters for detailed methodology.

TABLE 5
Commercially Available Protein A Derivatives[a]

Free protein
  Wild type protein A
  Recombinant protein A

Tracer forms
  Radiolabeled protein A (^{125}I, ^{131}I, ^{3}H, ^{35}S)
  Enzyme-labeled protein A derivatives
  Alkaline phosphatase
  β-galactosidase
  Urease
  Horseradish peroxidase
  Peroxidase
  Glucose oxidase

Immobilized protein A for use in immunoglobulin isolation and purification
  Agarose
  Silica
  Sepharose
  Acrylic

Immunoelectron microscopy/immunohistochemicals
  Biotinylated
  Gold-labeled
  Silver-labeled
  Ferritin-labeled

Fluorescent protein A derivatives
  Fluorescein isothiocyanote (FITC)-labeled
  Texas red-labeled
  Phycoerythrin-labeled
  Rhodamine-labeled

Immobilized protein A suitable for use in immunoprecipitation
  Formalin-fixed protein A positive *Staphylococcus aureus*
  Protein A-coated magnetic microspheres
  (See also reagents for immunoglobulin isolation and purification)

---

[a] For a list of commercial suppliers, see *Linscott's Directory of Immunological and Biological Reagents, Fifth Edition* (1989) or *Am. Chem. . . .* , The American Chemical Society, Washington, D.C., *American Chemical Society Guide to Biotechnology* (1990).

B. Type II

The type II immunoglobulin-binding activity is associated with certain group A strains. Unlike the type I-binding protein (protein A), relatively little information is available on type II IgG-binding proteins. The type II proteins appear to be a family of immunoglobulin-binding molecules associated with group A strains (Boyle *et al.*, 1990). Some isolates display surface binding proteins capable of binding all four human IgG subclasses, while others display more limited reactivity (Faulmann and Boyle, 1990; Ravdonikas *et al.*, 1984; Wagner *et al.*, 1983). The isolated proteins from group A strains also display heterogeneity. A single protein responsible for all of the IgG-binding activities of the bacteria has been isolated from several group A strains (Grubb *et al.*, 1982; Havlicek, 1978; Schalen and Christensen, 1990), while for other strains the reactivity has been shown to be the sum of two independently expressed surface proteins designated type IIa and type IIb. The IIa-binding protein reacts with human IgG_1, IgG_2, and IgG_4, in addition to rabbit and sheep IgG (Yarnall and Boyle, 1986a-c). The type IIb binds exclusively to human IgG_3 (Yarnall and Boyle, 1986b,c). Recently, a type II IgG-binding protein with the functional activities of a type IIa protein has been cloned (Heath and Cleary, 1987; Cleary and Heath, 1990; Heath *et al.*, 1990). The current state of IgG-binding proteins associated with group A streptococcal strains has been reviewed recently (Boyle *et al.*, 1990; Faulmann and Boyle, 1990; Schalen and Christensen, 1990). At this time there are no commercial sources of wild type or recombinant type II IgG-binding proteins and no studies describing the use of type II IgG-binding proteins for practical applications have been reported. The specificity of a bacterial binding protein for human IgG_3 (type IIb) does have potential applications for isolating and for quantifying IgG_3-specific immune responses.

C. Type III

The type III IgG-binding protein, frequently designated as streptococcal protein G, is found on the surface of most human groups C and G streptococcal isolates. This type III IgG-binding protein has the greatest range of species and subclass reactivity of any bacterial immunoglobulin-binding protein. (Figure 1; Tables 3 and 4). The wild type form of the protein has been isolated from both group C (Reis *et al.*, 1984a,b, 1985, 1986) and group G (Björck and Kronvall, 1984; Åkerström and Björck, 1986) streptococcal isolates and a number of investigators have cloned the gene for the type III immunoglobulin-binding protein from three separate human group G isolates (Fahnestock *et al.*, 1986; Guss *et al.*, 1986; Fipula *et al.*, 1987). For a comprehensive review of the molecular biology, chemistry, and functional activities of type III immunoglobulin-binding proteins, see Reis and Boyle (1990a), Björck and Åkerström (1990a), and Fahnestock et al. (1990).

The type III Fc-binding protein was first introduced commercially in 1987 as the wild type protein by Calbiochem (La Jolla, California). This material displays all of the species reactivity associated with the bacterial-bound type III Fc-binding proteins (Figure 1; Tables 3 and 4), in addition to showing affinity for human, baboon, and horse albumin (Table 6). This product shows no significant reactivity with goat, sheep, cow, or mouse albumin (Table 6). In an elegant series of experiments, Björck and colleagues have demonstrated that the albumin-binding domains are distinct from the IgG-binding domains on protein G (Björck et al., 1987; Åkerström et al., 1987; Sjöbring et al., 1988). Our own studies demonstrate that the presence of a 10–50 M excess of human serum albumin does not affect the ability of protein G to bind to IgG (Faulmann et al., 1989). In addition, Sjöbring et al. (1989) have reported that protein G has an affinity for human α_2 macroglobulin. The exact site on the molecule to which this serum protease inhibitor binds has not as yet been defined.

TABLE 6
Reactivity of Different Sources of Protein G with Various Species of Albumin[a]

Species of Albumin	Binding Reactivity		
	Wild type protein G (Calbiochem, La Jolla, California)	Recombinant protein G (Genex, Gaithersburg, Maryland)	Recombinant protein G (Pharmacia, Piscataway, New Jersey)
Human	++[b]	o[c]	o
Baboon	++	o	o
Guinea pig	++	o	o
Mouse	±[d]	o	o
Horse	±	o	o
Goat	o	o	o
Cow	o	o	o
Sheep	o	o	o

[a] (Reproduced from Faulmann et al., 1989, Journal of Immunological Methods **123**, 269–281, with permission.)
[b] ++, indicates a band on the autoradiograph could be detected after a 6 hr exposure to X-ray film at $-70°C$.
[c] o, indicates no reactivity following a 36 hr exposure to X-ray film at $-70°C$.
[d] ±, Indicates a weak band on the autoradiograph could be detected following a 36 hr exposure to X-ray film at $-70°C$.

In 1988, a number of forms of recombinant protein G became commercially available. Each of these products has been genetically engineered to eliminate or minimize the selective human albumin-binding properties of protein G. There is considerable variation in the size of the recombinant forms of protein G (M_r 56,000–28,000), as well as differences in their binding capacities for various species of IgG (Figure 2).

A second wild type protein G product was also introduced by Sigma Chemical Company (St. Louis, Missouri). This product was isolated by enzymatic digestion of a type III Fc-binding protein positive group C streptococcus and has a molecular weight of approximately 18,000 (Figure 2). This material was not as stable as either the original wild type product or any of the recombinant proteins (Faulmann *et al.*, 1989). The differences in physicochemical and functional properties of the two wild type products can be attributed to their methods of extraction. The N-terminal sequence of each form of the wild type protein is presented in Table 7. The higher molecular weight wild type protein available from Calbiochem contains the native N-terminal sequence predicted from analysis of the complete nucleotide sequence of the protein G gene of strain GX7809 (Fahnestock *et al.*, 1986). By contrast, the trypsin-extracted material from the group C strain 26RP66 represents a fragment of the molecule at starting amino acid residue #166. It is of interest that the amino acid sequences of the

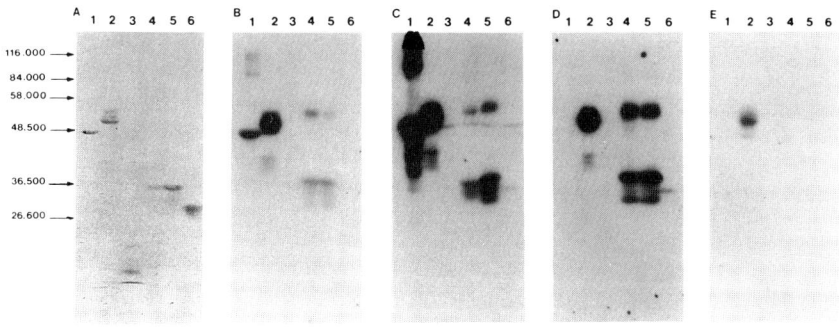

FIGURE 2
SDS-polyacrylamide gel electrophoresis (PAGE) analysis of various forms of protein G probed with radiolabeled IgG and human serum albumin. (A) Coomassie blue-stained gel. (B) Western blot probed with human IgG Fc. (C) Western blot probed with rabbit IgG Fc. (D) Western blot probed with goat IgG. (E) Western blot probed with human serum albumin. Lane 1, protein A. Lane 2, wild type protein G (Calbiochem, La Jolla, California). Lane 3, wild type protein G (Sigma, St. Louis, Missouri). Lane 4, recombinant protein G (Genex; Gaithersburg, Maryland). Lane 5, recombinant protein G (Perstorp, Lund, Sweden). Lane 6, recombinant protein G (Pharmacia, Piscataway, New Jersey). (Reproduced with permission from Faulmann *et al.*, 1989.)

TABLE 7
N-Terminal Sequence of Type III Fc-Binding Proteins and Fragments[a]

Wild type protein G
Val-Asp-Ser-Pro-Ile-Glu-Asp-Thr-Pro-Ile

Trypsin fragment from group C strain 26RP66
Ser-Glu-Thr-Pro-Ala-Glu-Asp-Thr-Val-Lys-Ser-Leu-Glu

Papain fragment from group G strain G148
Ser-Glu-Thr-Pro-Ala-Glu-Asp-Thr-Val-Lys-Ser-Leu-Glu

[a] Data compiled from Reis et al. (1986) and unpublished data from my laboratory.

trypsin fragment of group C streptococcus 26RP66 and the papain extract of strain G148 have been found to be identical (Reis et al., 1986).

In studying the various commercially available forms of protein G, we have observed some batch-to-batch variation, evidence for heterogeneity, and differences in stability on freezing and thawing. In our initial studies with the type III Fc-binding protein, we observed that the most homogeneous form of the protein, isolated by trypsin or papain digestion (Reis et al., 1985; von Mering and Boyle, 1986), was not as stable as the heterogeneous group of functionally and antigenically related proteins recovered following bacteriophage lysis of the group C streptococcus 26RP66 (Reis et al., 1984a,b). In general, there are considerable differences in the reactivities and properties of different sources of protein G and caution should be exercised in this regard. This is particularly important if protein G is to be used for mitogenic studies (Barrett, 1990). A detailed comparison of a number of commercially available forms of protein G has been published by Faulmann and colleagues (1989). It is advisable to consult this paper to determine the suitability of each different source of protein G for each potential application. In addition to free protein G, a variety of immobilized and tracer forms of the protein G molecule are commercially available. A representative listing of protein G-related products is presented in Table 8.

Although the practical applications of protein G have not been as extensively studied as protein A, this bacterial binding protein is now being used extensively for immunochemical applications. Based on its wider species and subclass reactivity (Tables 3 and 4), protein G is superior to protein A for many applications, in particular those involving sheep, goat, and cow immunoglobulins.

TABLE 8
Commercially Available Protein G Derivatives[a]

Free protein
  Wild type protein G
  Recombinant protein G

Tracer forms
  Radiolabeled protein G (^{125}I)

  Enzyme-labeled protein G derivatives

  Alkaline phosphatase
  Horseradish peroxidase

Immobilized protein G for use in immunoglobulin isolation and purification
  Agarose
  Sepharose

Immunoelectron microscopy/immunohistochemicals
  Biotinylated
  Gold-labeled

Fluorescent protein G derivatives
  FITC-labeled
  Phycoerythrin-labeled
  Rhodamine-labeled
  Phycocyanin

Immobilized protein G suitable for use in immunoprecipitation
  Heat-killed protein G-positive streptococci

  Protein G-coated magnetic microspheres
  (See also reagents for immunoglobulin isolation and purification.)

[a] For list of commercial suppliers see *Linscott's Directory of Immunological and Biological Reagents*, Fifth Edition (1989) or *American Chemical Society Guide to Biotechnology* (1990).

D. Type IV

The type IV IgG-binding protein is found on certain bovine, hemolytic streptococci (Myhre *et al.*, 1979; Reis *et al.*, 1990) and represents the narrowest range of species immunoglobulin reactivity (Figure 1). In view of this and the low affinity of the type IV immunoglobulin-binding proteins, little work has been done with these proteins, and based on the available data, this binding protein is not expected to be useful for immunochemical applications. For a review of type IV bacterial immunoglobulin-binding proteins, see Reis *et al.* (1990).

E. Type V

The type V bacterial immunoglobulin-binding protein is associated with certain strains of *Streptococcus zooepidemicus*. The existence of a type V bacterial Fc-binding protein is based on the IgG species and subclass reactivity of intact bacteria (Figure 1). The type V IgG-binding protein displays similar binding reactivities for human IgG subclasses as staphylococcal protein A, but displays subtle differences in that bacteria expressing the type V Fc-binding protein fail to bind canine and feline IgG (Boyle and Reis, 1987). Studies by Myhre and Kronvall (1980) indicate that type V bacterial Fc-binding proteins, like the other bacterial IgG-binding proteins, are stable to heating at 80°C for 5 min, but are destroyed by treatment with proteolytic enzymes. A type V receptor has recently been physicochemically characterized (Yarnall and Widders, 1990). Based on the similar IgG species and subclass reactivities of type V and the well characterized and readily available type I-binding protein (protein A), there is at present little practical value in isolating type V IgG-binding proteins as immunochemical reagents.

F. Type VI

Recently we have identified a strain of *Streptococcus zooepidemicus* that has a distinct immunoglobulin species-binding profile from that of the classical type V-binding protein (Reis *et al.*, 1988). We have designated this reactivity as type VI (Figure 1). The distinctive feature of the type VI IgG-binding protein is its reactivity with rat immunoglobulin. A stable, high expressing substrain of a type VI-positive *Streptococcus zooepidemicus* isolate has been identified that demonstrates 100-fold greater reactivity with rat immunoglobulin than the protein A positive *Staphylococcus aureus* Cowan strain, or a 30–40 fold higher reactivity than a type III-positive streptococcal isolate, G1400 (Reis *et al.*, 1988; Reis and Boyle, 1990b). At present, there is only limited information concerning the protein(s) responsible for the type VI immunoglobulin-binding activity (Reis and Boyle, 1990b). The availability of a bacterial IgG-binding protein with good reactivity for rat immunoglobulins would have practical value for studies involving rat monoclonal antibodies. Rat monoclonal antibodies have been reported to be superior to mouse monoclonal antibodies for certain applications and consequently, a selective binding protein for rat immunoglobulin is likely to have many practical applications for the detection and isolation of rat monoclonal antibodies.

G. Chimeric IgG-Binding Proteins

Recently, Eliasson and her colleagues have described the preparation of a protein A–protein G chimeric protein using genetic engineering approaches (Eliasson *et al.*, 1988, 1989). These studies demonstrate the use of gene fusion techniques for preparing immunochemical reagents containing immunoglobulin-binding characteristics of both protein A and protein G (Eliasson *et al.*, 1988, 1989). While this is an interesting approach, it does not provide any major, practical advantage over the combined use of protein A and/or protein G. For example, the chimera is superior to protein A in that it binds all four subclasses of human IgG; however, protein G alone has this property. The use of genetic engineering approaches to combine immunoglobulin-binding proteins with nonoverlapping specificities may however, prove extremely beneficial for therapeutic applications. For example, the ability to simultaneously remove IgG and IgA from serum may be advantageous. At this time a recombinant protein A–protein G hybrid is commercially available from InferGene (Benicia, California) and from Calbiochem (La Jolla, California).

IV. Second Generation Immunoglobulin-Binding Proteins

In addition to the original classification of IgG-binding proteins just described, a variety of new immunoglobulin selective binding activities not specific for IgG have been identified, associated with various bacterial isolates (Table 2). The properties and current understanding of these molecules have been reviewed in detail in the first volume of this series. The application of these proteins to immunochemical procedures is expected to follow a similar course to that of protein A and protein G, which are described in detail in this volume. At this time there is insufficient data to determine the many potential advantages, possible limitations, and technical difficulties that may be encountered using these reagents. Current advances in molecular biology and genetic engineering would suggest that each of these new selective immunoglobulin-binding proteins can be produced without any major difficulty. The properties of these nonIgG immunoglobulin-binding proteins are summarized in the following sections.

A. IgA Fc-Binding Proteins

The majority of practical applications of bacterial immunoglobulin-binding proteins have thus far been limited to proteins reactive with antibodies of the IgG isotype. Recent research has demonstrated that selective binding proteins that recognize the Fc region of other isotypes can be identified and isolated in a functionally homogeneous form (Russell-Jones et al., 1984; Cleaf and Timmis, 1987; Brady and Boyle, 1990; Lindahl et al., 1990). In particular, IgA Fc-binding proteins associated with group A and group B streptococci have been identified, isolated, and cloned (Russell-Jones et al., 1984; Lindahl and Åkerström, 1989). Jurgens et al. (1987) have reported that CAMP factor, a product of the group B streptococci, can bind IgG and IgM. In our studies of group B strains, we have been unable to demonstrate the presence of an IgG-binding protein expressed by any group B strain (Brady and Boyle, 1989, 1990; Coleman et al., 1990). For a complete review of bacterial IgA-binding proteins associated with group A and group B streptococci, see Brady and Boyle (1990) and Lindahl et al. (1990). At this time, there are no commercially available sources of bacterial IgA-binding proteins; however, we anticipate by the time this volume is published commercial sources of wild type and/or recombinant bacterial IgA-binding proteins will be available and will find broad applications for studies of mucosal immunity.

B. IgD-Binding Protein

A surface molecule that binds to IgD has been reported to be associated with certain isolates of *Branhamella catarrhalis* (Forsgren and Grubb, 1979). Little information is available on the physicochemical nature of this molecule(s) and the majority of studies have been directed toward understanding the effects of this functional binding activity on B cell function (Tedder, 1990). Since the biological activity of IgD seems to be involved in B cell differentiation, future studies are expected to be directed toward this area.

C. Protein L

In 1985 Myhre and Erntell described a strain of *Peptococcus magnus* that bound immunoglobulins via interaction with the light chain. This activity has subsequently been isolated and studied in detail by Björck (1988). Based on the high affinity of the isolated protein for immunoglobulin light chains, this protein has been designated as protein L (Björck, 1988). The current state of information on protein L has been reviewed recently by Björck and Åkerström (1990b). At this time, the practical use of protein L for detection and isolation of any isotype of immunoglobulin has not been fully developed. Experimental evidence indicates that protein

L can be iodinated without loss of light chain-binding capacity (Björck, 1988), and this finding would predict that protein L could be used as a tracer for antibody molecules. The recognition of light chains by protein L theoretically enables all isotypes of antibody to be detected and thus may have practical value for immunodiagnostic procedures requiring measurement of total antibody responses, irrespective of isotype. The practical applications of protein L for immunotechnology will emerge as more research is carried out with this protein and as it becomes commercially available as either the recombinant or wild type protein.

D. Protein P

Many investigators have attempted to find a bacterial binding protein that would display reactivity for constant regions of the μ heavy chain of IgM. To date, these approaches have met with limited success. Nielsen *et al.* (1981) have reported an IgM Fc-binding activity associated with *Brucella abortus*. This activity has not been observed with IgM from the majority of cattle serum tested and may represent an obscure allotype of IgM or some abnormal form of bovine IgM.

Lindahl and Kronvall (1988) have screened a large number of different bacteria for nonimmune reactivity with human IgM. Although a unique IgM-specific binding activity has not been identified, they have observed that certain strains of *Clostridium perfringens* preferentially bind IgM relative to IgG or IgA (Lindahl and Kronvall, 1988). Lindahl and his colleagues have extended these studies to isolate the protein responsible for this activity (Lindahl, 1990). This protein has been designated as protein P and displays selective binding to the $F(ab')_2$ region of the immunoglobulin. The reactivity of protein P is markedly reduced when the heavy and light chains are separated, which suggests the binding site for protein P is contributed by structures present on both heavy and light chains (Lindahl, 1990). "Alternative reactivity" with $F(ab')_2$ regions has been described for protein A (Erntell *et al.*, 1983) and protein G (Björck *et al.*, 1987). Whether the site on the immunoglobulin $F(ab')_2$ region that is recognized by protein P is the same as that recognized in the alternative reactivity of protein A or protein G remains to be established.

As the newest member of the bacterial immunoglobulin protein-binding family, the potential applications for protein P are hard to define. It is expected that the unique binding properties of protein P, protein L, and related molecules will find use either alone or in concert in a variety of applications for the isolation and quantitation of immunoglobulins or immunoglobulin fragments.

V. Summary

While the majority of applied studies using immunoglobulin-binding proteins have focused on the commercially available type I IgG-binding protein (staphylococcal protein A) and more recently on the type III protein (streptococcal protein G), a variety of other bacterial immunoglobulin-binding proteins have been recognized. In addition to proteins that recognize the Fc region of IgG, bacteria expressing surface receptors for certain species of IgM, IgA, IgD, and for light chain components of immunoglobulins have been described. At present, only protein A and protein G are readily available and consequently most of the applications described in this volume relate to use of these prototype bacterial immunoglobulin-binding proteins. It is anticipated that within the next few years many additional types of wild type and recombinant bacterial immunoglobulin-binding proteins will become available, and that the general methodology outlined in this volume can be expanded into a wider range of experimental and diagnostic procedures. The major focus of this volume will be on practical approaches for the detection, isolation, characterization, and use of bacterial immunoglobulin-binding proteins. These methods should be generally applicable to any bacterial immunoglobulin-binding protein, irrespective of its origin or immunoglobulin species, isotype, or subclass binding selectivity.

References

Åkerström, B., and Björck, L. (1986). *J. Biol. Chem.* **261**, 10240–10247.
Åkerström, B., Nielsen, E., and Björck, L. (1987). *J. Biol. Chem.* **262**, 1338–1339.
Ault, K. A. (1986). In "Manual of Clinical Laboratory and Immunology" (N. R. Rose, H. Friedman, and J. L. Fahey, edits.), 3rd Ed., pp. 247–253. A.S.M. Press, Washington, D.C.
Barrett, D. J. (1990). In "Bacterial Immunoglobulin-Binding Proteins," (M. D. P. Boyle, ed.), Vol. 1, pp. 279–294. Academic Press, San Diego.
Björck, L. (1988). *J. Immunol.* **140**, 1194–1197.
Björck, L., and Åkerström, B. (1990a). In "Bacterial Immunoglobin-Binding Proteins" (M. D. P. Boyle, ed), Vol. 1, pp. 113–126. Academic Press, San Diego.
Björck, L., and Åkerström, B. (1990b). In "Bacterial Immunoglobulin-Binding Proteins" (M. D. P. Boyle, ed), Vol. 1, pp. 267–278. Academic Press, San Diego.
Björck, L., and Kronvall, G. (1984). *J. Immunol.* **133**, 964–974.
Björck, L., Kastern, W., Lindahl, G., and Widebäck, K. (1987). *Mol. Immunol.* **24**, 1113–1122.
Boyle, M. D. P. (1984). *Biotechniques* **2**, 334–340.
Boyle, M. D. P. (1990). In "Bacterial Immunoglobulin-Binding Proteins" (M. D. P. Boyle, ed.). Vol. 1, pp. 17–28. Academic Press, San Diego.
Boyle, M. D. P., and Reis, K. J. (1987). *Biotechnology* **5**, 697–703.

Chapter 1. Introduction

Boyle, M. D. P., and Reis, K. J. (1990). *In* "Bacterial Immunoglobulin-Binding Proteins" (M. D. P. Boyle, ed.). Vol. 1, pp. 175–186. Academic Press, San Diego.
Boyle, M. D. P., Wallner, W. A., von Mering, G. O., Reis, K. J., and Lawman, M. J. P. (1985). *Mol. Immunol.* **220,** 1115–1121.
Boyle, M. D. P., Faulmann, E. L., Otten, R., and Heath, D. (1990). Microbial Determinants of virulence and Host Response (E. M. Ayoub, G. H. Cassell, W. C. Branche, and T. J. Henry, eds.) pp 19–44. A.S.M. Washington D.C.
Brady, L. J., and Boyle, M. D. P. (1989). *Infect. Immun.* **57,** 1573–1581.
Brady, J. L., and Boyle, M. D. P. (1990). *In* "Bacterial Immunoglobulin-Binding Proteins" (M. D. P. Boyle, ed.), Vol. 1. 201–225. Academic Press, San Diego.
Centers for Disease Control (1982). *Morbid. Mortal. Weekly Rep.* **31,** 577–580.
Chang, H. C., Takashima, I., Arikawa, J., and Hashimoto, N. (1984). *J. Virol. Methods* **9,** 143–151.
Cleary, P. P., and Heath, D. G. (1990). *In* "Bacterial Immunoglobulin-Binding Proteins" (M. D. P. Boyle, ed.), Vol. 1, pp. 83–100. Academic Press, San Diego.
Cleat P. H. and Timmis K. N. (1987) *Infect. Immun.* **55,** 1151–1155.
Coleman, S., Brady, L. J., and Boyle, M. D. P. (1990). *Infect. Immun.* **58,** 332–340.
Duboid-Dalcq, M., McFarland, H., and McFarlin, D. (1977). J. Histochem. Cytochem. **25,** 1201–1206.
Duggleby, C. I., and Jones, S. A. (1983). *Nucleic Acids Res.* **11,** 3065–3076–3076.
Eliasson, M., Olsson, A., Palmcrantz, E., Wiberg, K., Inganäs, M., Guss, B., Lindberg, M., and Uhlén, M. (1988). *J. Biol. Chem.* **263,** 4323–4327.
Eliasson, M., Anderson, R., Olsson, A., Wigzell, H., and Uhlén, M. (1989). *J. Immunol.* **142,** 575–581.
Engvall, E., and Perlmann, P. (1971). *Immunochemistry* **8,** 871–874.
Engvall, E., and Perlmann, P. (1972). *J. Immunol.* **109,** 129–135.
Erntell, M., Myhre, E. B., and Kronvall, G. (1983). *Scand. J. Immunol.* **17,** 201–209.
Fahnestock, S. R., Alexander, P., Nagle, J., and Filpula, D. (1986). *J. Bacteriol.* **167,** 870–880.
Fahnestock, S. R., Alexander, P., Filpula, D., and Nagle, J. (1990). *In* "Bacterial Immunoglobulin-Binding Proteins" (M. D. P. Boyle, ed.), Vol. 1, pp. 133–148. Academic Press, San Diego.
Faulmann, E. L., and Boyle, M. D. P. (1990). *In* "Bacterial Immunoglobulin-Binding Proteins" (M. D. P. Boyle, ed.), Vol. 1, pp. 69–82. Academic Press, San Diego.
Faulmann, E. L., Otten, R. A., Barrett, D. J., and Boyle, M. D. P. (1989). *J. Immunol. Methods* **123,** 269–281.
Filpula, D., Alexander, P., and Fahnestock, S. R. (1987). *Nucleic Acids Res.* **15,** 7210.
Forsgren, A., and Grubb, A. (1979). *J Immunol.* **122,** 1468–1472.
Forsgren, A., and Sjöquist, J. (1966). *J. Immunol.* **97,** 822–827.
Forsgren, A., Ghetie, V., Lindmark, R., and Sjöquist, H. (1983). *In* "Staphylococci and Staphylococcal Infections" (C. S. F. Easmon and C. Adlam, eds.), Vol. 2, pp. 429–480. Academic Press, London.
Gee, A. P., and Langone, J. J. (1981). *Anal. Biochem.* **116,** 524–530.
Giorgi, J. V. (1986). *In* "Manual for Clinical Laboratory Immunology" (N. R. Rose, H. Friedman, and J. L. Fahey eds.), 3rd Ed., pp. 236–246. A. S. M. Press, Washington, D.C.
Goding, J. W. (1978). *J. Immunol. Methods* **20,** 241–253.
Grubb, A., Grubb, R., Christensen, P., and Schalen, C. (1982). *Int. Arch. Allergy Appl. Immunol.* **67,** 369–376.

Guss, B., Eliasson, M., Olsson, A., Uhlén, M., Frej, A. K., Jornvall, H., Flock, J. I., and Lindberg, M. (1986). *EMBO J.* **5**, 1567–1575.
Guss, B., Lindberg, M., and Uhlén, M. (1990). In "Bacterial Immunoglobulin-Binding Proteins" (M. D. P. Boyle, ed.), Vol. 1, pp. 29–40. Academic Press, San Diego.
Haake, D. A., Franklin, E. C., and Frangione, B. (1982). *J. Immunol.* **129**, 190–192.
Harboe, M., and Fölliny, I. (1974). *Scand. J. Immunol.* **3**, 471–482.
Havlicek, J. (1978). *Exp. Cell Biol.* **46**, 146–151.
Heath, D. G., and Cleary, P. P. (1987). *Infect. Immun.* **55**, 1233–1238.
Heath, D. G., Boyle, M. D. P., and Cleary, P. P. (1990). Submitted.
Heidelberger, M., and Kendall, F. E. (1932). *J. Exp. Med.* **55**, 555–561.
Inganäs, M. (1981). *Scand. J. Immunol.* **13**, 343–352.
Jackson, A. L., and Warner, N. L. (1986). "Manual for Clinical and Laboratory Immunology" (N. R. Rose, H. Friedman, and J. L. Fahey, eds.), 3rd Ed., pp. 226–235. A. S. M. Press, Washington, D.C.
Jürgens, D., Sterzik, B., and Fehrenbach, F. J. (1987). *J. Exp. Med.* **165**, 720–732.
Kohler, G., and Milstein, C. (1975). *Nature (London)* **256**, 495–497.
Langone, J. J. (1978). *J. Immunol. Methods*, **24**, 269–285.
Langone, J. J. (1982a). *Adv. Immunol.* **32**, 157–252.
Langone, J. J. (1982b). *J. Immunol. Methods* **51**, 3–22.
Langone, J. J., Boyle, M. D. P., and Borsos, T. (1977). *J. Immunol. Methods* **18**, 281–293.
Langone, J. J., Boyle, M. D. P., and Borsos, T. (1979). *Anal. Biochem.* **93**, 207–215.
Lindahl, G. (1990). In "Bacterial Immunoglobulin-Binding Proteins" (M. D. P. Boyle, ed.), Vol. 1, pp. 257–266. Academic Press, San Diego.
Lindahl, G., and Åkerström, B. (1989). *Mol. Microbiol.* **3**, 239–247.
Lindahl, G., and Kronvall, G. (1988). *J. Immunol.* **140**, 1223–1227.
Lindahl, G., Åkerström, B., Frithz, E., Hedén, L. O., and Steinberg, L. (1990). In "Bacterial Immunoglobulin-Binding Proteins" (M. D. P. Boyle, ed.), Vol. 1, pp. 193–200. Academic Press, San Diego.
Linscott, W. D. (1989). "Linscott's Directory of Immunological and Biological Reagents (fifth ed.). Mill Valley, California.
Löfdahl, S., Guss, B., Uhlén, M., Philipson, L., and Lindberg, M. (1983). *Proc. Natl. Acad. Sci. U.S.A.* **80**, 697–701.
Myhre, E. B., and Erntell, M. (1985). *Mol. Immunol.* **22**, 879–885.
Myhre, E. B., and Kronvall, G. (1980). *Infect. Immun.* **27**, 808–816.
Myhre, E. B., and Kronvall, G. (1981). In "Basic Concepts of Streptococci and Streptococcal Diseases" (S. E. Holm and P. Christensen eds.), pp. 209–210. Reedbook, Chertsey, Surrey.
Myhre, E. B., Holmberg, O., and Kronvall, G. (1979). *Infect. Immun.* **23**, 1–7.
Nielsen, K., Stilwell, K., Stemshorn, B., and Duncan, R. (1981). *J. Clin. Microbiol.* **14**, 32–38.
Ravdonikas, L. E., Christensen, P., Burova, L. A., Grabovskaya, K., Björck, L., Schalen, C., Svensson, M. L., and Totolian, A. A. (1984). *Acta Pathol. Microbiol. Immunol. Scand. Sect. B* **92**, 65–69.
Reinherz, E. L., King, P. C., Goldstein, G., and Schlossman, S. F. (1979). *Proc. Natl. Acad. Sci. U.S.A.* **76**, 4061–4065.
Reis, K. J., and Boyle, M. D. P. (1990a). In "Bacterial Immunoglobulin-Binding Proteins" (M. D. P. Boyle, ed.), Vol. 1, pp. 101–112. Academic Press, San Diego.
Reis, K. J., and Boyle, M. D. P. (1990b). In "Bacterial Immunoglobulin-Binding Proteins" (M. D. P. Boyle, ed.), Vol. 1, pp. 165–174. Academic Press, San Diego.
Reis, K. J., Ayoub, E. M., and Boyle, M. D. P. (1984a). *J. Immunol.* **132**, 3091–3097.

Reis, K. J., Ayoub, E. M., and Boyle, M. D. P. (1984b). *J. Immunol.* **132**, 3098–3102.
Reis, K. J., Ayoub, E. M., and Boyle, M. D. P. (1985). *J. Microbiol. Methods* **4**, 45–58.
Reis, K. J., Hansen, H. F., and Björck, L. (1986). *Mol. Immunol.* **23**, 425–431.
Reis, K. J., Siden, E. J., and Boyle, M. D. P. (1988). *Biotechniques* **6**, 130–136.
Reis, K. J., Salpeter, J., and Boyle, M. D. P. (1990). *In* "Bacterial Immunoglobulin-Binding Proteins" (M. D. P. Boyle, ed.), Vol. 1, pp. 149–154. Academic Press, San Diego.
Richman, D. D. (1983). *Curr. Top. Microbiol. Immunol.* **104**, 159–576.
Rosenberg, Z. F., and Fauci, A. S. (1989). *Adv. Immunol.* **47**, 377–422.
Russell-Jones, G. J., Gotschlich, E. C., and Blake, M. S. (1984). *J. Exp. Med.* **160**, 1467–1475.
Schalen, C., and Christensen, P. (1990). *In* "Bacterial Immunoglobulin-Binding Proteins" (M. D. P. Boyle, ed.), Vol. 1, pp. 59–68. Academic Press, San Diego.
Schrezenmeier, H., and Fleischer, B. (1987). *J. Immunol. Methods* **105**, 133–137.
Shapiro, H. M. (1985). "Practical Flow Cytometry." Liss, New York.
Sjöbring, U., Falkenberg, C., Nielsen, E., Åkerström, B., and Björck, L. (1988). *J. Immunol.* **140**, 1595–1599.
Sjöbring, U., Trojnar, J., Grubb, A., Åkerström, B., and Björck, L. (1989). *J. Immunol.* **143**, 2948–2954.
Sjoquist, J., Meloun, B., and Hjelm, M. (1972) *Eur. J. Biochem.* **29**, 572–578.
Tedder, T. F. (1990). *In* "Bacterial Immunoglobulin-Binding Proteins" (M. D. P. Boyle, ed), Vol, 1. pp. 235–242. Academic Press, San Diego.
Towbin, H., Staehelin, T., and Gordon, J. (1979). *Proc. Natl. Acad. Sci. U.S.A.* **76**, 4350–4354.
Uhlén, M., Guss, B., Nilsson, B., Gatenbeck, S., Philipson, L., and Lindberg, M. (1984). *J. Biol. Chem.* **259**, 1695–1702.
Van der Merwe, J. P., and Stegeman, J. H. (1985). *Eur. J. Immunol.* **15**, 860–863.
Von Behring, E., and Kitasato, S. (1890). Ueber das Zustandekommen der Diptherie-Immunitaet urd Tetanus-Immunitaet bei Tieren. *Dtsch. Med. Wochenschr.* **16**, 1113–1117.
Von Mering, G., and Boyle, M. D. P. (1986). *Mol. Immunol.* **23**, 811–821.
Wagner, B., Wagner, M., and Ryc, M. (1983). *Zentralbl. Bakteriol. Hyg. A* **256**, 61–71.
Wallner, W. A., Lawman, M. J. P., and Boyle, M. D. P. (1987). *Appl. Microbiol. Biotechnol.* **27**, 168–173.
Widders, P. R., Stoke, C. R., Newby, T. J., and Bourne, F. J. (1985). *Infect. Immun.* **48**, 417–421.
Yallow, R. S., and Benson, R. S. (1960). *J. Clin. Invest.* **39**, 1157–1175.
Yarnall, M., and Boyle, M. D. P. (1986a). *Mol. Cell. Biochem.* **70**, 57–66.
Yarnall, M., and Boyle, M. D. P. (1986b). *J. Immunol.* **136**, 2670–2673.
Yarnall, M., and Boyle, M. D. P. (1986c). *Scand. J. Immunol.* **24**, 549–557.
Yarnall, M., and Widders, P. R. (1990). *In* "Bacterial Immunoglobulin-Binding Proteins" (M. D. P. Boyle, ed.), Vol. 1, pp. 155–164. Academic Press, San Diego.
Yarnall, M., Widders, P. R., and Corbeil, L. B. (1988). *Scand. J. Immunol.* **28**, 129–137.

CHAPTER 2

Detection and enhancement of expression of bacterial cell surface immunoglobulin-binding proteins

Kathleen J. Reis
Michael D. P. Boyle

I. Introduction

A variety of methods have been developed for the detection of immunoglobulin-binding proteins expressed on the surface of bacteria. The most critical aspect of any of these methods is assuring that one is detecting a selective, nonimmune reaction between the bacteria and the immunoglobulin rather than binding of specific antibodies to a bacterial surface component. One of the earliest methods used to detect immunoglobulin-binding proteins was agglutination, by strains of staphylococci bearing protein A, of sheep erythrocytes sensitized with a subagglutinating dose of rabbit antisheep red cell antibodies (Sjöquist and Stålenheim, 1969; Winblad and Ericson, 1973) and later on by certain strains of streptococci (Kronvall, 1973). By using antibodies directed against a known antigen and measuring reactivity with bound immune complexes only nonimmune interactions were detected. Later methods were based on the ability of bacterial strains to bind fluorescent-labeled (Lind *et al.*, 1970) or iodinated (Kronvall *et al.*, 1970) immunoglobulins or myeloma proteins. This chapter will describe the techniques used most commonly to detect bacterial cell surface immunoglobulin-binding proteins. Two methods for enhancing and/or selecting strains exhibiting high levels of immunoglobulin-binding proteins are also described.

II. Preparation of Bacteria

The method of preparation of the bacteria to be tested for expression of immunoglobulin binding-proteins depends on the growth requirements of the strains to be tested. The vast majority of bacterial immunoglobulin-binding proteins have been found on staphylococci and streptococci (for reviews see Langone, 1982; Boyle and Reis, 1987; and Vol. 1 of this series). In addition, immunoglobulin-binding proteins have been reported on strains of *Peptococcus magnus* (Myhre and Erntell, 1985; Björck, 1988), *Coprococcus comes* (van der Merwe and Stegeman, 1985), *Taylorella equigenitalis* (Widders *et al.*, 1985), *Clostridium perfringens* (Lindahl and Kronvall, 1988), and *Haemophilus somnus* (Yarnall *et al.*, 1988). Some strains of bacteria have been shown to alter expression of Fc-binding proteins during laboratory passage (Boyle and Reis, unpublished observation; Stjernquist-Desatnik *et al.*, 1984) or to consist of colonies exhibiting variable expression of Fc-binding proteins (Yarnall *et al.*, 1984; Reis *et al.*, 1988). In general, conditions for each bacteria will have to be established, but a number of general considerations applicable to any bacterial species will be described.

The bacteria should be grown in media and under conditions (e.g., aerobic vs. anaerobic) appropriate for the strain. Staphylococci can be grown in trypticase soy broth and streptococci in Todd-Hewitt broth. When screening both staphylococci and streptococci in a single experiment, we generally use Todd-Hewitt broth for both types of bacteria. The bacteria can be grown as stationary cultures and harvested by centrifugation during the late log phase of growth (18–24 hr at 37°C). Conditions should be optimized when growing larger volumes or for special needs; for example, staphylococci can be grown in higher yield by growing in trypticase soy broth with aeration provided by a stir bar or a more elaborate fermentor. Other specialized conditions or media, such as chemically defined media for streptococci (van de Rijn and Kessler, 1980), vitamin or mineral supplements (Müller and Blobel, 1983), or controlled pH may alter the expression of immunoglobulin-binding proteins or other bacterial products such as proteases. Bacteria are harvested routinely by centrifugation and washed 2–3 times in phosphate buffered saline (PBS), pH 7.2, containing 0.05% sodium azide. When large culture volumes are utilized, a variety of suitable ultrafiltration systems can be used.

It is convenient to work with killed bacteria, but until the stability of the immunoglobulin-binding protein is known, it is advisable to compare the activities of live and killed bacteria. Appropriate precautions should be exercised when working with live bacteria, particularly human pathogens, and care in the disposal of contaminated materials should be exercised.

Protein A on *Staphylococcus aureus* strains is stable to formalin fixation, which is necessary to kill the bacteria (Kessler, 1975). Formalin fixation may also be used for other strains of bacteria once it is established that the receptor is stable to this treatment. Streptococci can be killed by heating to 80°C for 5–15 min, followed by rapid cooling. IgG Fc-binding proteins on most strains of streptococci have been found to be stable to this treatment, but recently it was found that group B streptococci may lose their ability to bind human IgA Fc when heated in this manner (Brady and Boyle, unpublished observation).

III. Standardization of Bacteria

In order to compare the reactivities of different bacterial isolates it is necessary to standardize bacterial cell concentrations. This can be achieved by a variety of semiquantitative methods.

A. Standardization of Bacterial Cell Number Based on Wet Weight/Volume Ratio

The simplest method is to weigh the bacterial pellet following centrifugation and resuspend to 10% weight/volume (w/v). This method is most convenient for large volumes of bacteria and appears to give a consistent preparation from batch to batch. It is however, not the most quantitative measure of bacterial number.

B. Standardization of Bacterial Cell Number Based on Volume/Volume Ratio

This approach represents the most accurate method to standardize bacterial cell concentration. This can be achieved with the aid of an hematocrit centrifuge (Kessler, 1975). A capillary tube is filled with a thoroughly mixed suspension of bacteria (approximately 50% w/v) and the end is plugged. The tube(s) are centrifuged in an hematocrit centrifuge at full speed (12,000 rpm) for 5 min. The volume of bacteria is read as a percentage of the total suspension using an hematocrit reader. Based on these results, the bacterial suspension can be adjusted to a final concentration of 10% volume/volume (v/v). This method provides the greatest accuracy and reproducibility and can be used for all strains of bacteria, including aggregating strains. Small volumes of bacteria can be standardized by this procedure.

C. Standardization of Bacteria Based on Measurement of Turbidity

An estimate of bacterial cell concentration can be achieved by measuring light scatter at 550 nm. The OD_{550} (optical density) value can be related to cell number by comparison to a standard curve relating OD_{550} to cell numbers. This curve is determined experimentally by growing a number of dilutions on plates and counting the number of colonies formed. This procedure must be carried out for each strain and is extremely labor intensive. Another disadvantage of this method is that accuracy depends on the size of the bacteria and therefore not all bacteria can be standardized, e.g., self-agglutinating streptococci.

IV. Assays for the Detection of Immunoglobulin-Binding Proteins

A. Agglutination Assay

This method is based on the ability of bacteria with immunoglobulin Fc-binding proteins to agglutinate sheep red blood cells sensitized with subagglutinating doses of rabbit antibody prepared against sheep red blood cells.

Materials: Bacteria, prepared and standardized as described earlier

Buffers: The formulations for all buffers used are presented in the Appendix.

1. Sensitized Sheep Erythrocytes

Sheep erythrocytes (SRBC) are collected in Alsever's solution to be sensitized (after Anderson *et al.*, 1970), and stored at 4°C until use. One volume of cells is removed and centrifuged at approximately $500 \times g$ for 15 min and the plasma-containing supernatant is removed by aspiration. Resuspend the erythrocytes in PBS, centrifuge, and remove the supernatant. The wash procedure is repeated three times. Resuspend the washed red cell pellet to 1%. The supernatant should be free of hemoglobin following the final wash. If hemoglobin is still present, the cells should be discarded. Determine the concentration of sensitizing antibody by mixing an equal volume of doubling dilutions of rabbit anti-SRBC with the washed SRBC. Incubate at 4°C for 2 hr and inspect for agglutination. Use the antibody concentration at 25% of the concentration of the positive agglutination endpoint. At this concentration of antibody there should be no direct agglutination of sensitized red cells. The rabbit anti-SRBC may be either whole serum or an IgG fraction. IgG fractions can be prepared easily by either ion exchange chromatography or appropriate affinity purification (Boyle and Langone, 1980). Prior to each assay, a suitable quantity of sensitized SRBC is prepared by mixing equal volumes of washed SRBC with antibody at the predetermined sensitizing concentration, followed by incubation at ambient temperature for 15 min. After this period, the sensitized cells are centrifuged, and the supernatant is removed. The cell pellet is washed once in PBS and the sensitized erythrocytes are suspended to a final concentration of 1–3% in PBS.

2. Slide Agglutination Test for Bacterial-Binding Proteins

Mix one drop of two-fold dilutions of bacteria, prepared as described earlier, with one drop of 3% sensitized sheep red cells on a slide, using an applicator stick (Winblad and Ericson, 1973). The mixture on the slide is rocked back and forth and examined for agglutination for up to 5 min. A positive test is indicated by a strong agglutination reaction that develops rapidly. A bacterial sample known to have immunoglobulin IgG Fc receptors that are reactive with rabbit IgG should be included as a positive control. A negative control of unsensitized erythrocytes should also be included to control for any binding between bacteria and unsensitized red cells.

3. Tube Agglutination Test for Bacterial-Binding Proteins

Mix one drop of two-fold dilutions of bacteria, prepared as described previously, with one drop of 1% sensitized SRBC in a 12 × 75 mm glass tube (after Winblad and Ericson, 1973). Incubate for 2 hr at 37°C, then observe for agglutination by gently disrupting the cell pellet. Incubate the tubes an additional 16–18 hr at 4°C and reexamine for agglutination. Appropriate positive and negative control samples, as described earlier, should be included in each assay.

4. Microtiter Agglutination Test for Bacterial-Binding Proteins

This agglutination assay, adapted from Kronvall (1973) and Reis *et al.* (1983), can conveniently be performed in round-bottomed, 96-well microtiter plates by mixing an equal volume of 0.25% sensitized SRBC with two-fold dilutions of bacteria as described. A nonspecific protein such as gelatin, at a concentration of 0.5%, should be included in the PBS that is used as a diluent for all reagents. Incubate the plates at 4°C and examine for agglutination at 2 and 18 hr. A positive reaction will be noted by a mat of cells in the bottom of the well, while a negative reaction will be noted by a discreet red cell pellet.

For each of these assays, positive and negative controls should be included by testing a bacteria known to have immunoglobulin Fc receptors reactive with rabbit IgG, such as a protein A positive *Staphylococcus aureus* strain or a protein G positive group C or group G streptococcus. Any bacterial strain demonstrating reactivity should also be tested against unsensitized SRBC to ensure that the bacteria are reacting with the IgG on the red cells and not a surface component of the red cell itself. Reactivity of a bacteria with different species, classes, or subclasses of immunoglobulins can be determined by inhibition of agglutination or in a direct assay if the appropriate species of anti-red cell antibody is available.

5. Advantages

The agglutination assays are easy to perform and require no special equipment or reagents. Although the slide assay is simple and gives immediate results, Winblad and Ericson (1973) found the tube assay to be more sensitive. Since the antibody combining sites of the rabbit anti-SRBC are attached to the SRBC, any reaction with the rabbit IgG will be via a site remote from the antibody combining site and hence a nonimmune interaction. Although reactivity with different immunoglobulins can be determined in hemagglutination inhibition experiments as previously described, bacteria with immunoglobulin-binding proteins that are not reactive with rabbit IgG would not be detected by this assay.

6. Disadvantages

Many bacteria, particularly staphylococci and streptococci, produce red cell hemolysins, which can mediate hemolysis of the target cells during the incubation phase of tube and microtiter assays (Winblad and Ericson, 1973). Christensen and Kronvall (1974) have found that heating the bacterial suspension to 56°C for 30 min eliminates hemolysis and that use of the microtiter plate assay eliminates difficulties in interpretation of auto-agglutinating streptococci. In our initial studies on staphylococcal and streptococcal Fc immunoglobulin-binding proteins, we established an agglutination assay using microtiter plates as described earlier. We have found the assay to be suitable for screening staphylococci, but not for streptococci, since auto-agglutination by some strains prevented unequivocal identification of immunoglobulin-binding proteins on these strains. All of the agglutination assays were subjective and nonquantitative. For detailed studies, more objective assays such as those described in the next section are more suitable.

V. Direct Binding of Immunoglobulins to Bacteria

A variety of methods have been developed to detect immunoglobulin Fc-binding proteins based on direct binding of labeled immunoglobulins or selective depletion of immunoglobulins from solution (Reis et al., 1983; Kronvall et al., 1970). These methods are highly sensitive and are not subject to problems encountered in agglutination assays with hemolysins or auto-agglutinating bacteria. The most critical aspect of all of these assays is the preparation of a probe that detects interaction with the Fc region of immunoglobulin. This is particularly important when using polyclonal immunoglobulins, since both humans and animals are likely to have low levels of antibodies to many different bacterial antigens. Probes specific for the Fc region of immunoglobulin can be prepared in a variety of ways and will be discussed in the following section.

A. Preparation of Immunoglobulin Fc-Specific Probes
1. Fc Fragments

Fc fragments of immunoglobulins, such as human IgG or IgA Fc fragments, can be prepared by treatment with a variety of enzymes (Porter, 1959; Plaut, 1983) and many species of Fc fragments are commercially available. The use of purified Fc fragments ensures that any interaction of the tracer with the bacteria occurs via nonimmune constant regions rather than via specific antigenic recognition domains. We have found in our studies, using either whole bacteria or purified streptococcal Fc-binding proteins, that IgG Fc fragments from species such as human, rabbit, and guinea pig bind as well as whole IgG molecules. However, Fc fragments prepared from pig, goat, cow, or sheep IgG do not always bind as efficiently as nonimmune intact IgG molecules. This is most likely due to modification of the secondary or tertiary structure of the binding site on the immunoglobulin molecule during preparation of the Fc fragment. Alternative reactivity of bacterial IgG-binding proteins with the $F(ab')_2$ region has been reported (Erntell et al., 1983; Lindahl, 1990; Myhre, 1990); however, methods described in the next section using addition of unlabeled $F(ab')_2$ fragments enable this alternative reactivity to be distinguished from direct reactivity with Fc fragments.

2. Absorption of Immunoglobulins by Bacteria

An alternative method developed by Reis et al. (1983) measures the ability of bacteria to remove whole immunoglobulin from a solution containing a two to ten-fold molar excess of $F(ab')_2$ fragments. The $F(ab')_2$

fragments should be prepared from the same source of intact immunoglobulin that is tested for its ability to bind to bacteria. By adding a large molar excess of unlabeled F(ab')$_2$ fragments to the labeled whole IgG molecule, only nonimmune IgG Fc-binding is detected. Alternatively, removal of IgG in the presence of F(ab')$_2$ fragments can be quantified using an assay that measures only the presence of IgG Fc domains and is unaffected by the presence of F(ab')$_2$ fragments.

This form of Fc-specific probe is suitable for use with any species, class, or subclass of immunoglobulin for which purified F(ab')$_2$ fragments can be generated. A nonimmune reaction in the Fab region of the immunoglobulin molecule (e.g., within constant domains on the light chain) would not be detected by this method.

3. Use of Monoclonal Antibodies or Myeloma Proteins

Myeloma or monoclonal immunoglobulins make suitable probes for any type of nonimmune interaction with bacteria, once it has been established that the particular myeloma or monoclonal is not directed against a bacterial surface component. Caution should be exercised when using these immunoglobulins since not all monoclonal or myeloma immunoglobulins of a given subclass display the same reactivity. The best example of this is the interaction of staphylococcal protein A with IgG$_3$ immunoglobulins of the G3m (s^+t^+) allotype, but not with antibodies of other IgG$_3$ allotypes (Haake *et al.* 1982). This difference can be attributed to a single amino acid substitution at position 435 of the IgG$_3$ heavy chain (Haake *et al.*, 1982).

4. Iodination of Proteins

The preparation of iodinated probes is described fully in Chapter 7.

B. Detection of Bacterial IgG-Binding Proteins

The general assays described as follows can be used for detection of any bacterial Fc-binding protein for which a suitable probe can be prepared.

VI. Direct Binding Assay

A. Materials

Bacteria, prepared and standardized as described earlier in this chapter

^{125}I-labeled Ig Fc-specific probe prepared as described earlier

12 × 75 mm glass tubes

gamma counter

B. Buffers

VBS-gel-T: Veronal-buffered saline, pH 7.4, containing 1 mM Mg^{2+}, 0.15 mM Ca^{2+}, 0.1% gelatin, and 0.05% Tween 20

EDTA-gel-T: Veronal-buffered saline containing 0.01 M trisodium ethylenediaminetetraacetate, 0.1% gelatin, and 0.05% Tween 20

Note: PBS, containing gelatin and Tween 20 may be substituted. Buffers at other pH's may also be used to enhance binding (Åkerström and Björck 1986; Reis *et al.*, 1988).

The exact formulations for all buffers are presented in the Appendix.

C. Procedure

The general procedure measures the ability of different dilutions of bacteria to bind labeled Fc fragments or a suitable Fc-specific probe and is summarized in Figure 1. This reaction is usually carried out by adding approximately 30,000 cpm of tracer to the bacterial suspension in a total volume of 0.2 ml. All dilutions are carried out in VBS-gel-T. The mixture is incubated at 37°C for 1–2 hr and the unbound label is removed by washing. This is achieved by adding 2 ml of EDTA-gel-T to each tube and pelleting the bacteria by centrifugation at 3000 × g for 10 min. The washed bacterial pellets are counted in a gamma counter. Control tubes to which only labeled tracer is added are incubated and washed in an identical fashion and used to determine background levels of binding. (Note: if concentrated bacterial solutions are used, entrapment of tracer may present a problem. In such cases, a more appropriate background measure would be the counts associated with a similar number of bacteria from a related strain that is known to lack IgG-binding proteins.) An aliquot of tracer is counted to determine the number of counts added and to enable the percentage of counts bound to be calculated. This method is straightforward and provides a rapid, objective measure of the average distribution of Fc-binding proteins on bacteria.

VII. Absorption of IgG by Bacteria

The ability of bacteria to absorb IgG in a nonimmune fashion can be determined by measuring residual IgG in solution following incubation

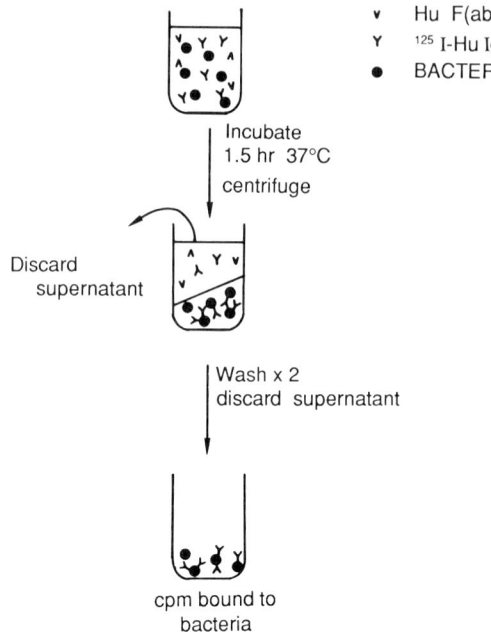

FIGURE 1
General procedure to detect IgG Fc-binding proteins using a radiolabeled Fc-specific probe.

with the bacteria (Reis et al., 1983). It is important in such assays to distinguish antigen-specific reactivities from nonimmune reactions. This is achieved by inclusion of excess F(ab')$_2$ fragments and by quantifying residual IgG using an assay that detects only the Fc region of the antibody molecule.

A. Materials

Bacteria, prepared and standardized as described earlier

Fc-specific probe (i.e., whole IgG containing a two to tenfold molar excess of F(ab')$_2$ fragments prepared from the same IgG source)

12 × 75 mm tubes

B. Buffers

VBS-gel-T (see Section VI)

EDTA-gel-T (see Section VI)

C. Procedure

The ability of differing dilutions of bacteria to absorb IgG from solution is determined by mixing 0.5 ml of a dilution of bacteria with 0.5 ml of a solution of IgG, containing 1 µg/ml of IgG and 5 µg of F(ab')$_2$ fragments, and incubating at ambient temperature for 1 hr. [In preliminary experiments, tenfold dilutions from the standardized bacteria stock should be prepared in VBS-gel-T to establish an appropriate concentration range to carry out the studies; usually between 10^9 and 10^{10} bacteria per ml prove satisfactory.] The bacteria are removed from the reaction mixture by centrifugation at 3000 × g for 5 min. An aliquot of the supernatant is removed and residual IgG is measured using the competitive binding assay described in the next section. Control samples containing the IgG/F(ab')$_2$ mixture incubated in the absence of bacteria are included in each assay.

1. Detection of Residual IgG in Bacterial Free Supernatant

Residual IgG in solution is quantified by the procedure of Langone *et al.* (1977), which uses a bacterial Fc-binding protein as tracer and can be used to measure IgG from any species reactive with protein A or protein G. Because these assays are based on reactivity with IgG Fc regions, F(ab')$_2$ fragments are not detected in this assay. Consequently, any F(ab')$_2$ fragments removed due to specific antibody–antigen interactions are not measured and only immunoglobulin removed by interaction with the Fc region will be quantified by this approach (Reis *et al.*, 1983).

In this assay, 0.2 ml of a test sample or buffer is mixed with 0.1 ml of a standard suspension of rabbit IgG covalently coupled to agarose beads (Immunobead, R-1 Bio-Rad Laboratories, Richmond, California) and 0.1 ml of ^{125}I-labeled protein A (PA) (approximately 20,000 cpm). After incubation at 37°C for 90 min, 2 ml of veronal-buffered saline containing 0.01 M trisodium ethylenediaminetetraacetate and 0.1% gelatin (EDTA-gel) is added to each tube and centrifuged at 1000 × g for 5 min and the supernatant fluid decanted. After an additional wash, the radioactivity associated with the beads is determined in a suitable Autogamma counter. The number of counts bound in the absence of fluid phase IgG is compared to the number of counts bound to the beads in the presence of known amounts of fluid phase IgG. The degree of inhibition is determined and a standard curve relating quantity of IgG to the percentage of inhibition is generated. The quantity of IgG in the test sample can be determined by comparing the percentage of inhibition with the standard curve. Fifty percent inhibition of binding of ^{125}I-labeled PA to the immunobeads is consistently achieved with 30–50 ng of fluid-phase IgG. By comparing the quantity of IgG offered with the quantity recovered after incubation with the bacteria, the Fc-binding capacity of the bacterial preparation can be determined. For representative examples of this procedure, see Chapter 3.

VIII. Dot Blot Procedure

The dot blot procedure to detect bacterial cell surface immunoglobulin-binding proteins is based on the property of nitrocellulose membranes to immobilize proteins and the ability to detect immunoglobulin-binding proteins using appropriately labeled tracers. This general procedure is described in detail in Chapter 14. We have found this procedure to be more sensitive by approximately 100-fold than the direct tube assay described. The procedure we have used utilizes iodinated tracers and autoradiography as the detection method (Yarnall *et al.*, 1986; Reis *et al.*, 1988); however, other forms of tracer such as enzyme, gold, or biotinylated tracers can be substituted.

A. Materials

Bacteria, prepared and standardized as described earlier

Iodinated probe prepared as described in Chapter 7

Nitrocellulose (NC) membranes and Dot Blot manifold containing 96 wells (Bio-Rad, Richmond, California)

Kodak XAR-5 X-ray film

X-ray film cassette with regular intensifying screens

B. Buffers

Tris-buffered saline (TBS): 20 mM Tris, 500 mM NaCl, pH 7.5

Tris-buffered saline-Tween (TBS-T): TBS, containing 0.05% Tween 20

Blocking buffer: 0.15 M veronal-buffered saline, containing 0.15% Tween 20 and 0.5% gelatin

Wash buffer: 0.01 M EDTA, 1.0 M NaCl, 0.25% gelatin and 0.15% Tween 20

The exact formulation for each buffer is provided in the Appendix.

C. Procedure

Dilute bacteria in TBS starting at 1×10^8 bacteria/0.1 ml, or make a 1:100 dilution of a 10% (wet weight/volume) bacterial stock. More concentrated bacterial suspensions tend to block the wells of the dot blot apparatus. Soak a NC membrane in TBS for 10–15 min prior to assembly into a suitable dot blot apparatus. (Bio-Rad dot blot apparatus or equivalent). Add 0.1 ml dilutions of bacteria to appropriate wells. Apply vacuum to promote contact between the bacteria and the nitrocellulose and to remove the liquid. When wells are drained of fluid, turn off the vacuum. Add 200 μl TBS-T per well to wash the bacteria and remove the wash liquid by applying the vacuum. Repeat this procedure two times. After the final wash, disassemble the apparatus and carefully remove the nitrocellulose while the vacuum is still applied to the lower chamber. The nitrocellulose membrane is washed three or four times in blocking buffer to ensure that any remaining active sites on the nitrocellulose membrane are blocked with nonspecific proteins. Each wash is carried out for 10–15 min in a tray containing 100–200 ml of wash buffer on a continuously shaking platform. After the final wash, the membrane is placed in a heat seal bag with 10 ml of blocking buffer containing 2×10^5 cpm/ml of ^{125}I-labeled ligand. The sealed bag is then rotated end over end to ensure uniform mixing for 2–3 hr at ambient temperature. Care should be taken to remove as many bubbles as possible from the bag prior to sealing, especially those bubbles stuck in the indentations made in the nitrocellulose membrane during the dot blot procedure. (Probing can be carried out overnight for convenience, but this frequently increases the background level of radioactivity that binds to the nitrocellulose membrane.) After probing, the membrane is washed four times in the wash buffer (250 ml/wash for 15 min each) and allowed to air dry. The film is wrapped in plastic wrap and exposed to X-ray film in a cassette containing regular intensifying screens at $-70°C$ for varying times. The length of exposure time for the autoradiograph will depend on the bacterial immunoglobulin-binding protein (avidity and number), the concentration of bacteria applied to the nitrocellulose membrane, and the specific activity of the iodinated probe.

This procedure can also be used to screen bacteria for expression of different types of immunoglobulin Fc-binding proteins by comparing the reactivity of a bacteria with different species or subclasses of immunoglobulin. A representative example of this procedure, in which a variety of human group A streptococcal isolates are probed with radioiodinated human IgG subclass proteins is presented in Figure 2.

Similar species reactivity profiles can be established by measuring inhibition of a single labeled probe. This inhibition assay is carried out by selecting a concentration of bacteria known to give a weak but detectable level of binding of the probe and adding that concentration of bacteria to all of the wells in the dot blot apparatus. Then varying concentrations of unlabeled competitor immunoglobulins are added directly to the wells of the apparatus, incubated for approximately 1–2 hr to permit binding to the

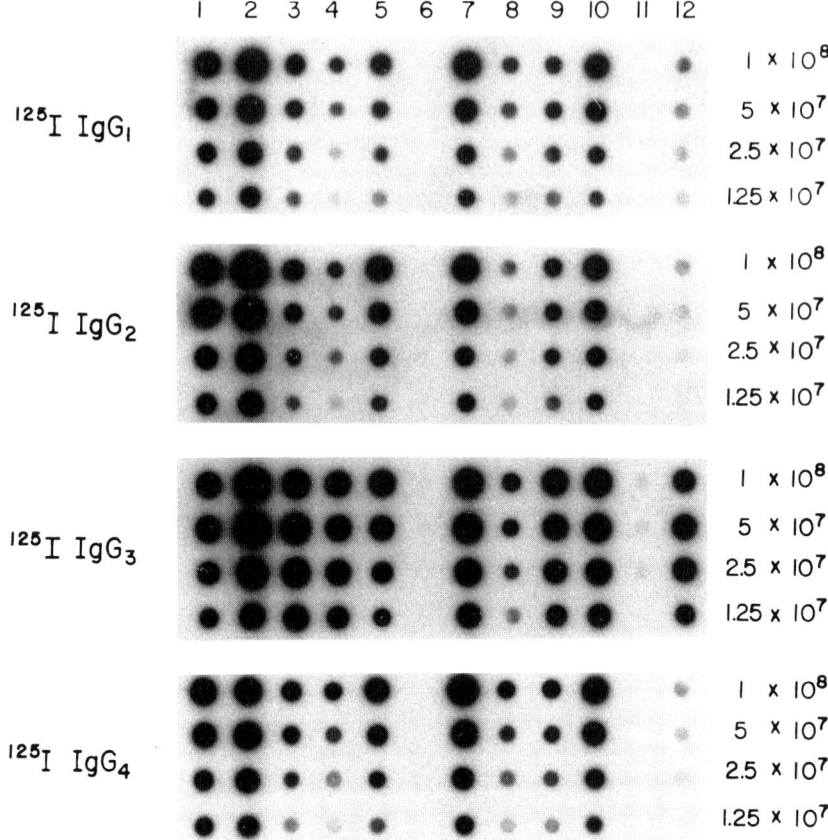

FIGURE 2
Representative dot blots of a number of group A streptococcal isolates probed with ^{125}I-labeled myeloma proteins representing each human IgG subclass. Lane 1, strain #64/14/P. Lane 2, strain #64/14/HRP. Lane 3, strain #64/14/43. Lane 4, strain #Hu13. Lane 5, strain #650. Lane 6, strain #G53. Lane 7, strain #SHS1. Lane 8, strain #SHS7. Lane 9, strain #SHS9. Lane 10, strain #SHS11. Lane 11, strain #B905. Lane 12, strain #B515.

bacterial protein and washed, blocked, and probed with a single labeled reactive immunoglobulin as described previously. Reactivity will be measured by a reduction in the intensity of the dot on the autoradiograph observed in the presence of unlabeled immunoglobulin when compared to no added immunoglobulin. The inhibition of tracer binding can be shown to be concentration dependent and a semiquantitative comparison of reactivity for different species or subclasses of IgG can be obtained. An example of this procedure to define the species reactivity of the type IIa immunoglobulin-binding protein is shown in Figure 7 of Chapter 4. The inhibition assay has the advantage that only a single labeled tracer is required.

Membranes other than nitrocellulose are available that may also be suitable. Manufacturers' directions for use of these products should be followed. Enzyme-labeled probes and suitable substrates, for example peroxidase-labeled IgG Fc and the substrate 4-chloro-1-naphthol, may be substituted for iodinated probes and autoradiography. Enzyme-labeled probes may be particularly advantageous for direct binding of multiple species of immunoglobulins since these probes can be stored for long periods of time without loss of activity. Similarly, biotinylated probes can be used, enabling a variety of avidin or streptavidin tracers to be used as the reporter molecule.

IX. Methods to Enhance Immunoglobulin-Binding Proteins

During our early studies of IgG Fc-binding proteins, we found that some immunoglobulin-binding proteins, particularly those on group A streptococci, are present only at low levels and frequently are lost during laboratory subculturing. Consequently, we sought ways to enhance or stabilize the binding proteins present on bacteria. We have found two methods that have resulted in strains with enhanced Fc-binding capabilities. The first method is by passage of strains of bacteria *in vivo* in mice. The second is a colony blot selection method that allows the expression of immunoglobulin-binding proteins by individual colonies of a given strain of bacteria to be monitored.

X. Mouse Passage

Previous studies have shown that passage of streptococci in mice results in increased expression of virulence and enhanced resistance to phagocytosis with concomitant enhanced expression of certain surface proteins. Burova *et al.* (1980) have found that during mouse passage of a group A streptococcus, mouse virulence increased along with IgG Fc-binding activity. Reis *et al.* (1984) have applied this procedure to two strains of group A streptococci. One strain (529) shows a highly variable response, fluctuating in the level of expression of immunoglobulin-binding proteins from one passage to the next, despite increasing mouse virulence following passage 5–6 (Figure 3A). The second strain (64) shows an initial decrease

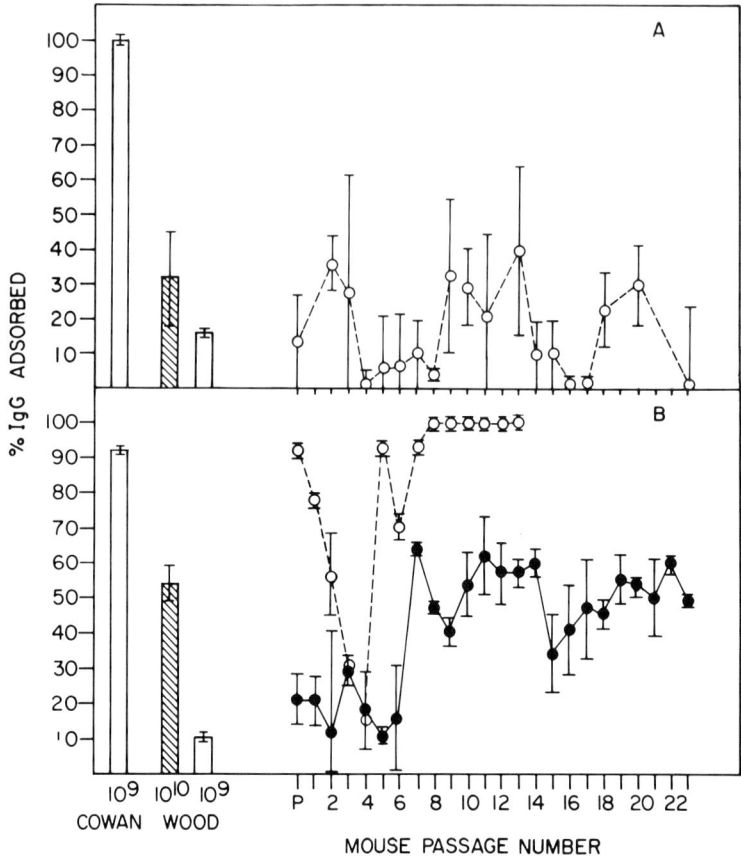

FIGURE 3
Effect of mouse passages on IgG Fc-binding protein expression of (A) the group A streptococcal strain 529, and (B) the group A streptococcal isolate 64. The IgG-binding capacity was measured with 10^{10} (0--0) or 0^9 (0-0) bacteria, respectively. *Staphylococcus aureus* Cowan I and Wood strains were included as reference high and low IgG-binding strains, respectively. (Reproduced from Reis *et al.*, 1984, with permission.)

in Fc-binding protein expression followed by an increased level of expression that parallels the virulence of this mouse-passed strain (Figure 3B). After 14 mouse passages, the level of Fc-binding associated with strain 64/14 had more than doubled when compared to the parent strain and this increased level of binding was found to be stable to laboratory passage on blood agar plates for over two years (Reis *et al.*, 1984). The level of immunoglobulin-binding protein expressed on this mouse-selected group

A streptococcus approaches that observed with the protein A-rich *Staphylococcus aureus*, Cowan I strain (Reis *et al.*, 1984).

A. Procedure for Mouse Passage of Bacteria

The procedure described next should be carried out in an appropriate isolation facility particularly when human pathogens are being used. This procedure has been used in the experiments reported by Reis et al. (1984) involving the mouse passage of two pathogenic group A streptococcal isolates. The selected strains to be mouse-passaged are grown overnight at 37°C in 10 ml of Todd-Hewitt broth. An aliquot of the overnight culture (0.5 ml) is injected intraperitoneally (i.p.) into 6–8 week old mice. When the mice die of septicemia or show signs of bacteremia, the animals are sacrificed and the spleen removed. Single-cell suspensions are prepared in a small volume of sterile saline (approximately 2 ml) by mashing the spleen through a series of sterile, fine mesh sieves. An aliquot (0.1 ml) of the resulting spleen cell suspension is injected i.p. into an uninfected mouse and the remaining portion is used to isolate the bacteria and to determine the bacterial cell number by performing colony counts on different dilutions. (The appropriate initial inoculation dose will depend on the virulence of the organism used and is expected to vary from isolate to isolate. Consequently, an initial titration of the bacteria to establish an appropriate LD_{100} is recommended.)

The length of time necessary for the mice to succumb to septicemia will depend on the virulence and number of infecting organisms injected. In our study, mice died 4–5 days after injection of the parent strain and a similar pattern was observed in mice injected with strains passed 1–3 times. Following the fourth or fifth passages, the injected spleen cell suspension resulted in mice becoming ill but the majority of animals did not die. It was therefore necessary to sacrifice these mice in order to recover bacteria from the spleen. After this initial decline in virulence, the mice became ill much more rapidly and death followed usually within 24 or 48 hr. By passage 18–20, the mice died within 12 hr following injection even with a markedly reduced inoculum. It should be noted that the passage of organisms through mice is expensive in terms of both the technical time involved and in animal costs. An alternative *in vitro* selection procedure is next described.

XI. Colony Blot Selection

We have found during our studies that many bacterial strains are heterogeneous in their expression of immunoglobulin-binding proteins. The colony blot selection procedure was developed to monitor the expression of immunoglobulin-binding proteins by individual colonies within a given bacterial isolate. We have successfully used this method to enhance the expression of a type II-binding protein on a group A streptococcus (Yarnall *et al.*, 1984) and a type VI-binding protein expressed by a *Streptococcus zooepidemicus* isolate (Reis *et al.*, 1988). This method is summarized in Figure 4 and will be described in this section. Although the example presented uses radiolabeled probes and autoradiography for visualization, enzyme-labeled probes and suitable substrates can also be used.

A. Materials

Stock strain of bacteria to be tested

Blood agar plates for replica plating

Todd-Hewitt agar plates or other suitable solid support media for electroblotting. These are made by pouring thin plates (approximately 10 ml/plate) made of Todd-Hewitt broth containing 1.5% agar.

RepliPlate™ Colony Transfer Pads (FMC Bioproducts, Rockland, Maine)

Nitrocellulose membranes (Bio-Rad, Richmond, California) cut in a circle to fit the plates

Filter paper (Whatman 3 MM), cut in a circle to fit the plates

Electroblot apparatus (Bio-Rad, Richmond, California)

Iodinated IgG Fc probe (see Chapter 7)

B. Buffers

Electroblot buffer: 25 m M Tris, 192 m M glycine (pH 8.3) and 20% (v/v) methanol

Blocking buffer: 0.15 M veronal-buffered saline, containing 0.15% Tween 20 and 0.5% gelatin

Wash buffer: 0.01 M EDTA, 1.0 M NaCl, 0.25% gelatin, and 0.15% Tween 20

Exact buffer formulations are presented in the Appendix.

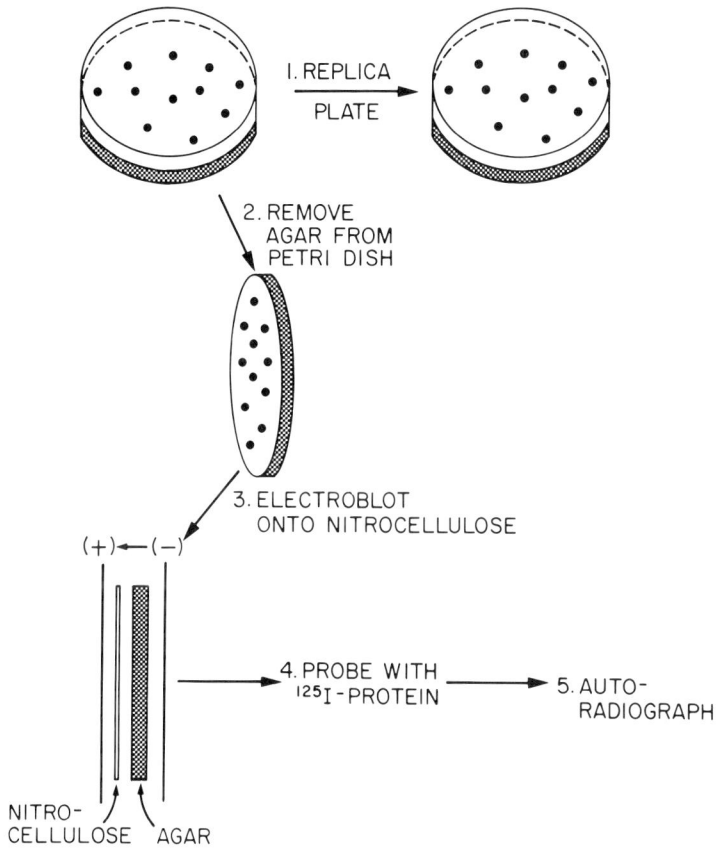

FIGURE 4
Schematic representation of the immunoblotting procedure for detection of Fc-binding proteins on the surface of bacteria. (Adapted from Yarnall et al., 1984, with permission.)

C. Procedure

This procedure is detailed diagrammatically in Figure 4 and is carried out as follows.

Essentially, a dilution of an overnight suspension of bacteria in sterile Todd-Hewitt broth is spread onto Todd-Hewitt agar plates to yield approximately 20–80 colonies following overnight incubation at 37°C. It is recommended that a series of dilutions be set up and plates that contain the appropriate size and number of well-spaced colonies be selected for further analysis.

Ideally, plates containing 20–80 distinct colonies are replica-plated onto blood agar plates using the colony transfer pads and incubated overnight at 37°C to serve as master plates for later selection of colonies expressing high or low reactivities. The plates are marked with either a series of needle stabs or by removal of a number of triangular notches to facilitate alignment of the replica plate and reactive colonies detected by autoradiography. The transfer of colonies to nitrocellulose membranes is achieved as follows. A circular piece of nitrocellulose that is the same size as the petri plate and two pieces of filter paper are soaked in electroblot buffer for approximately 10 min. The nitrocellulose is marked to allow orientation with the replica plate. This is most easily achieved by cutting a small "V" at the top and a "VV" on the right-hand side of the nitrocellulose and noting the position of these marks on the replica plate. The nitrocellulose membrane is carefully placed on top of the colonies followed by one piece of filter paper. Remove the agar from the petri dish by first rimming the edge of the agar with a spatula and carefully lifting one edge of the agar from the dish. Turn the dish upside down and allow the agar to gently fall from the dish. Place a second piece of filter paper on the underside of the agar so that the agar and nitrocellulose membrane are sandwiched between two pieces of filter paper. Assemble the complete nitrocellulose, agar, filter paper sandwich into an electroblot apparatus and transfer the colonies (and secreted proteins) to the nitrocellulose membrane by electrophoresis at 70 V for 3 hr in electroblot buffer. [Transfer of bacteria to nitrocellulose can be achieved by merely pressing nitrocellulose onto the surface of the bacterial agar without electroblotting. We have found, however, that inclusion of the electroblotting step results in more efficient transfer particularly of secreted proteins. This is of importance for the detection of Fc-binding proteins secreted by surface-negative strains.] After electrophoresis, wash the nitrocellulose membrane 3–4 times in blocking buffer to block the remaining protein-binding sites on the nitrocellulose membrane. Each wash is carried out for 10–15 min using 200 ml of buffer on a continuously shaking platform. After the final wash, the nitrocellulose is probed for 2–3 hr on an end-over-end rotating device in 10 ml of blocking buffer containing 2×10^5 cpm/ml of ^{125}I-labeled immunoglobulin probe. This is most easily carried out by sealing the blot in a heat seal bag of the appropriate size. Probing can be done overnight, but we have found that this increases the background level of radioactive probe that adheres to the nitrocellulose membrane. After probing, the membrane is washed four times in the wash buffer (250 ml/wash for 15 min each) and allowed to air dry. The nitrocellulose membrane is wrapped in plastic wrap and exposed to X-ray film in a cassette containing regular intensifying screens at −70°C for varying times (usually 1–3 days) before

Chapter 2. Detection and Enhancement of Bacterial Cell Surface 43

film development. Length of exposure time will depend on the nature of the bacterial immunoglobulin-binding protein (avidity and number), the number of bacteria in a given colony, the efficiency of transfer to the nitrocellulose membrane, and the specific activity of the iodinated probe. The resulting autoradiographs can be aligned with the blood agar replica plates and colonies of interest can be selected for further study. (Note: when blood agar plates were used in the electroblotting steps of this procedure for the nitrocellulose membrane, high nonspecific background binding was observed in the autoradiography.)

To obtain a high-expressing colony of a desired reactivity, a combination of selection methods can be used. For example, the group A streptococcus designated 64 was first mouse-passed to enhance the expression of type II Fc-binding proteins (Figure 3). The strain obtained following 14 mouse passages, 64/14, was then colony blotted and probed with a human IgG Fc-specific probe. As shown in Figure 5, the intensity of spots on the autoradiograph varied considerably, indicating heterogeneity in expression of Fc-binding proteins by individual colonies. This was in contrast to a similar blot of a protein A positive *Staphylococcus aureus* strain in which all of the colonies represented on the autoradiograph were of equiva-

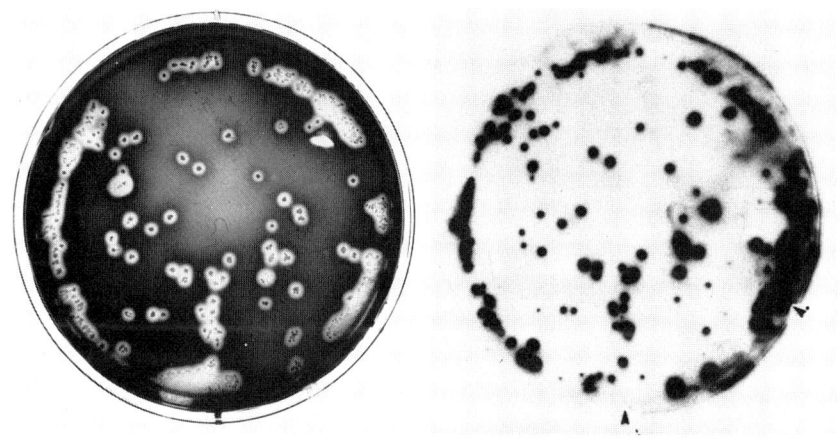

FIGURE 5
Fc-binding protein expression of a group A streptococcal strain. The left panel shows colonies of strain 64/14 on a blood agar replica plate. The right panel is an autoradiograph of a replica plate following probing with ^{125}I-labeled human IgG in the presence of unlabeled F(ab)$_2$ fragments. Autoradiography was carried out by exposure of the blot for 3 days at $-70°C$ to X-ray film using an intensifying screen. (Reproduced from Yarnall *et al.*, 1984, with permission.)

lent intensity (Yarnall et al., 1984). The heterogeneous expression of Fc-binding proteins on the group A strain could not be correlated with variations in size of individual colonies, compare Figures 5 A and B. A representative high intensity colony (Fc-binding protein rich) and a low intensity (Fc-binding protein poor) colony were selected from the replica plate and subcultured. The expression of Fc immunoglobulin-binding activity of the progeny is shown in Figure 6. The selected high-producing colony yielded progeny that expressed greater levels of Fc-binding protein than either the parent strain or the selected low-producing colonies; however, some heterogeneity of Fc-binding protein expression remained in the second generation strains. On repeated subculturing, the low and high producers retained these characteristics and the extent of heterogeneity declined on subsequent selections. This procedure has facilitated the isolation and characterization of group A (type II) immunoglobulin-binding proteins (Yarnall and Boyle, 1986a, b).

Similarly, colony blot selection can be carried out using more than one probe. The *Streptococcus zooepidemicus* strain S2-12 was first selected with a goat IgG Fc-probe to identify a high-expressing strain for goat IgG

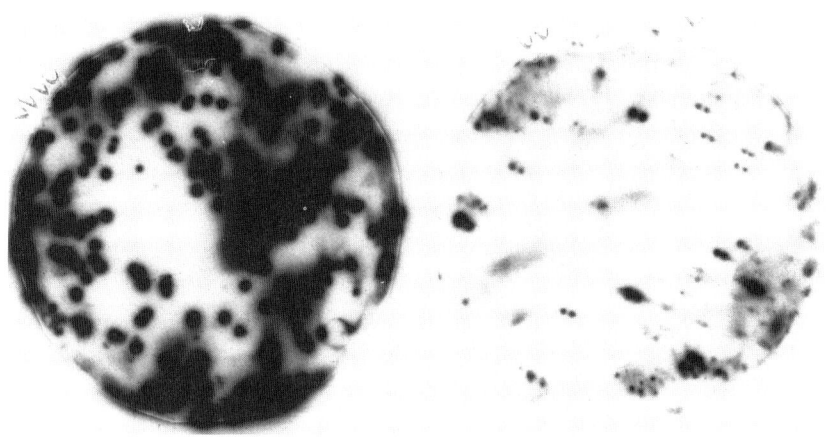

FIGURE 6
Fc-binding protein expression of two bacterial subpopulations selected from the original strain 64/14. The autoradiograph in the left panel was obtained by probing a high Fc receptor-producing substrain and the autoradiograph in the right panel was obtained by probing a low Fc receptor-producing colony. These colonies were selected and subcultured from individual colonies in the replica plate shown in Figure 5. Autoradiography was carried out by exposure of the blot for 3 days at −70°C to X-ray film using an intensifying screen. (Reproduced from Yarnall et al., 1984, with permission.)

binding (Reis and Boyle, 1990). However, this goat IgG-selected strain, when probed with polyclonal rat IgG displayed a high degree of colony heterogeneity. When this strain was further selected for reactivity with polyclonal rat IgG, a selected strain that demonstrated a high level of homogeneous binding with rat IgG was obtained following three rounds of colony selection (Reis *et al.*, 1988). The selection process resulted in a strain that exhibited a 10–20 fold increase in binding of ^{125}I- labeled rat IgG compared to the original goat-selected strain (Reis *et al.*, 1988). Interestingly, the rat-selected strain demonstrated enhanced binding with goat IgG.

The colony selection procedure has proven to be very efficient for selection of strains rich in a desired Fc-binding protein and this is a necessary first step to enable efficient isolation of the corresponding binding protein. This procedure has also been used to identify colonies secreting immunoglobulin-binding proteins (Yarnall *et al.*, 1984). For this application, the nitrocellulose is placed on the side of the Todd-Hewitt agar plate opposite from where the colonies are growing. The electrophoretic transfer enables secreted proteins to pass through the agar and bind to the nitrocellulose while preventing passage of the bacteria themselves. This approach has been used successfully in our laboratories to identify strains that secrete high levels of immunoglobulin-binding proteins.

XII. Storage of Strains

Bacteria can be stored by any number of common methods, including freezing in glycerol, lyophilization, or storage on solid media. In our work with staphylococci and streptococci, we have found the following methods to be most successful for the storage and recovery of strains expressing immunoglobulin-binding proteins.

A. Glycerol Stocks

We routinely prepare glycerol stocks of all strains. The isolated bacteria are grown overnight in 10 ml of suitable media. (Todd-Hewitt for streptococci and trypticase soy broth for staphylococci.) The culture is centrifuged and 8–9 ml of clear broth is removed with a sterile pipette, leaving 1–2 ml of concentrated bacteria. One milliliter of this suspension is added to an equal volume of a 25% suspension of glycerol in PBS, which has been previously autoclaved. The vials are thoroughly mixed and stored at −70°C. Some fresh isolates of streptococci, particularly animal isolates survive better in the presence of serum. For these strains, we add one volume of 50% sterile glycerol, one volume of heat-inactivated horse serum (56°C for 30 min), and two volumes of concentrated bacteria.

B. Recovery of Strains from Glycerol Stocks

Thaw the vial containing bacteria at room temperature and mix. A loopful of bacteria can be removed and inoculated into suitable media, such as Todd-Hewitt broth, trypticase soy broth, or blood broth (one of these media containing 1–2 drops/ml of sheep red blood cells), or directly onto a blood agar plate. The bacteria from any recovered bacterial stock should be streaked onto a blood agar plate to check for purity prior to use. The glycerol stock should be refrozen immediately after removal of an aliquot of the bacteria.

C. Storage on Blood Agar Plates

Bacteria can be stored on blood agar plates at 4°C, however they must be passed every 4–6 weeks. Once strains are isolated, they are passed by streaking through a heavy growth area on the first plate and then streaking onto a fresh plate. Selection of individual colonies should be avoided since a colony with low expression of immunoglobulin-binding proteins might be propagated by such a procedure. It is prudent to maintain glycerol and/or lyophilized strains selected for high immunoglobulin-binding activity in case the strain loses immunoglobulin-binding proteins following repeated *in vitro* passage or is lost or becomes contaminated.

XIII. Conclusions

In this chapter, we have described a number of assays that we have used to detect immunoglobulin-binding proteins found on the surface of bacteria. The most important aspect in detection of immunoglobulin-binding proteins is preparation of the probe to assure that the reaction between the bacteria and the immunoglobulin is not mediated by a specific antibody to a bacterial surface component, but is a genuine nonimmune interaction. Once a strain of interest is identified, colony blot selection or *in vivo* passage in mice can be used to enhance expression of the desired reactivity.

References

Åkerström, B., and Björck, L. (1986). *J. Biol. Chem.* **261**, 10240–10247.
Anderson, S. G., Bentzon, M. W., Houba, V., and Krag, P. (1970). *Bull. World Health Org.* **42**, 311–318.
Björck, L. (1988). *J. Immunol.* **140**, 1194–1197.
Boyle, M. D. P., and Langone, J. J. (1980). *J. Immunol. Methods* **32**, 51–58.
Boyle, M. D. P., and Reis, K. J. (1987). *Biotechnology* **5**, 697–703.
Burova, L. A., Christensen, P., Grubb, R., Jonsson, A., Samuelson, G., Schalen, C., and Svensson, M.-L. (1980). *Acta Pathol. Microbiol. Scand. Sect. B* **98**, 199–205.
Christensen, P., and Kronvall, G. (1974). *Acta Pathol. Microbiol. Scand. Sect. B* **82**, 19–24.
Erntell, M., Myhre, E. B., and Kronvall, G. (1983). *Scand. J. Immunol* **17**, 201–209.
Haake, D. E., Franklin, E. C., and Frangione, B. (1982). *J. Immunol.* **129**, 190–192.
Kessler, S. W. (1975). *J. Immunol.* **115**, 1616–1625.
Kronvall, G. (1973). *J. Immunol.* **111**, 1401–1406.
Kronvall, G., Quie, P. G., and Williams, R. C., Jr. (1970). *J. Immunol.* **104**, 273-278.
Langone, J. (1982). *Adv. Immunol.* **32**, 157–252.
Langone, J. J., Boyle, M. D. P., and Borsos, T. (1977). *J. Immunol. Methods* **18**, 281–293.
Lind, I., Live, I., and Mansa, B. (1970). *Acta Pathol. Microbiol. Scand. Sect. B* **78**, 673–682.
Lindahl, G. (1990). *In* "Bacterial Immunoglobulin-Binding Proteins" (M. D. P. Boyle, ed.), Vol. 1. pp. 257–265 Academic Press, San Diego.
Lindahl, G., and Kronvall, G. (1988). *J. Immunol.* **140**, 1223–1227.
Müller, H.-P., and Blobel, H. (1983). *Zentralbl. Bakteriol. Hyg. I Abt. Orig. A* **254**, 352–360.
Myhre, E. B. (1990). *In* "Bacterial Immunoglobulin-Binding Proteins" (M. D. P. Boyle, ed.), Vol. 1. pp. 243–256 Academic Press, San Diego.
Myhre, E. B., and Erntell, M. (1985). *Mol. Immunol.* **22**, 879–885.
Plaut, A. G. (1983). *Annu. Rev. Microbiol.* **37**, 603–622.
Porter, R. R. (1959). *Biochem. J.* **73**, 119–126.
Reis, K. J., and Boyle, M. D. P. (1990). *In* "Bacterial Immunoglobulin-Binding Proteins" (M. D. P. Boyle, ed.), Vol. 1. pp. 165–173 Academic Press, San Diego.
Reis, K. J., Ayoub, E. M., and Boyle, M. D. P. (1983). *J. Immunol. Methods* **59**, 83–94.
Reis, K. J., Yarnall, M., Ayoub, E. M., and Boyle, M. D. P. (1984). *Scand. J. Immunol.* **20**, 433–439.
Reis, K. J., Siden, E. J., and Boyle, M. D. P. (1988). *BioTechniques* **6**, 130-136.
Sjöquist, J., and Stålenheim, G. (1969). *J. Immunol.* **103**, 467–473.
Stjernquist-Desatnik, A., Kurl, D. N., and Christensen, P. (1984). *Acta Pathol. Microbiol. Scand. Sect. B* **92**, 223–227.
van de Rijn, I., and Kessler, R. E. (1980). *Infect. Immun.* **27**, 444–448.
van der Merwe, J. P., and Stegeman, J. H. (1985). *Eur. J. Immunol.* **15**, 860–863.
Widders, P. R., Stoke, C. R., Newby, T. J., and Bourne, F. J. (1985). *Infect. Immun.* **48**, 417–421.
Winblad, S., and Ericson, C. (1973). *Acta Pathol. Microbiol. Scand. Sect. B* **81**, 150–156.
Yarnall, M., and Boyle, M. D. P. (1986a). *Mol. Cell. Biochem.* **70**, 57–66.
Yarnall, M., and Boyle, M. D. P. (1986b). *Scand. J. Immunol.* **24**, 549–557.
Yarnall, M., Reis, K. J., Ayoub, E. M., and Boyle, M. D. P. (1984). *J. Microbiol. Methods* **3**, 83–93.
Yarnall, M., Ayoub, E. M., and Boyle, M. D. P. (1986). *J. Gen. Microbiol.* **132**, 2049–2052.
Yarnall, M., Widders, P. R., and Corbeil, L. B. (1988). *Scand. J. Immunol.* **28**, 129–137.

CHAPTER 3

Extraction and monitoring of soluble immunoglobulin-binding proteins

Michael D. P. Boyle
Kathleen J. Reis
Ronald A. Otten
Ervin L. Faulmann

I. Introduction

The usefulness of immunoglobulin-binding proteins for immunoassays is well documented by the wide range of applications described using staphylococcal protein A (Langone, 1978, 1982; Langone *et al.*, 1977, 1979; Boyle, 1984; Boyle and Reis, 1987; Goding, 1983). Protein A is the prototype of bacterial IgG-binding proteins and has been commercially available since 1978. Over the past decade other immunoglobulin-binding proteins have been studied in the research laboratory. The isolation of the type III Fc-binding protein, more frequently designated as protein G (Reis *et al.*, 1984a, b, 1985; Björck and Kronvall, 1984; Åkerström and Björck, 1986; Erntell *et al.*, 1988), and its subsequent cloning (Guss *et al.*, 1986; Fahnestock *et al.*, 1986, 1990; Fahnestock, 1988; Fipula *et al.*, 1987), have extended the immunotechnological applications of protein A to a wider range of species and subclasses of immunoglobulins (Boyle *et al.*, 1985; Wallner *et al.*, 1987; Reis *et al.*, 1984a, 1988). Protein G has the broadest species and subclass reactivity of any of the bacterial immunoglobulin-binding proteins thus far described and has enabled approaches pioneered using protein A to be extended into other systems (Boyle, 1984; Boyle and Reis, 1987). Other bacterial immunoglobulin-binding proteins that are more or less selective for different immunoglobulin isotypes have been described. For example, Myhre and Erntell (1985) and Björck (1988) have described a protein from *Peptococcus magnus* that demonstrates reactivity with immunoglobulin light chains. Russell-Jones *et al.*, (1984) have reported that an antigen associated with certain group B streptococci reacts with human IgA Fc fragments and our laboratory has reported a unique IgG-binding protein that reacts exclusively with human IgG_3 (Yarnall and Boyle, 1986a–c).

In Chapter 2, methods for screening bacteria for a given nonimmune IgG reactivity were described. These approaches are applicable to the selection of specific surface receptors or binding proteins on bacteria for any ligand and thus can be used to screen for any species, subclass, or isotype of immunoglobulin that is of interest. Methods for enhancing and selecting stable bacterial isolates displaying a desired reactivity are the most important prerequisites for isolation and characterization of the molecules responsible for the functional activity of interest (Chapter 2). It should be noted that many organisms, in particular the group A streptococcus, can change the expression of surface proteins during laboratory passage (Stjernquist-Desatnik *et al.*, 1984; Boyle *et al.*, 1990; Ravdonikas *et al.*, 1984; Faulmann and Boyle, 1990). As a first step in isolating a specific Fc-binding activity, it is important to establish that the desired activity is present as a stable characteristic of the strain selected for study.

The isolation of bacterial immunoglobulin-binding proteins requires both a method for solubilizing the product from the bacteria as well as a method for detecting the product once solubilized. Without a semiquantitative detection system for the solubilized material, it is impossible to compare the yields and efficiencies of different extraction procedures. In the remainder of this chapter a variety of extraction procedures are described and methods for quantifying soluble immunoglobulin-binding proteins are presented.

II. Extraction Procedures

The majority of immunoglobulin-binding proteins are detected as surface-expressed components of bacteria. Many of these molecules are also found to be secreted by the bacteria (von Mering and Boyle, 1986; Lämmler *et al.*, 1987), and indeed some bacteria have been found to secrete immunoglobulin-binding proteins in the absence of surface expression (Brady and Boyle, 1989). The recovery and detection of secreted immunoglobulin-binding proteins will be discussed later.

In our studies of streptococcal immunoglobulin-binding proteins, we have observed that no single extraction procedure is optimal for all strains. Indeed, differences in group-specific carbohydrates among streptococci, as well as differences in overall cell wall structure among other gram-positive and gram-negative organisms would predict such a finding. The choice of extraction procedure should be focused toward techniques that either have been shown to solubilize other surface proteins from similar bacteria or would be expected to affect the surface characteristics of the organisms under study. The extraction procedures we have used routinely to solubilize immunoglobulin-binding proteins from gram-positive organisms are outlined in the following sections.

A. Enzymatic Extraction Methods
1. *Mutanolysin Extraction*

Mutanolysin is a muramidase isolated from culture filtrates of *Streptomyces globisporus* (Yokogawa *et al.*, 1975). This enzyme is frequently found contaminated with proteases and care should be taken to remove this proteolytic activity before use. Mutanolysin has been used to prepare protoplasts of both *Streptococcus mutans* (Siegal *et al.*, 1981; Parks *et al.*, 1980) and group B streptococci (Calandra and Cole, 1980), as well as for the solubilization of various streptococcal surface proteins, including immunoglobulin-binding proteins (Reis *et al.*, 1985; Yarnall and Boyle, 1986c; Lämmler *et al.*, 1987; Tille *et al.*, 1986).

For the isolation of streptococcal Fc-binding proteins, we have found the following procedure to be successful. Approximately 6 g (wet weight) of bacteria to be extracted are suspended in 30 ml of 20 mM Tris–HCl, pH 7.5, 1 mM iodoacetic acid, and 1 mM benzamidine–HCl. To this suspension, add 100 µg/ml pancreatic DNase (Sigma Chemical Co., St. Louis, Missouri), and 100 µg/ml mutanolysin. A commercial preparation of mutanolysin is available from Sigma. This preparation is known to be contaminated with a protease. This undesirable activity can be separated from the glycolytic enzyme on an ion exchange column as described by Siegel *et al.* (1981). The protease-free mutanolysin preparation is incubated at 37°C with the bacteria in a shaking water bath for 4 hr. The mixture is then centrifuged at 10,000 × g for 10 min and the resulting supernatant filtered through a 0.2 µm filter to remove the remaining bacteria. The filtrate is dialyzed against 20 mM Tris–HCl, pH 7.5, containing 1 mM iodoacetic acid, 1 mM benzamidine–HCl, and 1 mM phenylmethyl sulfonyl fluoride (PMSF). This procedure has been shown to solubilize type II and type III IgG-binding proteins from group A and group C streptococci, respectively (Yarnall and Boyle, 1986b, c; Reis *et al.*, 1985). This procedure tends to result in a high yield of soluble immunoglobulin-binding proteins; however, in most cases the immunoglobulin-binding activity is associated with multiple molecular forms of the binding protein(s) (Yarnall and Boyle, 1986c; Reis *et al.*, 1985; Tille *et al.*, 1986).

2. Hyaluronidase Extraction

Hyaluronidase is an enzyme that will hydrolyze hyaluronic acid that is present in the capsule of certain streptococcal species. A variety of sources of hyaluronidase are available both from bacterial and mammalian origins. We have used hyaluronidase to solubilize type II IgG-binding proteins from group A streptococci (Yarnall and Boyle, 1986c). This procedure is carried out as follows. Approximately 6 g (wet weight) of bacteria to be extracted are suspended in 30 ml of 0.15 M phosphate-buffered saline (PBS), pH 7.2. To this suspension, 10 mg type IV hyaluronidase (Sigma) is added and incubated at room temperature for 30 min. The bacterial-free supernatant is recovered as described previously.

3. Trypsin Digestion

Trypsin is a highly selective protease, hydrolyzing peptide bonds involving the basic amino acids lysine and arginine. Treatment of bacteria with trypsin, under suboptimal conditions of ionic strength and pH for enzyme activity, has been used to isolate type III Fc-binding protein fragments from groups C and G streptococci (Reis *et al.*, 1985, 1986; von Mering and Boyle, 1986). Lämmler *et al.* (1987) have also used trypsin extraction to solubilize Fc-binding proteins from group C streptococci.

The procedure we have used to solubilize type III Fc-binding fragments is as follows. Approximately 2 g (wet weight) of bacteria to be extracted are suspended in 20 ml of 50 mM KH_2PO_4,5 mM ethylenediaminetetraacetic acid (EDTA), 0.02% NaN_3, pH 6.1, and incubated at 37°C for 1 hr with 80 μg pancreatic DNase and 400 μg trypsin (Sigma). These buffer conditions are not optimal for trypsin activity and facilitate the extraction of surface proteins without concomitant proteolysis of the solubilized material. Benzamidine–HCl is added to a final concentration of 100 mM to stop the reaction. Kinetic studies should be carried out since prolonged trypsin treatment results in the destruction of the solubilized proteins (Reis *et al.*, 1985). Proteins solubilized following trypsin treatment are removed from residual bacteria by centrifugation. Benzamidine–HCl, PMSF, or other serine protease inhibitors should be added to inhibit further enzymatic digestion by trypsin.

4. Papain Digestion

Papain is a proteolytic enzyme that hydrolyzes amides and esters, particularly those of basic amino acids that are not substituted on the side chain amino group. This specificity is similar to that of trypsin, but the specificity of papain is not as precise and hydrolysis at other residues can occur (Dixon and Webb, 1979). Papain digestion has been used to obtain a homogeneous, functionally active type III Fc-binding protein fragment from groups C and G streptococci (Björck and Kronvall, 1984; Reis *et al.*, 1985, 1986: von Mering and Boyle, 1986).

The procedure we use to isolate a type III Fc-binding protein from a group C strain is as follows. Approximately 6 g (wet weight) of the bacteria to be extracted are suspended in 20 ml of 10 mM Tris–HCl, pH 8.0 and 0.02% NaN_3. Two milliliters of 0.4 M cysteine and 1.6 mg papain are added to this suspension and allowed to incubate at 37°C for 1 hr. The reaction is stopped by addition of iodoacetic acid to a final concentration of 30 mM. Complete enzyme inactivation is achieved following a further 15 min incubation on ice with iodoacetic acid. The samples should be neutralized and bacteria and baterial debris removed by centrifugation at 10,000 × g for 10 min.

5. Treatment with the Bacteriophage-Associated Lysin

An enzyme activity released by group C streptococci infected by C1 bacteriophage has been reported by Krause (1957) and Maxted (1957). Fischetti *et al.*, (1971) subsequently isolated and characterized this phage-associated lysin activity. This enzyme activity has been found to be useful for the isolation of group A streptococcal cell wall components and in the preparation of protoplasts. We have used this enzyme, prepared as described by Fischetti *et al.*, (1971), for the solubilization of immunoglobulin-binding proteins from group A and group C streptococci (Reis *et al.*, 1984a; Yarnall and Boyle, 1986c).

The procedure we have used is carried out as follows. Approximately 2 g (wet weight) of the bacteria to be extracted are suspended in 20 ml of 50 mM KH_2PO_4, 5 mM EDTA, and 0.02% NaN_3, pH 6.1, and 0.2 ml of previously activated phage lysin is added and incubated at 37°C for 1 hr (Fischetti *et al.*, 1971). The bacteria-free supernatant is recovered as previously described. This phage-associated lysin enzyme is not commercially available and in most of our studies appears to solubilize a similar series of proteins to those solubilized by mutanolysin.

6. Lysostaphin Extraction Treatment

This procedure has been used successfully by Sjöquist *et al.*, (1972) to isolate protein A from *Staphylococcus aureus* and is carried out as follows. The lysostaphin preparation used in that study contained three distinct enzymatic activities: (1) an amidase, (2) a peptidase, and (3) an N-acetylglucosaminidase. In this study, the enzyme preparation contained high amidase and peptidase activities and a low glucosaminidase activity, and resulted in the solubilization of a homogeneous 42,000 dalton form of protein A. We have carried out a similar procedure using a commercial preparation of lysostaphin and obtained similar results.

The procedure we have used is as follows. Approximately 2 g (wet weight) of bacteria are suspended in 20 ml of 0.05 M Tris–HCl, 0.015 M NaCl, pH 7.5, containing 0.2 mg lysostaphin and 10 μg DNase (Sigma). Following a 4 hr incubation at 37°C the extracts are recovered by centrifugation, followed by filtration through a 0.2 μm filter.

7. General Comments Regarding Enzymatic Procedures

The conditions for any enzymatic digestion need to be carefully controlled to prevent degradation of the product once solubilized. Consequently, it is worth carrying out kinetic studies to determine the optimal time of enzyme treatment for solubilization of the desired reactivity. For example, in earlier studies using trypsin to solubilize an IgG-binding fragment from the group C streptococcus, 26RP66, we had initially found that a single functional species was solubilized. As the digestion continued, a second molecular weight fragment with IgG-binding activity was generated (Reis *et al.*, 1985). Following a 10–12 hr incubation with trypsin under the conditions described, the functional activity was destroyed.

B. Nonenzymatic Extraction Procedures

A variety of nonenzymatic procedures have been described for solubilization of bacterial membrane proteins (Poxton and Blackwell, 1984). A number of the general procedures used to solubilize bacterial Fc-binding proteins are described.

1. Acid, Alkaline, and Neutral Heat Extractions

Hot acid, alkali, or neutral extractions have been popular methods for solubilizing streptococcal antigens for serological typing assays (Lancefield, 1928). We and others have used the basic Lancefield extraction procedure to isolate a variety of different immunoglobulin-binding proteins (Reis *et al.*, 1985; Havlicek, 1978; Grubb *et al.*, 1982; Brady and Boyle, 1989). In this procedure, bacteria are suspended in PBS to form a 10% suspension and the pH is adjusted to 2 (or 10) with 0.5 M HCl (or 0.5 M NaOH). The bacterial suspension is boiled for 10 min and the pH neutralized. The neutral extraction is carried out as previously described, by heating bacteria suspended in PBS at pH 7.0. The bacterial-free supernatants are recovered by removal of bacteria by centrifugation as described earlier.

2. Acetone/Detergent Extraction

Extraction procedures utilizing detergents or organic solvents have also been utilized for solubilizing Fc-binding proteins. The procedure we have found to be most successful with streptococcal isolates is a modification of that described by Bhaduri and Demchick (1983).

Approximately 1 g (wet weight) of bacteria to be extracted is suspended in 10 ml of ice-cold acetone (Fisher Certified A.C.S. grade, Fair Lawn, New Jersey), allowed to stand on ice for 5 min., and then collected by centrifugation at 10,000 × g for 10 min. The supernatant is discarded and residual acetone is evaporated under a stream of air. The pellet is resuspended, with vortexing, in 25 ml of 1% (v/v) Triton X-100 in PBS, pH 7.3, containing 0.02% NaN_3 and incubated at room temperature for 5 min. [This procedure can be carried out using 0.1% sodium dodecyl sulfate (SDS) in place of the nonionic detergent Triton X-100.] The bacteria are removed by centrifugation and the detergent is removed by dialysis against 20 mM Tris–HCl, pH 7.5, or use of an appropriate column (e.g., Polyprep columns, Bio-Rad, Richmond, California or Extracti-gel, Pierce, Rockford, Illinois). Detergent extraction has been used to extract IgA-binding proteins from group B streptococci (Russell-Jones *et al.*, 1984).

3. General Comments on Nonenzymatic Procedures

Heat extractions at acid, alkali, or neutral pH have been successful in extracting IgG-binding proteins from certain streptococcal isolates. It should be noted that variations in the stability of type II Fc-binding proteins extracted from group A streptococci as a function of pH have been noted from isolate to isolate. For example, Grubb, *et al.* (1982) have isolated a type II Fc-binding protein from a T15 group A streptococcus using extraction with hot alkali. This procedure did not result in solubilization of a functional type II Fc-binding protein from group A isolate 64/14 (Yarnall and Boyle, 1986c). Similarly, the yield of soluble material following detergent extraction can be influenced by the phase of growth in which the bacteria are harvested. In general, it is necessary to establish optimal extraction conditions on a strain-by-strain basis.

III. Secreted IgG-Binding Proteins

Bacterial immunoglobulin-binding proteins can be secreted into the culture fluid during growth of bacteria. Previous studies with *Staphylococcus aureus* have demonstrated levels of 1850 ± 200 ng/ml of protein A in overnight cultures of the Cowan strain, while culture supernatants from the Wood 46 strain contained 162 ± 7 ng of protein A (Reis *et al.*, 1983).

The composition of the culture medium has been shown to markedly influence the quantities of protein A secreted into the culture fluid by various strains of *Staphylococcus aureus* (Lind, 1972) and this has proven to be a valuable source of wild type protein A for isolation and characterization. Other bacteria have been shown to secrete IgG-binding proteins (Brady and Boyle, 1989; Müller and Blobel, 1983; von Mering and Boyle, 1986). The level of reactive material varies from isolate to isolate, and considerable size heterogeneity is also observed in the binding proteins recovered from the culture fluid. For example, Figure 1 displays the pattern of IgG-binding proteins in the culture fluid of five group C and group G streptococci.

The cell-free supernatants from each strain were collected from an overnight culture of each isolate grown in Todd-Hewitt broth. The bacterial-free supernatants were concentrated ten-fold, extensively dialyzed against PBS containing 0.02% NaN_3, and analyzed by Western blotting. Fc-binding protein activity was detected using ^{125}I-labeled human IgG as probe. When equal volumes of concentrated supernatant from each

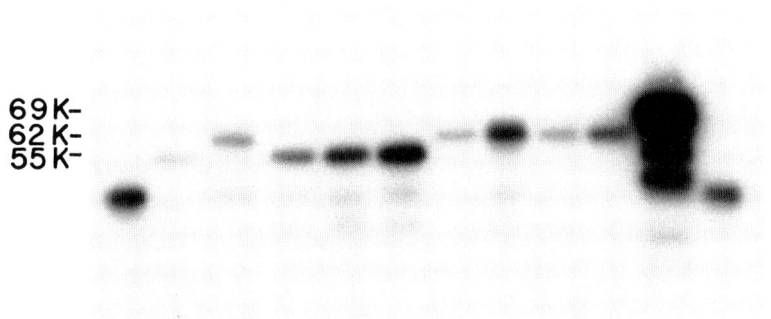

FIGURE 1
Western blot analysis of concentrated supernatants from overnight cultures of five group C and five group G streptococci. Samples were electrophoresed on 10% SDS-PAGE gels, electroblotted onto nitrocellulose, and probed with ^{125}I-labeled human IgG. Lanes B–F contain equal volumes (100 μl) of a sample from a tenfold concentrated supernatant from group C strains C6, C782, C281, C350, and 26RP66, respectively. Lanes G–K contain equal volumes (100 μl) of a ten-fold concentrated sample from the group G strains G60, G78, G493, G1070, and G1400, respectively. Lanes A and L contain the type I Fc receptor, staphylococcal protein A, as a positive control. (Reproduced from Von Mering and Boyle 1986, with permission.)

strain were analyzed by Western blotting, varying levels of Fc-binding protein activity were detected (Figure 1). Each strain was found to secrete detectable levels of Fc-binding protein activity, with the group C strain 26RP66 and the group G strain G1400 secreting the highest levels. All forms of Fc-binding activity secreted appeared to be functionally and antigenically related (von Mering and Boyle, 1986).

The heterogeneity in Fc-binding proteins is influenced by the culture conditions (e.g., length of culture, time, source of media, etc.). Many streptococci produce acid proteases that become active when the pH falls below 6.5, and activation of this activity can destroy or modify IgG-binding proteins (Elliot and Dole, 1947; Liu and Elliott, 1965). However, under controlled growth conditions reproducible patterns of secreted IgG-binding proteins can be recovered in culture supernatants and this is a valuable source of soluble material for purification. If a secreted form of bacterial immunoglobulin-binding protein is to be studied, the use of chemically defined media such as the medium formulation for group A streptococci, devised by van de Rijn and Kessler (1980), can be used. This medium can be concentrated readily and isolation of secreted protein is easier than from complex medium, which already contains high concentrations of heterogeneously sized proteins. When using chemically defined media, it is important to control both the pH of the culture and to carry out kinetic studies to determine the optimal time to harvest cultures to ensure maximal yield and minimal heterogeneity.

A. Detection of Solubilized Immunoglobulin-Binding Proteins

A variety of methods have been developed to detect immunoglobulin-binding proteins once in solution. These include agglutination of red cells sensitized with subagglutinating doses of anti-red cell antibodies, immunodiffusion methods, competitive inhibition assays, or following immobilization by measuring their interaction with a suitable, labeled IgG or IgG Fc fragment. All of these methods have proven to be capable of detecting bivalent Fc-binding proteins. The hemagglutination assay has been described in Chapter 2 using intact bacteria and can be readily adapted to measure soluble immunoglobulin-binding proteins. This procedure is semiquantitative, subjective, and is not practical if there are bacterial hemolysin present in the extracts. Similarly, the immunodiffusion assays are not very sensitive and reactivities due to bacterial antigen–antibody complexes cannot be distinguished readily from nonimmune IgG Fc-binding protein complexes. Consequently, the use of competitive inhibition assay and dot blot procedures are recommended for quantifying

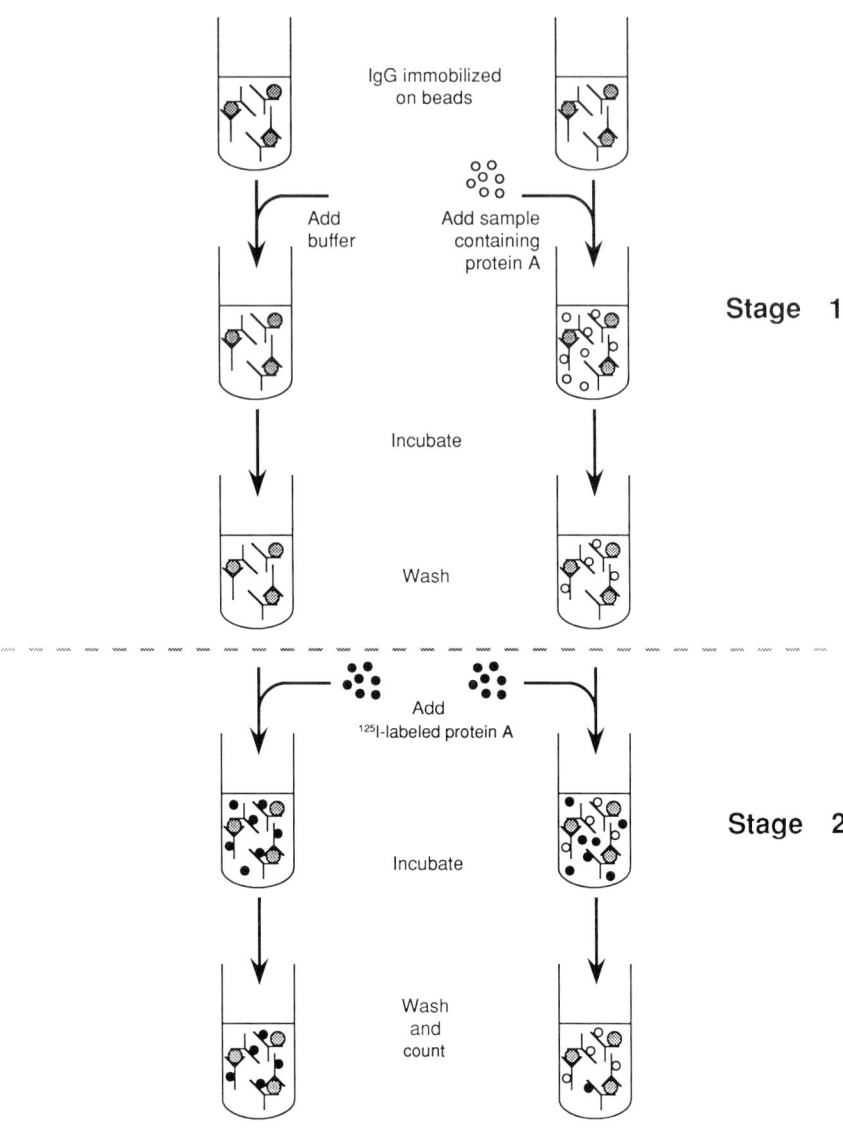

FIGURE 2
Schematic representation of a two-stage immunoassay selective for protein A or any IgG Fc-binding protein that binds to a similar or identical site on the Fc region of IgG. In Stage 1, the sample containing immunoglobulin-binding proteins is mixed with immobilized IgG and incubated for 1–2 hr at 37°C. At this time, the immobilized IgG beads are pelleted and the supernatant discarded. The IgG beads, with any complexed Fc-reactive material, are washed twice with 2 ml of 0.01 M EDTA-gel buffer and

soluble IgG-binding protein activities. These assays depend upon the functional activity of the IgG-binding protein; however, detection of epitopes on these proteins can also be used if suitable, specific antibodies are available (Chapter 6).

1. Competitive Binding Radioimmunoassays for Soluble Fc-Binding Proteins

A variety of competitive binding assays have been developed to measure soluble immunoglobulin-binding proteins (Langone *et al.*, 1977; Fey and Burkhard, 1981; Olsvik and Betdal, 1981; Reis *et al.*, 1983). These assays are based on the ability of the soluble Fc-binding protein to compete with a purified, labeled tracer form of the molecule for binding to immobilized IgG. This assay is essentially similar to the one stage assay for the detection of IgG described in Chapter 2, except that the immunoglobulin-binding protein, rather than IgG is the competitor. For this procedure to be of value, there must be an appropriate tracer molecule available. Since this one-step assay can measure either IgG or Ig-binding proteins, we have developed a two-stage assay, which is specific for immunoglobulin-binding proteins (Reis *et al.*, 1983). This assay is summarized for the type I Fc-binding protein in Figure 2. By carrying out the procedure in two stages, nonspecific inhibition by constituents of complex bacterial growth media has not been found to be a problem (Figure 3), and consequently this approach is of particular value for studying secreted immunoglobulin-binding proteins.

Frequently, when new immunoglobulin-binding activities are being isolated for the first time, suitable, purified tracers may not be available and the dot blot procedure described later in this chapter can be used. To date, all of the streptococcal IgG Fc-binding proteins that have been isolated bind either to the same or to a closely proximal site within the C_H2–C_H3 domain of reactive immunoglobulin molecules (Boyle and Reis, 1987; Woof and Burton, 1989). This property enables the use of a previously purified tracer, e.g., protein A or protein G, to detect the activity of an Fc-binding protein from different bacteria. Consequently, this competitive binding immunoassay is not restricted to only those immunoglobulin-binding proteins that have already been isolated. The basic procedure for this assay is outlined as follows.

---

resuspended in 0.1 ml VBS-gel. In Stage 2, 0.1 ml of ^{125}I-labeled protein A (approximately 20,000 cpm) is added to the washed bead suspension and incubated for an additional 60 min at 37°C. At this time the beads are washed twice with 0.01 M EDTA-gel buffer as described and the quantity of ^{125}I-labeled protein A associated with the beads determined in an automatic gamma counter. The example shown at the left of the figure determines maximal binding in the absence of any fluid-phase competitor.

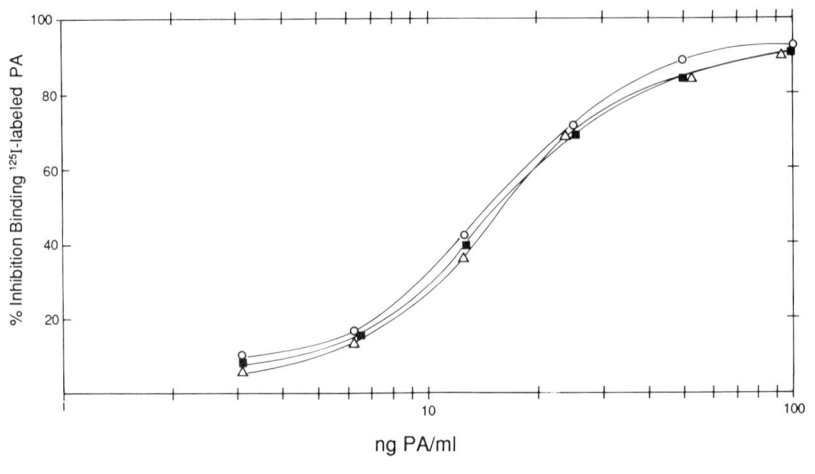

FIGURE 3
Effects of different bacterial culture media on the efficiency of detection of staphylococcal protein A (PA) using the two-stage immunoassay described in Figure 2. In this assay, immobilized rabbit IgG is used and the tracer is ^{125}I-labeled protein A. 50% inhibition ng PA/ml. ○—○ Veronal-buffered saline 15.0; ■—■ Todd–Hewitt broth 15.9; △—△ Trypticase soy broth 18.8.

a. Materials

Samples containing solubilized immunoglobulin-binding proteins

Rabbit IgG immunobeads (Bio-Rad, Richmond California (An activated immunobead support to which any desired species of IgG can be coupled is also available from this company, in case the binding protein to be measured is not reactive with rabbit IgG.)

^{125}I-labeled type I-binding protein (protein A) (See Chapter 7 for iodination procedures.)

VBS-gel is used for all dilution steps.

EDTA-gel is used for all washing steps.

For exact formulations of buffers, see Appendix.

b. Procedure. In the first stage, 0.1 ml of a dilution of immunobeads (immobilized rabbit IgG) is mixed with 1.0 ml of a solution containing a dilution of the soluble immunoglobulin-binding protein. (The appropriate dilution of immunobeads should be determined in preliminary experiments, in which 0.1 ml of bead dilutions are mixed with 0.1 ml of tracer for 1 hr at 37°C. The beads are washed twice as described in this section and the number of counts bound in the absence of any competitor is determined. Usually, we use a dilution of immobilized IgG immunobeads that will result in approximately 33% of the total offered counts being bound to the immobilized IgG at the end of the assay.) The reactants are mixed and incubated for an appropriate time (usually 30–60 min at 37°C) and then washed twice by centrifugation and resuspension in 2 ml of VBS-gel. The immobilized IgG pellet is then resuspended in 0.1 ml of EDTA-gel and 0.1 ml of radiolabeled tracer is added and incubated for an appropriate time (usually 1–2 hr) at 37°C. The quantity of labeled tracer associated with the immobilized IgG beads is determined, following two washes of 2 ml of EDTA-gel, by counting in a gamma counter. The presence of immunoglobulin-binding proteins is determined by a reduction in the radioactivity associated with the pelleted material compared to the maximum number of counts bound to immobilized IgG in the absence of any unlabeled competitor. Background binding is measured by the quantity of radioactivity associated with washed tubes to which tracer is added without addition of immunoglobulin beads. (If the background counts are high, i.e., $>5\%$ of the total counts offered, the labeled tracer should be centrifuged in a microfuge or filtered through a $0.2\ \mu$ filter.) If a pure source of the immunoglobulin-binding protein is available, a series of samples containing known concentrations of the protein can be included in the inhibition assay. The degree of inhibition resulting from known amounts of the binding protein can then be used to generate a standard inhibition curve and can be related to the absolute concentration of IgG-binding protein present in the sample. Like any competitive binding immunoassay, the absolute concentration of an unknown sample should be calculated from at least two dilutions. This will ensure that the observed inhibition behaves in a similar manner to the standard. If there is a significant difference in the calculated concentration for each dilution, following appropriate correction for the dilution factor, then the assay is not valid and the reason for the deviation from ideal behavior will need to be established.

In developing a competitive binding assay for any given immunoglobulin-binding protein, a series of preliminary studies should be conducted to optimize the assay conditions. An example of the effect of varying the incubation times for the first and second stages of an immunoassay for protein A is shown in Figure 4. Differences are seen in the sensitivity of detection of protein A, depending on the assay conditions. In all of our studies, we have carried out assays in which the first stage is between 1 and 2 hr at 37°C and the second stage is carried out for at least

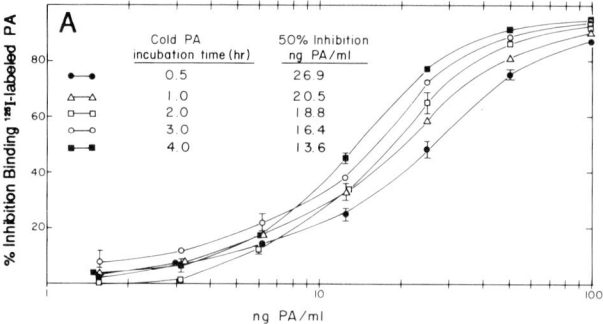

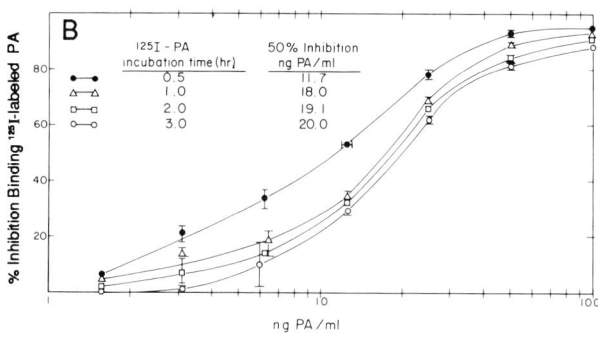

FIGURE 4
Optimization of times of incubation for the two-stage immunoassay for staphylococcal protein A. This assay follows the outline in Figure 2 using immobilized human IgG beads and ^{125}I-labeled protein A as tracer. The panel A shows the kinetics of the first stage of the reaction outlined in Figure 2. The panel B shows the kinetics of the second stage of the reaction outlined in Figure 2.

1 hr at 37°C. These conditions result in good day-to-day reproducibility. The two-stage assay is of value for detecting IgG-binding proteins in complex mixtures, especially those which contain IgG capable of binding to the radiolabeled tracer and thus inhibiting its binding to the beads. As shown in Figure 5, IgG is not detected efficiently in the two-stage assay described here.

The two-stage assay can be carried out with sample volumes as great as 3 ml, which enables quantitation of low levels of immunoglobulin-

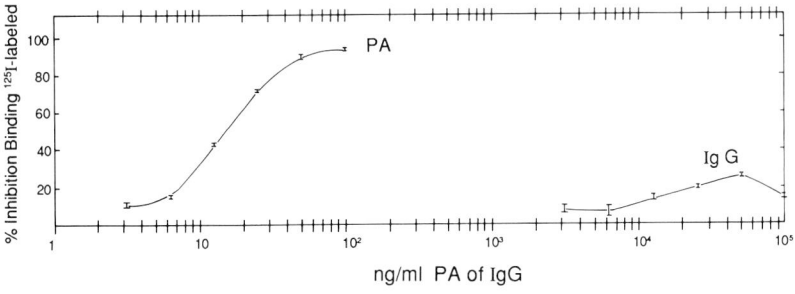

FIGURE 5
Selectivity of the two-stage immunoassay for protein A (PA). Note the absence of reactivity of IgG in this assay. In a one-stage assay, 50% inhibition of ^{125}I-labeled protein A binding could be achieved on addition of 25–50 ng of a reactive species of immunoglobulin (Langone et al., 1977). 50% inhibition by PA 15.0 ng/ml; 50% inhibition by IgG > 100 μg/ml. (Reproduced from Reis et al., 1983, with permission.)

binding proteins without having to use highly concentrated extracts or bacterial culture fluids. This assay will detect any immunoglobulin-binding protein that binds to the same or to a closely proximal location on IgG as the site recognized by the labeled tracer. To date, we have found that all such types of IgG-binding proteins can be detected with differing efficiencies in this type of competitive binding assay. The procedure described here can also be carried out with enzyme-labeled tracers (Olsvik and Berdal, 1981). However, the use of microtiter plates in the enzyme-linked immunosorbent assay (ELISA) limits the volumes of sample that can be tested.

2. Detection of Low Affinity Bacterial IgG-Binding Proteins

The types I (protein A) and III (protein G) Fc-binding proteins have been reported to bind IgG with affinities of approximately 10^{-10} M for human and rabbit IgG (Langone, 1982; Åkerström and Björck, 1984). The types IV, V, and VI bacterial Fc-binding proteins appear to display lower affinities in direct binding assays using intact bacteria (Boyle and Reis, 1987). In particular, the type IV-binding protein is found to display the lowest affinities for rabbit and human IgG of any of the streptococcal IgG-binding proteins (Reis et al., 1989). Consequently, we have been concerned that the competitive binding methods we have described might not be practical for detection of low-affinity binding proteins when either radioiodinated protein A or protein G is used as tracer.

To address this potential problem, we have compared the efficiency of detection of a low-affinity form of protein G, containing a single IgG-binding domain, in a standard competitive binding assay using two forms of radiolabeled protein G. One form of protein G contained a single IgG-binding domain (low-affinity) while the second contained two IgG-binding domains (high-affinity). These different forms of protein G were prepared by recombinant DNA procedures by Genex Corporation (Gaithersburg, Maryland) and kindly made available to us for these studies. The single binding domain form of protein G could be iodinated without loss of its binding ability for immobilized human IgG. As expected, it was necessary to increase the concentration of immobilized IgG in the reaction mixture to maintain the maximal tracer binding at 30% of the counts offered. This in turn decreased the sensitivity of the inhibition assay. The results presented in Figure 6 compare the inhibitory potential of the two recombinant forms of protein G when tested in competitive binding assays using as tracer either the low-affinity form of protein G (containing a single IgG-binding domain) or the high-affinity form (with two IgG-binding domains). As expected, the protein G with the single IgG-binding domain was less inhibitory than the protein G molecule containing two IgG-binding domain forms, using the high-affinity tracer (Figure 6A). When these experiments were repeated using the low-affinity tracer, similar inhibition curves were obtained when either the one IgG-binding or two IgG-binding domain forms of protein G were used as competitors (Figure 6B). Although the sensitivity of this assay was decreased for the detection of the two IgG-binding domain forms of protein G, the single domain form of protein G (low-affinity) was detected with increased sensitivity. The availablility of different affinity immunoglobulin-binding protein tracers will enable the development of assays for new immunoglobulin-binding proteins that may display lower affinity reactivities than protein A and protein G.

3. *Dot Blot Procedure to Detect Soluble Bacterial Immunoglobulin-Binding Protein*

This procedure is essentially similar to that described for detection of immunoglobulin-binding proteins on whole bacteria described in Chapter 2, with the exception that solubilized bacterial proteins rather than intact bacteria are immobilized to nitrocellulose. All other blocking and probing reactions are identical (for complete methodological details, see Chapter 14). As noted for all methods that utilize antibody probes as tracers, it is important to ensure that any reactivity being detected is not mediated by specific antibody binding, but is due to a nonimmune interaction. For a discussion of Fc-specific probes, see Chapter 2. The dot blot assay has been used to compare the efficiencies of different extraction conditions and has proven to be of value when the Fc-binding protein being studied is of low affinity, e.g., type IV Fc-binding protein (Reis *et al.*, 1990), and fails

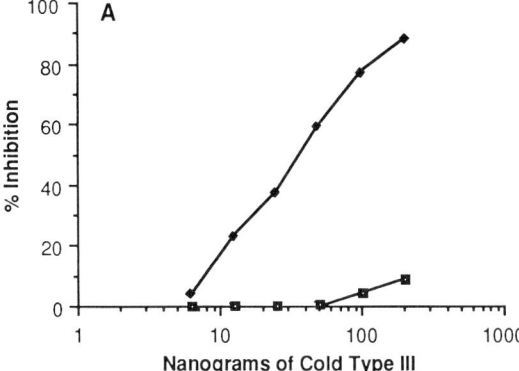

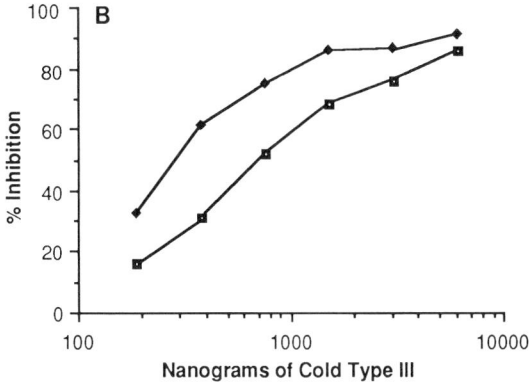

FIGURE 6
Competitive inhibition of a high-affinity form (A) and a low-affinity form (B) of radiolabeled protein G tracer by the corresponding unlabeled forms of protein G. GammaBind® G, Type 5: Protein G fragment containing a single IgG-binding domain (B_2, —□—). GammaBind® G, Type 2: Protein G fragment containing two IgG-binding domains (B_1-B_2 —◆—). These forms of protein G were prepared using recombinant DNA technology by the Genex Corporation (Gaithersburg, Maryland).

to compete efficiently with the available tracers in the two-stage competitive binding assay that we have described. An example of the use of the immunoblotting procedure to compare the efficiencies of extraction methods to solubilize a type IV positive, bovine group G streptococci, BG5, is shown in Figure 7.

The dot blot procedure and the competitive binding assay can be used to obtain semiquantitative data for soluble immunoglobulin-binding proteins; however, these assays give no indication of the number of distinct molecular species contributing to this reactivity. In order to determine the extent of heterogeneity in Fc-binding proteins in extracts, Western blotting techniques have proven to be of great value.

B. Analysis of Immunoglobulin-Binding Protein Heterogeneity by Western Blot Analysis

In this technique, extracted, soluble binding proteins are electrophoresed in polyacrylamide gels and transferred electrophoretically to nitrocellulose membranes (Western blot). Proteins on the nitrocellulose

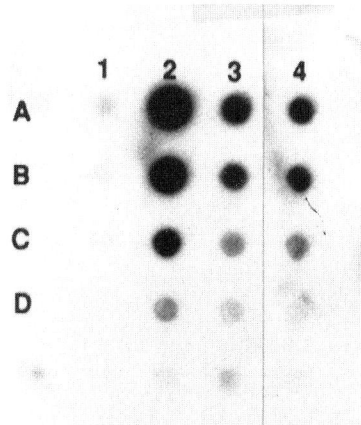

FIGURE 7
Comparison of extraction methods to solubilize type IV Fc-binding proteins from a bovine group G streptococcus, BG5. The extraction procedures were carried out as described in this chapter and reactivity was determined by probing with ^{125}I-labeled rabbit Fc fragments. The washed blots were autoradiographed at −70°C for 20 hr with an intensifying screen. Lane 1 contains a hot-alkaline extract. Lane 2, a hot-acid extract. Lane 3, a detergent (Triton X-100) extract. Lane 4, a mutanolysin extract. (A) Undiluted extracts. (B) Extracts diluted 1:3. (C) Extracts diluted 1:9. (D) Extracts diluted 1:27.

Chapter 3. Solubilization of IgG-Binding Proteins

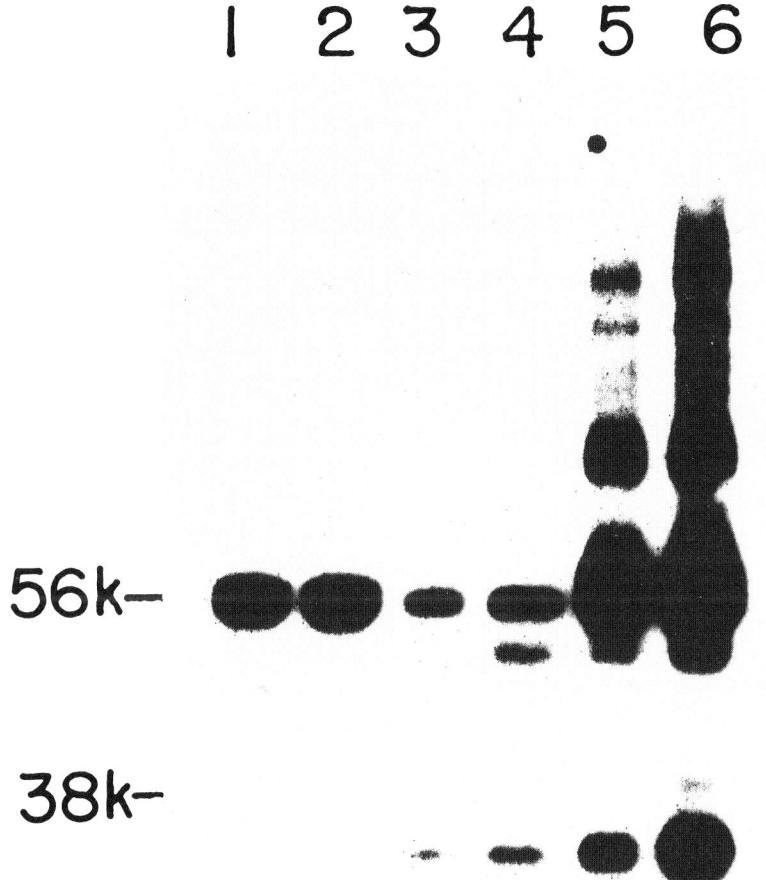

FIGURE 8
Western blot autoradiograph of affinity-purified extractions of 64/14/HRP. Lanes 1 and 2 contain 1.8 µg and 4.2 µg of heat-extracted, Fc-reactive material, respectively. Lanes 3 and 4 contain 4 µg and 12 µg of hyaluronidase-extracted, Fc-reactive material. Lanes 5 and 6 contain 5 µg and 1.2 µg mutanolysin-extracted, Fc-reactive material. The affinity-purified samples were electrophoresed on an SDS-polyacrylamide gel, electroblotted onto nitrocellulose, and probed with an ^{125}I-labeled Fc-specific probe. Autoradiography was for 20 hr at −70°C with an intensifying screen. [Reproduced from Yarnall and Boyle (1986), with permission.]

membrane are probed with labeled Fc-specific probes and immunoglobulin-binding proteins are detected according to the type of labeled tracer used (*e.g.*, color change as a result of substrate cleavage for enzyme-labeled immunoglobulins or autoradiography for iodinated immunoglobulins). This technique allows the number of differently sized molecules with immunoglobulin-binding properties to be identified. The technical details of how this procedure is carried out are described in detail in Chapter 14.

In our laboratory, we routinely analyze secreted or extracted bacterial immunoglobulin-binding proteins by Western blot analysis following the general procedures of Laemmli (1970) and Towbin *et al.*, (1979). An example of the results of this procedure, when used to compare a number of extraction techniques for solubilization of type II immunoglobulin-binding proteins from a group A streptococcal isolate, 64/14, is shown in Figure 8. This procedure demonstrates that each extraction procedure solubilizes a distinct range of immunoglobulin-binding proteins or fragments.

Until the properties of a new immunoglobulin-binding protein, have been established, it is advisable to include a reactive immunoglobulin-binding protein, (e.g., protein A or protein G), as a positive control. Molecular weight standards should be included on each gel to allow molecular weights to be assigned to reactive bands. This procedure can be used for both crude extracts as well as purified samples. By comparing reactive bands at each step in the purification protocol, any new molecular species of immunoglobulin-binding protein generated during the purification procedure can be identified. Methods for characterizing isolated bacterial immunoglobulin-binding proteins are described in detail in Chapter 4.

IV. Summary

The methods described in this chapter enable the optimal extraction procedure for solubilization of a given bacterial immunoglobulin-binding protein to be established. In general, we have used the methods that result in the highest yield of functional activity contained in the lowest number of molecular-sized forms. It should be noted however, that the most homogeneous forms of the protein are not always optimal for all purposes. For example, the type III Fc-binding protein isolated by treatment of a group C streptococcus with papain or trypsin does not retain all of its original, functional activity after either iodination or following storage (Boyle and Reis, 1987; Faulmann *et al.*, 1989). This is in marked contrast to the heterogeneous material isolated from a phage lysate of the same group C streptococcus (Reis *et al.*, 1984a).

Acknowledgment

The authors would like to thank the Genex Corporation, Gaithersburg, Maryland, for providing us with the two defined forms of recombinant protein G used in the assays described in Figure 6.

References

Åkerström, B., and Björck, L. (1986). *J. Biol. Chem.* **261,** 10240–10247.
Bhaduri, S., and Demchick, P. H. (1983). *Appl. Environ. Microbiol.* **46,** 941–943.
Björck, L. (1988). *J. Immunol.* **140,** 1194–1197.
Björck, L., and Kronvall, G. (1984). *J. Immunol.* **133,** 964–974.
Boyle, M. D. P. (1984). *Biotechniques* **2,** 334–340.
Boyle, M. D. P., and Reis, K. J. (1987). *Biotechnology* **5,** 697–703.
Boyle, M. D. P., Wallner, W. A., von Mering, G. O., Reis, K. J., and Lawman, M. J. P. (1985). *Mol. Immunol.* **22,** 1115–1121.
Boyle, M. D. P., Faulmann, E. L., Otten, R., and Heath, D. H. (1990). *In* "Microbial Determinants of Virulence and Host Response" (E. M. Ayoub, G. H. Cassell, W. C. Branche and T. J. Henry, eds.). pp. 19–44. ASM, Washington, D.C.
Brady, L. J., and Boyle, M. D. P. (1989). *Infect. Immun.* **57,** 1573–1581.
Calandra, G. B., and Cole, R. M. (1980). *Infect. Immun.* **28,** 1033–1037.
Dixon, N., and Webb, E. C. (1979). *Enzymes,* 3rd Edition. Academic Press, New York.
Elliott, S. D., and Dole, V. P. (1947). *J. Exp. Med.* **85,** 305–310.
Erntell, M., Myhre, E. B., Sjöbring, V., and Björck, L. (1988). *Mol. Immunol.* **25,** 121–126.
Fahnestock, S. R. (1988). *Trends Biotechnol.* **5,** 79–84.
Fahnestock, S. R., Alexander, P., Nagle, J., and Filpula, D. (1986). *J. Bacteriol.* **167,** 870–880.
Fahnestock, S. R., Alexander, P., Filpula, D., and Nagle, J. (1990). *In* "Bacterial Immunoglobulin-Binding Proteins" (M. D. P. Boyle, ed.), Vol. 1. pp. 133–148. Academic Press, San Diego.
Faulmann, E. L., and Boyle, M. D. P. (1990). *In* "Bacterial Immunoglobulin-Binding Proteins" (M. D. P. Boyle, ed.), Vol. 1. 69–81. Academic Press, San Diego.
Faulmann, E. L., Otten, R. A., Barrett, D. J., and Boyle, M. D. P. (1989). *J. Immunol. Methods* **123,** 269–281.
Fey, H., and Burkhard, G. (1981). *J. Immunol. Methods* **47,** 99–107.
Fipula, D., Alexander, P., and Fahnestock, S. R. (1987). *Nucleic Acids Res.* **15,** 7210.
Fischetti, V. A., Gotschlich, E. C., and Bernheimer, A. W. (1971). *J. Exp. Med.* **133,** 1105–1117.
Goding, J. W. (1983). "Monoclonal Antibodies: Principles and Practice," pp. 113–116. Academic Press, London.
Grubb, A., Grubb, R., Christensen, P., and Schalén, C. (1982). *Int. Arch. Allergy Appl. Immunol.* **67,** 369–376.
Guss, B., Eliasson, M., Olsson, A., Uhlén, M., Frej, A. K., Jornvall, H., Flock, J. I., and Lindberg, M. (1986). *EMBO J.* **5,** 1567–1575.
Havlicek, J. (1978). *Exp. Cell Biol.* **46,** 146–151.
Krause, R. M. (1957). *J. Exp. Med.* **106,** 365.
Lämmler, C., Schaufuβ, P., Frede, C., and Blobel, H. (1987). *Can. J. Microbiol.* **34,** 1–5.
Laemmli, U. K. (1970). *Nature (London)* **227,** 680–685.

Lancefield, R. C. (1928). *J. Exp. Med.* **47,** 91–103.
Langone, J. J. (1978). *J. Immunol. Methods* **23,** 269–285.
Langone, J. J. (1982). *J. Immunol. Methods* **51,** 3–22.
Langone, J. J., Boyle, M. D. P., and Borsos, T. (1977). *J. Immunol. Methods* **18,** 281–293.
Langone, J. J., Boyle, M. D. P., and Borsos, T. (1979). *Anal. Biochem.* **93,** 207–215.
Lind, I. (1972). *Acta Pathol. Microbiol. Scand. Sect. B* **80B,** 702–708.
Liu, T.-Y., and Elliott, S. D. (1965). *J. Biol. Chem.* **240,** 1138–1144.
Maxted, W. R. (1957). *J. Gen. Microbiol.* **16,** 584.
Müller, H.-P., and Blobel, H. (1983). *Zentralbl. Bakteriol. Hyg., I. Abt. Orig. A* **254,** 352–360.
Myhre, E. B., and Erntell, M. (1985). *Mol. Immunol.* **22,** 879.
Olsvik, Ø., and Berdal, B. P. (1981). *Acta Pathol. Microbiol. Scand. Sect. B* **89,** 289–290.
Parks, L. C., Shockman, G. D., and Higgins, M. L. (1980) *J. Bacteriol.* **143,** 1491–1497.
Poxton, I. R., and Blackwell, C. C. (1984). *In* Handbook of Experimental Immunology, Vol. I. Immunochemistry'' (D. N. Weir, ed.). Blackwell, Oxford.
Ravdonikas, L. E., Christensen, P., Burova, L. A., Grabovskaya, K., Björck, L., Schalén, C., Svensson, M. L., and Totolian, A. A. (1984). *Acta Pathol. Microbiol. Immunol. Scand. Sect. B* **92,** 65–69.
Reis, K. J., Ayoub, E. M., and Boyle, M. D. P. (1983). *J. Immunol. Methods* **59,** 83–94.
Reis, K. J., Ayoub, E. M., and Boyle, M. D. P. (1984a). *J. Immunol.* **132,** 3091–3097.
Reis, K. J., Ayoub, E. M., and Boyle, M. D. P. (1984b). *J. Immunol.* **132,** 3098–3102.
Reis, K. J., Ayoub, E. M., and Boyle, M. D. P. (1985). *J. Microbiol. Methods* **4,** 45–58.
Reis, K. J., Hansen, H. F., and Björck, L. (1986). *Mol. Immunol.* **23,** 425–431.
Reis, K. J., von Mering, G. O., Karis, M. A., Faulmann, E. L., Lottenberg, R., and Boyle, M. D. P. (1988). *J. Immunol. Methods* **107,** 273–280.
Reis, K. J., Salpeter, J., and Boyle, M. D. P. (1990). *In* "Bacterial Immunoglobulin-Binding Proteins" (M. D. P. Boyle, ed.), Vol. 1. pp. 149–154. Academic Press, San Diego.
Russell-Jones, G. J., Gotschlich, E. C., and Blake, M. S. (1984). *J. Exp. Med.* **160,** 1467–1475.
Siegal, J. L., Hurst, S. F., Liberman, E. S., Coleman, S. E., and Bleiweis, A. S. (1981). *Infect. Immun.* **31,** 808–815.
Sjöquist, J., Meloun, B., and Hjelm, H. (1972). *Eur. J. Biochem.* **29,** 572–578.
Stjernquist-Desatnik, A., Kurn, D. N., and Christensen, P. (1984). *Acta Pathol. Microbiol. Immunol. Scand. Sect. B* **92,** 223–227.
Tille, D., Chhatwal, G. S., and Blobel, H. (1986). *Med. Microbiol. Immunol.* **175,** 35–41.
Towbin, H., Stachelin, T., and Gordon, J. (1979). *Proc. Natl. Acad. Sci. U.S.A.* **76,** 4350–4354.
Van de Rijn, I., and Kessler, R. E. (1980). *Infect. Immun.* **27,** 444–448.
von Mering, G., and Boyle, M. D. P. (1986). *Mol. Immunol.* **23,** 811–821.
Wallner, W. A., Lawman, M. J. P., and Boyle, M. D. P. (1987). *Appl. Microbiol. Biotechnol.* **27,** 168–173.
Woof, J. M., and Burton, D. R. (1989). *In* "Bacterial Immunoglobulin-Binding Proteins" (M. D. P. Boyle, ed.), Vol. 1. pp. 305–316. Academic Press, San Diego.
Yarnall, M., and Boyle, M. D. P. (1986a). *J. Immunol.* **136,** 2670–2673.
Yarnall, M., and Boyle, M. D. P. (1986b). *Scand. J. Immunol.* **24,** 549–557.
Yarnall, M., and Boyle, M. D. P. (1986c). *Mol. Cell. Biochem.* **70,** 57–66.
Yokogawa, K., Kawata, S., Takesmura, T., and Yoshimura, Y. (1975). *Agric. Biol. Chem.* **39,** 1533–1543.

CHAPTER **4**

Isolation and functional characterization of bacterial immunoglobulin-binding proteins

Michael D. P. Boyle
Kathleen J. Reis
Ervin L. Faulmann

I. Introduction

The procedures described in Chapter 3 document methods for solubilizing immunoglobulin-binding proteins and quantifying them once solubilized. The focus of this chapter is to describe methods for the isolation and characterization of bacterial immunoglobulin-binding proteins. A variety of methods, including ion-exchange chromatography, molecular sieving, and affinity chromatography have been used to purify immunoglobulin-binding proteins (Sjöquist *et al.*, 1972; Reis *et al.*, 1984a). The most effective way of purifying these molecules is by affinity chromatography on columns of immobilized IgG (Hjelm *et al.*, 1972; Reis *et al.* 1984a, 1985; Björck and Kronvall, 1984; Yarnall and Boyle, 1986a,b). A number of considerations need to be addressed in designing the optimal affinity purification strategy including the following.

1. The source of IgG for immobilization
2. The nature of the sample to be purified
3. The methods of recovering the protein from the immobilized IgG matrix

As with any purification procedure, methods to quantitate the protein of interest and determine its purity are essential. The procedures described in Chapter 3 to detect soluble immunoglobulin-binding proteins can be used to detect and quantify the functional activity of the binding proteins during purification.

II. Selection of Immunoglobulin Source to Prepare Affinity Columns

The ability of antibody molecules to bind selectively through their $F(ab')_2$ regions has been used successfully as a method of affinity purification of a variety of bioactive molecules (Levy and Eveleigh, 1978; Kristiansen, 1978; Kaplan and Kabat, 1966; Cheng *et al.*, 1973). Use of immobilized IgG for the purification of IgG Fc-binding proteins, however, may result in the copurification of other undesired bacterial antigens, if specific antibodies to these antigens are present in the IgG pool used to prepare the immobilized affinity column. These contaminants can be minimized by the use of Fc fragments, but the purification of Fc fragments is time consuming, and frequently the immobilization of just the Fc fragment is not as efficient as the use of whole IgG. The problems associated with affinity purification of other bacterial products can be minimized in a number of ways. First, if there are similar bacteria that do not express the IgG-binding proteins or a strain is available that has lost IgG-binding properties during subculture, the non-IgG-binding form of the bacteria can be used to preabsorb the IgG preparation prior to immobilization. This approach is strongly recommended for studies with recombinant proteins expressed in, for example, *Escherichia coli*. The immunoglobulin to be immobilized should first be absorbed with the intact *E. coli* host strain as well as with immobilized lysates or sonicates of the bacteria. (Note, these preabsorption procedures will be counterproductive if an Fc-binding protein is expressed in the absorbing mixture.)

Other methods of minimizing bacterial antigen contamination include the use of differential elution conditions or by carrying out the affinity purification procedure twice, using a different immobilized species of IgG on each occasion. The latter approach is based on the assumption that the distribution of natural antibodies in two different species is unlikely to be the same, and hence the number of common bacterial contaminants copurified would be minimal. Additional purification steps based on molecular sieving or ion-exchange chromatography can be included to obtain a pure form of the desired bacterial immunoglobulin-binding protein.

A major consideration in the purification of any bacterial immunoglobulin-binding protein is the choice of species of IgG to use for immobilization. For example, in studies of type II immunoglobulin-binding proteins associated with a group A streptococcus, strain 64/14, we discovered that the major functional activity in heat extracts was a 56,000 dalton protein (Yarnall and Boyle, 1986b,c). However, following affinity purification, a minor 38,000 dalton protein was present on Coomassie-stained gels (Yarnall and Boyle, 1986a,b). This lower molecular weight protein proved not to be a contaminant, but rather a binding protein specific for human IgG_3 (Yarnall and Boyle, 1986a–c). Western blot analysis of the crude, heat extract of group A strain 64/14 did not reveal this activity because the specific activity of IgG_3 in the labeled human Fc pool used as the tracer was too low (Yarnall and Boyle, 1986c). The immobilized human IgG column however, contained sufficient IgG_3 to purify this activity. It is, therefore, important to determine that all of the IgG-binding activity associated with the intact bacteria can be accounted for in the affinity-purified material.

With these considerations in mind, there are a number of methods available to immobilize immunoglobulins, as well as a number of commercial sources of immobilized immunoglobulin supports. The choice of matrix used for immobilization of IgG should be determined by the chromatography system in use in an individual laboratory. For example, a variety of noncompressible matrices are available for use with high-pressure chromatographic systems.

Methods that result in covalent attachment of the immunoglobulin to the matrix should be used. There are a variety of available supports to which immunoglobulins can be coupled to prepare stable, immobilized IgG reagents. Suitable, activated supports that couple via amino groups or carboxyl groups on the immunoglobulins are available from a number of companies including Pharmacia (Piscataway, New Jersey), Bio-Rad Laboratories (Richmond, California), and the Pierce Chemical Company (Rockford, Illinois). Each of these companies offers a variety of activated, high-capacity gels suitable for immobilization of immunoglobulins. The use of the hydrazine method of immobilization of IgG via glycosylated residues in the Fc region (Little *et al.*, 1988) is not recommended for purifying bacterial Fc-binding proteins. In addition, a variety of matrices with different species of immunoglobulin covalently coupled to them are commercially available.

III. Nature of the Sample to Be Purified

Depending on the source of soluble bacterial Fc-binding protein, it is sometimes beneficial to carry out some form of pretreatment to debulk the undesired proteins from the sample. This is particularly relevant if the

IgG-binding protein is recovered as a secreted product present in a complex bacterial growth medium, such as Todd-Hewitt broth. In general, we have not had any difficulty with the direct application of bacterial extracts to affinity columns, and thus only the secreted products have been subjected to a debulking procedure. In general, the volumes of bacterial supernatants are large and the classical salting out approaches using $(NH_4)_2 SO_4$ (ammonium sulfate), polyethylene glycol, ethanol, or similar agents are not practical. In our experience, the use of batch absorption with ion-exchange resins has proven to be the most successful. For these procedures, a number of pilot studies should be carried out using DE52 (Whatman or equivalent) or CM52 (Whatman or equivalent) at a variety of pHs. The ion-exchange resin is mixed in a test tube with an aliquot of the bacterial culture fluid and incubated at room temperature with constant mixing for 30 min. The resin is allowed to settle, the culture fluid removed, and residual particles of the ion-exchange resin are removed by centrifugation. The supernatant is then monitored for functional immunoglobulin-binding activity and for protein content. Conditions that remove a high percentage of total protein and a low percentage of immunoglobulin-binding protein activity or vice versa, are established.

Once suitable conditions of pH have been determined for either an anion- or cation-exchange resin, the procedure can be easily scaled up by adding an excess of the resin to a large volume of culture supernatant, with constant stirring. The resin can then be separated from the culture fluid by vacuum filtration through a sintered glass filter. This approach is amenable for use with large volumes of bacterial culture fluid or any other source of soluble immunoglobulin-binding protein. The active material can either be recovered in the flow-through liquid and further concentrated or, if it is bound to the resin, be selectively eluted by washing the ion-exchange resin with an appropriate salt solution or a buffer of a suitable pH that facilitates dissociation of the bound proteins. Ideally, if the functional activity can be bound in the presence of low levels of other proteins, the desired reactivity can be recovered from the ion-exchange matrix in a more concentrated form by addition of a low volume of an appropriate buffer. The immunoglobulin-binding protein is then ready to be applied to an appropriate column of immobilized immunoglobulin.

IV. Selection of Eluting Agent

A number of different methods have been suggested for eluting immunoglobulin-binding proteins from columns of immobilized IgG. These include high or low pH (Reis *et al.*, 1984a), high salt (Yarnall and Boyle, 1986a), a variety of dipeptides (Bywater *et al.*, 1978, 1983; Yarnall and Boyle, 1986d), and chaotrophic agents (Bywater *et al.*, 1983). All of these approaches have proven satisfactory for isolation of certain immunoglobulin-binding proteins, but caution should be exercised since not all immunoglobulin-binding proteins are stable at extremes of pH. It is recommended that the crude preparation containing the immunoglobulin-binding protein be dialyzed into the eluting reagent and stored under these conditions for a few hours before returning the solution to phosphate-buffered saline at neutral pH. The functional activities of the treated and untreated samples should be compared to determine whether the conditions proposed for eluting the column are detrimental to the functional activity of the immunoglobulin-binding protein. It should also be noted that the susceptibility of purified binding proteins to proteolytic digestion appears greater after affinity purification. The addition of protease inhibitors to the eluting buffer or immediately following affinity purification may be desirable. We and others have observed the loss of functional activity of immunoglobulin-binding proteins on storage and with some types of Fc-binding proteins these effects are even more pronounced following affinity purification (Yarnall and Boyle, 1986c; Schalén and Christensen, 1990; Schalén *et al.*, 1982).

V. Affinity Purification of a Type III Fc-Binding Protein Solubilized by Bacteriophage Lysis of the Group C Streptococcus 26RP66

In this section, the purification of a crude bacteriophage lysate of a group C streptococcus, 26RP66, on a column of immobilized human IgG is described. Normal human IgG was immobilized onto the high-capacity Affi-gel 10 support (Bio-Rad, Richmond, California). Affi-gel 10 is a high-capacity, activated agarose support that forms stable covalent bonds with reactive amino groups on the immunoglobulin via N-hydroxysuccinimide ester functional groups. The coupling reaction was carried out according to the manufacturer's instructions. A 1×5 cm column containing the immobilized IgG support was poured and washed, first with $0.1\ M$ glycine–HCl, pH 2.0, to remove any noncovalently coupled IgG, and then it was equilibrated in $0.1\ M$ phosphate-buffered saline (PBS), pH 7.35.

A sample of a crude phage lysate from the group C streptococcus 26RP66 was then applied to the column in $0.1\ M$ PBS, pH 7.35, and eluted in the same buffer. The majority of the protein, as detected by monitoring the optical density at 280 nm (OD_{280}), flowed directly through the column. Once the OD_{280} of the fractions returned to base line values, the column was eluted with 0.1 M glycine–HCl, pH 2.0. A small protein peak was eluted from the column and this corresponded to the first fractions in which the pH fell below 3.0 (Figure 1). The starting sample and the various fractions that passed directly through the column or the fractions eluted from the column at low pH, following neutralization, were tested for the presence of Fc-binding proteins using the competitive binding radioimmunoassay described in Chapter 3. As shown in Figure 1, there was no Fc-binding activity associated with the fractions that passed directly through the column. This indicated that the capacity of the immobilized immunoglobulin to react with the binding protein had not been exceeded. It is important to measure the total functional activity applied and the total functional activity recovered in the affinity-purified fractions to establish the percentage of recovery. Estimates of the specific activity (i.e., the quantity of functional activity per amount of protein) should also be made to determine the degree of purification. In general, we have been able to recover about 60–70% of the Fc-binding protein applied to a column of immobilized IgG with a 150–200-fold increase in purity. The affinity-purified proteins may not be homogeneous, since this purification strategy will lead to the recovery of any form of binding protein or fragment with functional activity.

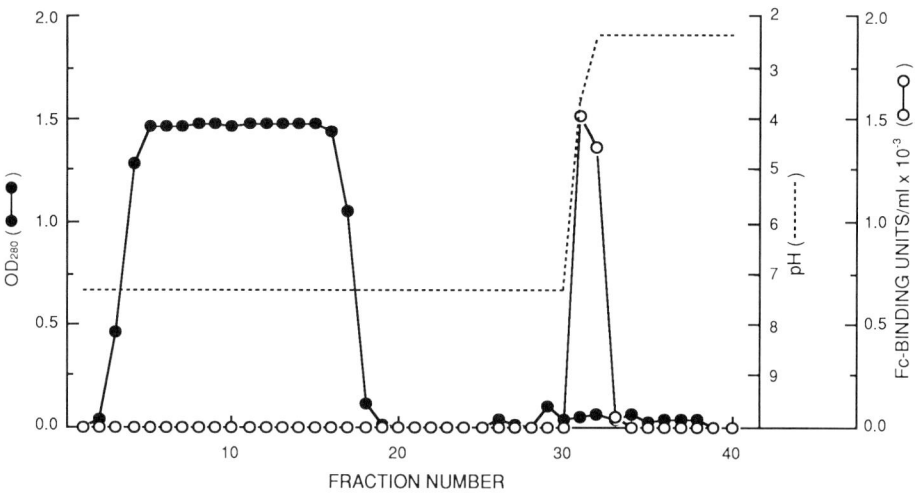

FIGURE 1
Representative affinity purification of the bacteriophage lysate of streptococcal strain 26RP66 on a column of immobilized IgG. Elution of bound IgG Fc-binding proteins was achieved using 0.1M glycine–HCl, pH 2.0.

The affinity columns can be reequilibrated and used again. It has been our experience that an immobilized IgG column can be used 10–15 times before a significant loss in capacity is apparent. It is important to store columns in the presence of azide or some other preservative. It is not recommended to use the same column for isolation of bacterial-binding proteins of different types, since a low level of cross-contamination can occur. This may be particularly problematic if a low-affinity binding protein is purified on the same column that was used previously to purify a high-affinity protein.

Affinity purification has proven to be the most efficient procedure for isolating bacterial immunoglobulin-binding proteins. This procedure has the additional advantage that it can be carried out with large volumes containing low levels of IgG-binding proteins. The active material binds to the column and can then be selectively recovered in a low volume of elution buffer, thereby facilitating both purification and concentration in a single step.

VI. Characterization of Affinity-Purified Immunoglobulin-Binding Proteins

The affinity-purification approaches just described result in the recovery of functionally related molecules that may not be homogeneous proteins. Indeed, many of the enzymatic extraction procedures described in the previous chapter result in the solubilization of a variety of differently sized molecules with immunoglobulin-binding activity. The purpose of this section is to describe methods that enable isolated immunoglobulin-binding proteins to be compared for purity and also facilitate analysis of different molecular forms of the binding proteins.

A. Physicochemical Analysis of Immunoglobulin-Binding Proteins

The most straightforward way to analyze immunoglobulin-binding proteins is by Western blotting techniques (also see Chapter 3). This enables a direct comparison of proteins present in a preparation by staining of a sodium dodecyl sulfate (SDS)–polyacrylamide gel, as well as a determination of functional activity by transfer of the proteins in a parallel gel to nitrocellulose or other suitable membrane and probing with radiolabeled or enzyme-labeled Fc fragments (Chapter 14). By comparing the crude extract to the affinity-purified material, it is possible to determine whether all of the active bands present in the starting material are represented in the affinity-purified sample. This is important since certain forms of the binding protein may display different affinities or different susceptibilities to the eluting agent. In addition, any molecular form of the binding protein present in the affinity-purified sample that is not present in the starting material must have been generated as a consequence of the purification procedure. We have found that many functionally active IgG-binding proteins can be detected by Western blot analysis; however, corresponding silver-stained bands on a parallel SDS–gel cannot be detected (Reis *et al.*, 1985; Boyle and Reis, 1987; Yarnall and Boyle, 1986b). If the gel is stained with Coomassie Blue R-250, the stained protein bands on the SDS–polyacrylamide gel can be shown to match with the IgG-binding activity (Reis *et al.*, 1985; Boyle and Reis, 1987; Yarnall and Boyle, 1986b). This inability to stain Fc-binding proteins efficiently with silver has been noted for types I, II, and III immunoglobulin-binding proteins (Boyle and Reis, 1987).

Also, it cannot be assumed that all the different species and subclass reactivities associated with a given bacteria are the result of the presence of a single immunoglobulin-binding protein. For example, in the case of at least one group A streptococcus, the IgG-binding activities have been shown to be the net result of expression of two distinct proteins, designated type IIa and type IIb. These proteins differ in their reactivities with human IgG subclasses. The type IIa protein binds IgG_1, IgG_2, and IgG_4 and the type IIb protein binds exclusively to human IgG_3 (Yarnall and Boyle, 1986a–c).

An example of the use of Western blot analysis to study Fc-binding proteins is provided in Figure 2. The group C streptococcus, 26RP66, was subjected to a variety of extraction procedures including phage lysis, hot-acid extraction, and treatment with the enzymes trypsin or mutanolysin (for precise conditions of time, temperature, and pH, see Reis *et al.*, 1985). The extraction of Fc-binding proteins was monitored in two ways in order to follow (1) the total quantity of Fc-binding proteins extracted, and (2) the heterogeneity of Fc-binding proteins extracted. The Fc-binding protein activity extracted was measured using the competitive binding assay we have described previously (Chapter 3 and Reis *et al.*, 1983). Heterogeneity of Fc-binding proteins was monitored by electrophoresing crude extracts on 10% SDS–PAGE gels and then transferring the separated proteins by electroblotting to nitrocellulose membranes. The blots were then probed for functional Fc-binding protein activity using an ^{125}I-labeled human Fc-specific probe. The results obtained, using a series of different extraction procedures are shown in Table 1 and Figure 2. These results indicate that Fc-binding protein activity can be solubilized by any of the extraction procedures tested (Table 1). A comparison of total Fc-

Chapter 4. Isolation and Functional Characterization

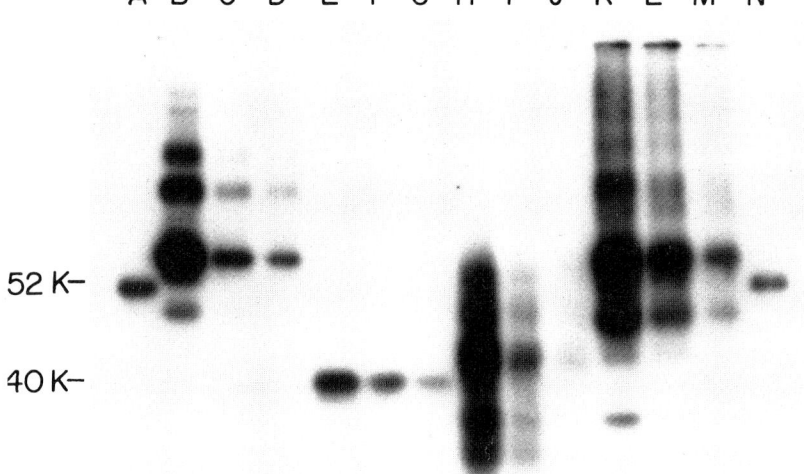

FIGURE 2
Western blot of extracts from the group C streptococcus, 26RP66. Extracts were electrophoresed on 10% SDS–PAGE gels, electroblotted onto nitrocellulose, and probed for Fc-binding proteins using ^{125}I-labeled human Fc fragments. Lanes B, C, and D contain material from phage-lysed bacteria with approximately 250, 125, and 63 ng of functional Fc-binding protein activity, respectively. Lanes E, F, and G contain material from trypsin-extracted bacteria with approximately 250, 125, and 63 ng of Fc-binding protein activity, respectively. Lanes H, I, and J contain material from hot acid-extracted bacteria with approximately 250, 125, and 63 ng of Fc-binding protein activity, respectively. Lanes K, L, and M contain material from mutanolysin-extracted bacteria with approximately 250, 125, and 63 ng of Fc-binding protein activity, respectively. Lanes A and N contain molecular weight standards and 40 ng staphylococcal protein A. The molecular weights shown were obtained from a parallel, silver-stained gel using the functional activity of protein A, lanes A and N as an internal standard on the silver-stained and Western blotted gels. (Reproduced from Reis *et al.* (1985) with permission.)

binding proteins recovered indicates that phage lysis resulted in the maximum yield of Fc-binding proteins and that the mutanolysin extract demonstrated the highest Fc-binding protein activity per A_{280} unit (Table 1). However, the most physicochemically homogeneous product was observed in the extracts obtained by treatment of bacteria with trypsin at suboptimal pH (Figure 2).

Phage lysis of the group C streptococcus 26RP66 yields four distinct proteins with Fc-binding activity (Reis *et al.*, 1984a,b, 1988). When the

TABLE 1
Comparison of Extraction Procedures to Solubilized Fc-Binding Proteins (FcRc) from a Group C Streptococcus (26RP66)

Method of Extraction	FcRc[a] (μg/g Bacteria Extracted)	FcRc[b](μg/A$_{280}$)	Number of Functional Fc Receptor Classes[c]
Phage lysis	1060 + 102	2.9	5
Hot-acid	78 + 18	2.6	4
Trypsin	129 + 10	3.2	1 (2)[d]
Mutanolysin	502 + 86	4.4	4

[a] Functional FcRc activity was determined using the competitive binding assay described by Reis *et al.* (1983).
[b] The specific activities of the FcRc preparations were calculated as the quantity of functional Fc receptor activity (μg/ml) divided by the A_{280} of the extract.
[c] Determined by SDS–PAGE followed by Western blotting (see Figure 2).
[d] One or two functional Fc-binding protein forms are detected depending on the time of trypsin treatment. (Reproduced from Reis *et al.* 1985, with permission.)

affinity-purified phage lysate is radioiodinated >98% of the radioactivity can be removed by incubation with immobilized human IgG (Reis *et al.*, 1984a,b). When these proteins are separated on nondenaturing polyacrylamide disc gels, four protein-staining bands can be observed and each protein has the ability to bind to IgG (Figure 3). These studies indicate that, depending on the extraction conditions, more than one molecular form of IgG-binding protein may be purified. Obviously, for protein sequence studies a homogeneous product is desirable and additional protein purification procedures that separate on the basis of size, charge, or hydrophobicity can be included to obtain a homogeneous fragment. Alternatively, a careful selection of the extraction procedure may help to minimize the heterogeneity observed. It should be noted that the most homogeneous form of immunoglobulin-binding protein may not always be the most useful for immunochemical applications. For example, the trypsin-solubilized type III Fc-binding protein is much more homogeneous than the family of proteins obtained following phage lysis (Figure 2). However, the smaller trypsin fragment loses functional activity following iodination and does not appear to be stable on storage or to display as high an average affinity for IgG as the material isolated following phage lysis of the bacteria (Reis *et al.*, 1985; Faulmann *et al.*, 1989).

B. Functional Characterization of Immunoglobulin-Binding Proteins

The characterization of immunoglobulin-binding proteins involves defining the species and subclass reactivity profiles as well as comparing the

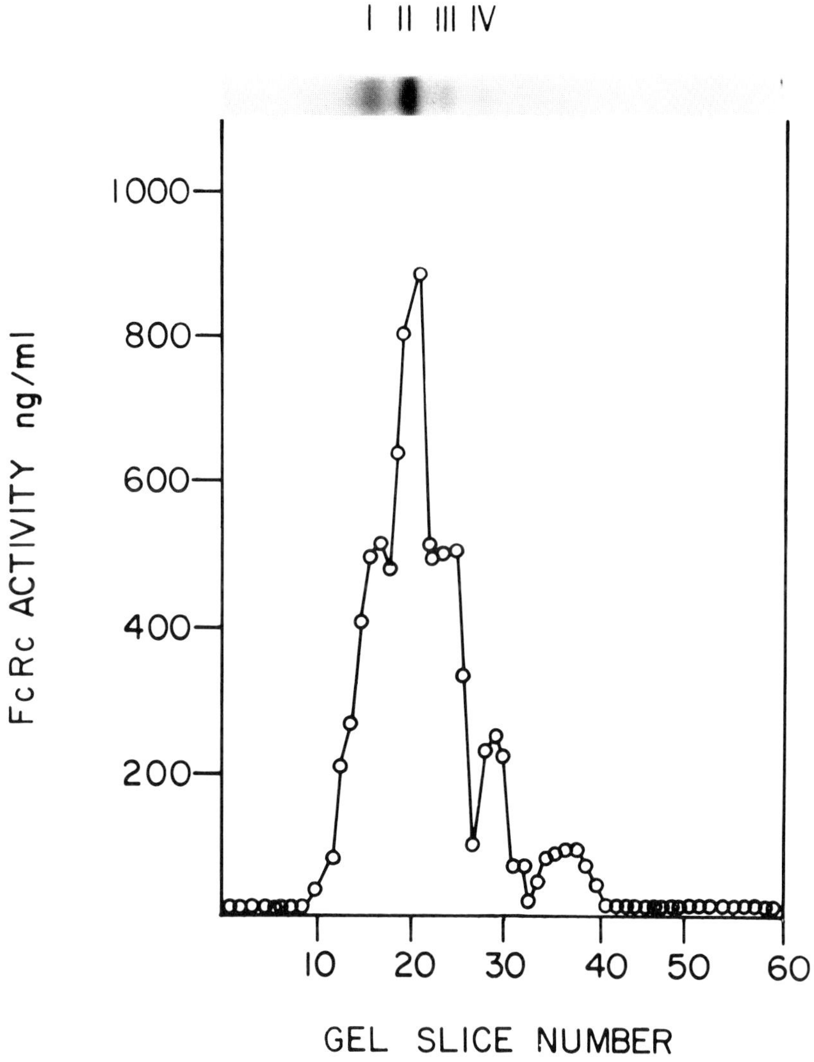

I II III IV

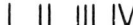

FIGURE 3
Nondenaturing polyacrylamide gel electrophoresis of affinity-purified type III Fc-binding proteins from the phage lysate of group C streptococcus, 26RP66. An aliquot containing affinity-purified type III Fc-binding protein (30 ng) was applied to parallel gels. One gel was stained with Coomassie Blue. The second gel was stained, the proteins eluted, and the functional activity determined by a competitive binding radioimmunoassay (Langone et al., 1977). Four protein bands were identified by staining and each protein displayed IgG-binding potential. (Adapted from Reis et al.(1984a) with permission.)

different functional types, with respect to antigenicity and the site on the reactive IgG molecule to which these molecules bind. It should be remembered that the initial classification of bacterial immunoglobulin-binding proteins was based on the reactivity of intact bacteria with different species, classes, and subclasses of IgG (Myhre and Kronvall, 1981). As noted earlier, all of these species reactivities may be accounted for by the expression of a single protein or may be the result of two or more distinct surface proteins. It is therefore important, in characterizing purified immunoglobulin-binding proteins, to determine whether they display all of the reactivities associated with the intact bacteria. There are a variety of methods to characterize the species reactivities of isolated IgG-binding proteins, including direct reactivity with various labeled IgG tracer sources or competitive inhibition assays with different species of IgG. All of the basic procedures, e.g., Western blot analysis or dot blot analysis (Chapter 14) and competitive binding assays (Chapter 3), are described elsewhere in this volume. In the remainder of this chapter a number of examples are presented to illustrate the types of results that might be expected.

VII. Comparison of Functional Activities of Fc-Binding Proteins

A. Western Blot Analysis

Western blotting techniques allow the physicochemical and functional heterogeneities of Fc-binding proteins to be compared. Fc-binding protein samples are electrophoresed on SDS–polyacrylamide gels (either under reducing or nonreducing conditions). The separated proteins on one gel are stained to identify the number of distinct molecular-weight-protein species that are present. The proteins on the second gel are transferred to nitrocellulose or some other suitable membrane by electroblotting and can then be probed for reactivity with a suitable Fc tracer probe. (The detailed procedures for carrying out Western blot analysis are presented in Chapter 14.) A representative example of Western blot analysis of types I, II, and III Fc-binding proteins, probed with each of the labeled human IgG subclasses, is presented in Figure 4. Protein A (the type I Fc-binding protein), shown in Lane 1 of each panel, displays the expected reactivity with IgG_1, IgG_2, and IgG_4 at an M_r of approximately 45,000. No reactivity is observed with protein A when the IgG_3 allotype is used as the probe. Lane 2 of each panel contains the homogeneous trypsin fragment of a group C streptococcus and reacts with all four IgG subclasses at an M_r of approximately 30,000. The affinity-purified type II receptor is present in Lane 3 of each

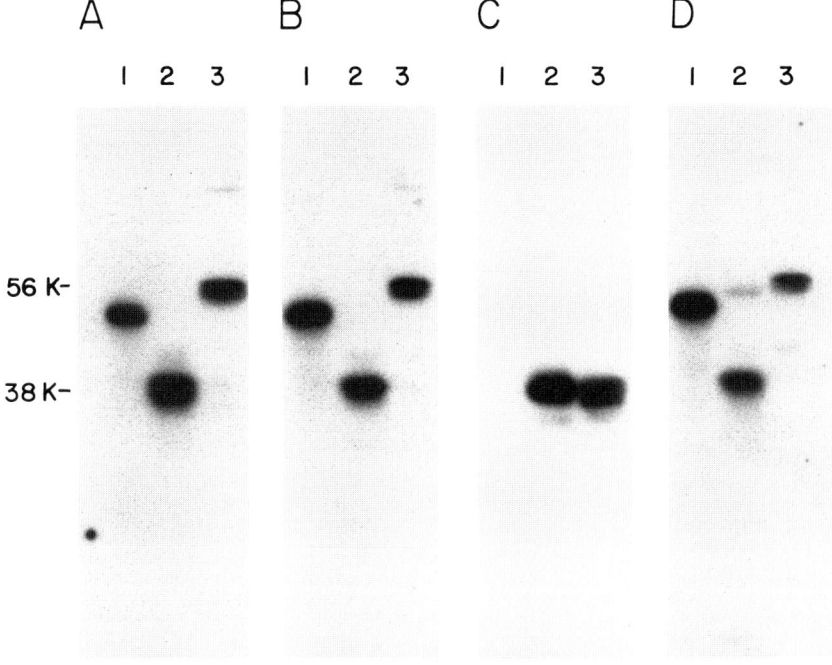

FIGURE 4
Comparison of human IgG subclass reactivities of isolated types I, II, and III Fc-binding proteins. Lane 1 in all panels contains the type I protein (protein A). Lane 2 contains a trypsin fragment of the type III protein (protein G) isolated from a group C streptococcus. Lane 3 contains the type II Fc-binding protein(s) isolated from strain 64/14 by heat extraction at neutral pH. Panel A was probed with ^{125}I-labeled human IgG$_1$ myeloma. Panel B was probed with ^{125}I-labeled human IgG$_2$ myeloma. Panel C was probed with ^{125}I-labeled human IgG$_3$ myeloma. Panel D was probed with ^{125}I-labeled human IgG$_4$ myeloma. (Reproduced from Yarnall and Boyle, 1986c, with permission.)

panel and shows reactivity at an M_r of 56,000 with human IgG$_1$, IgG$_2$, and IgG$_4$. Lane 3 of panel C demonstrates that the 56,000-dalton protein in the heat extract of group A strain 64/14 is not reactive with IgG$_3$, however a 38,000-dalton protein in this extract binds IgG$_3$ and none of the other subclasses. These findings indicate that all of the human IgG subclass properties of a protein A positive *Staphylococcus aureus* can be accounted for by a single protein molecule. Similarly, the human IgG subclass reactivity of the type III positive group C streptococcus, 26RP66 can also be accounted for by a single bacterial protein. By contrast, the group A strain 64/14 requires two proteins to account for its interaction with human IgG subclasses. Other group A strains have been identified that produce a single IgG-binding protein reactive with all four human IgG subclasses (Boyle *et al.*, 1990; Faulmann and Boyle, 1990; Grubb *et al.*, 1982; Nardella *et al.*, 1987).

In order to determine how many distinct bacterial proteins are required to account for all of the species and subclass reactivities of any bacterial immunoglobulin-binding protein, this approach can be extended using probes of different species of IgG. For example, when heat extracts of group A strain 64/14 (types IIa and IIb positive) were probed with ^{125}I-labeled rabbit, pig, dog, or cow IgG by a Western blotting procedure, only the rabbit and pig probes were reactive and that reactivity was associated only with the M_r 56,000 type IIa-binding protein (Yarnall and Boyle, 1986b).

B. Fluid-Phase Competitive Inhibition Assays

Comparison of the reactivity of Fc-binding proteins can be achieved using a competitive inhibition assay, provided a functionally active tracer form of the binding protein can be prepared. This approach is more quantitative than Western blotting and can also be used to compare the relative species reactivities of different immunoglobulin-binding proteins. An example of this approach is presented in Figure 5 using an enzyme-labeled tracer. In this experiment, the ability of fluid-phase sheep IgG_1 or IgG_2 to prevent binding of either enzyme-labeled protein A or protein G to immobilized sheep IgG is compared. In agreement with previous studies, protein G displays a greater reactivity towards sheep IgG than protein A. The predominant reactivity of protein A is found to be with the IgG_2 subclass (Langone, 1982a: Reis *et al.*, 1984b, 1988). Similar studies with other species of IgG have defined the profile of reactivities for each isolated immunoglobulin-binding protein (Langone *et al.*, 1977; Langone, 1982b; Boyle, 1984; Björck and Kronvall, 1984; Reis *et al.*, 1984b; Faulmann *et al.*, 1989).

This competitive binding assay can also be used to compare the binding properties of different, isolated bacterial IgG-binding proteins for reactive immunoglobulins. For example, addition of unlabeled protein A to a mixture of immobilized rabbit IgG and ^{125}I-labeled protein G can prevent binding of the labeled tracer to rabbit IgG and vice versa (Figure 6). This finding indicates that the sites on the rabbit IgG molecule to which the type I (protein A) and type III (protein G) immunoglobulin-binding proteins interact are either identical or in close proximity. In similar studies using immobilized human IgG, a comparable pattern of cross-inhibition has been observed (Reis *et al.*, 1984b). Schröeder *et al.* (1986) and Stone *et al.*(1989) have used isolated IgG fragments to map the region of the IgG molecule

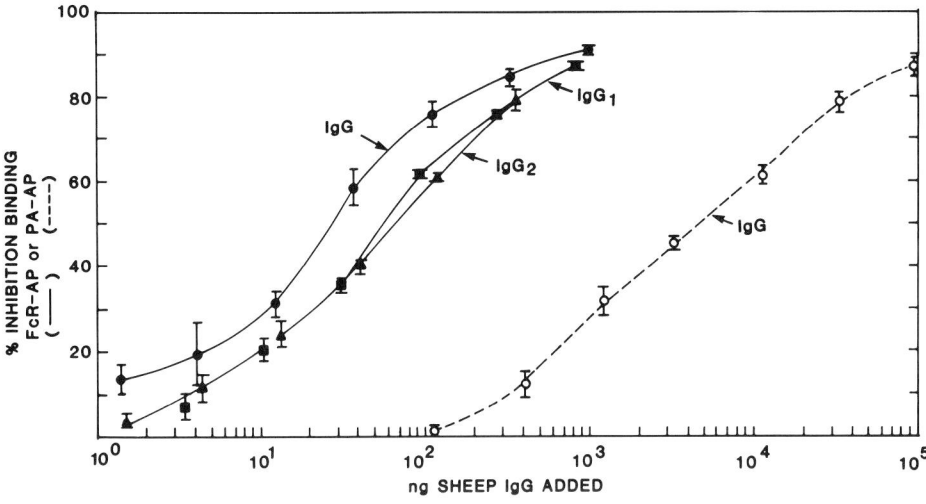

FIGURE 5
Reactivity of sheep IgG subclasses with alkaline phosphatase-conjugated bacterial Fc-binding protein. Type III Fc-binding protein–alkaline phosphatase with sheep IgG (●); with sheep IgG$_1$ (■); with sheep IgG$_2$ (▲). Protein A–alkaline phosphatase with sheep IgG (○). (Reproduced from Reis *et al.*, 1988, with permission.)

with which various cell-bound and soluble bacterial IgG-binding proteins interact. Taken together, these studies suggest that the types I, II, and III immunoglobulin-binding proteins all bind to a similar region in the C_H2–C_H3 interface of the IgG molecule (Stone *et al.*, 1989; Nardella *et al.*, 1987; Nardella and Opplinger, 1990; Reis *et al.*, 1984b; Woof and Burton, 1990).

C. Competitive Inhibition Dot Blot Assay

A modification of the fluid-phase, competitive binding assay can be carried out using a dot blotting procedure. In this procedure, the binding protein is immobilized to nitrocellulose and the ability of unlabeled IgG from various species to inhibit binding of a labeled, tracer form of IgG is determined. An example of this procedure is presented in Figure 7. In this assay the group A streptococcus, 64/14, expressing both type IIa- and type IIb-binding proteins, was immobilized onto nitrocellulose and then incubated with different concentrations of unlabeled IgG from different species. The blots were then blocked and probed with radiolabeled human IgG Fc fragments (shown previously to detect only type IIa-binding protein).

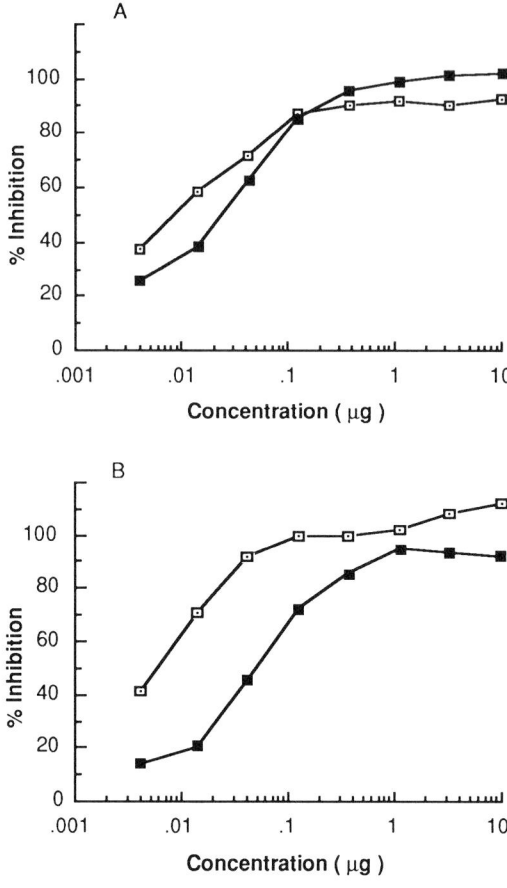

FIGURE 6
Inhibition of binding of ^{125}I-labeled protein G (Panel A), or ^{125}I-labeled protein A (Panel B) to immobilized rabbit IgG by unlabeled protein A (▫ – ▫) or protein G (■ – ■). This assay was carried out as described in detail in Chapter 3.

The blots were washed and exposed to X-ray film. A decrease in the intensity of a dot on the autoradiograph indicates competition between the unlabeled immunoglobulin and the labeled tracer. In agreement with the Western blot analyses (Yarnall and Boyle, 1986a, c), the dot-blot inhibition studies shown in Figure 7 support the conclusion that the type IIa-binding protein reacts with human, pig, and rabbit IgG.

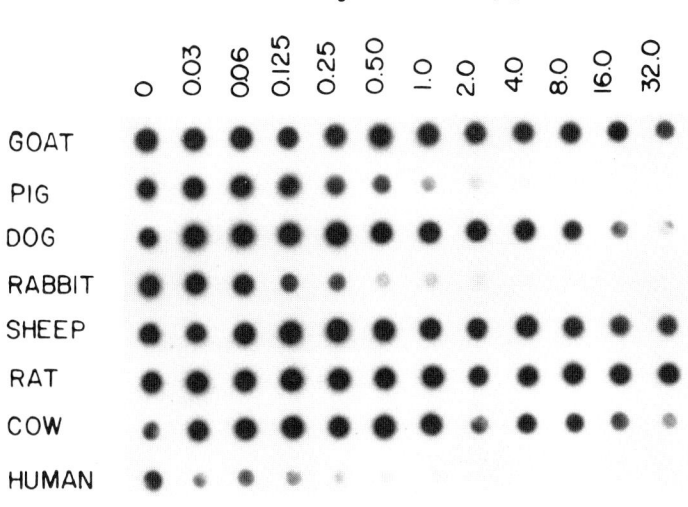

FIGURE 7
Inhibition of ^{125}I-labeled human IgG to group A strain 64/14 by IgG from a variety of mammalian species. A standard number of group A bacteria was incubated at 37°C for 1 hr with the indicated quantity of goat, pig, dog, rabbit, sheep, rat, cow, or human IgG. Following incubation, each mixture was dotted onto nitrocellulose. The nitrocellulose was washed and probed with ^{125}I-labeled human IgG and the washed blot autoradiographed for 16 hr at −70°C with an intensifying screen. (Reproduced from Yarnall and Boyle, 1986, with permission.)

D. Antigenic Characterization

Isolated immunoglobulin-binding proteins can also be compared antigenically using monospecific polyclonal antibodies. This approach is discussed in detail in Chapter 6.

VIII. Summary

The methods outlined in this chapter are designed to enable the purification and characterization of bacterial immunoglobulin-binding proteins, once solubilized. There are a number of important factors that influence the purification strategy of an individual bacterial immunoglobulin-binding protein. In general, affinity purification provides the most efficient purification strategy. The choice of species of IgG to immobilize and the optimal eluting agent are important considerations and may vary for each immunoglobulin-binding protein type.

The general approach to analyzing purified immunoglobulin-binding proteins and relating their activities to those of the organism from which they were isolated should be applicable to any strain. It should be noted that the type I (protein A) and type III (protein G) Fc-binding proteins are not typical protein molecules. They are stable to extremes of pH, retain activity after heating at 80°C for 10 min or lyophilization and show no loss of functional activity following Western blotting procedures. These properties may not be common to all bacterial immunoglobulin-binding proteins and adjustments in procedures may be necessary in order to purify or characterize immunoglobulin-binding proteins expressed by other microorganisms.

By combining the various approaches described in this chapter, it is possible to isolate, compare, and contrast the activities of bacterial immunoglobulin-binding proteins isolated from different organisms as well as comparing different forms of immunoglobulin-binding activities recovered from a single strain.

References

Björck, L., and Kronvall, G. (1984). *J. Immunol.* 133, 964–974.
Boyle, M. D. P. (1984). *Biotechniques* 2, 334–340.
Boyle, M. D. P., and Reis, K. J. (1987). *Biotechnology* 5, 697–703.
Boyle, M. D. P., Faulmann, E. L., Otten, R. A., and Heath, D. G. (1990). Microbial Determinants of Virulence and Host Response. (E. M. Ayoub, G. H. Cassell, W. C. Branche and T. J. Henry, eds.). pp. 19–44. A. S. M. Washington, D.C.
Bywater, R. (1978). *In* "Chromatography of Synthetic and Biological Polymers" (R. Epton, ed.), pp. 337–340. Ellis Horwood, Chichester, U. K.
Bywater, R., Eriksson, G. B., and Ottosson, T. (1983). *J. Immunol. Methods* 64, 1–6.
Cheng, W. C., Fraser, K. J., and Haber, E. (1973). *J. Immunol.* 111, 1677–1689.
Faulmann, E. L., and Boyle, M. D. P. (1990). *In* "Bacterial Immunoglobulin-Binding Proteins" (M. D. P. Boyle, ed.), Vol. 1. pp. 69–81. Academic Press, San Diego.
Faulmann, E. L., Otten, R. A., Barrett, D. J., and Boyle, M. D. P. (1989). *J. Immunol. Methods*, 123, 269–281.
Grubb, A., Grubb, R., Christensen, P., and Schalen, C. (1982). *Int. Arch. Allergy Appl. Immunol.* 67, 369–376.
Hjelm, H., Hjelm, K., and Sjöquist, J. (1972). *FEBS Lett.* 28 73–76.
Kaplan, M. E., and Kabat, E. A. (1966). *J. Exp. Med.* 123, 1061–1081.
Kristiansen, T. (1978). *In* "Affinity Chromatography" (O. Hoffman-Ostenhof, ed.) pp.191–206. Pergamon, Oxford.
Langone, J. J. (1982a). Adv. Immunol. 32, 157–252.
Langone, J. J. (1982b). *J. Immunol. Methods* 51, 3–22.
Langone, J. J., Boyle, M. D. P., and Borsos, T. (1977). *J. Immunol. Methods* 18, 281–293.
Levy, D. E., and Eveleigh, J. W. (1978). *J. Immunol. Methods* 22, 131–142.

Little, M., Siebert, C., and Matson, R. (1988). *Biochromatography* **3,** 156–160.
Myhre, E. B., and Kronvall, G. (1981). *In* "Basic Concepts of Streptococci and Streptococcal Diseases" (S. E. Holm and P. Christensen, eds), pp. 209–210. Redbook, Chertsey, Surrey.
Nardella, F. A., Schröder, A. K., Svensson, M.-L., Sjöquist, C. B., and Christensen, P. (1987). *J. Immunol.* **138,** 922–926.
Nardella, F. A., and Oppliger, I. R. (1990). *In* "Bacterial Immunoglobulin-Binding Proteins" (M. D. P. Boyle, ed.), Vol. 1. pp. 317–334. Academic Press, San Diego.
Reis, K. J., Ayoub, E. M., and Boyle, M. D. P. (1983). *J. Immunol. Methods* **59,** 83–94.
Reis, K. J., Ayoub, E. M., and Boyle, M. D. P. (1984a). *J. Immnol.* **132,** 3091–3097.
Reis, K. J., Ayoub, E. M., and Boyle, M. D. P. (1984b). *J. Immunol.* **132,** 3098–3102.
Reis, K. J., Ayoub, E. M., and Boyle, M. D. P. (1985). *J. Microbiol. Methods* **4,** 45–58.
Reis, K. J., von Mering, G. O., Karis, M. A., Faulmann, E. L., Lottenberg, R., and Boyle, M. D. P. (1988). *J. Immunol. Methods* **107,** 273–280.
Schalén, C., and Christensen, P. (1990). *In* "Bacterial Immunoglobulin-Binding Proteins" (M. D. P. Boyle, ed.), Vol. 1. pp. 347–364. Academic Press, San Diego.
Schalén, C., Svensson, M.-L., and Christensen, P. (1982). *Acta Pathol. Microbiol. Scand. Sect. B* **90B,** 347–351.
Schröder, A. K., Nardella, F. A., Mannik, M., Svensson, M.-L., and Christensen, P. (1986). *Immunology* **57,** 305–309.
Sjöquist, J., Meloun, B., and Hjelm, H. (1972). *Eur. J. Biochem.* **29,** 572–578.
Stone, G. C., Sjöbring, U., Björck, L., Sjöquist, J., Barber, C., and Nardella, F. A. (1989). *J. Immunol.* **143,** 565–570.
Woof, J. M., and Burton, D. R. (1990). *In* "Bacterial Immunoglobulin–Binding Proteins" (M. D. P. Boyle, ed.), Vol. 1. Academic Press, San Diego.
Yarnall, M., and Boyle, M. D. P. (1986a). *Mol. Cell. Biochem.* **70,** 57–66.
Yarnall, M., and Boyle, M. D. P. (1986b). *Scand. J. Immunol.* **24,** 549–557.
Yarnall, M., and Boyle, M. D. P. (1986c). *J. Immunol.* **136,** 2670–2673.
Yarnall, M., and Boyle, M. D. P. (1986d). *Biochem. Biophys. Res. Commun.* **135,** 1105–1111.

CHAPTER 5

Determination of protein-binding activities among bacterial cell surface proteins

Lars Björck
Bo Åkerström

I. Introduction

The studies of the two immunoglobulin-binding molecules, protein G and protein L, are largely based on various methods for assaying protein–protein binding and binding strength. The different stages of the increasingly detailed analyses of these proteins require methodologies that are specifically adjusted to each individual case. Thus, for the detection of such proteins on the bacterial cell surface, there is a need for a rapid screening-type method. The solubilization and subsequent purification should be monitored by simple, sensitive, and specific assays, which determine the concentration of the immunoglobulin-binding molecule in the solubilizate and in various chromatographic fractions. Once the protein is purified, its binding specificities and binding strength can be estimated by methods that are preferably accurate without consuming much of the purified protein.

In *Bacterial Immunoglobulin-Binding Proteins, Volume 1*, we reviewed the work on protein G and protein L, two immunoglobulin-binding, bacterial cell wall proteins that interact with IgG and kappa-type Ig light chains, respectively. In those reviews, the results of the work have been emphasized. In this chapter, we will summarize the methods that we have used to detect the binding of various plasma proteins to bacterial proteins such as proteins G and L. We will also describe methods used for the determination of both binding specificity and strength. In this review, we have not had the ambition to cover all of the various techniques used by us and our research colleagues, but merely describe some of the methods we have used in order to identify and characterize bacterial proteins capable of interacting with host proteins.

II. Binding of Mammalian Proteins to Bacterial Surfaces: Screening Procedures

The nonimmune interaction between staphylococcal protein A and IgG was originally investigated in a gel precipitation system, which, however, demands the presence of soluble bacterial immunoglobulin-binding components in the growth medium. The identification of a putative, surface-bound bacterial molecule interacting with a mammalian protein requires a direct binding assay. If a large number of bacterial strains, perhaps belonging to different bacterial species, are to be tested, the screening procedure should be easy and reliable. Such a procedure has been developed by Myhre and Kronvall (1977) for the identification of IgG-binding surface structures among gram-positive cocci. In this assay, 200 μl of a bacterial suspension (2×10^8 cells) in PBS, pH 7.4, containing 0.02% NaN_3 and 0.05% Tween 20 (PBSAT) is mixed with 25 μl of ^{125}I-labeled protein solution (1–10 ng of protein, corresponding to about 10^4 cpm). After a 1-hr incubation at 37°C, 2 ml of PBSAT is added to the tube, cells are spun down, and the radioactivity in the pellet is expressed as a percentage of the total radioactivity added. A binding of less than 10% is regarded as negative. Nonspecific adsorption to test tubes and bacteria can be a problem, especially at low protein concentrations. However, the addition of a nonionic detergent such as Tween 20, at a low concentration, does not interfere with the protein–protein interactions we have studied, but efficiently eliminates nonspecific binding.

The assay just described has proven to be a powerful tool. The sensitivity of the assay is dependent on the ratio of the amount of tested protein and the number of bacterial cells used in the experiment. High sensitivity is accomplished with small amounts of protein and a large number of cells, whereas a relative excess of binding protein molecules will reflect quantitative aspects of protein reactivity, a set-up that can be used when determining the maximum binding capacity of the tested bacterial cells. The purity of tested proteins and bacterial strains is, of course, crucial for the binding assay. With a high degree of purity, it is also possible to gain valuable information by inhibiting the binding of radiolabeled protein to the bacteria with unlabeled protein. If this is done with a protein identical or similar to the radiolabeled protein, the competitive nature of the system makes it possible to compare different protein preparations (for instance IgG from different animal species) and to estimate the specificity of the binding. Inhibition experiments can also be used to compare the binding of different proteins to a bacterial strain. For instance, if another protein can block the binding of the radiolabeled molecule, it indicates that the responsible binding site(s) at the bacterial surface are identical or, if the sites are separate, are located close enough to each other to cause steric hindrance. Finally, inhibition of the binding of radiolabeled protein to the bacteria by material solubilized from the bacteria, can be used to detect and assay the bacterial-binding molecule during its purification (Björck and Kronvall, 1984).

During the last few years, several different, highly purified immunoglobulin-binding proteins have been isolated and tested in various protein interaction assays. In retrospect, it is amazing how compatible the results obtained with the simple binding and inhibition assays that we have just described are with those obtained using more complicated and sophisticated experimental systems.

III. Solubilization of Immunoglobulin-Binding Bacterial Surface Proteins

In direct binding experiments with whole bacteria, it is possible to identify bacterial strains that, for instance, express surface IgG-binding proteins. In order to isolate such a protein, the next step requires solubilization of the molecule. We and others have successfully used proteolytic enzymes for this purpose. The efficiency of different proteolytic enzymes in releasing IgG-binding proteins from the bacterial cell surface can be measured with the direct binding assay. Thus, bacteria are incubated with proteolytic enzymes at different concentrations and for different time periods. The digestion is blocked, cells are washed, and tested for binding of radiolabeled IgG. By diluting the cells and comparing the dilution curve with the corresponding curve obtained with untreated bacteria, it is possible to estimate to what extent the IgG-binding protein has been solubilized.

To solubilize protein G from group G streptococci, we originally used papain (Björck and Kronvall, 1984). Figure 1 shows that at a concentration of 100 μg papain per ml of a 10% bacterial suspension, the binding of IgG starts to decrease. The binding assay is run with an excess of bacteria and does not give any quantitative information. However, if the papain-treated cells are tested in dilutions and compared with untreated cells, it is evident from Figure 2 that the IgG-binding capacity is reduced about 1000-fold by the papain digestion. This suggests that a large part of the bacterial surface proteins responsible for IgG binding have been solubilized. These experiments with papain represent an example, and other protein-cleaving en-

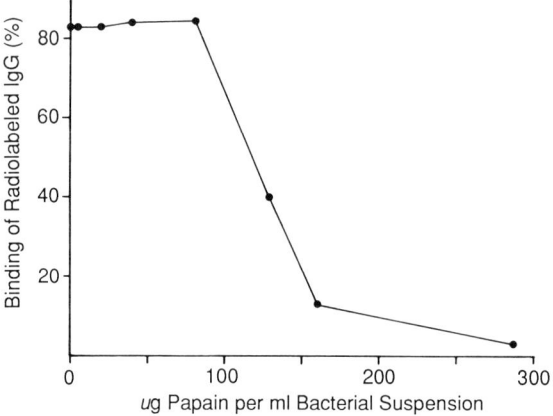

FIGURE 1
Binding of radiolabeled human polyclonal IgG to group G streptococci (strain G148) after pretreatment of the bacteria with papain. Different amounts of papain were added to 10% suspensions of G148 bacteria in 0.01 M Tris–HCl, pH 8.0. One hundred microliters of 0.4 M L-cysteine and 10 μl papain (of varying concentrations) in the same buffer were added per ml bacterial suspension. The mixture was incubated for 1 hr at 37°C. Iodoacetamide was added to a final concentration of 6 mM to block the activity of the enzyme. Bacteria were spun down, washed, and analyzed for IgG binding by the direct binding assay. (Reproduced from Björck and Kronvall, 1984, with permission.)

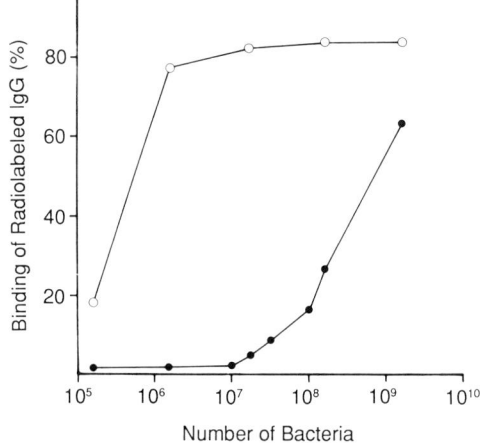

FIGURE 2
Binding of radiolabeled, human polyclonal IgG to different dilutions of group G streptococci, preincubated in buffer alone (○—○) or in buffer containing 100 μg papain (●—●) per ml 10% bacterial suspension. (Reproduced from Björck and Kronvall, 1984, with permission.)

zymes and chemicals could, of course, be tested and perhaps used in a similar way.

In order to solubilize functionally active molecules, in this case IgG-binding peptides, it is important to find experimental conditions that release but do not degrade the binding protein. Thus, following enzyme digestion, bacteria are spun down and the resulting supernatants are analyzed for Ig-binding activity. This analysis can be performed in four ways:

1. The capacity of the supernatants to inhibit binding of radiolabeled IgG to the bacterial cells can be measured (Björck and Kronvall, 1984).
2. Gel precipitation systems can be used (Kronvall and Williams, 1969).
3. Supernatants can be applied to nitrocellulose filters and probed with radiolabeled IgG (Reis *et al.*, 1983).
4. Supernatants can be subjected to sodium dodecyl sulfate–polyacrylamide gel electrophoresis (SDS–PAGE) and analyzed on Western blots using radiolabeled IgG as the probe. (Reis *et al.*, 1986; Björck, 1988).

Of these techniques, Western blotting is the most informative. Thus, both the molecular weight and the homogeneity of the released material can be assessed. However, the method requires that the binding activity is not destroyed by boiling in SDS and/or by separation on SDS–PAGE and electrotransfer to nitrocellulose. Fortunately, most immunoglobulin-binding bacterial proteins have proven to be very resistant to this kind of treatment, and much valuable information has been obtained from Western blot experiments. In this context, it could also be mentioned that much work on these immunoglobulin-binding proteins has been done with ^{125}I-labeled proteins, and routine labeling procedures have mostly functioned well, which suggests that the interacting protein regions are not denatured by these procedures.

Over the last five years, molecular biology has made it possible to clone and express genes encoding immunoglobulin-binding proteins from gram-positive bacteria in *Escherichia coli,* which has greatly facilitated research work on these proteins. For instance, papain only solubilizes a fragment of protein G, whereas when the gene was cloned and expressed in *E. coli,* the entire protein could be isolated (Björck *et al.*, 1987). In many situations, however, it is still a great advantage to have access to the protein isolated from its original source as well.

IV. Determination of Immunoglobulin-Binding Protein in Low Concentrations

A. Competitive Binding Assay

An estimate of the concentration of a bacterial immunoglobulin-binding protein during its purification has been determined by either a competitive binding assay (CBA) or by a microtiter plate-based assay, which will also be described (Section IV, B). Both assays are sensitive and suitable for a large number of samples. The CBA was first described by Langone *et al.* (1977), who used it to determine IgG concentrations. The method, as we have adapted it for the determination of streptococcal protein G concentrations, has been described in detail by Åkerström and Björck (1986).

The principle of the method is a competition between a constant amount of radiolabeled protein G (or any other immunoglobulin-binding protein) and various amounts of unlabeled protein G for the binding sites on matrix-coupled IgG. ^{125}I-labeled protein G (0.1 ml), 0.1 ml Immunobead-coupled IgG, and 0.2 ml unlabeled standard protein G are mixed in a dilution series with known concentrations and incubated for 3 hr at 37°C. The IgG has been coupled to polyacrylamide beads (Immunobeads, Bio-Rad, Richmond, California). The beads are washed, centrifuged, and the radioactivity of the washed beads is measured. The proper amount of Ig-beads is determined in advance by incubating ^{125}I-labeled protein G with a dilution series of the Ig-beads, measuring the bound radiolabeled protein G, and choosing a dilution of the Ig-beads that binds protein G just less than maximally. Radiolabeled and unlabeled protein G compete for binding to the IgG-beads, and a displacement curve is plotted with unlabeled protein G on the x-axis and radioactivity bound to the IgG-beads on the y-axis. A high concentration of unlabeled protein G thus gives a small amount of ^{125}I-labeled protein G on the IgG-beads. Protein G concentrations in unknown samples can then be measured by substitution of the standard protein G with proper dilutions of bacterial solubilizates, chromatographic fractions, etc. In our hands, the sensitivity of this method is approximately 0.3–1 nM (20–50 μg/liter) protein G.

B. Solid Phase Radioassay or Enzyme-Linked Immunosorbent Assay

The competitive binding assay described in the previous section has several advantages. However, it is unnecessarily laborious and its application to, for instance, chromatographic fractions can lead to handling a large number of samples. Thus, to monitor the purification of protein G by high-performance liquid affinity chromatography (HPLAC), we have developed a microtiter-based assay (Falkenberg *et al.*, 1987), which is called solid-phase radioassay (SPRA) or enzyme-linked immunosorbent assay (ELISA).

The principle of this method is a competition between labeled and unlabeled protein G for IgG that has been immobilized to plastic walls. In the three-step SPRA, an antigen (human α_1-microglobulin), 0.1 μg, in 100 μl PBS (phosphate-buffered saline: 30 mM sodium phosphate buffer, pH 7.4, 0.12 M NaCl) is coated to the wells of microtiter plates for 1–3 hr. After washing three times with a mixture of 0.9% NaCl and 0.05% Tween 20, 100 μl goat anti-α_1-microglobulin serum, diluted in PBS and 0.05% Tween 20, is added and incubated for 1 hr. The goat antibodies bind to the antigen, exposing their Fc regions. After another washing, 50 μl unlabeled protein G, either in a known standard concentration or an unknown, diluted sample, and 50 μl ^{125}I-labeled protein G (1–5 ng), both in PBS and 0.05% Tween 20, are added. These are then allowed to compete for the goat antibodies for at least 2 hr at room temperature. After a final washing, the plates are dried and the wells counted for radioactivity.

In the two-step SPRA, unlabeled and ^{125}I-labeled protein G compete for human IgG (0.5 μg) coated directly to the plastic walls. The radiolabeled protein can also be substituted with protein G conjugated to alkaline phosphatase (Nilson *et al.*, 1988). This variation of the assay is called an ELISA.

The radioactivity bound either to the antibodies or to IgG is plotted against the logarithm of the concentration of unlabeled protein G (Figure 3), and the concentration of protein G in unknown samples can be deduced from this standard curve. The sensitivity of the three-step SPRA, where goat antibodies bind to their antigen (Figure 3B), is much increased compared to the two-step SPRA, coating IgG directly to the walls (Figure 3A). Approximately 20–50 pM protein G (1–3 μg/liter) can be detected.

V. Analysis of the Binding of Immunoglobulins and Other Host Proteins to Purified, Bacterial Surface Proteins

With a suitable solubilization procedure and a sensitive and reliable assay for detection, the purification of an immunoglobulin-binding protein is usually not difficult. Conventional methods of protein chemistry, such as affinity chromatography, gel filtration, and ion-exchange chromatography are sufficient to obtain highly purified samples of these molecules. Once purified, there are several different ways of studying the interaction of an immunoglobulin-binding protein with Ig or with other proteins. Some of

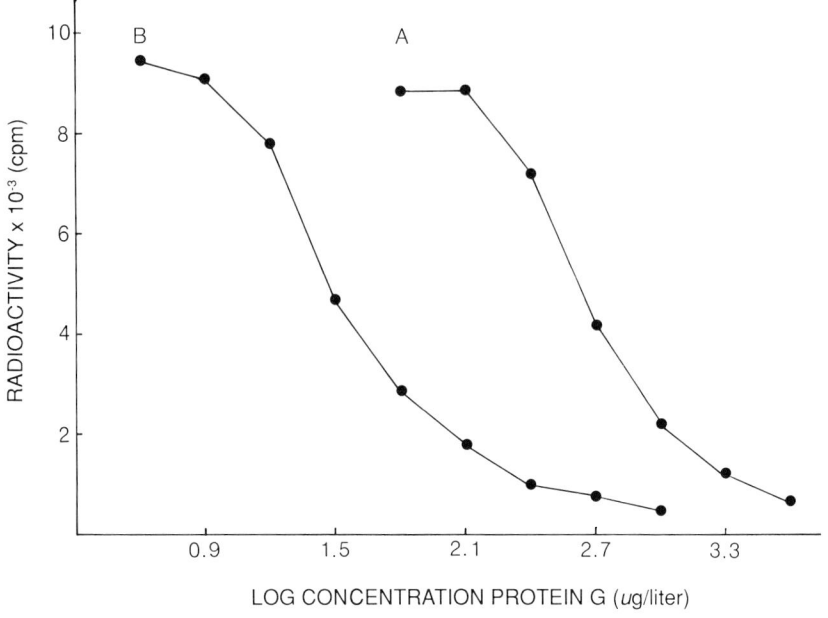

FIGURE 3
Standard plots from the protein G SPRA, either coating directly with human IgG (two-step SPRA, A) or first with an antigen followed by its antibody (three-step SPRA, B). (A) 0.5 μg human IgG in 100 μl PBS was coated to microtiter plate wells for 1–3 hr. Unbound IgG was washed away with 0.9% NaCl + 0.05% Tween 20. Cold protein G in different concentrations and ^{125}I-labeled protein G, diluted in PBS + 0.05% Tween 20 (50 μl of each) were then incubated for 2 hr before washing, cutting, and counting the radioactivity of the wells. (B) 0.1 μg human α_1-microglobulin in 100 μl PBS was coated to microtiter plate wells. After washing, goat anti-α_1-microglobulin serum, diluted 1000 times, was then incubated for 1 hr. The final incubation with protein G and ^{125}I-labeled protein G was the same as for the two-step SPRA. (Reproduced from Falkenberg *et al.*, 1987, with permission.)

the methods will be discussed in this chapter and all of them have the advantage of requiring very small amounts of purified bacterial protein.

A. Gel Filtration

A radiolabeled sample of the purified bacterial protein and a sample of unlabeled host protein (IgG, albumin, α_2-macroglobulin, or any protein to be analyzed for interaction with the radiolabeled molecule) are separately run on a suitable column (we have mostly used Sephadex or Sepharose). The two proteins are then incubated for at least 1 hr at 37°C, the mixture is run on the same column, and the radioactivity of the fractions is measured. If the radioactivity moves toward the void fractions, it is a clear indication of a physical association between the two proteins. This procedure represents an easy, sensitive, and physiological way of studying protein–protein interactions, which we have used several times (Björck and Kronvall, 1984; Sjöbring *et al.*, 1989).

B. Dot Binding

Host proteins are applied to nitrocellulose filters, which are subsequently incubated with labeled bacterial protein or vice versa. By preincubating the proteins together prior to probing the filters, this binding assay can also be used as a sensitive inhibition assay (Sjöbring *et al.*, 1989).

C. Binding to Host Proteins on Solid Phase

The interaction between a purified bacterial protein and host proteins can also be studied with host proteins coupled to Sepharose, polyacrylamide beads, or plastic surfaces. This can be done both analytically and quantitatively (Section IV).

D. Western Blot Analysis

As mentioned previously, the Western blot is a powerful method to study immunoglobulin-binding bacterial proteins. Also, in this case, either the bacterial protein or the immunoglobulin can be used as the probe. In combination with amino acid sequence determinations of Immunoglobulin-reactive bands on Imobilon filters (Millipore Corp., Massachusetts), Western blots can also be utilized to map the binding sites of bacterial immunoglobulin-binding proteins Åkerström *et al.*, 1987).

The binding specificity of the purified bacterial proteins can be studied in different ways.

1. To analyze whether a given protein at the bacterial surface interacts with one or more plasma proteins, we have used the following experimental approach. Bacteria are incubated with human plasma followed by extensive washing of the cells, which are then boiled in SDS–PAGE sample buffer containing SDS and 2-mercaptoethanol. As a negative control, the bacteria are incubated with buffer prior to boiling. Cells are spun down and the resulting supernatants are analyzed on Western blots using the purified, bacterial surface protein as the labeled probe. The number of extra protein bands appearing in the

SDS–PAGE gel following plasma absorption gives an indication of the total number of plasma proteins adsorbed to the bacteria. Probing with a certain purified, bacterial cell surface protein indicates which of these adsorbed proteins are present in the supernatant as a result of binding to this certain protein. Figure 4 gives an example of this approach, which has enabled us to locate the binding of albumin to streptococcal protein G.

2. A mixture of proteins, for instance human plasma, is separated by agarose gel electrophoresis and the proteins are transferred to nitrocellulose filters, which are then probed with a labeled sample of bacterial protein. This procedure can pick up protein interactions that are sensitive to the denaturing conditions during SDS–PAGE (Sjöbring et al., 1989).

3. A more direct way of analyzing the protein-binding specificity of an isolated bacterial protein is the application of a number of different proteins to nitrocellulose and a subsequent probe of these filters with a labeled sample of the bacterial protein (Sjöbring et al., 1989). However, this screening demands a collection of highly purified proteins and is perhaps most suitable when there is reason to believe that a certain protein can interact with the bacterial protein.

VI. Determination of the Affinity Constant for Binding between a Bacterial Cell Wall Protein and Its Ligand

A. Theoretical Considerations

After purification of a bacterial cell wall protein, we have tried to estimate the binding affinity for immunoglobulins by determination of the equilibrium constant for the binding reaction:

$$BP + Ig \rightleftharpoons BPIg, \tag{1}$$

where BP is the bacterial protein, Ig the immunoglobulin, and BPIg the binding reaction product. [BP], [Ig], and [BPIg], represent the concentrations of the reactants and products, respectively. The affinity constant, K_a (the equilibrium constant for this reaction), is defined by the formula

$$K_a = [BPIg]/[BP][Ig], \tag{2}$$

or

$$K_a = [\text{Bound BP}]/[\text{Free BP}][\text{Total Ig} - \text{Bound Ig}], \tag{3}$$

or

$$\text{Bound BP}/\text{Free BP} = K_a (\text{Total Ig} - \text{Bound Ig}). \tag{4}$$

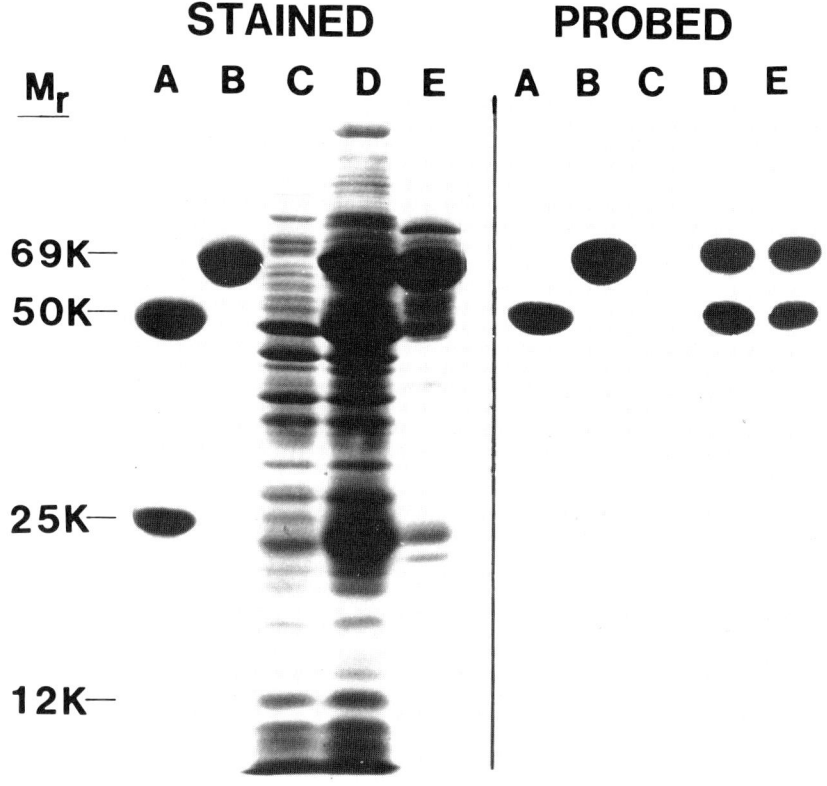

FIGURE 4
Binding of streptococcal protein G to human plasma proteins adsorbed by group G streptococci (strain G148). Lane (A), Human IgG (1 mg/ml in PBS). Lane (B), Human albumin (1 mg/ml in PBS). Lane (C), 5×10^9 heat-killed G148 bacteria were incubated with 5 ml of PBS for 2 hr at 37°C. The cells were washed five times in PBS and boiled for 3 min in 1 ml of SDS–PAGE sample buffer containing 2% SDS and 5% 2-mercaptoethanol. The cells were spun down and the sample in lane C represents 50 μl of the supernatant. Lane (D), As in lane C, but the bacteria were incubated with 5 ml of human plasma instead of PBS. Lane (E), Human plasma diluted 1 : 100 in PBS. Fifty microliters of samples A, B, and E were mixed with 50 μl of SDS-PAGE sample buffer and boiled. Fifty microliters of each mixture were then submitted to SDS–PAGE (T = 10%, C = 3.3%). The left half of the figure shows the gel stained with Coomassie Brilliant Blue. In the right half of the figure, an identical gel was electroblotted onto nitrocellulose and probed with ^{125}I-labeled protein G (2×10^5 cpm/ml). The membrane was autoradiographed for 24 hr. (Reproduced from Björck *et al.*, 1987, with permission.)

K_a is determined according to the principle described by Scatchard (1949). A constant amount of Ig in a series of test tubes is incubated with different amounts of the BP. The total concentration of the added Ig does not have to be known. After the reaction has reached equilibrium, the amount of bound BP is determined. A Scatchard plot is drawn (Figure 5), with the ratio of Bound BP/Free BP plotted on the y-axis as a function of the Bound BP on the x-axis. The K_a is then equal to the absolute value of the slope of the curve, according to equation (4) since Bound Ig is equal to Bound BP.

We have performed such a Scatchard analysis with the immunoglobulins coupled to an insoluble matrix. This approach should give a theoretical advantage—a binding to only one of the binding sites on the bacterial protein. Thus we have tried to avoid complications caused by enhancement of the binding strength, which has been described for multiple-point binding of antibodies to a single molecule (Ehrlich *et al.*, 1982). Also, from

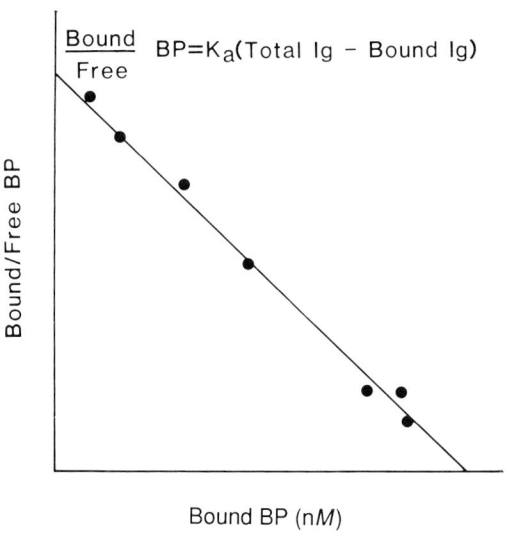

FIGURE 5
Scatchard plot of the binding reaction between an immunoglobulin-binding bacterial cell wall protein (BP) and immunoglobulin (Ig). Different concentrations of BP are mixed with a constant amount of Ig in a series of incubations. After equilibrium has been reached, the concentration of BPIg complexes is determined (bound BP or bound Ig). Free BP is then calculated by subtracting bound BP from the added total BP. Bound/Free BP is plotted against bound BP, and the affinity constant is equal to the absolute value of the slope according to the formula (see text). The concentration of added binding sites on the Ig is equal to the x-axis intercept.

a practical point of view, it is much easier to determine the amount of BP that is bound to immobilized Ig, rather than a soluble BPIg complex.

Equation (4) also shows that the x-axis intercept of the Scatchard plot gives the total concentration of Ig. This can be used to estimate the amount of BP on the bacterial cell walls. In this case, a known amount of whole bacteria, carrying the immunoglobulin-binding BP, is mixed with different amounts of radiolabeled Ig. The affinity constant and the total number of binding sites for the Ig can be determined from the Scatchard plot. The number of BP per bacterial cell can then be calculated. For example, the determination of both the affinity constant of cell wall protein A (binding of a human myeloma globulin: $4 \times 10^7 \ M^{-1}$) and the number of protein A molecules on *Staphylococcus aureus* strain Cowan I have been described by Kronvall *et al.* (1970).

B. Procedure

Åkerström and Björck (1986) have described a procedure to determine the affinity constants of streptococcal protein G for the binding of IgG from different species. The procedure has gone through a number of modifications and has been used for several other applications. The method is modified from the competitive binding assay described in Section IV (A).

^{125}I-labeled protein G (0.5–5 ng) and Ig are mixed in 0.2 ml in a series of tubes. The immunoglobulin has been coupled to polyacrylamide beads (Immunobeads, Bio-Rad, Richmond, California). Different dilutions of unlabeled protein G (0.2 ml) are added to the Ig-beads and ^{125}I-labeled protein G. After incubation at 37°C for 1–24 hr, the beads are washed, centrifuged, and the radioactivity of the washed beads is then measured. The proper amount of Ig-beads to add is determined in advance by incubating ^{125}I-labeled protein G with a dilution series of the Ig-beads, measuring the bound, radiolabeled protein G, and choosing a dilution of the Ig-beads that binds protein G just less than maximally. The exact amount and specific radioactivity of the total protein G added to each tube is known from the experimental protocol, and bound protein G (nM) can be derived from the radioactivity on the Ig-beads. Free protein G is then calculated by subtracting bound protein G from total protein G. When calculating the specific radioactivity and bound protein G, the ^{125}I-labeled protein G that does not bind to beads with a 500-fold molar excess of human polyclonal IgG is subtracted from the added ^{125}I-labeled protein G.

This procedure has been used for the determination of the affinity constants of protein G for polyclonal IgG from rabbit, goat, rat, and mouse, and for human IgG subclasses (Åkerström and Björck, 1986). The human IgG subclasses were coupled to Sepharose 4B-CL after cyanogen bromide (CNBr) activation. However, higher background binding with the Sepharose and practical difficulties in handling this reagent make the polyacrylamide beads preferable for this type of experiment. The affinity constants of different fragments of protein G to human serum albumin–beads have been obtained following this procedure (Åkerström et al., 1987; Sjöbring et al., 1988). Finally, the equilibrium constants for the binding of protein L to immunoglobulin light chains, immunoglobulins of various classes, or IgG from different species have been measured using this method (Åkerström and Björck, 1989).

Acknowledgments

This work was financially supported by Swedish Medical Research Projects 7480 and 7144, Excorim KB, HighTech Receptor, King Gustav V:s 80-year Foundation, the Medical Faculty of the University of Lund, and the Österlund, Kock, and Tesdorpfs Foundations.

References

Åkerström, B., and Björck, L. (1986). J. Biol. Chem. **261**, 10240–10247.
Åkerström, B., and Björck, L. (1989). J. Biol. Chem., J. Biol. Chem. **264**, 19740–19746.
Åkerström, B., Nielsen, E., and Björck, L. (1987). J. Biol. Chem. **262**, 13388–13391.
Björck, L. (1988). J. Immunol. **140**, 1194–1197.
Björck, L., and Kronvall, G. (1984). J. Immunol. **133**, 969–974.
Björck, L., Kastern, W., Lindahl, G., and Widebäck, K. (1987). Mol. Immunol. **24**, 1113–1122.
Ehrlich, P. H., Molyle, W. R., Moustafa, Z. A., and Canfield, R. E. (1982). J. Immunol. **128**, 2709–2713.
Falkenberg, C., Björck, L., Åkerström, B., and Nilsson, S. (1987). Biomed. Chromatogr. **2**, 221–225.
Kronvall, G., and Williams, Jr., R. C. (1969). J. Immunol. **103**, 828–833.
Kronvall, G., Quie, P., and Williams, Jr., R. C. (1970). J. Immunol. **104**, 273–278.
Langone, J. J., Boyle, M. D. P., and Borsos, T. (1977). J. Immunol. Methods **18**, 281–293.
Myhre, E. B., and Kronvall, G. (1977). Infect. Immun. **17**, 475–482.
Nilson, B., Björck, L., and Åkerström, B. (1988). J. Immunoassay **9**, 207–225.
Reis, K. J., Ayoub, E. M., and Boyle, M. D. P. (1983). J. Immunol. Methods **59**, 83–94.
Reis, K. J., Hansen, H. F., and Björck, L. (1986). Mol. Immunol. **23**, 425–431.
Scatchard, G. (1949). Ann. N.Y. Acad. Sci. **51**, 660–672.
Sjöbring, U., Falkenberg, C., Nielsen, E., Åkerström, B., and Björck, L. (1988). J. Immunol. **140**, 1595–1599.
Sjöbring, U., Trojnar, J., Grubb, A., Åkerström, B., and Björck, L. (1989). J. Immunol., **143**, 2948–2954.

CHAPTER **6**

Production of polyclonal antibodies to immunoglobulin-binding proteins

Kathleen J. Reis
Michael D. P. Boyle

I. Introduction

The availability of antibodies to bacterial immunoglobulin-binding proteins provides an additional resource with which to detect, identify, compare, and even purify these receptors (Boyle and Reis, 1987, 1990). Important considerations in the production of any antibody are: (1) selection of the species of animal to immunize, (2) preparation of the immunogen and immunization schedule, (3) kinetics of antibody production, and (4) methods to detect the antibody. These points will be addressed specifically as they apply to the production of antibodies to bacterial immunoglobulin-binding proteins.

II. Selection of the Species of Animal to Immunize

The functional nature of bacterial immunoglobulin-binding proteins (*i.e.*, their ability to bind to immunoglobulin (Ig) molecules at a site remote from the antigen-combining site) makes selection of the animal species for immunization a prime consideration when attempting to produce antibodies to these proteins. Use of an animal for antibody production whose normal immunoglobulin(s) react with the immunogen (immunoglobulin-binding protein) complicates detection and purification of specific antibodies. In the case of IgG Fc-binding proteins, distinguishing nonimmune interactions between the immunogen and the Fc portion of the IgG molecule from specific immune reactions involving the antibody-combining site in the Fab region would necessitate the use of $F(ab')_2$ fragments for all antibody preparations. Ideally, the species used for antibody production should be one whose immunoglobulin(s) does not react with the immunoglobulin-binding protein. The intended use of the antibody should also be considered when selecting a suitable species to immunize. For example, if large quantities of antibody to the type II IgG Fc-binding protein were required, goats could be immunized since goat IgG does not react with this protein (Myhre and Kronvall, 1981; Yarnall and Boyle, 1986a). There is also concern over the biological effects of injection of immunoglobulin-binding proteins. In many animal studies, it has been shown that injection of these proteins leads to a variety of immediate hypersensitivity reactions ranging from mild skin inflammation to fatal anaphylactic shock (Gustafson *et al.*, 1968; Lawman *et al.*, 1984). Consequently, the selection of an animal whose IgG is nonreactive with the immunoglobulin-binding protein is desirable for preparation of specific antibodies.

A. Use of the Chicken for Antibody Production

We have found in our studies of the antigenic relationships of types I, II, III, IV, V, and VI Fc-binding proteins that the chicken is a suitable host for producing antibodies to these proteins (Boyle and Reis, 1990). The advantages of using chickens are twofold: (1) chicken immunoglobulins have minimal-to-no reactivity with any bacterial immunoglobulin-binding proteins identified to date, thus making it easier to distinguish immune from nonimmune reactions; (2) the chicken is easy to maintain in most conventional animal facilities; and (3) large amounts of IgG are present in the egg yolk, thereby providing a convenient source of antibody.

Rose *et al.* (1974) have reported that IgG concentrations of approximately 25 mg/ml are present in egg yolks compared to 6 mg/ml in serum. The egg yolk does not contain detectable levels of IgM or IgA. Immunization of egg-laying hens for antibody production eliminates the need to continually draw blood with the incumbent stress on the animals and difficulties in maintaining veins free of hematomas in animals subjected to frequent bleeding.

Prior to immunization, some chicken serum or egg yolk extracts are found to react in sensitive assays for antibodies to bacterial Fc-binding proteins. This may be due to low-affinity, nonimmune binding to a chicken immunoglobulin allotype or preexisting natural antibodies to the immunogen present as a result of a previous bacterial infection. It is therefore recommended that a number of chickens be screened prior to immunization to identify animals with preimmunization serum or egg-derived IgG that shows no antibody activity.

III. Preparation of Immunogen and Immunization

A wide variety of successful immunization protocols have been reported. Variables to be considered include (1) the age and size of the animal, (2) immunization schedule, (3) route of administration, (4) choice of adjuvants, (5) concentration of immunogen and its preparation, and (6) individual animal response. Although many approaches may be used to produce antibodies to bacterial immunoglobulin-binding proteins, we have found the following protocol to be successful.

Mature, white leghorn, egg-laying hens should be maintained for 2–4 weeks prior to immunization. We have found that some chickens stop laying during transportation, but generally resume laying eggs within 1–2 weeks. Prior to immunization, serum and/or eggs should be obtained and assayed for antibody activity. An emulsion of purified immunoglobulin-binding protein (25–50 μg) is prepared by emulsifying with a suitable adjuvant, e.g., Freund's complete adjuvant or one of the synthetic Ribi-type adjuvants. If large quantities of the purified proteins are not readily available, alternative sources of the antigen can be used as immunogen. Immunoglobulin-binding proteins can be electrophoresed on polyacrylamide gels, stained with Coomassie Blue, and individual, functionally active bands cut out of the gel. Gel slices can be mixed with a small volume of saline and mashed through a fine mesh sieve. The mashed gel should be passed through a series of progressively smaller needles until the mixture will easily flow through a 21 gauge needle. A sample of the mashed gel containing 25–50 μg of the immunoglobulin-binding protein is emulsified with adjuvant and injected intramuscularly (i.m.) at 2–4 sites. At 2–4 week intervals, chickens should be boosted i.m. at multiple sites with an appropriate source of the antigen (containing approximately 25–50 μg), emulsified in incomplete Freund's adjuvant or an equivalent adjuvant. Antibody titers can be followed conveniently by collecting eggs and monitoring antibody in egg yolk extracts as described later in this chapter or by monitoring serum antibody in a similar fashion. Periodic boosts with 25–50 μg of antigen in incomplete adjuvant should be continued until desired quantities of the specific antibody are obtained. This basic protocol has been used to produce monospecific antibodies to isolated type I, type II, and type III Fc-binding proteins (Reis *et al.*, 1984a,b; von Mering and Boyle, 1986; Yarnall and Boyle, 1986b).

IV. Kinetics of Antibody Production

Using the protocol outlined in the preceding section, we immunized two hens with isolated type III Fc-binding protein and monitored the production of antibodies over time. A gel slice containing approximately 50 μg of the type III Fc-binding protein was emulsified with Freund's complete adjuvant, as described. Both chickens were boosted on day 14 and day 35 with the same source of immunogen emulsified in incomplete Freund's adjuvant and the chickens were exsanguinated 40 days after the primary injection with immunogen.

The time course of antibody production was followed in extracts of egg yolks collected daily. The yolks were extracted in phosphate-buffered saline (PBS) as described in the next section and assayed for anti-type III activity in a competitive binding radioimmunoassay. One unit of activity was defined as the reciprocal of the dilution of serum or PBS–egg yolk extract that would inhibit binding of ^{125}I-labeled type III Fc-binding protein to immobilized human IgG by 50%. This assay is described in detail later in this chapter.

The quantities of antibody produced per egg yolk during the course of immunization are shown in Figure 1. Both chickens initially stopped laying eggs following the primary immunization, but resumed egg laying by day 10 and continued laying eggs throughout the immunization schedule. High levels of antibody were detected in egg yolks by day 21, approximately 1 week after the first boost. Titers dropped rapidly and leveled off at about day 26. Following the second boost, antibody titers again rose rapidly in egg yolks and the chickens were exsanguinated on day 40. Serum samples obtained prior to immunization and samples obtained on days 14, 21, and 40 postimmunization were also tested and displayed similar responses to that shown in Figure 1. The antibody titer in serum samples appeared to rise steadily over the course of the immunization schedule, however, this result may be somewhat misleading since only four serum samples were obtained during this time. Egg yolks extracted with PBS were found to be a suitable source of antibody, without further purification, in the assay we used. In some cases it may be desirable to further purify the egg yolk-derived antibody to remove lipids and undesired proteins.

A. Isolation of Antibody from Eggs

A number of protocols have been devised for the purification of IgG from chicken egg yolks (Aulisio and Shelokov, 1967; Bar-Joseph and Malkinson, 1980; Jensenius, *et al.*, 1981; Bade and Stegemann, 1984). We

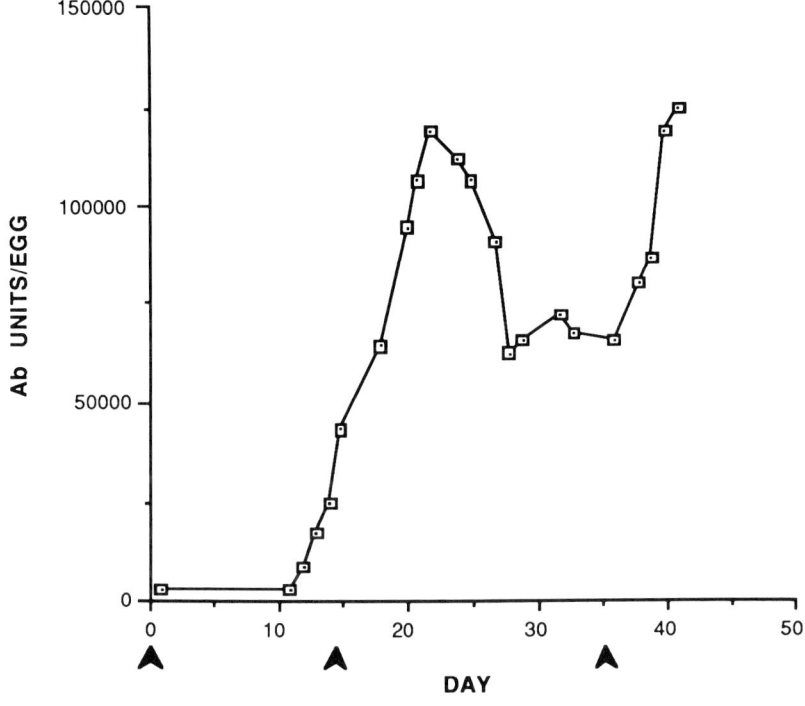

FIGURE 1
Time course of production of antibody to type III Fc-binding protein in chickens, monitored in egg yolk extracts. Antibody units were quantitated using the competitive binding assay described in this chapter and shown diagrammatically in Figure 3A. One unit of activity is defined as the reciprocal of the dilution of chicken egg yolk extract that could inhibit the binding of radiolabeled, type III Fc-binding protein to human IgG immobilized on immunobeads by 50%. Arrows indicate days of immunization. (See text for details.)

have found the following protocol to be straightforward, reproducible, and efficient.

1. Collection of Egg Yolks and PBS Extraction

Eggs can be collected and stored at 4°C for 2–3 weeks prior to extraction. The egg yolks are first separated from the whites. Adhering egg white-containing albumin can be removed by gently rinsing with saline prior to rupturing the yolk membrane. The PBS extract containing antibody is obtained by adding an equal volume (usually about 20 ml) of PBS to each yolk in a centrifuge tube and mixing thoroughly by shaking. The mixture is centrifuged at 12,000 × g for 20 min and the supernatant collected (Bar-Joseph and Malkinson, 1980). The antibody is recovered in the supernatant, usually in a volume of 25–35 ml. This source of antibody can be used for certain studies or further purified as described in the next section.

2. Chloroform Extraction

An equal volume of chloroform is added to the PBS extract just described (adapted from Auliso and Shelokov, 1967). The extract and chloroform are mixed by inversion and allowed to stand at ambient temperature for 30 min. This procedure is repeated at least five times. After storage at 4°C overnight, the mixture is centrifuged at approximately 3000 × g for 10 min and a biphasic solution is apparent. The PBS layer containing antibody is found in the upper layer and can easily be separated from the lower, pigmented, chloroform layer. (Note: Chloroform extraction can be carried out in a single step in a separating funnel by adding the chloroform directly to the yolk–PBS mixture. In this case, a middle layer may form containing yolk constituents, which are normally not present when the mixture has been subjected to centrifugation.) In our hands the inclusion of a centrifugation step in the procedure results in a better separation.

Approximately 50–60% of the antibody found in PBS–yolk extracts can be recovered following chloroform extraction. Based on a comparison of specific antibody activity per unit of protein this procedure results in an approximately 400-fold purification. The chloroform-extracted antibody mixture can be concentrated by ammonium sulfate precipitation (45%) or by ultrafiltration.

V. Detection of Antibody to Immunoglobulin-Binding Proteins

Antibody to bacterial immunoglobulin-binding proteins can be monitored in a variety of assays. Three types of assays will be described. The first two approaches use assay systems that are based on the inhibition of functional activity of the immunoglobulin-binding proteins; that is, the ability of the antibody to prevent binding of the immunoglobulin-binding protein to the Fc region of IgG. The third approach detects the ability of the antibody to bind to epitopes on the immunoglobulin-binding proteins regardless of whether these sites are involved in IgG binding or not. These assays are described in the following sections and use radioiodinated tracers, but the general principle can be carried out with any form of tracer molecule that can be readily quantified.

A. Inhibition of Functional Activity by Antibody
1. Using Whole Bacteria as a Source of Immobilized Immunoglobulin-Binding Protein

This assay is based on the ability of antibodies to a specific immunoglobulin-binding protein to combine with the immunoglobulin-binding protein on a bacterial surface and thereby inhibit the binding of a labeled tracer, usually an ^{125}I-labeled IgG Fc fragment. This assay can be used when limited quantities of the purified binding protein are available or in cases where the purified binding protein loses functional activity when labeled. Using chicken antibodies to Fc-binding proteins of types I, II, and III, Yarnall and Boyle (1986b) have used this type of assay to demonstrate that the type II Fc-binding protein on the group A strain 64/14/HRP was antigenically distinct from types I and III Fc-binding proteins (Figure 2).

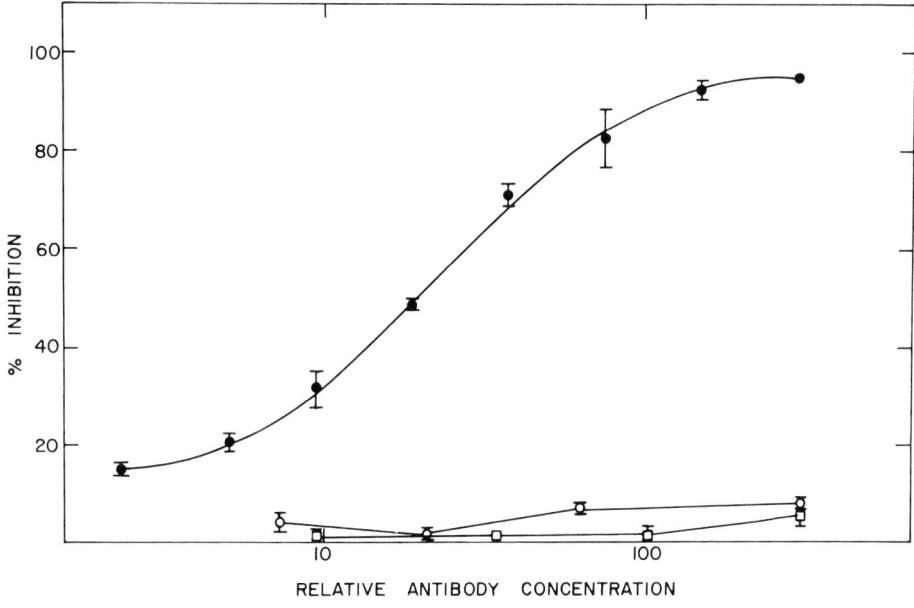

FIGURE 2
Inhibition of binding of ^{125}I-labeled human IgG to the type II Fc-binding protein positive group A streptococcal isolate 64/14/HRP, by antibody against the type I-binding protein (□-□), the type II-binding protein (●-●), or the type III-binding protein (○-○). (Reproduced from Yarnall and Boyle, 1986a, with permission.)

This general type of assay can be used to monitor antibody production in serum or egg yolk extracts to any binding protein by using the bacterial strain from which the binding protein was isolated as the source of immobilized binding protein. An example of this procedure follows, describing the titer of a chicken antibody prepared against a type III Fc-binding protein isolated from group C strain 26RP66 and using ^{125}I-labeled rabbit IgG Fc fragments as probe.

a. Materials

Stock solution of bacteria, group C strain 26RP66 (For method of standardization of bacterial number, see Chapter 2.)

^{125}I-labeled rabbit IgG Fc fragments

Source of antibody from immunized chickens expected to contain antibodies to type III Fc-binding proteins (anti-III)

Control antibody from the chicken prior to immunization (Control)

Buffers:

VBS-G-T; Veronal-buffered saline, 0.15 M, containing 0.1% gelatin, 0.15 mM Ca^{2+}, 1.0 mM Mg^{2+}, and 0.05% Tween 20, pH 7.4

EDTA-G-T; Veronal-buffered saline, 0.15 M, containing 0.01 M trisodium ethylenediaminetetraacetate, 0.1% gelatin, and 0.05% Tween 20, pH 7.4

The exact formulations for all buffers are presented in the Appendix.

b. Procedure. Preliminary experiments are necessary to determine the optimal ratio of bacteria to radiolabeled IgG Fc fragments to establish conditions under which a suitable number of counts bind to the bacteria in the absence of antibody (i.e., maximal binding). This is achieved by incubating 0.1 ml of a dilution (ten-fold) of bacteria, with 0.1 ml of ^{125}I-labeled rabbit IgG Fc fragments (or other suitable probe) containing approximately 30,000 cpm. The time and temperature for this incubation step are arbitrary. For most experiments, we have found 1 hr at 37°C to be convenient while still maintaining a suitable level of sensitivity. After this incubation period, the bacteria are washed twice with 2 ml of EDTA-G-T. The bacterial pellet is recovered by centrifugation at 3000 × g for 10 min and the radioactivity associated with each dilution of bacterial pellet is determined. For experimental purposes, a dilution of the bacterial stock that will bind approximately 33% of the counts offered is usually satisfactory.

The background binding of radioactivity in the absence of bacteria should be less than 5% of the total counts offered. Under these conditions, inhibition of binding of tracer to bacteria can be measured readily. Once these assay conditions have been established, assays for antibodies that recognize bacterial IgG-binding proteins are carried out as follows (Table 1):

2. Detection of Anti-Immunoglobulin-Binding Protein Antibodies

a. General Procedure. The general protocol for this assay is detailed in Table 1. First, prepare a working suspension of bacteria in VBS-G-T so that 0.1 ml/tube will bind approximately 33% of the offered ^{125}I-labeled IgG Fc probe. [If stored bacteria are used, they should be washed twice in VBS-G-T to remove any immunoglobulin-binding protein that may have been shed from the bacteria during storage.]

Prepare three-fold dilutions of samples of antibody from chickens

TABLE 1
Protocol for Quantifying Anti-Fc-Binding Protein Antibodies Using Whole Bacteria as the Source of Immobilized Fc-Binding Proteins[a]

Tube #	Anti-III antibody dilution (0.1 ml/tube)	Control serum (0.1 ml/tube)	Bacteria (ml)	VBS-G-T (ml)	^{125}I-labeled rabbit IgG Fc
1,2	1:10	—	0.1	—	0.1
3,4	1:30	—	0.1	—	0.1
5,6	1:90	—	0.1	—	0.1
7,8	1:270	—	0.1	—	0.1
9,10	1:810	—	0.1	—	0.1
11,12	—	1:10	0.1	—	0.1
13,14	—	1:30	0.1	—	0.1
15,16	—	1:90	0.1	—	0.1
17,18	—	1:270	0.1	—	0.1
19,20	—	1:810	0.1	—	0.1
21,22[b]	—	—	0.1	0.1	0.1
23,24[c]	—	—	—	0.2	0.1
25,26[d]	—	—	—	—	0.1

[a] This protocol is designed to measure anti-type III antibody present in immunized chickens. The protocol will recognize the IgG-binding protein on the type III Fc-binding protein positive group C strain (26RP66) and prevent it from binding radioiodinated rabbit IgG Fc fragment.
[b] Counts bound in tubes 21 and 22 represent the maximum binding.
[c] Counts bound in tubes 23 and 24 represent background binding.
[d] Tubes 25 and 26 are not used in the calculation but should be included to ensure that the expected percentage of IgG bound by the bacteria alone (tubes 21 and 22) is achieved.

immunized with type III IgG-binding proteins or the appropriate preimmunization control sample. The lowest dilution should not be greater than 1 : 10 and VBS-G-T should be used as diluent.

To a series of appropriately labeled tubes, add 0.1 ml of each antiserum dilution to duplicate tubes (Note: for antiserum with low titers, the volume of diluted antibody added can be increased up to 1.0 ml per tube.)

Mix the bacteria at the working concentration prepared in step one and dispense 0.1 ml/tube. Two additional tubes, containing 0.1 ml of VBS-G (no Tween 20) rather than antibody, and 0.1 ml of bacteria are included in each assay (tubes #21 and 22) to determine the maximum binding (max), of tracer to the bacteria. Two other tubes, containing 0.2 ml VBS-G and no bacteria are included (tubes #23 and 24) to determine background binding, (bkg).

Mix all tubes and incubate at 37°C for approximately 30 min to allow interaction between antibodies and bacteria. After this time, add 0.1 ml of ^{125}I-labeled rabbit IgG Fc (containing approximately 30,000 cpm) directly to all tubes and mix. [Note: The bacteria are *not* washed free of antibody at this point in the assay.] The reaction mixture is then incubated for an additional 1 hr at 37°C. [Two additional tubes, to which 0.1 ml of tracer alone is added are prepared and set aside. These tubes (#25 and 26) are used to determine the total cpm added to each tube and are not carried through any further steps in the procedure.]

At the end of the incubation period, 2 ml of EDTA-G-T are added to each tube and the contents of each tube centrifuged at 3000 × g for 10 min. The bacterial-free supernatant is discarded into a suitable radioactive waste container. Keeping the tubes upside down so the bacterial pellet is not disturbed, the remaining liquid associated with the test tubes is blotted onto adsorbent paper. This washing procedure is carried out twice and separates unbound, labeled Ig Fc tracer from tracer associated with the bacterial pellet.

Finally, the quantity of labeled tracer (in this example ^{125}I-labeled rabbit Fc fragments) associated with the bacterial pellet is quantified in a gamma counter and the percentage of inhibition of tracer binding to the bacteria by specific or control antibody is determined as follows:

$$\text{Inhibition of binding } (\%) = 1 - \frac{(\text{test cpm} - \text{bkg cpm})}{(\text{max cpm} - \text{bkg cpm})} \times 100$$

In addition to using this assay to monitor antibody production, we have also found this procedure to be an efficient way to screen many different bacterial isolates for expression of antigenically related immunoglobulin-binding proteins (Boyle and Reis, 1987). For example, this type of assay was used to demonstrate that type III Fc-binding proteins expressed on the surfaces of groups C and G streptococci were antigenically related (von Mering and Boyle, 1986).

3. Quantitation of Specific Antibodies Using a Competitive Binding Assay

This assay is essentially similar to that described in the preceding section, except in this example the probe is a purified, radiolabeled immunoglobulin-binding protein and inhibition of its binding to immobilized IgG is quantified. In this assay, specific antibodies compete with immobilized IgG for binding of the labeled Fc-binding protein (Figure 3A).

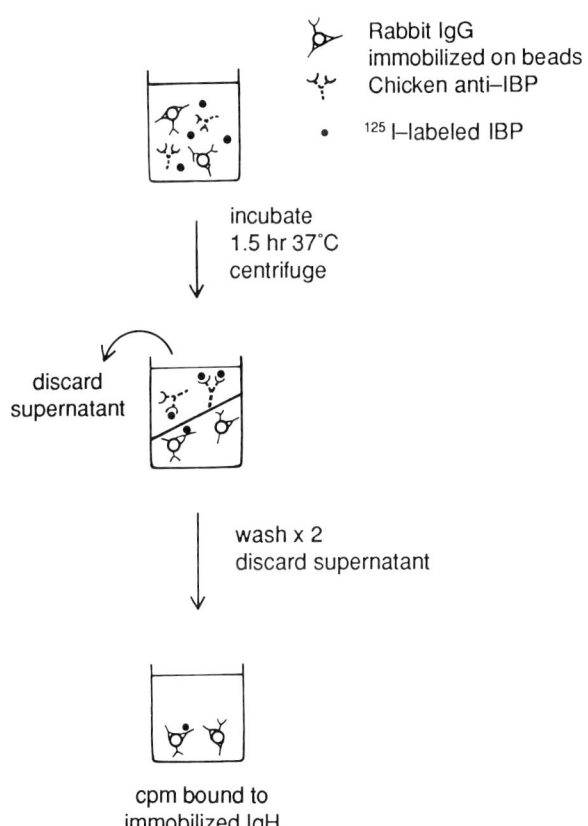

FIGURE 3A
Competitive binding assay for the quantitation of chicken anti-immunoglobulin Fc-binding proteins (IBP). Flow chart of assay, in which chicken antibody competes for the radiolabeled Fc-binding protein tracer with immobilized rabbit IgG.

TABLE 2
Protocol for Quantifying Anti-Fc-Binding Protein Antibodies Using Competition Between Antibody and Labeled Tracer for Binding Immobilized IgG

Tube#	Chicken anti-III dilution (0.1 ml/tube)	Normal chicken serum dilution (0.1 ml/tube)	IgG immunobeads (ml)	VBS-G (ml)	^{125}I-labeled type III Fc-binding protein
1,2[a]	1:100	—	0.1	—	0.1
3,4	300	—	0.1	—	0.1
5,6	900	—	0.1	—	0.1
7,8	2700	—	0.1	—	0.1
9,10	8100	—	0.1	—	0.1
11,12	24,300	—	0.1	—	0.1
13,14	72,900	—	0.1	—	0.1
15,16	—	1:100	0.1	—	0.1
17,18	—	300	0.1	—	0.1
19,20	—	900	0.1	—	0.1
21,22[b]	—	—	0.1	0.1	0.1
23,24[c]	—	—	—	0.2	0.1
25,26	—	—	—	—	0.1

[a] Counts per minute (cpm) bound to immunobeads in the presence of a given dilution of antisera or preimmune serum (NCS, tubes 15–20).
[b] cpm bound to immunobeads in the presence of buffer alone (tubes 21, 22).
[c] cpm bound when no beads or serum are present (tubes 23, 24).

The advantages of this assay are increased sensitivity, selectivity, and standardization compared with the previous assay. This approach is, however, limited to systems in which the IgG-binding protein of interest has been isolated and a functionally active tracer form is available.

The protocol, summarized in Table 2, describes the competitive binding assay for the detection of anti-type III-binding proteins using iodinated type III-binding protein as tracer.

a. Materials

Chicken anti-type III-binding protein antiserum (anti-III)

Preimmunization chicken serum (NCS)

Rabbit or goat IgG Immunobeads (These sources of immobilized IgG beads are commercially available from Bio-Rad, Richmond, California, and an activated immunobead support that allows any species of IgG to be coupled efficiently to this support is also available from this company.)

^{125}I-labeled type III-binding protein (protein G).

VBS-G (no Tween) (used for all dilution steps)

EDTA-G (no Tween) (used for all washing steps)

For exact formulations of buffers, see the Appendix.

b. Procedure. This assay is similar in principle to that previously described using bacteria as the source of immobilized binding protein. In this procedure, the target for the binding protein, i.e., immunoglobulin Fc regions, is immobilized and the soluble tracer is a radioiodinated bacterial IgG-binding protein (Figure 3A). As described previously, preliminary experiments need to be carried out to establish conditions under which binding of tracer to the immobilized target allows approximately 33% of the total counts offered to be bound and also that the specific binding is at least ten times the background level observed when only tracer is added to the tubes. The dilution of immobilized IgG immunobeads to be used in this assay is determined in preliminary experiments by incubating differing dilutions of the beads with approximately 30,000 cpm of the labeled tracer for 1 hr at 37°C. The quantity of tracer associated with the beads after two washes with EDTA-G is determined in a gamma counter.

Prepare three-fold serial dilutions of samples of antibody from chickens immunized with type III-binding protein or the appropriate preimmunization control sample in VBS-G. Diluted samples, 0.1 ml, should be added to duplicate tubes containing 0.1 ml of a suitable dilution of immobilized IgG immunobeads.

Two additional tubes, containing 0.1 ml of VBS-G rather than an antibody sample, are included in each assay (tubes #21 and 22) to determine the maximum cpm bound to immobilized IgG and two other tubes containing 0.2 ml of VBS-G and no immobilized IgG are included to determine background binding (tubes #23 and 24).

A dilution containing 0.1 ml of ^{125}I-labeled type III-binding protein, which contains approximately 30,000 cpm per 0.1 ml is added to each tube and mixed. All samples are mixed and incubated for 1 hr at 37°C. [Two additional tubes, to which 0.1 ml of tracer alone is added, are prepared and set aside. These tubes (#25 and 26) are used to determine the total cpm added per tube and are not carried through any further steps in the procedure.]

At the end of the 1-hr incubation period, 2.0 ml of EDTA-G is added to each tube, and centrifuged at 3000 × g for 5 min. The supernatant is decanted into a liquid radioactive waste container. Keeping the tubes upside down so the immunobead pellet is not disturbed, the remaining liquid is removed by blotting the test tube onto adsorbent paper. This washing step to remove unbound tracer is carried out twice using EDTA-G and then the quantity of labeled tracer associated with the IgG immunobeads is determined by counting in a gamma counter. The percentage of binding inhibition of ^{125}I-labeled type III-binding protein is calculated as follows:

$$\text{Inhibition of binding } (\%) = 1 - \frac{(\text{test cpm} - \text{bkg cpm})}{(\text{max cpm} - \text{bkg cpm})} \times 100$$

The results of a typical experiment are shown in Figure 3B. This assay can also be used to test bacteria for antigenic activity by mixing a standard amount of antibody with an excess of bacteria and then testing for depletion of the antisera in the competitive binding assay previously described. Purified immunoglobulin-binding proteins with similar functional activity can also be compared in this type of competitive binding assay.

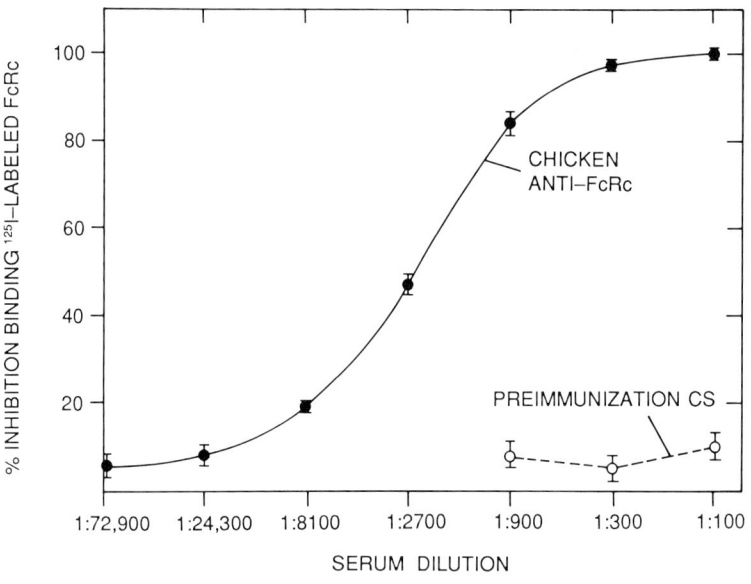

FIGURE 3B
Inhibition of binding of purified ^{125}I-labeled type III Fc-binding protein to immobilized rabbit IgG by chicken antibody prepared against the affinity-purified type III Fc-binding protein (FcRc) (●-●) or preimmunization chicken serum (CS) (○-○). (Adapted from Reis et al., 1984b, with permission.)

Examples of these applications have been described elsewhere (Reis *et al.*, 1984b,c; von Mering and Boyle, 1986).

B. Detection of Antigenic Determinants on Immunoglobulin-Binding Proteins

The assays described thus far are based on the ability of antibodies to the bacterial IgG-binding proteins to inhibit the functional activity of these molecules. Assays that detect classical antigen–antibody reactions that are independent of the functional properties of these proteins can also be performed. Because of the nature of these IgG-binding proteins, caution must be exercised in devising methods to detect the antigen–antibody reaction. For example, if a second antibody is used to detect the primary antibody, appropriate controls must be included to ensure that any positive reactivity is mediated by antigenic-specific interaction. In most cases, preparation of $F(ab')_2$ fragments of the second antibody can eliminate these problems. However, nonimmune binding to the $F(ab')_2$ region of some immunoglobulins by bacterial Fc-binding proteins has been described (Milon *et al.*, 1978; Inganäs *et al.*, 1980; Erntell *et al.*, 1983).

A more definitive approach to the antigenic analysis of bacterial immunoglobulin-binding proteins is the use of a nonantibody-dependent technique to separate antigen–antibody complexes from free antigen as outlined in the assays described in this chapter. These assays can be divided into those that detect soluble binding proteins and those that detect binding proteins immobilized on the surface of bacteria or on nitrocellulose.

1. Antigenic Assays to Detect Soluble Immunoglobulin-Binding Proteins

a. Precipitation in Agarose. Immunoprecipitation assays (Ouchterlony, radial immunodiffusion, or immunoelectrophoresis) have not generally been successful in our hands. This is most probably due to the use of chicken immunoglobulins, which do not generally precipitate well. The use of aged chicken serum, polyethylene glycol (2–4%) or high salt concentrations (3 M) have been reported to enhance the efficiency of chicken immunoglobulins in the formation of insoluble immune complexes. Other investigators have been successful in demonstrating immunoprecipitation reactions with bacterial immunoglobulin-binding proteins; however, the resulting patterns have not always been easy to interpret (Kronvall and Williams, 1971; Lind, 1974; Heath and Cleary, 1988).

b. Farr Assay. A variety of methods for separating antigen–antibody complexes from free antigen have been devised for use in radioimmunoassays. The Farr technique involves the use of an $(NH_4)_2SO_4$ (ammonium sulfate) solution to differentially precipitate immune complexes, while leaving the free, tracer antigen in solution (Farr, 1958). We have used this approach successfully to separate complexes of chicken anti-type I antibodies and labeled protein A in a radioimmunoassay to quantify free protein A.

Essentially, 0.1 ml of a fixed concentration of chicken anti-type I antibody is incubated with 0.1 ml of ^{125}I-labeled protein A tracer (approximately 50,000 cpm) in the presence or absence of fluid-phase competitor. The final reaction mixture in each tube is 0.3 ml and VBS-G is used as diluent for each reactant. The mixture is incubated at 37°C for 1 hr and then all tubes are transferred to ice. Two ml of 35% saturated ice-cold $(NH_4)_2SO_4$ is added to each tube, mixed, and left to stand on ice for 2 hr. The tubes are then centrifuged at 10,000 $\times$ g for 30 min at 4°C and the supernatant discarded. The pellets are washed once with 2 ml of 35% saturated ice-cold $(NH_4)_2SO_4$ and recentrifuged at 10,000 $\times$ g for 30 min at 4°C. The radioactivity associated with the pellet is counted. In each assay, a series of standard protein A samples are included and the degree of inhibition of binding for each known sample is calculated and used to generate a standard curve. The concentration of unknown sample can then be determined from the standard curve. This assay is quite sensitive, with 50% inhibition of binding occurring in the 10–20 ng range. The use of $(NH_4)_2SO_4$ or an equivalent reagent to separate antigen–antibody complexes from free antigen avoids many of the complications inherent in using second antibody reagents in systems in which the antigen is potentially capable of nonimmune interaction with the second antibody. For this type of immunoassay to be of value, it is necessary to have a pure antigen to use as a tracer.

c. Antigenic Analysis of Soluble Immunoglobulin-Binding Proteins by Western Blotting Techniques. In this technique, soluble binding proteins, either crude preparations or purified proteins, are electrophoresed on polyacrylamide gels and transferred electrophoretically to nitrocellulose (Western blot) or other suitable membranes. Proteins on the nitrocellulose membrane are probed with labeled, affinity-purified antibody to the binding protein and the antibody is visualized according to the type of label (e.g., color change as a result of substrate cleavage for enzyme-labeled antibodies or autoradiography for iodinated antibodies). This technique allows both the number of antigenically related molecules in a soluble preparation of binding proteins and the molecular weight of these proteins to be identified. A duplicate membrane, probed with labeled IgG Fc probe permits direct comparison of functionally and antigenically related molecules. The advantages of this sensitive assay are the ability to detect immunoglobulin-binding proteins in a crude mixture and to relate the molecular weight to the antigenic or functional activity.

A general outline of the method that we use follows, using ^{125}I-labeled affinity-purified antibody to type I Fc-binding proteins. Antigen reactivity is detected by use of autoradiography. This assay can also be carried out with biotinylated or enzyme-labeled probes or carried out as a two-stage sandwich-type assay, provided the second antibody is carefully selected to avoid any nonimmune reactivity with the antigen being probed.

d. Procedure. Samples to be tested are electrophoresed on duplicate SDS–polyacrylamide gels under either reducing or nonreducing conditions. (For technical details of this procedure, see Chapter 8.) In our studies, we normally run SDS–polyacrylamide gels according to the method of Laemmli (1970). A positive control of a reactive immunoglobulin-binding protein and molecular weight markers should be included on each gel. After electrophoresis, the gels are soaked in 25 mM Tris, 192 mM glycine and 20% ethanol, pH 8.3, for approximately 30 min. The gel is then placed next to a sheet of nitrocellulose or other suitable membrane and assembled into a Transblot apparatus and the separated proteins are transferred to the nitrocellulose membrane by electrophoresis for 3 hr at 70 V (volts). [Note: We use the Bio-Rad transblot system and a modification of the method of Towbin *et al.* (1979). A variety of other procedures, including a semi-dry blotting system have been shown to facilitate the transfer of proteins from the gel to a nitrocellulose membrane.] Following the transfer, the nitrocellulose membrane is washed four times with 250 ml of VBS, pH 7.4, containing 0.5% gelatin and 0.25% Tween 20 to block any residual protein-binding sites on the membrane. The blocked nitrocellulose membranes are then probed for antigenic reactivity by incubating with 20 ml of the ^{125}I-labeled affinity-purified chicken anti-Fc-binding protein probe (approximately 2×10^5 cpm/ml) diluted in VBS-G-T. A parallel membrane prepared from an identical gel can be probed for functional Fc-binding activity by incubating in a similar fashion with a suitable reactive ^{125}I-labeled IgG Fc specific probe. This probing step is carried out most efficiently by sealing the nitrocellulose membranes in plastic bags with the probe and mixing end-over-end for 3 hr at ambient temperature. Care should be taken to avoid air bubbles and it is not recommended to attempt to probe more than one membrane in a single bag. At the end of the probing reaction, unbound tracer is removed by washing the nitrocellulose membrane four times (15 min each wash) with 250 ml of 0.01 M EDTA, pH 7.2, containing 1 M NaCl, 0.25% gelatin, and 0.25% Tween 20. Following the washing procedure, the nitrocellulose membranes are air dried and wrapped in plastic wrap and exposed to Kodak XAR-5 X-ray film in a cassette containing regular intensifying screens for 1–3 days at −70°C. The exposure time for autoradiography will vary according to the quantity of Fc-binding proteins electrophoresed, the efficiency of protein transfer to the nitrocellulose membrane, and the specific activity of the labeled probe.

An example of this approach, in which Fc-binding proteins from concentrated, overnight culture supernatants of canine *Staphylococcus intermedius* isolates and purified *Staphylococcus aureus* protein A are compared, is presented in Figure 4.

These approaches can also utilize a sandwich-type assay in which a suitable tracer second antibody is used to react with immobilized antigen–antibody complexes on the nitrocellulose membrane. This procedure requires the inclusion of a variety of different controls to ensure that only the specific antibody to the bacterial immunoglobulin-binding protein is detected. An example of this approach, used to relate the group B streptococcal β antigen with IgA Fc-binding activity can be found in Brady and Boyle (1989).

The availability of radiolabeled, affinity-purified antibodies allows

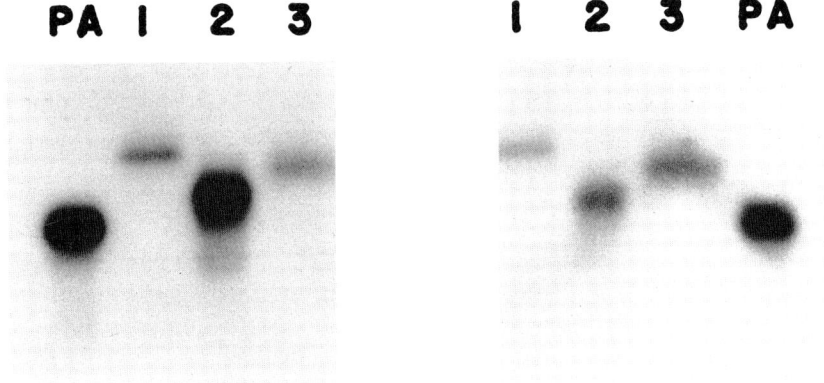

FIGURE 4
Western blot analysis of immunoglobulin-binding proteins from three canine *Staphylococcus intermedius* isolates. The left panel displays the functional activity and the right panel the antigenic activity. Lanes 1, 2, and 3 contain 100 μl of tenfold concentrated supernatants of overnight cultures of *Staphylococcus intermedius* isolates from acral lick granuloma (lane 1), callus pyoderma (lane 2), and superficial pyoderma (lane 3). The lane designated PA contains 40 ng of the type I Fc-binding protein, protein A. The left panel was probed with a ^{125}I-labeled human IgG Fc-specific probe and the right panel was probed with ^{125}I-labeled affinity-purified chicken antibody against protein A. (Reproduced from Fehrer *et al.* (1988), with permission.)

immunoglobulin-binding proteins on the surface of bacteria to be probed directly. For this application, labeled, affinity-purified antibodies are substituted for IgG Fc-specific probes in the procedure used to detect bacterial-bound, functional Fc-binding proteins detailed in Chapter 2.

VI. Conclusion

In this chapter, we have described a number of procedures to prepare antibodies to immunoglobulin-binding proteins and to monitor antibody production. A few examples of how these antibodies can be used to compare different types of bacterial-binding proteins have also been presented. Because of the functional activity of these proteins, i.e., their ability to bind to immunoglobulin molecules in a nonimmune manner, extreme caution must be exercised in selecting the animal species used for antibody production and in devising assays to measure the immune reaction of the antibody with the Fc-binding protein versus the functional activity of the binding protein itself. It is essential in all studies to include preimmunization serum or yolk extracts from the same animal, since subtle variation in immunoglobulin-binding proteins has been documented with different allotypes, and strain-to-strain and animal-to-animal variations may occur. The serological approach to characterizing bacterial surface markers has proven to be of great value for defining different groups and subtypes of microorganisms. Finally, the use of antibodies to compare bacterial Fc-binding proteins will be of value in developing a complete classification of these important, biologically active, bacterial molecules.

References

Aulisio, C. G., and Shelokov, A. (1967). *Proc. Soc. Exp. Biol. Med.* **126**, 312–315.
Bade, H., and Stegemann, H. (1984). *J. Immunol. Methods* **72**, 421–426.
Bar-Joseph, M., and Malkinson, M. (1980). *J. Virol. Methods* **1**, 179–183.
Boyle, M. D. P., and Reis, K. J. (1987). *Biotechnology* **5**, 697–703.
Boyle, M. D. P., and Reis, K. J. (1990). In "Bacterial Immunoglobulin-Binding Proteins" (M. D. P. Boyle, ed.), Vol. 1. pp 175–186. Academic Press, San Diego.
Brady, L. J., and Boyle, M. D. P. (1989). *Infect. Immun.* **57**, 1573–1581.
Erntell, M., Myhre, E. B., and Kronvall, G. (1983). *Scand. J. Immunol.* **17**, 201–209.
Farr, R. S. (1958). *J. Infect. Dis.* **103**, 239–262.
Fehrer, S. L., Boyle, M. D. P., and Halliwell, R. E. W. (1988). *Am J. Vet. Res.* **49**, 697–701.
Gustafson, G. T., Stülenheim, G., Forsgren, A., and Sjöquist, J. (1968). *J. Immunol.* **100**, 530–534.
Heath, D. G., and Cleary, P. P. (1988). *Infect. Immun.* **55**, 1233–1238.

Inganäs, M., Johansson, S. G. O., and Bennich, H. H. (1980). *Scand. J. Immunol.* **12,** 23–31.
Jensenius, J. C., Andersen, I., Hau, J., Crone, M., and Koch, C. (1981). *J. Immunol. Methods* **46,** 63–68.
Kronvall, G., and Williams, R. C. (1971). *Immunochemistry* **8,** 577–580.
Laemmli, U. K. (1970). *Nature (London)* **227,** 680–685.
Lawman, M. J. P., Boyle, M. D. P., Gee, A. P., and Young, M. (1984). *J. Immunol. Methods* **69,** 197–206.
Lind, I. (1974). *Scand. J. Immunol.* **3,** 689–696.
Milon, A., Houdayer, M., and Metzger, J.-J. (1978). *Dev. Comp. Immunol.* **2,** 699–711.
Myhre, E. B., and Kronvall, G. (1981). *In* "Basic Concepts of Streptococci and Streptococcal Diseases" (S. E. Holm and P. Christensen, eds.), pp. 209–210. Redbook, Chertsey, Surrey.
Reis, K. J., Boyle, M. D. P., and Ayoub, E. M. (1984a). *J. Clin. Immunol.* **13,** 75–80.
Reis, K. J., Ayoub, E. M., and Boyle, M. D. P. (1984b). *J. Immunol.* **132,** 3091–3097.
Reis, K. J., Ayoub, E. M., and Boyle, M. D. P. (1984c). *J. Immunol.* **132,** 3098–3102.
Rose, M. E., Orlans, E., and Buttress, N. (1974). *Eur. J. Immunol.* **4,** 521–523.
Towbin, H., Staehelin, T., and Gordon, J. (1979). *Proc. Natl. Acad. Sci. U.S.A.* **76,** 4350–4354.
von Mering, G. O., and Boyle, M. D. P. (1986). *Mol. Immunol.* **23,** 811–821.
Yarnall, M., and Boyle, M. D. P. (1986a). *Mol. Cell. Biochem.* **70,** 57–66.
Yarnall, M., and Boyle, M. D. P. (1986b). *Scand. J. Immunol.* **24,** 549–557.

CHAPTER 7

Use of radiolabeled bacterial Fc-binding proteins as tracers for soluble antigens

Ervin L. Faulmann

I. Introduction

Bacterial Fc-binding proteins have been shown to bind specifically to many species of mammalian immunoglobulin with a very high affinity, even in the presence of high concentrations of unrelated proteins (Langone and Levine, 1979; Reis *et al.*, 1984). The binding to the constant regions of IgG molecules by these bacterial proteins does not interfere with the association of the antibody with specific antigen (Langone *et al.*, 1978). The selectivity and affinity of this interaction allows bacterial Fc-binding proteins to be used effectively as tracers for the detection of immunoglobulin (antibodies) bound to cells and in immunoassays (Langone *et al.*, 1977). Labeled bacterial Fc-binding proteins have been used as tracers in immunoassays for immunoglobulins (Gee and Langone, 1981; Langone, 1978, 1980a; Langone *et al.*, 1977), drugs (Langone and Levine, 1979; Langone, 1980b), and antibodies to specific bacterial (Christensen *et al.*, 1976; Lambden and Watt, 1978; Zeltzer *et al.*, 1978; Marier *et al.*, 1979), viral (Atanasiu and Perrin, 1979; Cleveland *et al.*, 1979; Columbatti and Hilgers, 1979; Crowther and Abu Alzein, 1980; Nicolaieff *et al.*, 1980; Callis and Ritzi, 1980, 1981; Richman *et al.*, 1981; Yolken and Leister, 1981), and parasitic (Hamilton *et al.*, 1981; Avraham *et al.*, 1980) antigens (for an extensive review, see Langone, 1982). This chapter focuses on the practical approaches used in setting up radioimmunoassays for soluble antigens using radiolabeled bacterial Fc-binding proteins as tracer.

The basis for any radioimmunoassay is the specificity of the antibody for its cognate antigen. Initially, radioimmunoassays were performed by detecting labeled antigens complexed with specific antibody using a nonspecific protein precipitation procedure to separate complexed from free antigen. This is the basis of the Farr assay (Farr, 1958). Though very specific for soluble antigen, this assay requires that a pure sample of the antigen is available to be radiolabeled and that the radiolabeling process does not alter the antigenic properties of the antigen. When using the procedure to detect a number of different antigens (each of which has to be separately labeled), this approach is cumbersome. Furthermore, some antigens can themselves be precipitated in the procedure and thus must be modified as well as radiolabeled in order to to be suitable tracers in this assay (Jensenius *et al.*, 1983). The use of labeled, second antibody tracers specific for immunoglobulin associated with antigen–antibody complexes has since gained broad acceptance. This enables the detection of the antigen–antibody complexes using a specific antibody to the species of antibody used in the primary stage of the assay to detect the specific antigen. Thus a single labeled tracer can be used to monitor a number of different antigen-specific assays involving primary antibodies from the same species.

Labeled bacterial Fc-binding proteins, as reporter molecules for antibodies in antigen–antibody complexes, have many advantages over radiolabeled secondary antibodies (Langone, 1978). These advantages include (1) bacterial Fc-binding proteins display less nonspecific binding than many secondary antibody tracers, (2) bacterial Fc-binding proteins are more economic to use than purified, secondary antibody preparations, (3) bacterial Fc-binding proteins display less batch-to-batch variability in binding affinity than secondary antibody preparations, (4) bacterial Fc-binding proteins can be labeled to a higher specific activity than normal secondary antisera, and (5) bacterial Fc-binding proteins allow for greater flexibility in choosing the appropriate primary antibody because they react with a wide range of species of mammalian immunoglobulin (Kronvall, 1973; Langone, 1980a; Myhre and Kronvall, 1981; Reis *et al.*, 1984; Boyle and Reis, 1987).

The practical considerations in using radiolabeled tracers for measuring antigen–antibody complexes require that the labeled tracer bound to the antigen–antibody complex can be separated easily from the unbound tracer. This can be achieved by first immobilizing the antigen, allowing the antibody to react, and then monitoring the immunoglobulin associated with the immobilized antigen–antibody complex with the labeled tracer. Thus, most immunoassays currently use some form of immobilized antigen. This chapter will focus on the use of particulate antigens or antigens covalently coupled to beads in radioimmunoassays utilizing bacterial Fc-binding proteins for the detection of the antigen–antibody complexes.

Other chapters will deal with the use of antigens immobilized on charged membranes (Chapter 14) or immobilized on cells (Chapters 9 and 10).

II. Competitive Inhibition Radioimmunoassay

Competitive inhibition radioimmunoassays, using antigen coupled to particles, have been developed and are capable of quantifying soluble antigens and haptens in complex solutions in the nanogram range (Langone *et al.*, 1977). The critical step in establishing any sensitive, competitive immunoassay is in determining the antiserum:solid-phase antigen ratio, such that the addition of very low concentrations of soluble antigen effectively blocks the binding of the antibody to the solid-phase support. Unbound antibodies are removed by a series of centrifugation and washing steps. The quantity of antibody complexed with the solid-phase antigen support is then determined by measuring the amount of radiolabeled, bacterial Fc-binding protein that will bind to the pelleted material. Using dilutions of a pure preparation of a soluble antigen of known concentration, a standard inhibition curve can be generated, relating the degree of inhibition of binding of the radiolabeled tracer to the absolute concentration of soluble antigen in the primary reaction mixture. The standard curve can then be used to determine the concentration of antigen in the unknown samples.

The key reagents needed to set up a competitive inhibition radioimmunoassay are as follows.

1. Soluble antigen (a source of antigen (10–20 mg) to be immobilized and to serve as a standard for subsequent assays)
2. Specific antiserum (antiserum that is monospecific for the soluble antigen of interest and of a species and isotype that is reactive with the Fc-binding protein tracer to be used)
3. Radiolabeled tracer (a radiolabeled bacterial Fc-binding protein that binds to the specific antiserum)

The overall scheme of the two-stage inhibition radioimmunoassay is shown in Figure 1.

A. Immobilizing the Antigen

The initial step in developing an inhibition radioimmunoassay is to immobilize the antigen onto a solid matrix. There are a variety of suitable solid supports available to which protein and carbohydrate antigens can be

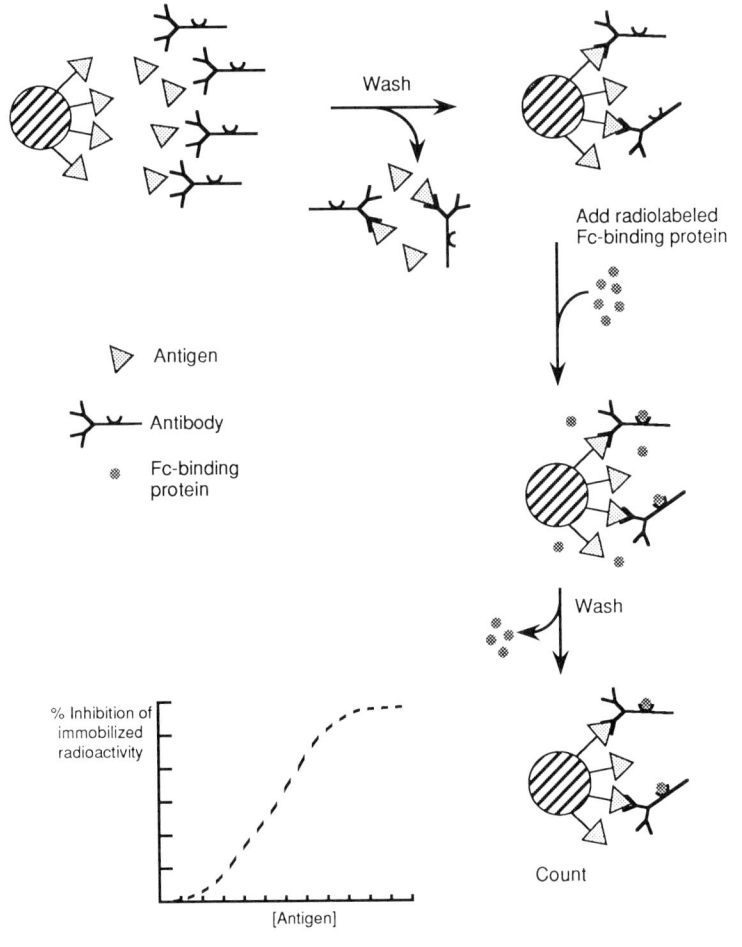

FIGURE 1
Schematic of inhibition radioimmunoassay using specific antibody and a bacterial Fc-binding protein as tracer.

effectively immobilized. Most of these reagents react with primary amino groups or carboxylic groups on the termini or amino acid side chains of protein antigens or with hydroxy residues of carbohydrate antigens. We have achieved good results in coupling a variety of proteins to Immunobeads (Bio-Rad, Richmond, California) via carbodiimide coupling (Reis *et al.*, 1984; Faulmann *et al.*, 1989). The bead material in this product is polyacrylamide and is resistant to fragmentation under the forces applied by the repeated centrifugation steps. The carbodiimide coupling procedure is relatively mild (pH 6.3) and many proteins thus coupled retain their function and antigenicity. The antigen preparation used to couple to the beads does not need to be completely free from contaminants, provided the antiserum is monospecific and does not bind with any of the contaminants in the antigen preparation. Similarly, if a pure antigen is immobilized, the antibody preparation need not be monospecific, because only the antibody specifically bound to the immobilized antigen will be detected in the immunoassay.

The procedure we have used to couple the protein to the beads is essentially that suggested by the manufacturer. The antigen (8–10 mg) is dialyzed into coupling buffer (3 mM KH_2PO_4, pH 6.3) and added to 200 mg of Immunobeads. The solution is rotated in the cold (4°C) for 1 hr, after which 40 mg of EDAC (1-ethyl-3-[dimethylaminopropyl] carbodiimide HCl) is added, and the solution is mixed vigorously. The reaction is allowed to proceed overnight with rotation in the cold. Phosphate-buffered saline (PBS: 10 mM KH_2PO_4, 0.15 M NaCl, pH 7.2) is then added to the bead suspension and centrifuged for 10 min at 1000 × g. The beads are then washed a second time in PBS, followed by two washes in high salt buffer (10 mM KH_2PO_4, 1.4 M NaCl, pH 7.2), followed by two more washes in PBS. The beads are finally resuspended in veronal-buffered saline with gel (VBS-gel; for formulation of all buffers used, see Appendix), containing 0.02% NaN_3. Antigen-coupled Immunobeads may be kept at 4°C for more than a year. A variety of other suitable supports for immobilizing antigens are commercially available (including magnetic microspheres, glass beads, etc.). Any matrix to which an antigen can be covalently bound, and which displays uniform properties in the washing steps outlined in Figure 1, can be substituted in the procedure described.

B. Radiolabeling the Tracer

Radioiodinated bacterial Fc-binding proteins from a number of sources have been shown to be suitable tracers in radioimmunoassays (Langone, 1978; Faulmann et al., 1989). The appropriate bacterial Fc-binding protein to use as a radiolabeled tracer in a specific assay depends upon a number of factors. Of primary concern is the reactivity of the bacterial Fc-binding protein with the species of immunoglobulin used as the specific antiserum in the assay. For assays utilizing rabbit, human, pig, or dog antiserum, either protein A (isolated from *Staphylococcus aureus*) or protein G (isolated from group G or group C streptococcal species) would be suitable tracers. If goat, sheep, cow, or horse antisera are used to detect the specific antigens, protein G is the bacterial Fc-binding protein of choice. Suitable bacterial Fc-binding protein tracers for immunoassays using specific monoclonal rat or mouse antibodies need to be determined individually, because the binding of Fc-specific reagents to different monoclonal antibody preparations is highly variable. Another consideration in producing a suitable radiolabeled tracer is the choice of the radioisotope to label the bacterial Fc-binding protein. Radiolabeled protein A and protein G products are currently commercially available from Amersham (Arlington Heights, Illinois), Dupont New England Nuclear (Wilmington, Delaware), and ICN (Costa Mesa, California). Radiolabeling of bacterial Fc-binding tracers is not difficult, however a number of considerations must be addressed in order to choose an appropriate labeling procedure, including, (1) the capabilities of the laboratory (fume hood, gamma counter, scintillation counter, etc.), (2) the chemistry of the tracer, (3) the anticipated use in the laboratory (e.g., number of assays per month), and (4) the sensitivity of the assay for which the tracer will be used (which relates to specific activity of the labeled probe). In our laboratory, we routinely use ^{125}I (in the Na-salt form) for tracer labeling, due to its relative ease of use, relatively long shelf-life, and the ability to radiolabel proteins to a high specific activity (typically ~0.3 mCi/mg protein) (Reis *et al.*, 1984). Other researchers (Wilder *et al.*, 1979) have reported labeling bacterial Fc-binding proteins with ^{3}H with good results. Use of ^{131}I to radioiodinate a protein probe may be indicated for double label assays, in which two different probes (one labeled with ^{125}I and the other with ^{131}I) are used to assay a single sample and the energy profile of the emissions from each probe can be separately determined. However, the short half-life of ^{131}I limits its utility. Protein A and protein G, as well as other bacterial Fc-binding proteins, can be labeled with ^{125}I using lactoperoxidase, chloramine-T, or Bolton-Hunter reagent with good results using the procedures described in the following sections.

Important Note

Manipulations of radioactive materials are potentially dangerous and all precautions for personal and public safety must be recognized and practiced. Unbound radioactive iodine (usually supplied as the Na-salt in NaOH) is volatile, therefore all labeling procedures must be conducted in a fume hood. Appropriate testing for correct air flow and hood leakage must be completed before initiating any labeling procedure. Whenever possible, use lead shielding to protect from direct radioactive emissions during the radioiodination procedure. All contaminated solid waste should be disposed of carefully so that the volatile radioisotope does not contaminate the immediate air space (i.e., use disposable tubes with air-tight caps to collect pipette tips, etc.). Fluid radioactive waste from protein iodinations should be diluted with one-tenth volume of iodination neutralization solution (0.1 M NaOH, 0.1 M NaI, and 0.1 M NaS$_2$O$_3$) and stored separately from normal radioactive waste. The radioactivity associated with the protein at the end of the procedure is no longer volatile and further manipulations do not need to be carried out in a fume hood, though standard precautions regarding contamination and disposal of radioactive wastes must be observed.

1. Iodinating Proteins with Chloramine-T

The tyrosine residues on proteins can be radiolabeled using the oxidizing agent chloramine-T (Glover *et al.*, 1967). This is accomplished as follows:

1. Add 50 μg of the protein in 200 μl 50 mM phosphate buffer (pH 7.2) into a tube on ice.
2. Add 0.5 mCi ^{125}I or ^{131}I (Na-salt solution from Amersham, ICN, etc.).
3. Add 0.2 ml of cold chloramine-T (0.4 mg/ml in 50 mM phosphate buffer).
4. Incubate 5 min on ice.
5. Add 0.2 ml cold sodium metabisulfite (0.4 mg/ml in 50 mM phosphate buffer).
6. Incubate 5 min on ice.
7. Separate proteins from unbound radiolabel (discussed later in this chapter).

This reaction is initiated by the oxidizing action of the chloramine-T, which is subsequently stopped by the reducing action of the sodium metabisulfite. This procedure is relatively harsh, and can affect protein function. In our hands, protein A and protein G can be effectively radioiodinated by this procedure, however the functional activity of other proteins may be destroyed by the oxidation and reduction in this process (Fraker and Speck, 1978).

A milder modification of the chloramine-T iodination procedure involves the use of immobilized oxidizing agent on beads (Iodobeads, Pierce, Rockford, Illinois), which allows the reaction to be terminated without the addition of reducing agents by simply removing the protein solution from the beads (Markwell, 1982). The procedure is as follows:

1. Incubate 2 Iodobeads with 1 mCi ^{125}I or ^{131}I (Na-salt) in 0.2 ml iodination buffer for 5 min at ambient temperature.

2. Add 50 μl of the protein to be labeled (1 mg/ml in iodination buffer).
3. Incubate mixture for 15 min at ambient temperature.
4. Remove protein solution from the beads.
5. Separate labeled proteins from free radiolabel.

The formulation for the iodination buffer is provided in the Appendix.

2. Iodinating Proteins with Lactoperoxidase

Bacterial Fc-binding proteins can be radiolabeled readily (via their tyrosine residues) by use of lactoperoxidase in the presence of ^{125}I-labeled Na salt and glucose (Marchalonis *et al.*, 1971). Use of the lactoperoxidase linked to beads (Enzymobeads, Bio-Rad, Fremont, California) allows for the rapid removal of the enzyme from the radiolabeled tracer solution (Reis *et al.*, 1984). The protein to be iodinated is extensively dialyzed against PBS and stored at a concentration of 1 mg/ml at −70°C. The iodination reaction is carried out at room temperature and proceeds as follows:

1. Add:
   0.1 ml iodination buffer
   0.1 ml Enzymobead solution
   50 μl of protein solution (1 mg/ml)
   1 mCi ^{125}I or ^{131}I (Na-salt)
   0.1 ml 2% glucose [weight/volume (w/v) in H_2O]
2. Incubate 15 min at ambient temperature.
3. Separate proteins from unbound radiolabel and Enzymobeads, as described in a later section of this chapter.

This procedure is a relatively mild treatment of the protein to be labeled, yet we have achieved specific activity levels similar to those seen using the chloramine-T procedures (Reis *et al.*, 1984). Note that the lactoperoxidase labeling reaction is inhibited by NaN_3 and buffers containing primary amines (e.g., Tris) and it is essential that such agents be removed from the protein solution prior to iodination by this method.

3. Iodinating Proteins with Bolton-Hunter Reagent

Bacterial Fc-binding proteins may also be iodinated by the Bolton-Hunter technique of reacting an ^{125}I-labeled acylating agent with the epsilon amino groups on the protein, forming amide bonds (Bolton and Hunter, 1973). This reaction is carried out under mild conditions and does not affect the tyrosine residues on the proteins. Consequently, any form of bacterial IgG-binding protein that requires tyrosine residues for its function can be radiolabeled by this procedure and will retain its IgG-binding activity. The reaction proceeds as follows:

1. Dialyze the protein extensively against 50 mM phosphate buffer (pH 8.0) and store at 0.5 mg/ml at $-70°C$.
2. Add 0.2 mCi of Bolton-Hunter reagent (^{125}I-labeled 3-(4-hydroxyphenyl) propionic acid N-hydroxysuccinimide ester [Amersham/Searle, Arlington Heights, Illinois (specific activity >1400 Ci/mM)] in 150 μl of benzene to a tube and evaporate the solvent with a gentle stream of air.
3. Add 100 μl of the protein solution (500 μg/ml) and incubate for 15 min at ambient temperature.
4. Add 100 μl of a 100 mM solution of glycine in 50 mM phosphate buffer (pH 8.0) and incubate for a further 15 min at ambient temperature.
5. Separate proteins from low molecular weight reactants (discussed in the following section).

This procedure can result in the generation of very high specific activity tracers without any loss of IgG-binding function (Langone *et al.*, 1977).

4. Separating Proteins from Free Iodine

A number of methods are available to separate radiolabeled proteins from free radioactive products. Dialysis has been used for this purpose, but dialysis of radioactive solutions is time consuming and increases the volume of radioactive waste that must be disposed of. A more effective method to separate unbound ^{125}I or ^{131}I from labeled proteins is to pass the reaction solution over a disposable, desalting column [PD-10 (Pharmacia, Piscataway, New Jersey), Econo-Pak 10DG (Bio-Rad, Richmond, California), or equivalent]. The procedure is rapid and efficiently separates the volatile, free radioactive iodine from the radiolabeled protein (greater than 10,000 daltons) with the generation of a minimal volume of radioactive waste. The procedure must be carried out in a fume hood and is as follows:

1. The column is equilibrated in VBS-gel containing 0.02% NaN$_3$.
2. The radiolabeling solution is added to the column and eluted from the column with VBS-gel containing 0.02% NaN$_3$ and 1 ml fractions are collected.
3. Small aliquots (e.g., 10 μl) from each fraction are counted in capped tubes in a gamma counter.

The radiolabeled protein is recovered in the void volume fractions of the column and the free radioactive iodine is in the inclusion volume (Figure 2). Fractions from the first peak containing high levels of radioactivity are pooled, centrifuged, and filtered through a 0.2 μm filter to remove residual Enzymobeads and nonspecific binding agents, and the percentage of radioactivity associated with the protein is determined by nonspecific precipitation. A simple precipitation procedure is to add 10 μl of the pooled, radiolabeled protein, 10 μl of a concentrated, nonspecific protein solution (i.e., human serum, 10% bovine serum albumin, etc.), and 1 ml of ice-cold, 10% (w/v) trichloroacetic acid (TCA). Allow the precipitate to form for 10 min on ice, centrifuge (3000 × g for 10 min), discard the supernatant, wash the pellet in 10% TCA, and count the pelleted material in a gamma counter. In most labeling procedures, more than 95% of the radioactivity from the pooled fractions of the first peak can be precipitated by 10% TCA.

In our studies, we have found that protein A and protein G solutions labeled by any of these procedures retain functional activity (Reis *et al.*, 1984; Faulmann *et al.*, 1989). The effective shelf-life of any bacterial IgG

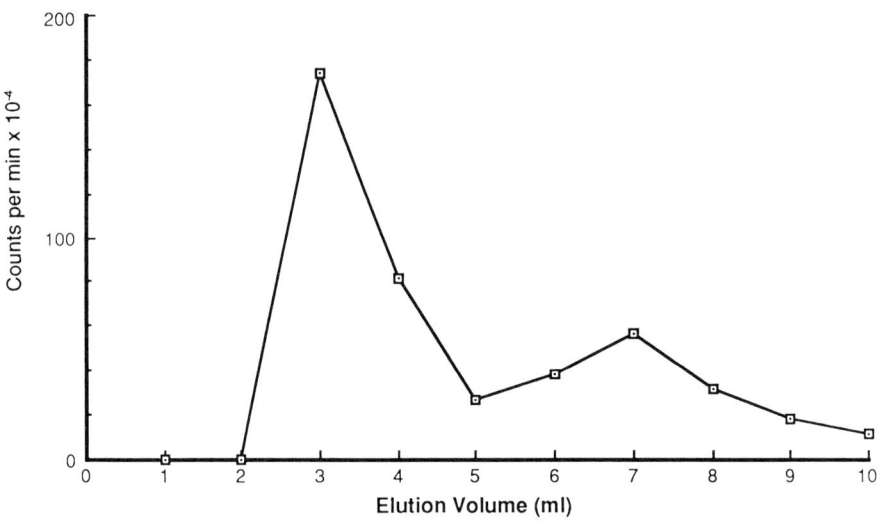

FIGURE 2
Elution of radiolabeled protein G on a Sepharose G-25 column. Protein G (50 μg) was labeled with ^{125}I using the lactoperoxidase method described in the text. The protein solution was applied to a Sepharose G-25 column (10 ml bed volume), equilibrated in VBS-gel containing 0.02% NaN$_3$, and 1 ml fractions were collected. A 10 μl sample of each fraction was counted in a gamma counter (Beckman 5500B). Fractions 3 and 4 were pooled and used as tracer for subsequent immunoassays.

Fc-binding protein tracer is dependent in part on the shelf-life of the radioisotope used to label. We have observed that bacterial Fc-binding proteins labeled with ^{125}I can be used as effective probes for immunoglobulin in immunoassays for 1–2 months without significant loss of sensitivity in the assay.

C. Development of a Competitive Binding Immunoassay

The first step in developing a competitive inhibition radioimmunoassay is to establish conditions for detection of the interaction of the specific antibody and the immobilized antigen. This is carried out in two stages using a checkerboard approach, in which each reactant is varied independently. The purpose of these preliminary experiments is to determine the optimal concentrations of antigen-coupled beads, antiserum, and radiolabeled tracer that will allow sufficient radioactivity to be associated with the pelleted beads at the end of the assay to facilitate easy quantitation. An experiment is set up using a checkerboard of varying concentrations of antigen-coupled beads and varying concentrations of specific antiserum in the first step and the quantity of immobilized antigen–antibody complex determined in a second step by quantifying the amount of bound radiolabeled bacterial Fc-binding protein. Initially the concentration of the labeled tracer added to each tube is kept constant.

Antigen-coupled beads and primary antiserum are diluted separately in VBS-gel. One hundred μl of each dilution of the antigen-coupled beads and primary antiserum is added to duplicate tubes. Three hundred μl of VBS-gel is added and the antibody is allowed to bind to the immobilized antigen for 1 hr at 37°C. The time, temperature, pH, and ionic strength of this reaction can be varied depending on the characteristics of each antigen–antibody combination used in the assay. Unbound immunoglobulin is washed from the antigen-coupled beads by adding 2 ml ethylenediaminetetraacetic acid (EDTA) with gelatin (EDTA-gel, for precise formulation, see Appendix), pelleting the beads by centrifugation at 1000 × g for 8 min, and decanting the supernatant. The beads are resuspended and washed with EDTA-gel once more. The pelleted beads are then resuspended in 300 μl of VBS-gel and 100 μl ^{125}I-labeled bacterial Fc-binding protein (containing between 20,000–50,000 counts per minute (cpm)) is added and allowed to bind for 1 hr at 37°C. Unbound, radiolabeled tracer is removed by washing the beads twice in EDTA-gel, as previously described. The quantity of radioactivity associated with the antigen-coupled beads is then determined by counting disintegrations in a scintillation gamma spectrometer. By plotting the measured radioactivity against the dilution of antigen-coupled beads added to the assay, curves similar to

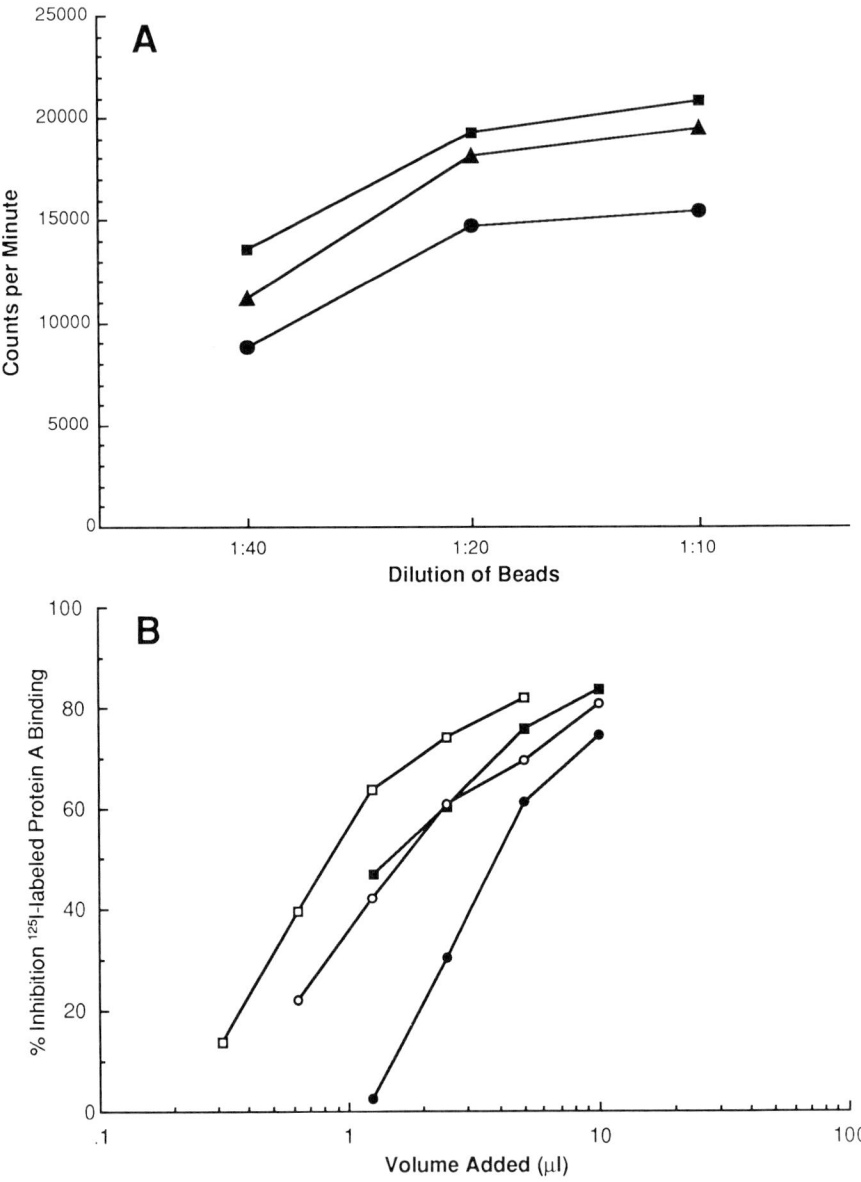

FIGURE 3
Development of a competitive binding radioimmunoassay for human C1 esterase inhibitor. Human C1 esterase inhibitor was partially purified from human serum by a two-step process. Human serum (10 ml) was applied to a CIBACRON-Blue agarose column (50 ml bed volume) and eluted with 0.15 M phosphate-buffered saline (PBS),

Chapter 7. RIAs Using Bacterial Fc-Binding Protein

those shown in Figure 3A can be generated for each dilution of primary antiserum.

In the example shown in Figure 3A, human C1 esterase inhibitor was partially purified from human serum (Faulmann, 1985) and immobilized on Immunobeads (as previously described). Various dilutions of the bead suspension were aliquoted and dilutions of monospecific rabbit antiserum to the human C1 esterase inhibitor (Organon Teknika-Cappel, Malvern, Pennsylvania) were added. After incubation at 37°C, the beads were washed twice in EDTA-gel and the bead aliquots were then probed with ^{125}I-labeled protein G (approximately 40,000 cpm per tube). The protein G was obtained as the wild type protein from Calbiochem (La Jolla, California) and labeled by the lactoperoxidase method described earlier. Unbound, radiolabeled tracer was removed by washing the beads twice in EDTA-gel. The bead pellets were then counted in a gamma counter and the radioactivity associated with each dilution of bead and antiserum was plotted (Figure 3A). The plateau associated with each resulting curve represents a situation in which the antibody reagent is limiting and the addition of further immobilized antigen does not result in the generation of additional antigen–antibody complexes that can be detected by the binding of radiolabeled tracer. Addition of soluble antigen to tubes containing these dilutions of antisera and beads would not cause an appreciable decrease in binding of the primary antiserum to the beads. As the concen-

---

pH 7.3. Fractions reactive with monospecific rabbit anti-human C1 esterase inhibitor, detected by double diffusion immunoprecipitation, were pooled and applied to a concanavalin A–agarose column equilibrated in PBS. Unbound proteins were washed from the column with PBS and the C1 esterase inhibitor for protein was eluted with 25 mM α-methyl-mannose in PBS. The partially purified C1 esterase inhibitor eluted from the lectin column was dialyzed against PBS and coupled to Immunobeads (Bio-Rad, Richmond, California) by the method described in the text. (A) Various dilutions of C1 esterase inhibitor-coupled beads were added to dilutions of the rabbit anti-C1 esterase inhibitor, incubated for 1 hr at 37°C, and washed to remove unbound antibodies. The amount of rabbit immunoglobulin associated with the pelleted material was determined by incubating with ^{125}I-labeled protein G for 1 hr at 37°C and washing free of unbound tracer. The radioactivity associated with the bead pellets was counted in a gamma counter. (—■—) 1:250 dilution of rabbit anti-human C1 esterase inhibitor antiserum. (—▲—) 1:500 dilution of rabbit anti-human C1 esterase inhibitor antiserum. (—●—) 1:1000 dilution of rabbit anti-human C1 esterase inhibitor antiserum. (B) Dilutions of human serum samples inhibit the binding of rabbit anti-C1 esterase inhibitor (1:500) to C1 esterase inhibitor-coupled beads (1:25). The absolute concentration of C1 inhibitor in each serum sample was determined by measuring inhibition of ^{125}I-labeled protein G bound to the beads and comparing the inhibition to the standard curve generated using the purified C1 esterase inhibitor protein standard. (—□—) Purified C1 esterase inhibitor protein standard. (—○—) Serum from individual #1. (—■—) Serum from individual #2. (—●—) Serum from individual #3.

tration of beads is reduced, the antibody is no longer limiting, but rather the amount of bead-bound antigen becomes the limiting factor in determining the amount of radioactivity associated with the final bead pellet. The conditions under which the tracer binding is found to change with dilution of immobilized antigen, in the presence of a constant dilution of antibody, represent the situation at which the immobilized antigen becomes limiting. At these dilutions, addition of soluble antigen will markedly inhibit the amount of antibody associated with the pellet of immobilized antigen, therefore inhibiting the amount of radioactive tracer bound. This represents the conditions necessary to be able to measure fluid-phase antigen with good sensitivity.

In choosing the appropriate dilutions of the antigen-coupled beads and primary antibody for use in subsequent two-stage inhibition assays, a number of considerations must be weighed. The sensitivity of the inhibition assay is determined by the ability of the soluble antigen to compete for a limited quantity of specific antibody. Consequently, the detection of antigen will be most sensitive when the minimum amount of antibody is used. Attempts to reduce the quantity of specific antibody used in the assay in order to increase the sensitivity must be balanced with the theoretical and technical difficulties of quantifying low numbers of radioactive disintegrations. For reproducibility of the assay, therefore, the number of counts bound in the absence of soluble antigen should be at least 4000 cpm and the ratio of maximum binding to background binding (i.e., binding of tracer to immobilized antigen in the absence of specific antibody or in the presence of nonimmune antibody) should be at least five-fold. As mentioned previously, the amount of radiolabeled Fc-binding protein added in the last stage of the assay must be optimized. Using the labeling procedures outlined earlier, the specific activity of the resulting tracer is sufficient such that addition of 20,000–50,000 cpm in 100 μl to each tube provides sufficient tracer to be detected in this immunoassay. However, different species of antibody or different specific activity tracers will influence the quantity of radiolabeled tracer that needs to be added. In general, we have found a dilution of antibody and immobilized antigen that results in approximately 30% of the offered ^{125}I-labeled bacterial Fc-binding protein being bound to the immobilized antigen at the end of the assay is optimal (Reis *et al.*, 1984). Under these conditions, we have found that inhibition by nanogram levels of soluble antigen can be reproducibly measured.

D. Quantitation of Antigens in a Two-Stage Competitive Radioimmunoassay

The procedure for optimizing the reagents is a necessary first step in developing any competitive binding radioimmunoassay. The optimal reaction conditions may vary for antibodies from different species or for certain antigen–antibody pairs. For each system it will be necessary to establish these conditions empirically by following the procedure just outlined.

Once conditions of immobilized antigen concentration, antibody concentration, tracer concentration, time, and buffer conditions have been established, the next step in the procedure is to test the specificity and sensitivity of the procedure for the detection of soluble antigen. This is achieved by determining the inhibition of binding of radiolabeled tracer to immobilized antigen at the end of the assay, when different dilutions of specific antigens are added to the immobilized antigen and specific antibody in the first stage of the procedure depicted in Figure 1. It is essential that 100% inhibition of binding of the tracer can be achieved when high concentrations of specific antigen are added. If this cannot be achieved then the assay is not completely specific for the antigen of interest.

An assay was developed to quantify human C1 esterase inhibitor in serum and results from a representative experiment are shown in Figure 3B. From the results shown in Figure 3A, 0.1 ml of a dilution of 1:25 for the antigen-coupled beads (human C1 esterase inhibitor) and 0.1 ml of a dilution of 1:500 for the antiserum (rabbit anti-human C1 esterase inhibitor) were added to tubes containing 0.1 ml of various dilutions of individual serum samples. As a control, dilutions of a known concentration of human C1 esterase inhibitor, purified from human serum by the method of Harrison (1984), were included in this assay. After incubation for 1 hr at 37°C and washing twice in EDTA-gel, the beads were probed by incubation with ^{125}I-labeled protein G (approximately 25,000 cpm per tube). Unbound tracer was removed by washing and the pellets were counted in a gamma counter. The amount of radioactivity associated with antigen-coupled beads in the absence of any competitor was compared to tubes containing various dilutions of human serum. Any serum C1 esterase inhibitor antigen present in the serum samples would compete with the specific antiserum and inhibit it from binding to the beads (Figure 3B). The resulting curves show remarkable similarities in shape, level of final inhibition, and slope for all solutions tested (Figure 3B). Curves generated in this assay that differ in any one of these categories imply that either (1) the antigens in the solutions assayed have different affinities for the antiserum, (2) the antigens in the solutions do not contain all of the epitopes recognized by the antiserum, or (3) some samples may contain other components that are affecting the assay. In the graph shown in Figure 3B, the curves are similar and the results from serum sample 3 indicate that it contains approximately 0.2 mg/ml, while serum samples 1 and 2 contain approximately 0.6 mg/ml of C1 esterase inhibitor, which is within the normal range (Rosen *et al.*, 1971). It is of interest to note that all of the sera

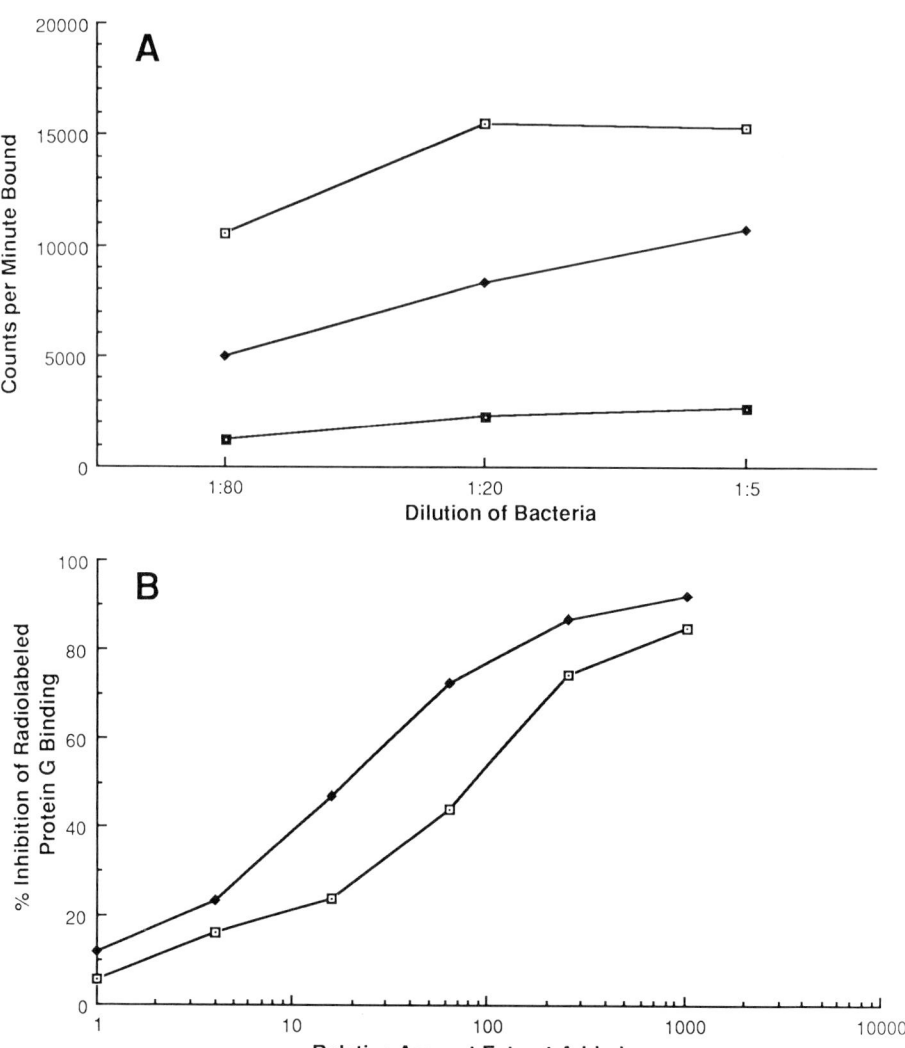

FIGURE 4
Development of a competitive binding immunoassay for soluble group B streptococcal β antigen using bacterial surface antigen as the solid phase. (A) Various dilutions of the rabbit anti-β antiserum added to dilutions of a 10% solution (wet weight bacteria/volume PBS) of group B streptococci β antigen positive strain TC 795. The quantity of rabbit immunoglobulin associated with the pelleted bacteria was determined by measuring the quantity of ^{125}I-labeled protein G associated with bacterial bound antigen–antibody complexes. (—□—) 1:200 dilution of rabbit anti-β antiserum. (—◆—) 1:1000 dilution of rabbit anti-β antiserum. (—■—) 1:5000 dilution of rabbit anti-β antiserum. (B) Dilutions

Chapter 7. RIAs Using Bacterial Fc-Binding Protein   141

tested contain normal levels of human IgG (~10 mg/ml). Human IgG binds with a high affinity to protein G and could cause inhibition in this assay. However, as shown in Figure 3 of Chapter 3, IgG is not detected in a two-stage assay, indicating the low nonspecific binding of proteins to the immobilized antigen matrix and the efficiency of the washing procedure.

The inhibition radioimmunoassay described in this section can also utilize antigens on bacterial surfaces as the solid phase of the assay (Chapter 9). Solubilized bacterial antigens can then be quantified using a modification of the general procedure outlined in Figure 1, in which specific immobilized antigen is replaced by a "naturally" immobilized form of the antigen. In this case, the specificity of antigen detection is based on the availability of a suitable monospecific or monoclonal antibody. An example of this is shown in Figure 4. In these experiments, an antiserum that contained antibodies specific for the β antigen expressed on the surface of certain group B streptococci (Brady and Boyle, 1989) and a corresponding group B strain expressing the β antigen were used in the presence of various extracts containing the soluble antigen. The presence of soluble β antigen could be detected by inhibition of binding of the specific antibody to the antigen-positive bacterial surface. Initial experiments (Figure 4A) were carried out to determine the appropriate concentrations of antiserum and bacteria to use in subsequent inhibition assays. In the inhibition assay, bacteria, antiserum, and dilutions of soluble antigen (extracts from group B streptococci) were added together and incubated at 37°C. After unbound immunoglobulin was removed by centrifugation, the amount of antibodies remaining associated with the bacteria was measured by incubation with radiolabeled protein G (approximately 25,000 cpm per tube), followed by washing, and counting in a gamma counter. The presence of soluble β antigen inhibited the binding of the primary antibody to the bacteria, as can be seen by the inhibition of radioactive protein G binding to the bacterial pellet (see Figure 4B), and the results show that there was approximately fourfold more β antigen in the SDS-extracted material than in the heat-extracted material.

---

of soluble extracts of group B streptococcal strain TC 795 containing β antigen were added to tubes containing β antigen surface positive bacteria (1:50 dilution of a 10% solution) and rabbit anti-β antiserum (1:1000). The relative amount of soluble β antigen in the extracts was determined by measuring inhibition of ^{125}I-labeled protein G bound to bacteria incubated with antibody in the absence of added soluble antigen. (—□—) Heat extract of group B streptococcus TC 795. (—◆—) SDS extract of group B streptococcus TC 795.

III. Summary

The information presented in the preceding sections provides a practical approach to setting up and interpreting immunoassays for soluble antigens using radiolabeled bacterial Fc-binding proteins. These assays are simple, specific, economical, and can be used to quantify a variety of soluble antigens.

References

Atanasiu, P., and Perrin, P. (1979). *Ann. Microbiol.* **130A,** 257.
Avraham, H., Spira, D. T., Gorsky, Y., and Sulitzeanu, D. (1980). *J. Immunol. Methods* **32,** 151.
Bolton, A. E., and Hunter, W. H. (1973). *Biochem. J.* **133,** 529–539.
Boyle, M. D. P., and Reis, K. J. (1987). *Biotechnology* **5,** 697–703.
Brady, L. J., and Boyle, M. D. P. (1989) Infect. Immun. **57,** 1573–1581.
Brady, L. J., Daphtary, U. D., Ayoub, E. M., and Boyle, M. D. P. (1988). *J. Infect. Dis.* **158,** 965–972.
Callis, A. H., and Ritzi, E. M. (1980). *J. Virol.* **35,** 876.
Callis, A. H., and Ritzi, E. M. (1981). *Intervirology* **15,** 111.
Christensen, K. K., Christensen, P., Mardh, P. A., and Weström, L. (1976). *J. Infect. Dis.* **134,** 317.
Cleveland, P. H., Belnap, L. P., Knotts, F. B., Nayak, S. K., Baird, S. M., and Pilch, Y. H. (1979). *Int. J. Cancer* **23,** 380.
Columbatti, A., and Hilgers, J. (1979). *J. Gen. Virol.* **43,** 395.
Crowther, J. R., and Abu Alzein, E. M. E. (1980). *J. Immunol. Methods* **34,** 261.
Farr, J. S. (1958). *J. Infect. Dis.* **103,** 239–262.
Faulmann, E. L. (1985). Doctoral dissertation, University of Florida.
Faulmann, E. L., Otten, R. A., Barrett, D. J., and Boyle, M. D. P. (1989). *J. Immunol. Methods, J. Immunol. Methods* **123,** 269–281.
Fraker, P. J., and Speck, J. C. (1978). *Biochem. Biophys. Res. Commun.* **80,** 849–857.
Gee, A. P., and Langone, J. J. (1981). *Anal. Biochem.* **116,** 524.
Glover, J. S., Salter, D. N., and Shepherd, B. P. (1967). *Biochem. J.* **103,** 120–128.
Hamilton, R. G., Hussain, R., Ottesen, E. A., and Adkinson, Jr., N. F. (1981). *J. Immunol. Methods* **44,** 101.
Harrison, R. A. (1984). *Biochemistry* **22,** 5001–5007.
Jensenius, J. C., Siersted, H. C., and Johnstone, A. P. (1983). *J. Immunol. Methods* **56,** 19–32.
Kronvall, G. (1973). *J. Immunol.,* **11,** 1401–1406.
Lambden, P. R., and Watt, P. J. (1978). *J. Immunol. Methods* **20,** 277.
Langone, J. J. (1978). *J. Immunol. Methods* **24,** 269–285.
Langone, J. J. (1980a). *J. Immunol. Methods* **34,** 93.
Langone, J. J. (1980b). *Biochem. Biophys. Res. Commun.* **94,** 473.
Langone, J. J. (1982). *J. Immunol. Methods* **51,** 3–22.
Langone, J. J., and Levine, L. (1979). *Anal. Biochem.* **95,** 472–478.
Langone, J. J., Boyle, M. D. P., and Borsos, T. (1977). *J. Immunol. Methods* **18,** 281–293.
Langone, J. J., Boyle, M. D. P., and Borsos, T. (1978). *J. Immunol.* **121,** 327–332.
Langone, J. J., Boyle, M. D. P., and Borsos, T. (1979). *Anal. Biochem.* **93,** 207.

Marchalonis, J. J., Cone, R. E., and Santer, V. (1971). *Biochem. J.* **124,** 921–927.
Marier, R., Jansen, M., and Andriole, V. T. (1979). *J. Immunol. Methods* **28,** 41.
Markwell, M. A. K. (1982). *Anal. Biochem.* **125,** 427–432.
Myhre, E. B., and Kronvall, G. (1981). *In* "Basic Concepts of Streptococci and Streptococcal Diseases" (S. E. Holm and P. Christensen, eds.). pp. 209–210. Redbook, Chertsey, Surrey.
Nicolaieff, A., Obert, G., and Van Regensmortel, M. H. V. (1980). *J. Clin. Microbiol.* **12,** 101.
Reis, K. J., Ayoub, E. M., and Boyle, M. D. P. (1984). *J. Immunol.* **132,** 3098–3102.
Richman, D. D., Cleveland, P. H., Oxman, M. N., and Zaia, J. A. (1981). *J. Infect. Dis.* **143,** 693.
Rosen, F. S., Alper, C. A., Pensky, J., Klemperer, J., and Donaldson, V. H. (1971). *J. Clin. Invest.* **50,** 2143–2149.
Yolken, R. H., and Leister, F. J. (1981). *J. Immunol. Methods* **43,** 209.
Wilder, R. C., Yuen, C. C., Subbartao, B., Woods, V. L., Alexander, C. B., and Mage, R. G. (1979). *J. Immunol. Methods* **28,** 255–266.
Zeltzer, P. M., Peprose, J. S., Bishop, N. H., and Miller, J. N. (1978). *Infect. Immun.* **21,** 163.

CHAPTER 8

Application of enzyme-labeled IgG-binding proteins in immunoassay

Kathleen J. Reis
Michael D. P. Boyle

I. Introduction

Immunoassays using enzyme-labeled tracers are playing an increasing role in both research and diagnostic laboratories. Enzyme-linked immunosorbent assays (ELISA) are now widely used in place of radioimmunoassay tracers for the detection and quantitation of soluble antigens or antibodies. Like radioimmunoassays, ELISAs are highly sensitive and easily automated. Enzyme-labeled tracers have a long shelf-life, thereby eliminating the need for frequent tracer labeling. Furthermore, use of enzyme-labeled tracers eliminates the need for training and approval for use of radioactive materials and the problems associated with radioactive waste disposal.

The combination of enzyme technology with bacterial IgG Fc-binding proteins provides a powerful tool for immunoassay, encompassing all the advantages of ELISA with the added advantage of being able to use a single tracer for a variety of applications. A large number of reports have been published that utilize the type I Fc-binding protein, protein A, labeled with the enzymes alkaline phosphatase or horseradish peroxidase as the tracer for the detection of a variety of antigens and antibodies. A partial list of these assays is presented in Table 1. For additional examples, see reviews by Langone (1982) and Forsgren *et al.* (1983).

Reis *et al.* (1988) and Nilson *et al.* (1988) have demonstrated the usefulness of an alkaline phosphatase-labeled, type III IgG Fc-binding protein, protein G, for the detection of sheep, goat, rabbit, and mouse antibodies to a variety of antigens (Table 1). Recently, the type III-binding

TABLE 1
Assays Utilizing Enzyme-Labeled Fc-Binding Protein

Enzyme probe	Antibody species	Antigen detected	Reference
PA[a]-AP[b]	rabbit	mouse hepatoma	Engvall (1978)
PA-AP	rabbit	human AFP[c]	Engvall (1978)
PA-AP	goat	mouse AFP	Engvall (1978)
PA-AP	rabbit	human IgE	Gee and Langone (1981)
PA-AP	rabbit	5-methyltetrahydrofolate	Gee and Langone (1981)
PA-HRP[d]	llama	*Mycobacterium bovis*	Thoen *et al.* (1980)
PA-HRP	rhinoceros	*M. bovis*	Thoen *et al.* (1980)
PA-HRP	elephant	*M. bovis*	Thoen *et al.* (1980)
PA-HRP	pig	pseudorabies virus	Potgieter *et al.* (1980)
PA-HRP	horse	equineherpes virus	Potgieter *et al.* (1980)
PA-HRP	cow	IBR[e] virus	Potgieter *et al.* (1980)
PA-HRP	cat	feline calicivirus	Potgieter *et al.* (1980)
PA-HRP	dog	canine adenovirus	Potgieter *et al.* (1980)
PA-HRP	rabbit	herpesvirus hominis	Potgieter *et al.* (1980)
PA-HRP	human	herpesvirus hominis	Potgieter *et al.* (1980)
PA-HRP	human	human rotavirus	Yolken and Leister (1981)
PA-HRP	human	*Haemophilus influenza*, type b polysaccharide	Yolken and Leister (1981)
PG[f]-AP	sheep	mouse IgG	Reis *et al.* (1988)
PG-AP	goat	human plasminogen	Reis *et al.* (1988)
PG-AP	rabbit	streptokinase	Reis *et al.* (1988)
PG-AP	goat	human-α-1-microglobulin	Nilson *et al.* (1988)
PG-AP	rabbit	human-α-1-microglobulin	Nilson *et al.* (1988)
PG-AP	monoclonal mouse γ1	human-α-1-microglobulin	Nilson *et al.* (1988)
PG-AP	monoclonal mouse γ2a	human-α-1-microglobulin	Nilson *et al.* (1988)
PG-AP	monoclonal mouse γ2b	human-α-1-microglobulin	Nilson *et al.* (1988)

[a] PA=protein A.
[b] AP=alkaline phosphatase.
[c] AFP=α-fetoprotein
[d] HRP=horseradish peroxidase
[e] IBR=infectious bovine rhinotracheitis virus
[f] PG=protein G

protein, protein G, has become commercially available and a variety of enzyme-labeled forms of the IgG Fc-binding proteins have been prepared.

The purpose of this chapter is to describe the preparation and use of enzyme-labeled IgG Fc-binding proteins in immunoassays for the measurement of antigens and antibodies. Although these assays are described using 96-well polystyrene plates for immobilization of antigen, a variety of other supports are possible (e.g., polypropylene tubes, magnetic microspheres, and nitrocellulose). A comprehensive description of the principle of an ELISA can be found in a variety of published sources (Engvall, 1978, 1980; Engvall and Perlmann, 1971, 1972; Nakamura *et al.*, 1986; Harlow and Lane, 1988).

II. Types of Assays

There are two general types of assays that can be developed using enzyme-labeled Fc-binding proteins: (1) a direct binding assay for the detection of IgG antibody to a given antigen and (2) a competitive binding assay for the detection of soluble antigen. Examples of each type of assay and how they are carried out are provided in the next sections.

A. Direct Binding Assay for the Detection of Antibody

The basic principle of these assays is that specific antibodies are allowed to bind to immobilized antigen and following removal of unbound, irrelevant antibodies, the number of immune complexes formed are quantified using an appropriate, enzyme-conjugated IgG Fc-binding protein as tracer. This general procedure is summarized schematically in Figure 1.

In this type of assay, antigen is bound to a solid support such as a 96-well microtiter plate. Unbound antigen is washed away and any remaining active sites are blocked with a nonspecific protein such as albumin or gelatin. Samples to be assayed for the presence of IgG antibodies are added to the wells and incubated to allow binding to the antigen. After washing to remove unbound antibodies and other immunoglobulins, any antibody complexed to the immobilized antigen is detected by the addition of IgG-binding protein coupled to enzyme as tracer. Unbound, enzyme-labeled tracer is removed by washing, while enzyme-labeled tracer bound to IgG in antibody–antigen complexes is detected by the addition of a suitable substrate. The enzyme cleaves the substrate resulting in a color change, which can be measured spectrophotometrically. Under standardized conditions the assay is quantitative for antibody since the degree of color change is proportional to the quantity of enzyme-labeled tracer, which in turn, is proportional to the amount of antibody bound to antigen.

This type of assay is suitable for the detection of antibodies whose Fc regions are reactive with the immunoglobulin Fc-binding protein–enzyme tracer. Antibody of a class or subclass that is nonreactive with the immunoglobulin Fc-binding protein would not be detected and furthermore, large quantities of such an antibody, e.g., IgM or IgA, would compete for

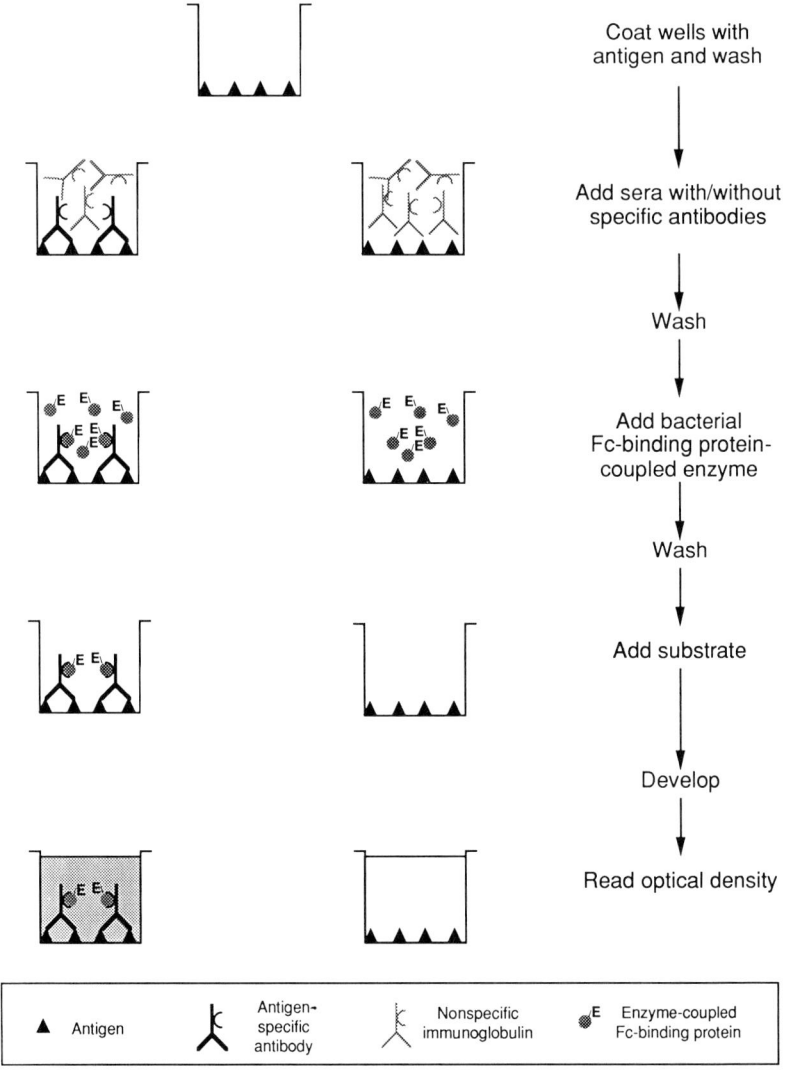

FIGURE 1
Schematic representation of the use of enzyme-linked IgG Fc-binding protein tracer to detect specific antibodies.

antigen and prevent binding of reactive antibodies. This may lead to an underestimation of reactive antibody or possibly false, negative results. The use of IgG Fc-binding proteins for the detection of antibodies to soluble and cell surface antigens is discussed in detail in Chapters 9 and 10.

B. Two-Stage Competitive Binding Assay for the Detection of Soluble Antigen

The two-stage competitive binding assay is carried out as depicted schematically in Figure 2. In this assay, antigen is coated onto microtiter plates as described in the previous section. A sample containing soluble antigen is added to appropriate wells followed by a predetermined, optimal amount of specific antibody of an immunoglobulin class that is able to bind to the enzyme-conjugated, immunoglobulin-binding protein tracer. After a suitable incubation phase and a washing step to remove unbound proteins, any remaining bound antibody is detected in a second step by the addition of an enzyme-labeled, Fc-binding protein conjugate. Unbound tracer is removed by washing and the quantity bound determined by addition of substrate as described earlier. Soluble antigen is detected based on its ability to compete with the immobilized antigen for binding of a fixed, limited quantity of specific antibody. By comparing the absorbance that results when no soluble antigen is added to the decrease in absorbance in the presence of known quantities of soluble antigen, a standard inhibition curve can be generated and this information can be used to quantitate the concentration of antigen in unknown samples.

A variety of modifications of the ELISA have been developed, including antigen-capture techniques in which specific antibody rather than antigen is coated on the plate. These techniques can also be used with enzyme-conjugated, Fc immunoglobulin-binding tracers, provided only the second, or tracer antibody is reactive with the binding protein. All of these assays are based on a similar principle; i.e., that free tracer antibody can be separated from antibody in antigen–antibody complexes and the bound antibody can be quantified.

The remainder of this chapter describes the development of an ELISA to measure human IgA using the type III Fc-binding protein (protein G)–alkaline phosphatase conjugate as the tracer. The general procedure outlined as follows is readily adaptable to any other system for which suitable antigen and antibody preparations are available.

III. Preparation of Immunoglobulin Fc-Binding Protein–Enzyme Conjugate Tracers

Appropriate immunoglobulin Fc-binding protein–enzyme conjugates (tracers) can be prepared as described in the following procedure. In addition, both the type I-binding protein, protein A, and the type III-binding protein, protein G, are commercially available, conjugated to a variety of enzymes suitable for use in ELISA procedures. We have used a

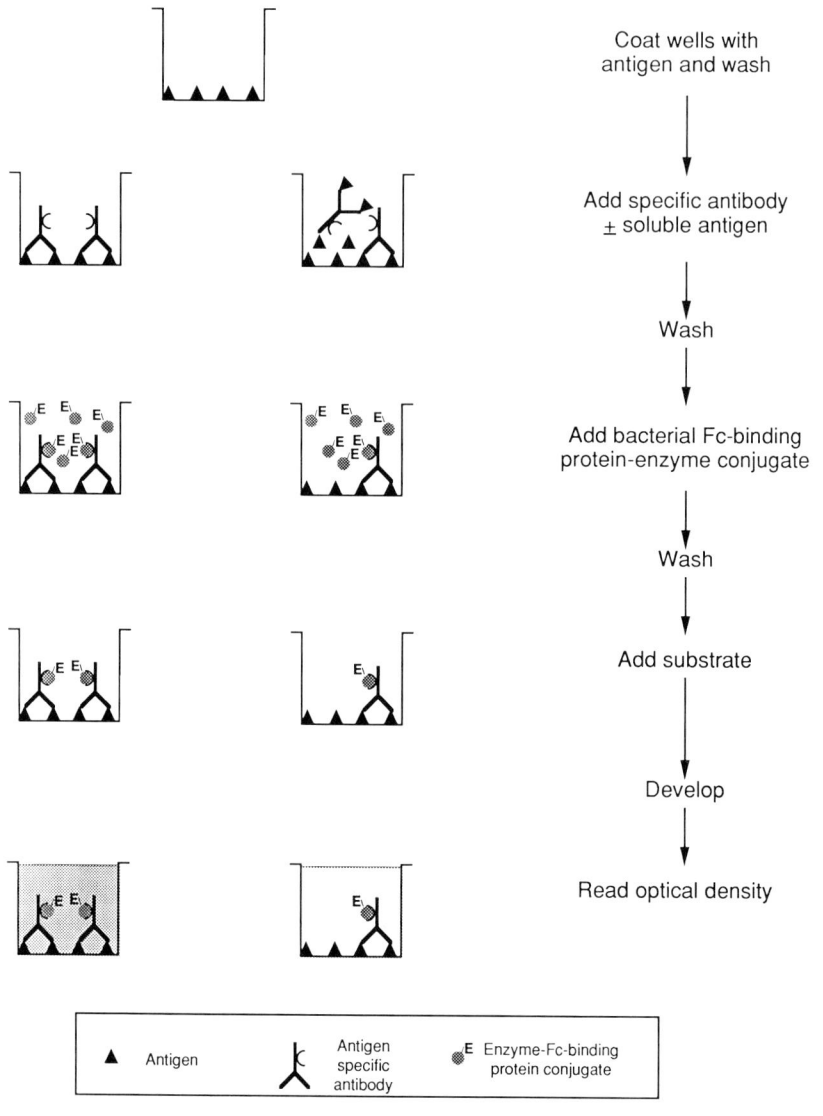

FIGURE 2
Schematic representation of an ELISA for the quantitation of antigen using an enzyme-linked IgG Fc-binding protein tracer as the probe.

number of reported methods to couple these enzymes to appropriate tracer molecules (Reis *et al.*, 1988; Engvall, 1978).

A. Conjugation of the Type III Fc-Binding Protein to Alkaline Phosphatase

1. Materials

Type III Fc-binding protein (purified as described in Reis *et al.*, 1984)

(Note: A variety of forms of purified immunoglobulin Fc-binding proteins are commercially available, see Chapter 1.)

Alkaline phosphatase, type VII-S, 5 mg/ml (Sigma, St. Louis, Missouri)

Glutaraldehyde, 25%, grade II (Sigma, St. Louis, Missouri)

Phosphate-buffered saline (PBS), 0.01 M phosphate, containing 0.15 M NaCl, pH 7.2

Superose 12 molecular sieving column (Pharmacia, Piscataway, New Jersey), or equivalent gel filtration column

2. Procedure

One ml of alkaline phosphatase (2.5 mg/ml) is dialyzed against PBS, pH 7.2, to remove ammonium sulfate (adapted from Reis *et al.*, 1988). The enzyme is then dialyzed against 0.2% glutaraldehyde overnight at ambient temperature, followed by overnight dialysis in PBS to remove excess glutaraldehyde.

The glutaraldehyde-treated alkaline phosphatase is mixed with 0.5 mg of type III

Fc-binding protein (5 mg/ml) in PBS and allowed to stand at ambient temperature overnight.

Fractionate the mixture on a Superose 12 molecular sieving column using the Pharmacia FPLC (Fast Protein Liquid Chromatography) system (Pharmacia, Piscataway, New Jersey) or other suitable molecular sieving chromatography support. Collect 1.0 ml fractions in PBS and test fractions for both alkaline phosphatase activity and for Fc-binding activity. The simplest way to do this is to coat a plate with human or rabbit IgG, 100 ng/ml (200 μl/well) as described later. An aliquot, 5–10 μl from each fraction containing protein (as determined by optical density at 280 nm) is added to individual wells of the microtiter plate. Incubate at ambient temperature for 1–2 hr, wash, add the appropriate substrate, and observe for substrate cleavage and color generation. Those wells displaying a color change will correspond to fractions containing functionally active, enzyme-labeled immunoglobulin-binding protein.

Pool the fractions containing both enzymatic and IgG-binding activities and add glycine to a final concentration of 0.02 M to block remaining active groups, bovine serum albumin (BSA) to a final concentration of 1.0% to serve as a stabilizer, and sodium azide to a final concentration of 0.02% as a preservative. (Note: Do not add sodium azide to peroxidase conjugates as azide inhibits this enzyme. A suitable alternative is 0.01% merthiolate.) Aliquot the enzyme-labeled conjugate and store at $-20°C$ or 4°C. Do not freeze-thaw aliquots as this tends to destroy enzyme activity.

IV. Development of an ELISA to Quantify Human IgA Using a Type III Fc-Binding Protein–Alkaline Phosphatase Conjugate as Tracer

The general procedure for developing any ELISA is similar. We present here a representative example of how an assay for human IgA was developed. This ELISA is a two-stage competitive binding assay that follows the basic outline detailed in Figure 2. As with all immunoassays, a series of preliminary studies are required to determine optimal concentrations of reagents and to establish sensitivity and specificity.

The first step in developing the assay is to immobilize the antigen by coating microtiter plates with varying concentrations of human IgA. These antigen-coated plates are then used in preliminary experiments to establish and optimize conditions of concentration, time, temperature, buffer, etc., for each reagent and each step of the procedure summarized in Figure 2.

A. Materials

96-well flat-bottomed microtiter plates (Nunc-Immunoplate II, USA/Scientific Plastics, Orlando, Florida)

Human serum IgA (Cappel, Malvern, Pennsylvania)

Goat anti-human IgA, α chain-specific (Sigma, St. Louis, Missouri)

Type III Fc-binding protein–alkaline phosphatase conjugate

P-nitrophenyl phosphate substrate tablets, 5 mg each (Sigma)

B. Buffers

Coating Buffer: 0.1 M carbonate-bicarbonate, pH 9.6

Mix 4.53 ml of 1.0 M NaHCO$_3$, 1.82 ml of 1.0 M Na$_2$CO$_3$ and 0.2 ml of 10% NaN$_3$, adjust to 100 ml with deionized H$_2$O. Store at 4°C for up to 2 weeks.

PBS-Tween, containing 0.02% NaN$_3$, pH 7.4:

To 800 ml deionized H$_2$O add: 8.0 g NaCl, 0.2 g KH$_2$PO$_4$, 2.9 g Na$_2$HPO$_4$ · 12H$_2$O, 0.2 g KCl, 0.2 g NaN$_3$, adjust pH to 7.4, and add 0.5 ml Tween 20, adjust to 1000 ml. Store PBS-T at 4°C.

Blocking Buffer: PBS-T, containing 0.1% gelatin

Slowly add 0.1 g of gelatin per 100 ml of PBS-T, warm to dissolve.

Diethanolamine Buffer, 1.0 M diethanolamine-HCl, pH 9.8, containing 0.5 mM MgCl$_2$

To 700 ml deionized H$_2$O, add: 97 ml diethanolamine, 0.2 g NaN$_3$, and 100 mg MgCl$_2$ · 6H$_2$O, adjust pH to 9.8 with 1 M HCl and adjust to 1000 ml. Store at 4°C in the dark.

Substrate for alkaline phosphatase:

1 mg/ml p-nitrophenyl phosphate in diethanolamine buffer. Add 1 tablet (5 mg) (Sigma, St. Louis, Missouri) per 5 ml of diethanolamine buffer at ambient temperature. Prepare immediately prior to use.

The exact formulation for each buffer is included in the Appendix.

In the initial preliminary experiments, optimal antigen-coating conditions and concentrations of specific antibody and tracer are determined by setting up a checkerboard titration. In the example next described, four different IgA coating concentrations, six goat anti-IgA dilutions, and four dilutions of enzyme-conjugated type III Fc IgG-binding protein will be compared.

C. Step 1: Immobilizing Antigen onto Microtiter Plates

Two hundred microliters of dilutions of human IgA in coating buffer at 250, 100, 50, 10, 5, or 0 ng/ml are added to duplicate, vertical columns of 96-well microtiter plates and incubated in a humidified, moist chamber at 4°C overnight. (A styrofoam cooler lined with moist paper towels makes a suitable chamber.) The next day the microtiter plates are washed three times with PBS-T by inverting the plates and shaking out the liquid and blotting onto a paper towel. Two hundred microliters of PBS-T is added to all wells, allowed to stand 1–2 min, the liquid shaken out, and blotted as before. This step removes all unbound antigen from the plate and should be repeated at least twice. Finally, the washed microtiter plates are blocked by adding 200 μl of blocking buffer to each well and incubating for 2 hr at ambient temperature or overnight at 4°C. The blocking buffer can then be removed and the plates stored either dry or in PBS-T at 4°C for up to six weeks. Once coating conditions have been established, it is convenient to prepare a large number of plates at one time and store them until needed.

D. Step 2: Establishing Optimal Concentration of Each Reagent

Antigen-coated plates, prepared with different concentrations of antigen as described in the preceding section, are used in preliminary experiments to determine optimal dilutions of the antibody and enzyme-tracer conjugate. Initially, 100 μl of twofold dilutions of goat anti-human IgA in PBS-T are added to horizontal rows of each plate and incubated for 1–2 hr at ambient temperature. Unbound antibody is removed by washing three times with PBS-T as described earlier. The quantity of antibody associated with the antigen is determined by adding a dilution of the type III Fc-binding protein–alkaline phosphatase or other appropriate enzyme–tracer conjugate. The initial dilution of a high titer, specific antibody should be at least 1:1000.

Two hundred microliters of a dilution of enzyme-conjugated, Fc-binding protein tracer is then added to each well of the microtiter plates that have previously been incubated with specific antibody and washed. The plates are incubated with the tracer for 1 hr at 37°C. This provides a sufficient time for the immunoglobulin-binding protein tracer to interact with the Fc region of any antibody–antigen complex associated with the immobilized antigen on the microtiter plate. The unbound enzyme tracer is removed by washing three times with PBS-T and the quantity of enzyme associated with the microtiter plate is quantified by addition of a suitable, freshly prepared substrate and monitoring product generation with time. Substrate cleavage can be measured by changes of absorbance at an appropriate wavelength using a multichannel spectrophotometer. Incubation at higher temperatures will result in more rapid substrate cleavage and conditions for the final enzyme reaction can be adjusted for the convenience of the individual performing the assay.

The results of a representative checkerboard titration are presented in Figure 3. In the preliminary studies, the microtiter plates have different

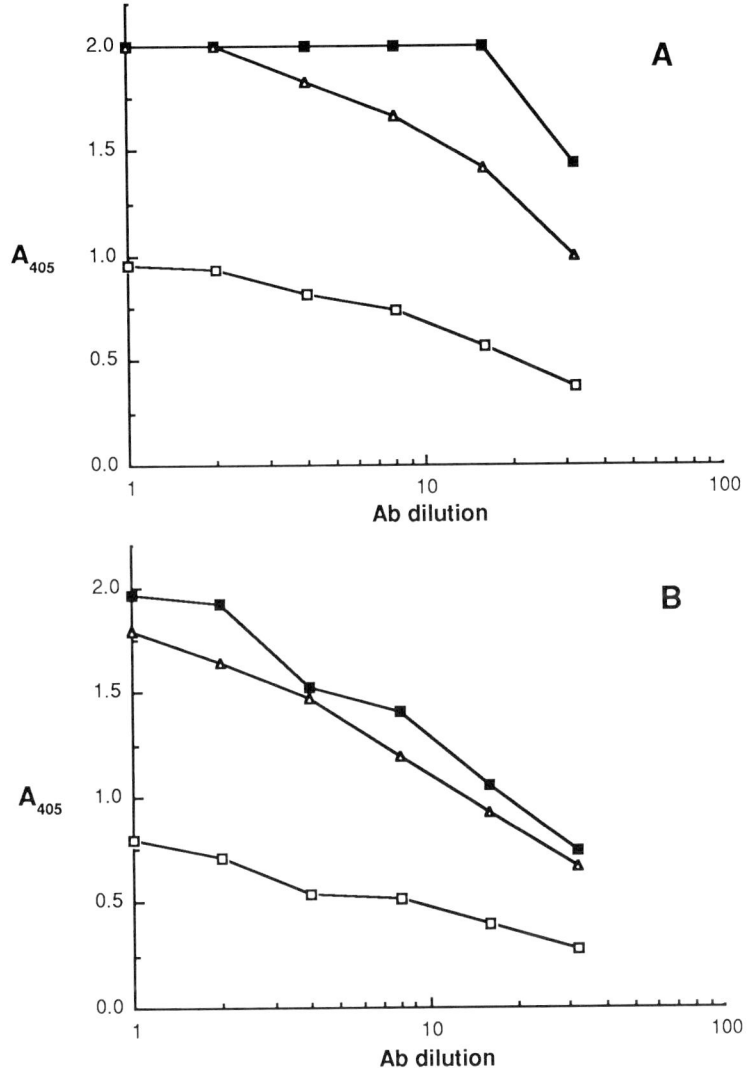

FIGURE 3
Results of a checkerboard titration used to develop an ELISA for human IgA. Panel (A) Coating conditions: 100 ng IgA/ml. Panel (B) Coating conditions: 50 ng IgA/ml. Relative concentration of 1 = 1:1000 dilution of goat anti-human IgA. In each assay, three different dilutions of the enzyme-conjugated Fc-binding protein tracer (protein G–alkaline phosphatase) were included. (■, 1:300 dilution of tracer; △, 1:900 dilution of tracer; □, 1:2700 dilution of tracer.) The A_{405} was determined following a 60 min incubation at 37°C. For precise experimental details, see text.

antigen concentrations in the vertical rows and different antibody dilutions in the horizontal rows. Consequently, for each dilution of tracer used in the checkerboard titration, a complete 96-well plate would be required. It is frequently more efficient to narrow the range of antigen-coating conditions and dilutions of specific antibody required by carrying out the first studies using excess enzyme-conjugated tracer. Once the conditions for two of the reactants have been narrowed, titration of the enzyme-conjugated tracer can be initiated. If the specific activity of the tracer is unknown, we usually start with 1:100 dilution and use a three-fold dilution series.

The checkerboard titrations can be repeated at a variety of dilutions until suitable conditions have been achieved. These preliminary studies are important to establish appropriate assay conditions for any antigen–antibody pair and should be repeated any time a new preparation of antigen, antibody, or enzyme-conjugated tracer is introduced into a previously standardized assay.

E. Optimization of Reaction Conditions for Detection of Human IgA

For the competitive binding assay we have developed for human IgA, we have selected an antigen coating concentration, a specific antibody dilution, and a dilution of the tracer conjugate that has resulted in an absorbance at 450 nm (A_{405}) reading of approximately 1.0–1.2 following a 1 hr incubation with the substrate at ambient temperature. As shown in Figure 3, this can be achieved using a number of combinations of reagents. Absorbance values using a 1:100 dilution of conjugate were too high and are not shown. Based on the initial preliminary experiments, we chose to use an IgA-coating concentration of 100 ng/ml, an antibody dilution in the range of 1:2000–4000, a conjugate dilution of 1:1000, and a substrate incubation phase of 30–45 min at ambient temperature.

The competitive binding assay is carried out in 96-well plates in which all but one row of wells are coated with the selected concentration of antigen (human IgA). One row of wells is not coated with antigen but is blocked as described earlier. These wells are used to control for nonspecific binding of antibody or tracer to the wells of the microtiter plate and to determine any spontaneous cleavage of the substrate. The assay is performed by adding 100 μl of sequential dilutions of human IgA to duplicate test wells and mixing with an equal volume of an appropriate dilution of the specific antibody. The selected antibody dilution is also added to duplicate antigen-coated wells in the absence of competition to establish maximal specific binding and to wells lacking antigen to establish background nonspecific binding. The plates are incubated for 1 hr at ambient temperature, washed three times with PBS-T, and then an appropriate dilution of enzyme-conjugated tracer is added to all wells, incubated for 1 hr at ambient temperature, and washed twice with PBS-T to remove unbound tracer. At this time, freshly prepared substrate is added to each well to determine the quantity of tracer bound and hence the number of antigen–antibody complexes bound to the plate. Product generation is monitored by reading the absorbance at 405 nm in each well using a multichannel spectrophotometer. Absorbance readings can be performed at various times and the reaction stopped when the absorbance reaches 1.0–1.5 units in any well.

The maximum binding of tracer should occur in wells containing antigen incubated with specific antibody in the absence of any fluid-phase competitor (maximum binding). The minimum binding of tracer and hence minimum substrate cleavage should occur in non-antigen-coated wells incubated with substrate alone. If this value is greater than 0.1 absorbance units, it would indicate spontaneous hydrolysis of the substrate. If this occurs, the assay should be repeated with freshly prepared diethanolamine buffer and care should be taken to ensure that the substrate solution is prepared immediately prior to its addition to the microtiter plates. Similarly, if high levels of substrate hydrolysis are observed in control wells containing antigen plus tracer but not in the wells with substrate alone, this would indicate binding of tracer either due to incomplete blocking of the plates or direct interaction of the tracer with a component present in the antigen preparation. This latter problem can occur when the antigen being studied might have been isolated with contaminating IgG, e.g., certain serum IgA preparations contain trace quantities of IgG as a contaminant. This problem can be alleviated by preabsorption of the antigen-coating solution with a suitable source of the immobilized Fc-binding protein. A second possible source of nonspecific antibody binding of tracer can occur when the antigen-coated plates have been blocked with a protein solution containing low levels of IgG. In this regard, we do not recommend bovine serum albumin (BSA) as a blocking reagent since many commercial sources of BSA contain bovine IgG, which can be readily detected with protein G tracers. We recommend the use of gelatin or ovalbumin as a nonspecific protein blocking agent for use in this system. Occasionally, antigen preparations, particularly those derived from bacteria, have been found to contain an enzyme activity that can cleave the substrate directly. These problems can be minimized by selecting a suitable enzyme for conjugation with the Fc-binding protein tracer.

Provided all of the control wells display low levels of substrate hydrolysis, the percentage of inhibition of binding of specific antibody can be calculated as follows:

$$\% \text{ inhibition} = [1 - (\text{test abs} - \text{bkg abs}/\text{max abs} - \text{bkg abs})] \times 100$$

where:

test abs = the A_{405} observed when the test sample is added to the standard assay.

max abs = the A_{405} observed when no inhibitor is added to the standard assay.

bkg abs = the A_{405} obtained in the absence of specific antibody.

In the assay developed here for human IgA, a standard inhibition curve has been generated using three different dilutions of the specific goat anti-human α chain-specific antibody. The results of a typical assay are shown in Figure 4. Fifty percent inhibition of binding of specific antibody

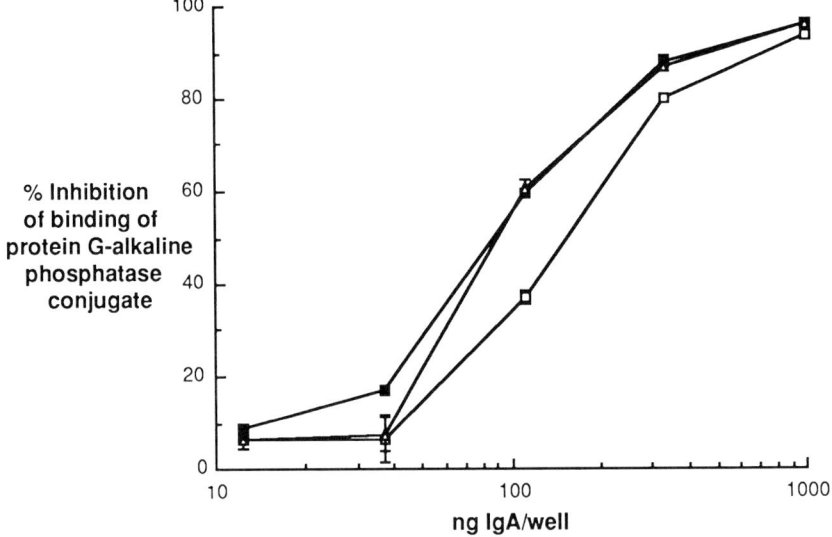

FIGURE 4
Standard inhibition curves generated in an ELISA for fluid-phase human IgA. In this assay, plates were coated with 100 ng/ml IgA, the specific antibody was used at a dilution of 1:2000 (-□-), 1:3000 (-■-), or 1:4000 (-△-). The protein G–alkaline phosphatase conjugate was used at a dilution of 1:1000. The assay was carried out in two stages using a similar procedure to that summarized in Figure 2. For precise experimental details on determining the optimal conditions for each reactant, see text.

was achieved on addition of approximately 70–80 ng of the corresponding antigen (human IgA) when either the 1:2000 or 1:3000 dilution of goat anti-human IgA antibody was used (Figure 4).

This assay, using an anti-IgA antibody dilution of 1:3000 was applied to quantifying IgA in human serum samples and the resulting values fell within the normal range. The assay was also capable of detecting secretory IgA and was shown to be specific for IgA as demonstrated by seeding known quantities of IgA into IgA-deficient cord serum samples. The observed and expected levels were found to be the same within experimental error. These findings indicate that there was no significant inhibition under these assay conditions by IgG or any other non-IgA serum component.

The steps required to develop any ELISA would follow the same sequence of preliminary studies as detailed here for the development of a specific assay for human IgA. In any immunoassay it is important to establish specificity. This sensitivity will depend on the selectivity, titer, and average affinity of the antibody used. It is also necessary to include controls for nonspecific binding of the specific tracer antibody and for nonspecific binding of the enzyme-conjugated tracer. In addition, appropriate control wells must be included to ensure that nonspecific hydrolysis of the substrate is not occurring.

V. Summary

The availability of a variety of enzyme-conjugated tracer forms of Fc-binding proteins allows these versatile tracers to be used for many immunoassays to detect either specific antibodies or antigens. The use of enzyme-labeled tracer has a number of practical advantages over the use of radiolabeled tracers. The inherent amplification associated with enzyme–substrate reactions provides the potential for increased sensitivity of detection of antigen–antibody complexes. Furthermore, the enzyme tracers have a long shelf-life, thereby eliminating the need for frequent tracer labeling and the many complications involved in the use and disposal of radioactive material can be avoided. In this chapter, we have provided an example of the use of enzyme-labeled immunoglobulin Fc-binding proteins for detection of human IgA. The application of enzyme-labeled tracers for the detection of immune complexes immobilized to nitrocellulose is discussed in Chapter 14 and the application of enzyme-labeled tracers to detect cell-surface antigens is described in Chapter 9.

References

Åkerström, B., Brodin, T., Reis, K. J., and Björck, L. (1985). *J. Immunol.* **135,** 2589–2592.
Boyle, M. D. P. (1984). *Biotechniques* **2,** 334–340.
Boyle, M. D. P., and Langone, J. J. (1979). *J. Natl. Cancer Inst.* **62,** 1537–1544.
Boyle, M. D. P., Wallner, W. A., von Mering, G. O., Reis, K. J., and Lawman, M. J. P. (1985). *Mol. Immunol.* **22,** 1115–1121.
Chang, H. C., Takashima, I., Arikawa, J., and Hashimoto, N. (1984). *J. Virol. Methods* **9,** 143–151.
Engvall, E. (1978). *Scand. J. Immunol.* **8,** 25–31.
Engvall, E. (1980). *In* "Methods in Enzymology" (H. van Vunakis and J. J. Langone, eds.), Vol. 70, pp. 419–439. Academic Press, New York.
Engvall, E., and Perlmann, P. (1971). *Immunochemistry* **8,** 871–874.
Engvall, E., and Perlmann, P. (1972). *J. Immunol.* **109,** 129–135.
Forsgren, A., Ghetie, V., Lindmark, R., and Sjöquist, J. (1983). *In* "Staphylococci and Staphylococcal Infections" (C. S. F. Easmon and C. Adlam, eds.), Vol. 2, pp. 420–480. Academic Press, London.
Gee, A. P., and Langone, J. J. (1981). *Anal. Biochem.* **116,** 524–530.
Gee, A. P., and Langone, J. J. (1983). *In* "Methods in Enzymology" (J. J. Langone and H. van Vunakis, eds.), Vol. 92, pp. 403–413. Academic Press, New York.
Harlow, E. and Lane, D. (1988). "Antibodies: A Laboratory Manual, pp. 553–612. Cold Spring Harbor Laboratory, Cold Spring Harbor, New York.
Langone, J. J. (1978). *J. Immunol. Methods* **24,** 269–285.
Langone, J. J. (1980a). *J. Immunol. Methods* **34,** 93–106.
Langone, J. J. (1980b). *Biochem. Biophys. Res. Commun.* **94,** 473–479.
Langone, J. J. (1982). *Adv. Immunol.* **32,** 157–252.
Langone, J. J., Boyle, M. D. P., and Borsos, T. (1977). *J. Immunol. Methods* **18,** 281–293.
Nakamura, R. M., Voller, A., and Bidwell, D. E. (1986). *In* Handbook of Experimental Immunology, Vol. 1 Immunochemistry" (D. N. Weir, ed.), pp. 27.1–27.20. Blackwell, Oxford.
Nilson, B., Björck, L., and Åkerström, B. (1988). *J. Immunoassay* **9,** 207–225.
Potgieter, L. N. D., Rouse, B. T., and Webb-Martin, T. A. (1980). *Am. J. Vet. Res.* **41,** 978–980.
Reis, K. J., Ayoub, E. M., and Boyle, M. D. P. (1984). *J. Immunol.* **132,** 3091–3097.
Reis, K. J., von Mering, G. O., Karis, M. A., Faulmann, E. L., Lottenberg, R., and Boyle, M. D. P. (1988). *J. Immunol. Methods* **107,** 273–280.
Thoen, C. O., Mills, K., and Hopkins, M. (1980). *Am. J. Vet. Res.* **41,** 833–835.
Wallner, W., Lawman, M. J. P., and Boyle, M. D. P. (1987). *Appl. Microbiol. Biotechnol.* **27,** 168–173.
Yolken, R. H., and Leister, F. J. (1981). *J. Immunol. Methods* **43,** 209–218.

CHAPTER 9

Use of Fc-binding proteins to identify cell surface and secreted antigens associated with group B streptococci

L. Jeannine Brady
Corey Musselman
Colleen Chun
Elia M. Ayoub
Michael D. P. Boyle

I. Introduction

Binding proteins that interact specifically with the Fc region of immunoglobulin molecules have been isolated from a variety of staphylococcal and streptococcal species (Forsgren and Sjöquist, 1966; Kronvall, 1973; Myhre and Kronvall, 1981; Langone, 1982a; Reis et al., 1983). These bacterial proteins bind specifically and with high affinity to the Fc regions of various immunoglobulin species, primarily of the IgG class (Boyle and Reis, 1987). Based on the reactivity of different species, classes, and subclasses of immunoglobulins with intact bacteria, Myhre and Kronvall proposed a functional classification of bacterial "Fc receptors" that included five patterns of reactivity (Myhre and Kronvall, 1981). The type I and type III bacterial Fc-binding proteins, commonly designated as protein A and protein G, are commercially available. These molecules have proven to be very useful as immunochemical reagents. The range of reactivities of bacterial Fc-binding proteins is expanding as additional interactions of bacterial products with immunoglobulins, [e.g., human IgA Fc-binding proteins expressed by certain group A (Christensen and Oxelius, 1975; Kronvall *et al.,* 1979; Myhre and Kronvall, 1979; Schalén, 1980; Schalén, *et al.,* 1980; Magliano and Ponzi, 1983; Lindahl and Åkerström, 1989; Lindahl, 1989)] and group B streptococci (Russell-Jones *et al.,* 1984) are identified.

The ability of bacterial Fc-binding proteins to react with IgG molecules from a number of species has been exploited by using the purified proteins for immunochemical applications, primarily for the purification and quantitation of reactive species and subclasses of IgG (Ey *et al.,* 1978; Goding, 1978; Langone, 1982b; Boyle, 1984; Boyle and Reis, 1987). One of the most valuable properties of staphylococcal and streptococcal IgG Fc-binding proteins is that they can be labeled to high specific activity with a variety of tracer molecules, for example, radioisotopes (Gee and Langone, 1981), enzymes (Duboid-Dalcq *et al.,* 1977; Gee and Langone, 1981; Reis *et al.,* 1988), biotin (Chang *et al.,* 1984), fluorescent tags (Sisson, Chapter 11, this volume), or colloidal gold (Lucocq and Baschong, 1986) with little, if any, loss in Fc-binding activity. The labeled molecules can then be used to detect and quantify antigens, antibodies, or antigen–antibody complexes (Langone *et al.,* 1979; Gee and Langone, 1981; Boyle, 1984; Boyle and Reis, 1987).

The use of radiolabeled and enzyme-labeled protein A and protein G to detect group B streptococcal cell surface antigens is detailed in this chapter. This is a specific example of a general procedure that could be used to detect any cell surface or immobilized antigen for which a monospecific antiserum or monoclonal antibody is available. However, caution must be exercised when applying this technique to the study of bacteria and other cells to ensure that the test samples themselves do not express immunoglobulin-binding proteins, which could react with the antibodies in a non-immune fashion. For this reason, normal serum or an irrelevant antibody should be included as a negative control in assays of this type.

II. Group B Streptococcal Typing Nomenclature

In order to enable the reader to appreciate the usefulness and practicality of the general assay procedure, some explanation of the classification of group B streptococci is warranted.

The nomenclature of type-specific antigens present on group B streptococci (GBS) has been revised through the years and the current terminology was reviewed by Henricksen *et al.,* in 1984. The current classification of GBS is based on the serological detection of antigens in hot-acid extracts of these bacteria (Wilkinson, 1978). In addition to the group-specific carbohydrate, the presence of one of four type-specific carbohydrate antigens designated Ia, Ib, II, and III is determined to assign the GBS serotype. Two additional carbohydrate antigens designated as type IV and provisional type V have also been reported (Jelínková and Matlová, 1985). Strains expressing only the group B-specific carbohydrate and no identifiable type-specific carbohydrates have been identified and are designated as "no type" (Johnson and Ferrieri, 1984). In addition to the carbohydrate antigens detected in hot-acid extracts, a protein marker called the c protein (formerly referred to as Ic or Ibc) has also been identified (Wilkinson and Moody, 1969; and Wilkinson and Eagon, 1971). The c protein has been reported to be expressed almost always on strains bearing the Ib carbohydrate antigen, frequently on strains bearing the Ia or II carbohydrate antigens, and rarely on strains expressing the type III carbohydrate antigen (Johnson and Ferrieri, 1984). The c protein has been reported to consist of at least two acid-extractable antigens, α (trypsin-resistant) and β (trypsin-sensitive) (Bevanger and Iverson, 1981, 1983; Bevanger, 1983, 1985; Johnson and Ferrieri, 1984; Ferrieri et al., 1985). These antigens are expressed independently of each other (Johnson and Ferrieri, 1984) and studies by Bevanger (1985) indicate that they exist on the bacterial surface as nonlinked molecules. Studies in our laboratory indicate that in addition to the α and β antigens, two other antigens designated as γ and δ, are expressed on the surfaces of certain GBS. These antigens are recognized by rabbit, polyclonal, anti-c protein-typing antiserum from the Centers for Disease Control (CDC) (Atlanta, Georgia) (Brady et al., 1988).

III. Two-Stage Radioimmunoassay for Detection of Group B Streptococcal Type-Specific Antigens

A two-stage radioimmunoassay (RIA) was developed to type GBS (Brady et al., 1988). Briefly, bacteria are reacted with appropriate dilutions of a battery of rabbit type-specific antisera. The bacteria are washed free of unbound antibodies and bacterial-bound antibodies are detected using either enzyme or radiolabeled protein A or protein G. Classical typing by the method of Lancefield (1928) involves reacting bacterial hot-acid extracts with type-specific antisera in capillary tubes or agarose gel (Jensen, 1979), followed by visual inspection for a zone of precipitation. The semiquantitative RIA requires less typing reagents than does classical precipitin testing of hot-acid extracts and is more objective, reproducible, and rapid. Results are obtained within three hours. The assay utilizes intact bacteria and does not require hot-acid extraction. Consequently, antigens are measured in a native, unmodified form on the cell surface. The classical precipitin test is dependent on optimal concentrations of both antigens and antibodies for precipitation to occur; it is difficult to score and there is the potential for false-negative results. This problem is not encountered with the more sensitive RIA procedure.

The two-stage radioimmunoassay procedure is as follows.

A. Bacterial Strains, Media, and Growth Conditions

All strains to be tested are confirmed as GBS by screening with the Phadebact® *Streptococcus* Test (Pharmacia Diagnostics, Piscataway, New Jersey). Bacteria are grown to stationary phase in Todd-Hewitt broth (BBL Microbiology Systems, Cockeysville, Maryland) for 18–24 hr at 37°C, under aerobic conditions. The bacteria are harvested by centrifugation, washed, and resuspended in 0.15 M phosphate-buffered saline (PBS), pH 7.4. Light-scatter, detected at 550 nm, is used to standardize the concentration of organisms used in subsequent tests.

B. Source of Group B Streptococcal-Typing Antisera

Rabbit anti-types Ia, Ib, II, and III carbohydrate antigens, as well as rabbit anti-c protein-typing antisera may be obtained from the Centers for Disease Control (CDC) (Atlanta, Georgia). Anti-c protein-typing antiserum is rendered monospecific for reactivity against single antigens, or depleted of reactivity against single antigens, by selective adsorption with appropriate group B streptococcal strains or combinations of strains as described by Brady *et al.* (1988). Briefly, the bacteria from 5 ml of a Todd-Hewitt overnight culture are pelleted by centifugation and washed once with 2 ml of PBS, pH 7.4. A 100 μl aliquot of anti-c protein antiserum is added to the washed bacterial pellet and rotated at 4°C for 1 hr. The bacteria are removed from the adsorbed antiserum by centrifugation at 10,000 × g for 15 min. The adsorption is repeated at least twice until all reactivity against the adsorbing strain is eliminated as detected by the two-stage RIA described later in this chapter.

C. Iodination of Protein A and Protein G

Protein A (Pharmacia Fine Chemicals, Piscataway, New Jersey) and protein G (Calbiochem, La Jolla, California) are radioiodinated by a modification of the mild lactoperoxidase method of Marchalonis *et al.* (1971) using Enzymobeads® (Bio-Rad, Richmond, California) (Reis *et al.*, 1983). The labeled protein is separated from free iodine by passage over a G25 column (PD 10, Pharmacia) and collected in 0.15 M veronal-buffered saline, pH 7.4, containing 1.0 mM Mg^{2+}, 0.15 mM Ca^{2+}, and 0.1% gelatin

(VBS-gel). Proteins labeled by this method routinely have a specific activity of approximately 0.3 mCi/mg (Reis *et al.*, 1983).

D. Two-Stage Radioimmunoassay for Determination of Subtypes of Group B Streptococcal Strains

Laboratory strains are inoculated into 10 ml Todd-Hewitt broth starter culture tubes and grown to late log phase at 37°C (18–24 hr). The bacteria are pelleted by centrifugation for 8 min at $1000 \times g$, and the bacterial pellets resuspended in approximately 2 ml PBS, pH 7.4, to a concentration of 1×10^{10} organisms per ml. Tubes containing 100 µl of bacterial suspension (approximately 1×10^9 bacteria) are incubated for 1 hr at 37°C with 100 µl of a 1:400 dilution (optimal concentration was predetermined by titration using serial two-fold dilutions in PBS) of each type-specific antiserum: anti-Ia, anti-Ib, anti-II, or anti-c protein antiserum before and after selective adsorption. Normal rabbit antiserum (also diluted 1:400 in PBS) is included in each assay as a control to insure against nonimmune binding of rabbit IgG molecules. Following incubation, the tubes are washed to remove unbound antibodies by addition of 2 ml PBS, followed by centrifugation for 8 min at $1000 \times g$. After the 2 ml of PBS wash buffer is decanted, the bacterial pellets are resuspended in the residual buffer (approximately 100 µl) by vortexing. Bacterial-bound antibody is quantitated by addition of 100 µl of ^{125}I-radiolabeled protein A or protein G containing approximately 30,000 cpm. The tubes are incubated for 1 hr at 37°C and the bacterial pellets washed twice with 2 ml of metal-free VBS containing 0.01 M ethylenediaminetetraacetic acid (EDTA) with 0.1% gelatin (EDTA-gel) to remove any labeled tracer not associated with a bacterial antigen–antibody complex. The amount of labeled tracer associated with the bacterial pellet is quantified using a gamma counter. The bacterial-associated radioactivity is determined in control tubes containing bacteria and radiolabeled protein A or protein G only. The exact formulation for each of the buffers used is presented in the Appendix.

E. Results of the Two-Stage Radioimmunoassay

Fifty-three group B streptococcal isolates were tested by the procedure just described for their reactivity with rabbit anti-types Ia, Ib, II, and III carbohydrate antigens and these data are illustrated in Figure 1. The height of each line depicts the amount of ^{125}I-labeled protein A associated with each isolate minus the background radioactivity, thus giving a measure of the quantity of each specific antiserum associated with each bacterial pellet. The lines represent the mean values of counts per minute (cpm)

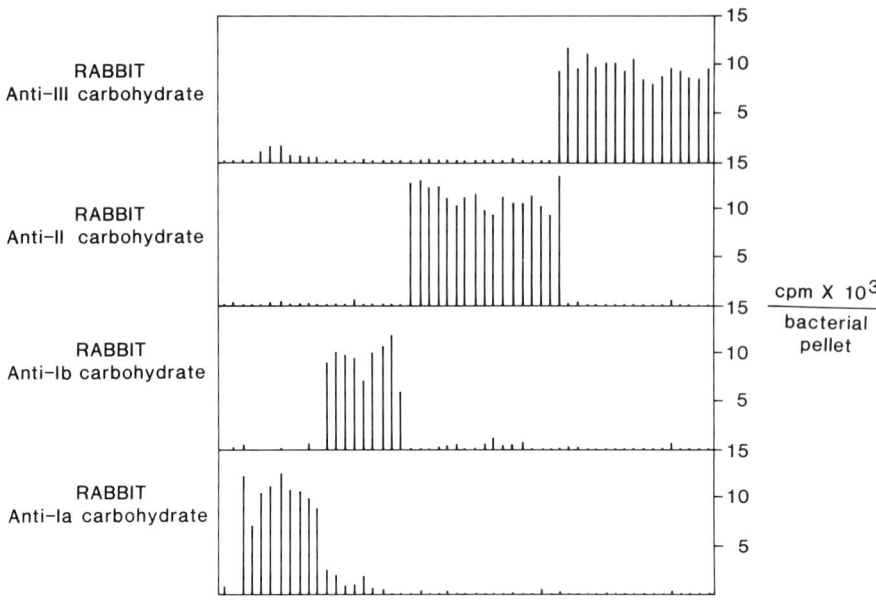

FIGURE 1
Analysis of type-specific carbohydrate antigens on the surfaces of group B streptococci using a two-stage radioimmunoassay. The two-stage radioimmunoassay procedure is detailed in the text. The height of each line depicts the amount of ^{125}I-labeled protein A associated with each strain minus the background radioactivity, thus giving a measure of the quantity of each specific antiserum associated with the bacterial pellet. Each line represents the mean value of cpm measured for duplicate tubes. There was less than 5% variation between duplicate tubes. The 53 GBS isolates tested are shown in the same order as listed in Table 1. (Reproduced from Brady, et al., (1988), with permission from Univ. of Chicago Press.)

measured for duplicate tubes. There was less than 5% variation between duplicate tubes. No bacteria expressing IgG Fc-binding proteins were identified based on a lack of reactivity with normal rabbit serum. To date, no group B streptococcus has been found to express an IgG Fc-binding protein (Russell-Jones et al., 1984; Boyle and Reis, 1987; Brady and Boyle, 1989; Lindahl, 1989). In these studies, we have found no evidence for the existence of the group B-associated "unspecific" antibody-binding factor that has recently been suggested (Jürgens et al., 1987). The fifty-three isolates were also typed by conventional precipitin testing of hot-acid extracts against type-specific antisera by double diffusion in agarose gel. There was an absolute correlation between typing results detected by precipitin testing and RIA (Table 1); however, the results presented in

Figure 1 demonstrate that variation in the quantities of type-specific carbohydrate antigens expressed on various strains was detected by the two-stage RIA. In contrast to the semiquantitative results obtained by RIA, precipitin testing of hot-acid extracts indicated only the presence or absence of a given carbohydrate.

When the RIA was compared with precipitin testing for detection of reactivity of the 53 GBS isolates with rabbit anti-c protein-typing antiserum, the results were not as straightforward as had been observed for detection of type-specific carbohydrate antigens. Reactivity with anti-c protein antiserum was detected with 36/53 isolates when assayed by two-stage RIA and with only 20/53 isolates when assayed by precipitin testing. In order to analyze the reasons for these differences, the two-stage RIA was repeated with a series of anti-c protein antisera, which had been selectively adsorbed with bacteria (or combinations of bacteria) showing different RIA reactivity profiles (Figure 2). Using this approach, a variety of distinct binding patterns were observed, which could be accounted for by a minimum of four distinct antigens. Analysis of hot-acid extracts by immunoelectrophoresis indicated that two of the four reactivities corresponded to the α and β antigens. The two previously unreported antigens were designated as γ and δ (Brady *et al.*, 1988).

The results presented in Figure 2, panel e show the reactivities of the 36 positive strains with unadsorbed rabbit anti-c protein-typing antiserum, while Figure 2, panel d demonstrates the lack of reactivity of those strains when the antiserum was exhaustively adsorbed with the CDC's immunizing strain, A909, which expresses α, β, γ, and δ antigens. Figure 2 (panels a, b, and c) shows the reactivities of the 36 isolates when the antiserum was adsorbed with GBS strains expressing only the δ, β, or α antigen. Hence, a lack of reactivity with an antiserum depleted of reactivity against a single antigen identifies those bacteria that express only a single c protein-typing antiserum-reactive antigen. The reactivities of the 36 isolates with antiserum that had been rendered monospecific for reactivity against δ, γ, and β antigens is shown in Figure 3 (panels b, c, and d). Monospecific antiserum against the α antigen could not be generated since no GBS strains were identified that expressed the γ antigen in the absence of the α antigen. Strains expressing α alone were identified by comparison of assay results using γ-specific (Figure 3, panel c) as opposed to α- plus γ-specific (Figure 3, panel e) antisera. All 36 isolates retained reactivity with anti-c protein-typing antiserum that had been adsorbed with the group A strain R-28 (Figure 3, panel a), demonstrating that none of the four reactivities were due to the previously described R protein antigen (Wilkinson, 1972; Flores and Ferrieri, 1985).

Since the precipitin test is a qualitative one and is dependent on optimal concentrations of antigens and type-specific antibodies, low levels

TABLE 1
Summary[a] of Precipitin Assay and Two-Stage RIA Typing Results[b]

	Reactivities	
GBS[c] strain	Ppt assay[d]	RIA[e]
N86K	No type	No type
NP1AR	No type	No type
HG824	Ia[d]	Ia
SS617	Ia	Ia
HG346	Ia,c	Ia,c(α)
PF534AR	Ia,c	Ia,c(α)
J46	Ia,c	Ia,c(α)
HG783	Ia	Ia,c(α)
HG784	Ia	Ia,c(α)
HG381	Ia,c	Ia,c($\alpha,\beta,\gamma,\delta$)
A909	Ia,c	Ia,c($\alpha,\beta,\gamma,\delta$)
HG812	Ib,c	Ib,c(α,γ)
HG806	Ib,c	Ib,c(α,γ)
2AR	Ib,c	Ib,c(α,γ)
TC795	Ib,c	Ib,c(β)
PF549AR-B	Ib,c	Ib,c(α,β,γ)
HG805	Ib,c	Ib,c(α,β,γ)
HG769	Ib,c	Ib,c(α,β,γ)
TC137	Ib,c	Ib,c(α,β,γ)
SS618	Ib,c	Ib,c(α,β,δ)
HG811	II	II
PF58AV	II	II
PF536AR	II	II
PF549AR-NB	II	II
PF541AR	II	II
J44	II,c	II,c(α)
PF65BV	II,c	II,c(α)
PF25AR	II,c	II,c(α)
PF610AR	II,c	II,c(α)
NPF1AV	II,c	II,c(α)
HG818	II	II,c(α,γ)
HG819	II	II,c(α,γ)
9B200	II,c	II,c(α,γ)
HG768	II	II,c(α,γ)
HG804	II	II,c(α,γ)
HG774	II	II,c(α,γ)
HG782	II	II,III,c(α,γ)
HG820	III	III
VC75	III	III
HG780	III	III
HG757	III	III
HG814	III	III

(*continued*)

TABLE 1 *(Continued)*

GBS[c] strain	Reactivities	
	Ppt assay[d]	RIA[e]
HG754	III	III
HG802	III	III
HG738	III	III
J48	III	III,c(δ)
J52	III	III,c(δ)
PEH	III	III,c(δ)
J51	III	III,c(δ)
HG786	III	III,c(δ)
HG828	III	III,c(δ)
HG770	III	III,c(δ)
HG771	III	III,c(δ)

[a] Reproduced from Brady *et al.* (1988), with permission from Univ. of Chicago Press.
[b] Results of either the precipitin assay or the radioimmunoassay indicate the cell-associated, type-specific antigens defected for each strain.
[c] GBS=Group B streptococcus
[d] Ppt=precipitin.
[e] RIA=radioimmunoassay

of one or more antigenic components may lead to false negative results. This is most likely to be the case with respect to detection of the γ antigen since a third precipitin line, in addition to those observed for the previously described α and β antigens, could be detected by immunoelectrophoresis when hot-acid extracts of GBS isolates were concentrated ten-fold or greater. Low levels of most surface antigens would be detectable using the more sensitive, semiquantitative RIA. The RIA has the added advantage of detecting unmodified, native antigens on the cell surface. The hot-acid extraction required for precipitin testing has the potential of modifying antigenic structures such that in many cases, only core antigens will be identified. In addition, some antigens may not be acid extractable or may be acid labile; therefore, they would only be detectable by a method that evaluates the reactivity of antibodies with intact bacteria. This may explain why the δ antigen was not detected by immunoelectrophoresis, even when hot-acid extracts were concentrated by as much as 50-fold. In addition, unlike hot-acid extracts of strains that expressed the δ antigen, solubilized antigens present in hot-acid extracts of α, β, and γ bearing strains could be detected by their ability to inhibit binding of the corresponding antibodies to cell-associated antigens when included as competi-

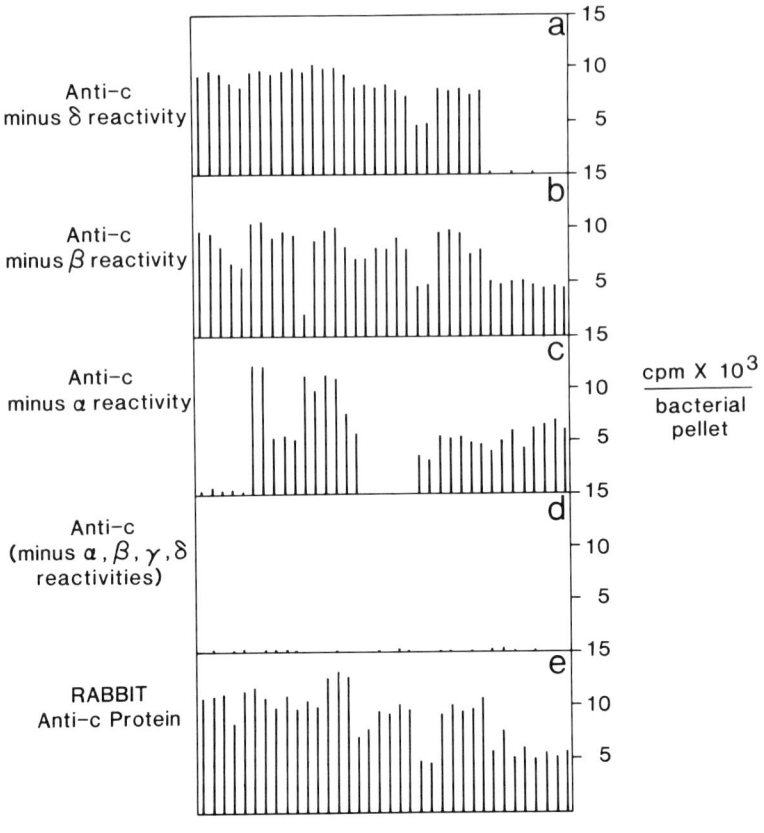

FIGURE 2
Analysis of c protein antigens on the surfaces of group B streptococci by two-stage radioimmunoassays. The antiserum used in the assays is either the unadsorbed anti-c antiserum or the same antiserum that had been adsorbed with bacteria demonstrating unique reactivities (for details of the preparation of specific antisera, see Brady et al., 1988). The height of each line depicts the amount of ^{125}I-labeled protein A associated with each strain minus the background radioactivity, thus giving a measure of the quantity of each specific antiserum associated with the bacterial pellet. Each line represents the mean value of cpm measured for duplicate tubes. There was less than 5% variation between duplicate tubes. The strain designations for the 36 GBS isolates are as follows: HG346, PF534AR, J46, HG783, HG784, HG381, A909, HG812, HG806, 2AR, TC795, PF549AR-B, HG805, HG769, TC137, SS618, J44, PF65BV, PF25AR, PF610AR, NPF1AV, HG818, HG819, 9B200, HG768, HG804, HG774, HG782, J48, J52, PEH, J51, HG786, HG828, HG770, HG771. For details of other characteristics of these strains, see Table 1. (Reproduced from Brady et al., (1988), with permission, from Univ of Chicago Press.)

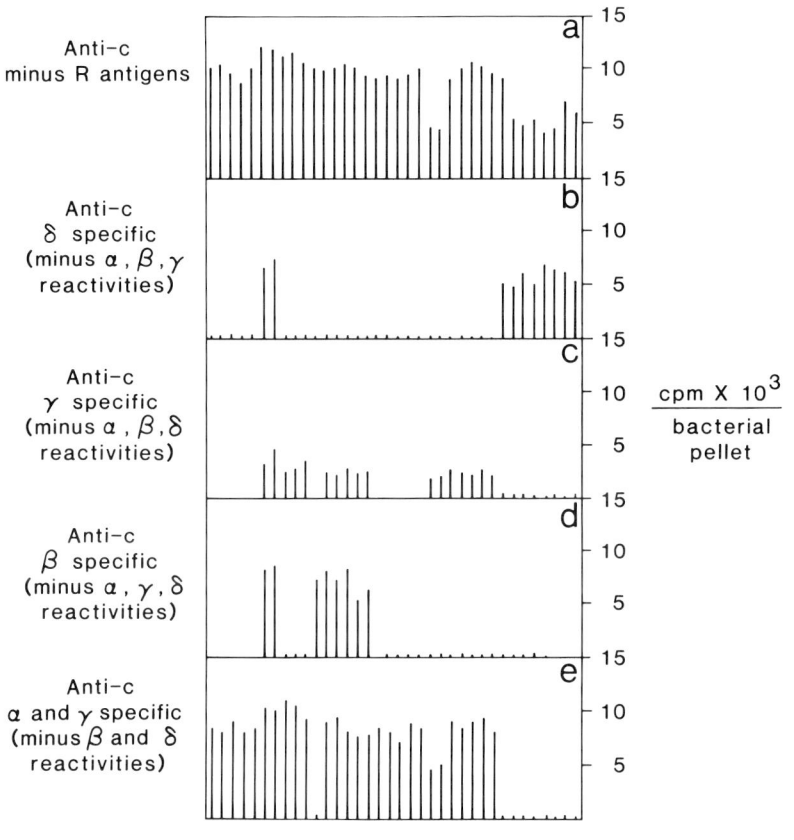

FIGURE 3
Further analysis of the distribution of α, β, γ, and δ antigens on group B streptococci. The monospecific typing antiserum was generated as described by Brady *et al.*, 1988. The experimental conditions and strain designations are identical to those described in Figure 2. (Reproduced from Brady *et al.*, (1988), with permission from Univ. of Chicago Press.)

tive inhibitors in the first stage of the two-stage RIA procedure (data not shown).

The use of a radiolabeled IgG Fc-binding protein tracer (i.e., protein A or protein G) to detect reactivity of rabbit antibodies with intact group B streptococcal bacteria enabled a systematic approach to dissect apart component antigens recognized by a polyclonal antiserum. This was feasible because of the sensitivity and objectivity of the assay, the ease and rapidity with which multiple isolates and multiple antisera could be tested, and the need for relatively small amounts of bacteria and typing antisera as compared to conventional precipitin testing.

IV. Adaptation of the Two-Stage RIA to a Dot Blot Assay

The two-stage radioimmunoassay described in the previous section can easily be adapted to a dot blot assay, in which intact bacteria or concentrated bacterial culture supernatants are immobilized on nitrocellulose, reacted with an appropriate dilution of type-specific antiserum, and probed with radiolabeled protein A or protein G. The advantages of this approach are that a large number of bacterial isolates can be screened rapidly in a single experiment and that culture supernatants can be tested for the presence of secreted antigens; however, the results obtained are somewhat less quantitative than those obtained using the tube assay procedure, in which radioactivity associated with a given number of bacteria is measured using a gamma counter.

A. Dot Blot Autoradiographic Procedure for Detection of Group B Streptococcal Antigens

Bacterial strains, media, and growth conditions, a source of group B streptococcal-typing antisera, and iodination of protein A and protein G have been described previously. Concentrated culture supernatants are prepared by pelleting bacteria by centrifugation, filtering out residual bacteria using 0.2 μ Acrodiscs® (Gelman Sciences, Ann Arbor, Michigan), and concentrating the filtered supernatants using Minicon® macrosolute concentrators (Amicon Corporation, Danvers, Massachusetts). Dot blots were performed using the Bio-Rad bio-dot microfiltration apparatus (Bio-Rad, Richmond, California) and a modification of the Bio-Rad procedure. A piece of nitrocellulose previously soaked in phosphate-buffered saline (PBS), pH 7.4, is placed in the apparatus. Fifty microliters of bacterial suspensions in PBS (containing approximately $2.5-5 \times 10^7$ organisms) or 25, 10, and 5 μl of 15-fold concentrated Todd-Hewitt broth culture supernatants are pipetted into the wells. The wells are washed twice with 200 μl of PBS and the nitrocellulose removed from the apparatus. The nitrocellulose filters are blocked by washing four times (15 min per wash) with 250 ml of 0.15 M veronal-buffered saline (VBS), pH 7.4, containing 0.25% gelatin and 0.25% Tween 20 (VBS-gel-Tween). The blocked filters are reacted with 5 ml of a 1:400 dilution of rabbit anti-c protein-typing antiserum or adsorbed, rabbit, monospecific anti-β antiserum (diluted in VBS-gel-Tween) for 3 hr at ambient temperature, washed four times with 250 ml of VBS-gel-Tween, and incubated with 5 ml of VBS-gel-Tween containing approximately 3×10^5 cpm/ml of ^{125}I-labeled protein A or ^{125}I-labeled protein G for 3 hr at ambient temperature. The filters are then washed four times with 250 ml of VBS-gel-Tween containing 0.01 M EDTA and 1 M NaCl, dried, and autoradiographed using Kodak XAR-5 film and a Kodak X-omatic intensifying screen at $-70°C$ for 6–12 hr.

B. Results of Dot Blot Autoradiographic Procedure to Detect Cell Surface and Secreted Group B Streptococcal Antigens

Figure 4 shows the autoradiograph of a dot blot assay in which suspensions of seven group B streptococcal strains were dotted onto nitrocellulose, reacted with rabbit polyclonal anti-c protein-typing antiserum, and the nitrocellulose filter probed with ^{125}I-labeled protein G. Six of the seven strains were reactive with the anti-c protein antiserum and therefore expressed at least one of the α, β, γ, or δ antigens on their surfaces (lanes 1, 3, 4, 5, 6, and 7). The surface antigenic profile for these strains, as determined by two-stage RIA, is detailed in the figure legend.

Figure 5 shows the autoradiograph from a dot blot assay in which 15-fold concentrated culture supernatants from ten group B streptococcal isolates were dotted onto nitrocellulose and reacted with anti-c protein-typing antiserum, which had been selectively adsorbed to render it mono-

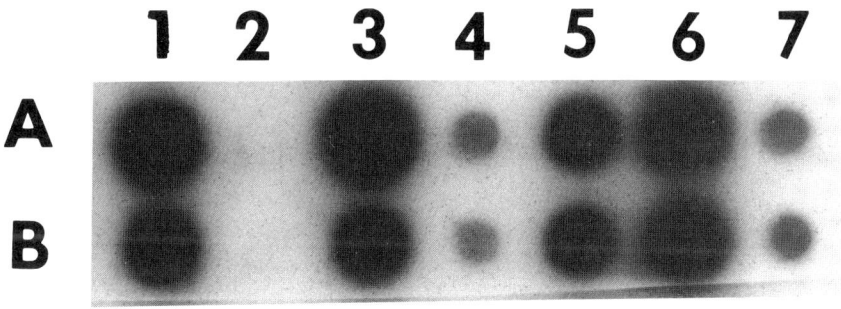

FIGURE 4
Dot blot autoradiograph to detect reactivity of group B streptococcal isolates with rabbit anti-c protein-typing antiserum. Bacterial suspensions in PBS containing approximately 2.5×10^7 (Row A) or 5.0×10^7 (Row B) cells were dotted onto nitrocellulose, reacted with anti-c protein-typing antiserum, and probed with ^{125}I-labeled protein G. Columns 1–7 correspond to GBS strains TC795 (Ib, β), HG738 (III), A909 (Ia, α, β, γ, δ), J48 (III, δ), HG782 (II/III, α, γ), J44(II, α), and HG818 (II, α, γ), respectively. The parentheses indicate the cell-associated type-specific antigens detected by two-stage RIA for each strain. Autoradiography was for 12 hr at $-70°C$ with an intensifying screen.

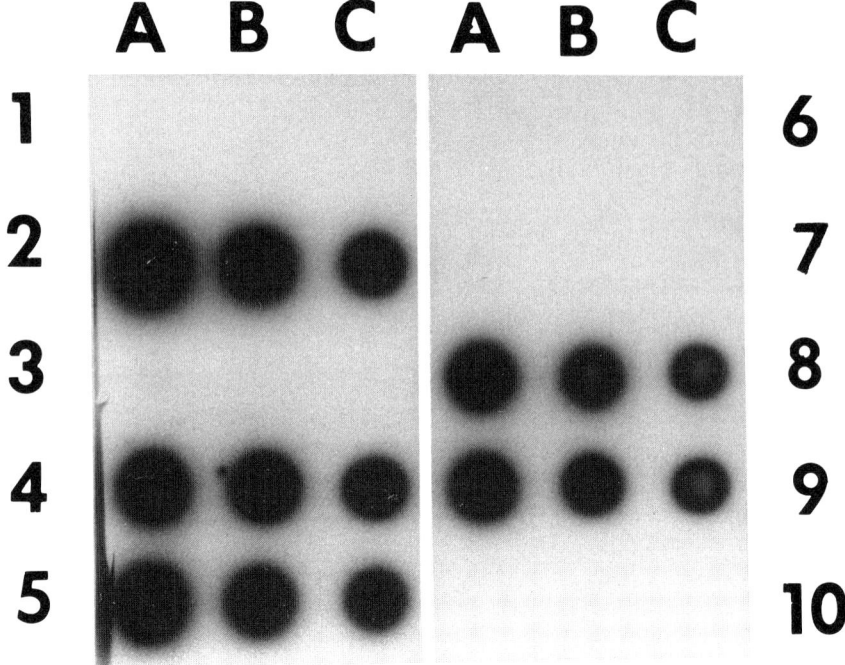

FIGURE 5
Dot blot autoradiograph to detect reactivity of GBS culture supernatants with rabbit monospecific anti-β antiserum. Twenty-five (column A), ten (column B), or five (column C) microliters of 15-fold concentrated Todd-Hewitt broth culture supernatants were dotted onto nitrocellulose, reacted with anti-β antiserum, and probed with ^{125}I-labeled protein A. Rows 1–10 correspond to GBS strains SS617 (Ia), A909 (Ia, α, β, γ, δ), HG812 (Ib, α, γ), HG806 (Ib, α, γ), 2AR (Ib, α, γ), DL413M (no type), DL414B (no type), DL469M (Ib, α, γ), DL471B (Ib, α, γ) and DL506M (Ia, α), respectively. The parentheses indicate the cell-associated, type-specific antigens detected by two-stage RIA for each strain. Autoradiography was for 6 hr at $-70°C$ with an intensifying screen.

specific for reactivity against the β antigen, and the filter probed with ^{125}I-labeled protein A. Five of the ten tested strains secreted β antigen into culture supernatants (rows 2, 4, 5, 8, and 9), while the remaining five did not (rows 1, 3, 6, 7, and 10). These results are interesting because only three of the ten strains demonstrated reactivity with anti-β antiserum when intact bacteria were tested using the two-stage RIA. The strains shown in rows 4 and 5, HG806 and 2AR, secreted the β antigen in the absence of surface expression. A more detailed analysis of secreted and cell surface forms of β antigen has been reported (Brady and Boyle, 1989).

Dot blot analysis of culture supernatants has also identified a GBS isolate, TC795, which secreted the α antigen in the absence of surface expression (data not shown). The results of these dot blot assays indicate that, at least for group B streptococci, secreted molecules as well as surface molecules should be analyzed in order to obtain a complete antigenic profile of a given organism.

V. Adaptation of the Two-Stage RIA to an ELISA Typing Procedure

In those situations in which the use of radiolabeled probes is not desirable, the two-stage RIA just described can be adapted to an ELISA (enzyme-linked immunosorbent assay) procedure, in which an enzyme-labeled conjugate is used in place of ^{125}I-labeled protein A or ^{125}I-labeled protein G. The procedure used to couple alkaline phosphatase to bacterial immunoglobulin Fc-binding proteins is described in Chapter 8. An ELISA typing procedure can be performed essentially the same way as described earlier for the two-stage RIA until the final steps to detect type-specific antibodies associated with bacterial pellets. After the bacteria are reacted with type-specific antisera, washed, and vortexed to resuspend the pellets, rather than adding a radiolabeled probe, 1 ml of an appropriate dilution of alkaline phosphatase-conjugated protein G (in this case 1:5000 in VBS-gel) is added to each tube. The tubes are incubated for 1 hr at 37°C and washed twice with 2 ml of VBS-gel to remove any unbound enzyme–protein G conjugate. Again, the pellet is vortexed to resuspend the bacteria and 0.5 ml of reconstituted Sigma 104 *p*-nitrophenylphosphate chromogenic substrate for alkaline phosphatase is added to each tube. The tubes are incubated at 37°C for 90 min to allow the enzyme-induced color formation to occur and the reaction stopped by the addition of 1.5 ml of ice-cold 0.1 M NaOH to each tube. The tubes are centrifuged at $1000 \times g$ for 8 min to pellet the bacteria and the cell-free supernatants are decanted. The optical density at 405 nm of the supernatant is proportional to the amount of specific antibody associated with the bacteria.

Figure 6 shows a comparison of the results of the ELISA and two-stage RIA procedures for detection of type-specific antigens expressed on the surface of the group B streptococcal strain PF25AR. The left panel shows the ELISA results, with the amount of reactivity of each individual typing antiserum indicated by the optical density at 405 nm. The right panel shows the RIA results, with cpm $\times 10^3$/bacterial pellet indicating the degree of reactivity of this strain with each individual typing antiserum. The results of the two assays are identical. In addition to the normal rabbit

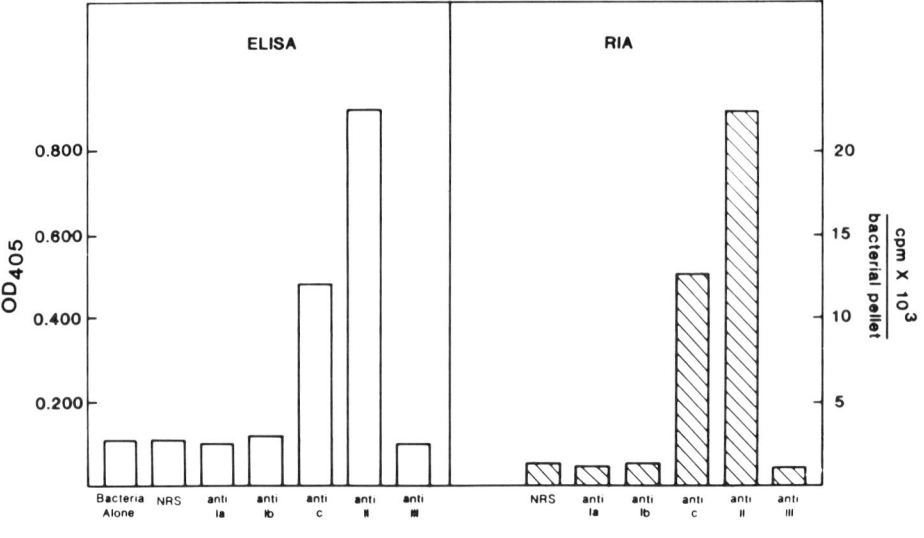

FIGURE 6
Comparison of ELISA versus RIA typing procedures for detection of cell-associated type-specific antigens of group B streptococcal strain PF25AR (type II, c). x-axis: Type-specific rabbit antisera reacted with intact bacteria. NRS = normal rabbit serum. y-axis: The amount of reactivity of each antiserum with the bacteria as determined by OD_{405} (optical density at 405 nm) for the ELISA procedure (left) or cpm $\times$ 10^3 per bacterial pellet for the RIA procedure (right). Each bar represents the mean value for duplicate tubes. Less than 5% variability was observed between duplicate samples.

serum control, included in each assay to ensure that the strain was not expressing immunoglobulin Fc-binding proteins, which could bind the rabbit antibodies in a nonimmune manner, a control with bacteria only (no antibodies or enzyme–protein G conjugate added prior to the substrate) was included in the ELISA procedure. This was done to ensure that this strain did not demonstrate any intrinsic alkaline phosphatase activity. Such activity was observed for several GBS isolates tested. The interference in the ELISA typing procedure due to intrinsic alkaline phosphatase-like activity associated with certain strains of GBS can be avoided by switching to a horseradish–peroxidase conjugate system.

The ELISA typing procedure can also be adapted to a slot blot assay analogous to the dot blot adaptation of the two-stage RIA. The procedure is similar to typing by the tube ELISA and uses the identical alkaline phosphatase-conjugated protein A or protein G probe. A precipitable substrate, 5-bromo-4-chloro-3-indolyl phosphate p-toluidine salt (BCIP)/p-nitro blue tetrazolium chloride (NBT) solution (Bio-Rad, Richmond, California) is used for color development. The relative amounts of precipitate can be quantitated by scanning the nitrocellulose filter with a laser densitometer.

VI. Summary

The two-stage radioimmunoassay (RIA) described in this chapter was used to identify type-specific antigens expressed by 53 laboratory isolates of group B streptococci. This assay utilizes the ability of radiolabeled, bacterial immunoglobulin Fc-binding proteins (i.e., protein A and protein G) to bind with high affinity to the Fc region of type-specific rabbit antibodies, which have been previously reacted with intact bacteria. There was an absolute correlation between carbohydrate antigens detected by the RIA and the classical precipitin assay; however, more isolates were reactive with the anti-c protein marker antiserum when assayed by the RIA rather than by precipitin testing. By selective adsorption of the rabbit polyclonal anti-c protein-typing antiserum, four distinct group B streptococcal surface antigens were detected by RIA.

The RIA tube assay has also been adapted to a dot blot autoradiographic procedure for detection of cell-associated as well as secreted antigens. Both the tube assay and the dot blot assay can be adapted to an ELISA system in which protein A or protein G is conjugated to an enzyme such as alkaline phosphatase and the degree of reactivity of a bacterial strain with each type-specific antiserum is assessed colorimetrically using a chromogenic substrate.

The two-stage RIA and all of its adaptations utilize small quantities of intact bacteria (or culture supernatants), require less type-specific antisera than conventional precipitin testing, and are rapid, semiquantitative, and objective. The use of intact bacteria enables detection of acid-labile antigens in their native, unmodified form. Labeled bacterial Fc-binding proteins such as protein A or protein G could be used to trace specific antibodies bound to any bacteria (or bacterial product), provided that the test bacteria themselves do not express Fc-binding proteins specific for the species of immunoglobulin being used in the assay system. The procedures described in this chapter have focused on detection of antigens on group B streptococci; however, this general approach can be used for the detection of any cell surface or immobilized antigen against which specific monoclonal or polyclonal antibodies are available.

References

Bevanger, L. (1983). *Acta Pathol. Microbiol. Immunol. Scand. B* **91**, 231–234.
Bevanger, L. (1985). *Acta Pathol. Microbiol. Immunol. Scand. B* **93**, 113–119.

Bevanger, L., and Iverson, O. J. (1981). *Acta Pathol. Microbiol. Immunol. Scand. B* **89**, 205–209.
Bevanger, L., and Iverson, O. J. (1983). *Acta Pathol. Microbiol. Immunol. Scand. B* **91**, 75–81.
Boyle, M. D. P. (1984). *Biotechniques* **2**, 334–340.
Boyle, M. D. P., and Reis, K. J. (1987). *Biotechnology* **5**, 697–703.
Brady, L. J., and Boyle, M. D. P. (1989). *Infect. Immun.* **57**, 1573–1581.
Brady, L. J., Daphtary, U. D., Ayoub, E. M., and Boyle, M. D. P. (1988). *J. Infect. Dis.* **158**, 965–972.
Chang, H. C., Takashima, I., Arikawa, J., and Hashimoto, N. (1984). *J. Virol. Methods* **9**, 143–151.
Christensen, P., and Oxelius, V. A. (1975). *Acta Pathol. Microbiol. Immunol. Scand. C* **83**, 184–188.
Duboid-Dalcq, M., McFarland, H., and McFarlin, D. (1977). *J. Histochem. Cytochem.* **25**, 1201–1206.
Ey, P. L., Prowse, S. J., and Jenkin, C. R. (1978). *Immunochemistry* **15**, 429–436.
Ferrieri, P., Johnson, D. R., and Flores, A. E. (1985). In "Recent Advances in Streptococci and Streptococcal Diseases" (Y. Kimura, S. Kotami, and Y. Shiokawa, eds), pp. 204–206. Reedbooks, Berkshire.
Flores, A. E., and Ferrieri, P. (1985). *Zentralbl. Bakteriol. Hyg. A* **259**, 165–178.
Forsgren, A., and Sjöquist, J. (1966). *J. Immunol.* **97**, 822–827.
Gee, A. P., and Langone, J. J. (1981). *Anal. Biochem.* **116**, 524–530.
Goding, J. W. (1978). *J. Immunol. Methods* **20**, 241–253.
Henricksen, J., Ferrieri, P., Jelínková, J., Köhler, W., and Maxted, W. R. (1984). *Int. J. Syst. Bacteriol.* **34**, 500.
Jelínková, J., and Matlová, J. (1985). *J. Clin. Microbiol.* **21**, 361–362.
Jensen, N. E. (1979). *Acta Pathol. Microbiol. Imunol. Scand. B* **87**, 77–83.
Johnson, D. R., and Ferrieri, P. (1984). *J. Clin. Microbiol.* **19**, 506–510.
Jürgens, D., Sterzik, B., and Fehrenbach, F. J. (1987). *Exp. Med.* **165**, 720–732.
Kronvall, G. (1973). *J. Immunol.* **11**, 1401–1406.
Kronvall, G., Björck, L., Myhre, E. B., and Wannamaker, L. (1979). In "Pathogenic Streptococci" (M. T. Parker, ed.), pp. 74–76. Reedbooks, Chertsey.
Lancefield, R. C. (1928). *J. Exp. Med.* **47**, 91–103.
Langone, J. J. (1982a). *Adv. Immunol.* **32**, 157–252.
Langone, J. J. (1982b). *J. Immunol. Methods* **51**, 3–22.
Langone, J. J., Boyle, M. D. P., and Borsos, T. (1979). *J. Immunol. Methods* **18**, 281–293.
Lindahl, G. (1989). *Mol. Gen. Genet.* **216**, 372–379.
Lindahl, G., and Åkerström, B. (1989). *Mol. Microbiol.* **3**, 239–247.
Lucocq, J. M., and Baschong, W. (1986). *Eur. J. Cell Biol.* **42**, 332–337.
Magliano, S. D., and Ponzi, N. A. (1983). *Microbiologica* **6**, 327–337.
Marchalonis, J. J., Cone, R. E., and Santer, V. (1971). *Biochem. J.* **124**, 921–927.
Myhre, E. B., and Kronvall, G. (1979). In "Pathogenic Streptococci" (M. T. Parker, ed.), pp. 76–78. Reedbooks, Chertsey.
Myhre, E. B., and Kronvall, G. (1981). In "Basic Concepts of Streptococci and Streptococcal Diseases" (S. E. Holm and P. Christensen, eds.), pp. 209–210. Reedbooks, Chertsey, Surrey.
Reis, K. J., Ayoub, E. M., and Boyle, M. D. P. (1983). *J. Immunol. Methods* **59**, 83–94.
Reis, K. J., von Mering, G. O., Karis, M., Faulmann, E. L., Lottenberg, R., and Boyle, M. D. P. (1988). *J. Immunol. Methods* **107**, 273–280.

Chapter 9. Antigens of Group B Streptococci

Russell-Jones, G. J., Gotschlich, E. C., and Blake, M. S. (1984). *J. Exp. Med.* **160,** 1467–1475.
Schalén, C. (1980). *Acta Pathol. Microbiol. Scand. C* **88,** 271–274.
Schalén, C., Christensen, P., Grubb, A., Samuelsson, G., and Svensson, M. L. (1980). *Acta Pathol. Microbiol. Scand. C* **88,** 77–82.
Wilkinson, H. W. (1972). *Appl. Microbiol.* **24,** 669–670.
Wilkinson, H. W. (1978). *Annu. Rev. Microbiol.* **32,** 41–57.
Wilkinson, H. W., and Eagon, R. G. (1971). *Infect. Immun.* **4,** 596–604.
Wilkinson, H. W., and Moody, M. D. (1969). *J. Bacteriol.* **97,** 629–634.

CHAPTER **10**

Application of Fc-binding proteins for the detection of specific antibodies

Michael D. P. Boyle
Michael J. P. Lawman
Adrian P. Gee

I. Introduction

Detection of specific antibodies is an important aspect of clinical immunology and blood banking. In addition, there are many research applications in which the ability to detect antibodies is of great importance, e.g., screening for production of monoclonal or polyclonal antibodies. The detection of specific antibodies requires both a pure source of antigen with which the antibody can be complexed and some method to physically separate antigen–antibody complexes from free antibody. In this chapter, a series of examples of the use of Fc-binding protein tracers for the detection of antibodies of both reactive, and unreactive immunoglobulin isotypes is presented. The general procedure is essentially similar and is summarized in Figure 1. (In these studies, the Fc-binding protein that is to be used as the tracer can be radiolabeled, biotinylated, or tagged with an enzyme or fluorescent dye.) Methods for preparation of each of these tracer forms have been described elsewhere in this volume.

In this chapter, three representative examples of procedures to measure antibodies are presented.

1. Detection of bovine antibodies to an antigen associated with *Brucella abortus*
2. Detection of antibodies to tumor-associated antigens
3. Detection of antibodies of isotypes or species that fail to react directly with the bacterial IgG-binding protein tracer

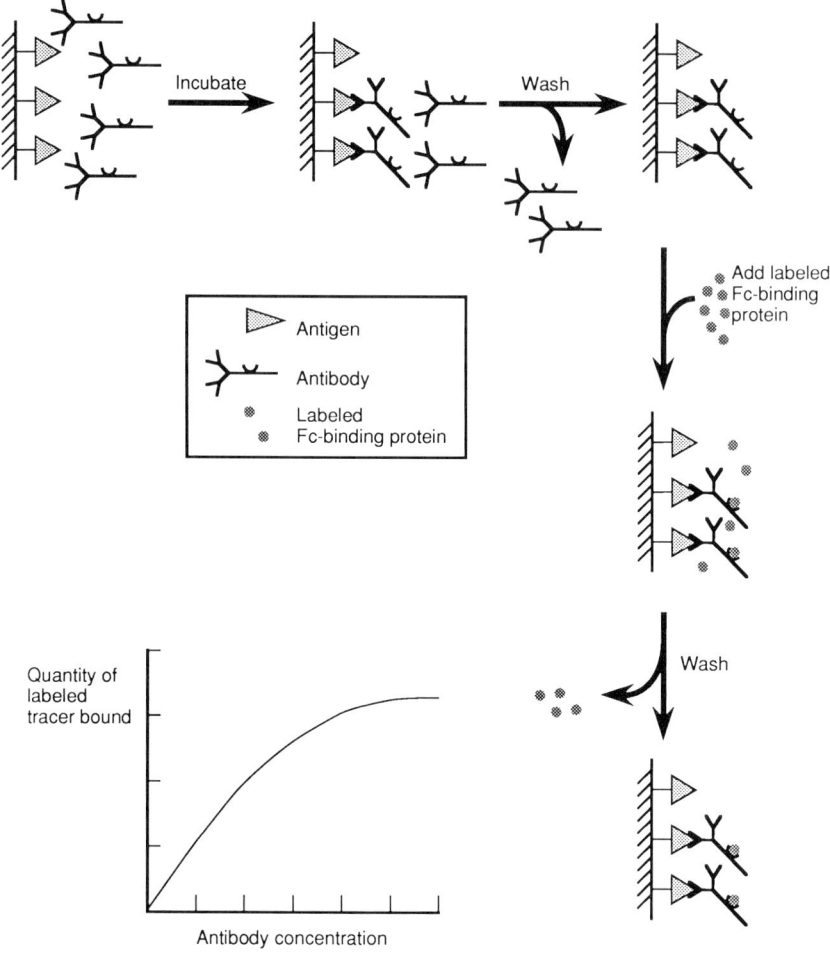

FIGURE 1
General schematic for detection of specific antibodies using an Fc-binding protein as tracer.

Although each of these assays follows a similar strategy, in which IgG complexed to an immobilized antigen is detected using an Fc-binding protein, there are a number of differences in the way each assay is developed, and these variations will be described.

II. Development of an Assay for Antibodies to a Soluble Antigen

The first example describes the development of an assay to measure bovine serum antibodies that specifically recognize an antigen solubilized from *Brucella abortus*. The procedure was first described by Lawman *et al.* (1984) and is carried out in three stages.

In stage one, the soluble *Brucella* antigen (BASA), obtained by autoclaving the intact organism as described by Kaneene *et al.* (1978), was immobilized by adding 100 µl volumes to each well of a 96-well, round-bottomed, disposable, flexible, polyvinyl chloride microtiter plate (Dynatech Laboratories Inc., Arlington, Virginia) (precise details will follow). In stage two, varying dilutions of bovine serum, suspected of containing antibody to *Brucella* antigens, were incubated in 100 µl volumes with the immobilized antigen. Unbound antibody was removed by washing three times with phosphate-buffered saline (PBS), pH 7.2, containing 0.1% Tween 20 and 0.1% bovine serum albumin (PBS-Tween-BSA). In stage three, the quantity of specific antibody bound to the antigen was determined by binding of 100 µl of ^{125}I-labeled protein A. Finally, the wells were washed three times in PBS-Tween-BSA to remove unbound ^{125}I-labeled protein A. The individual wells were cut out and placed in glass tubes, and the residual (bound) radioactivity measured. Although the assay described here utilizes a radioactive tracer, this method is readily adaptable for use with enzyme-labeled tracers.

Optimal conditions for each stage of the assay procedure were established in preliminary experiments as next described. For precise formulation of the buffers used, see the Appendix. The ^{125}I-labeled protein A tracer was prepared as described in Chapter 7.

A. Optimization of Conditions to Detect Anti-*Brucella* Antibodies

A variety of incubation times and temperatures for binding the *Brucella abortus* antigen to microtiter plates were compared. The antigen was diluted in 0.05 M carbonate buffer (pH 9.6) and was added in 100 µl volumes to each well of a 96-well microtiter plate. After incubation for varying times at 4°C or 37°C, the BASA-coated plates were washed three times with PBS-Tween-BSA. The plates were then tested for maximum antibody binding using a known positive serum. While all combinations of times and temperatures (37°C and 4°C) bound detectable levels of antibody, the optimal conditions for immobilization of the target antigen were found to be 2 hr at 37°C, or 1 hr at 37°C with a further 2 hr at 4°C (Lawman et al., 1984). Once the binding of antigen was complete, antigen-coated plates could be stored at 4°C for periods of up to 2 weeks without loss of antibody-binding capacity.

In the next series of preliminary experiments, optimal conditions for the second stage of the assay were established, (i.e., conditions for binding of bovine anti-*Brucella* antibody to immobilized antigen).

A series of twofold dilutions of a positive and a negative serum were incubated for various times at either 4°C or 37°C, in microtiter plates coated with antigen, and the degree of binding was measured following incubation with ^{125}I-labeled protein A for 1 hr at 37°C. The results of these preliminary studies indicated that a 1-hr incubation at 37°C of the positive test serum gave the best binding of specific immunoglobulins, with the least amount of nonspecific binding of the negative control serum.

In defining the optimal conditions for the third stage of the assay—the binding of ^{125}I-labeled protein A to immobilized *Brucella*-specific antibody—a number of buffers were used to dilute the ^{125}I-labeled protein A probe, differing in (1) detergent content (Tween 20 or 40) and (2) the concentration of nonspecific protein (bovine serum albumin; BSA). The time and temperature of incubation were also varied. The optimal time and temperature for binding of ^{125}I-labeled protein A were either 1 hr at 37°C or 2 hr at 4°C, and the optimal buffer condition was PBS, containing 0.1% Tween 20 and 5 mg of BSA/ml (Lawman et al., 1984). For the purposes of this assay, the time and temperature chosen were 2 hr at 4°C.

Once optimal assay conditions had been established, the assay procedure was applied to screening bovine serum for presence of antibodies that recognized soluble *Brucella*-associated antigens. In each assay, known positive and negative sera were included. The antibody concentrations were calculated from the highest serum dilutions in which the radioactivity was equal to that of the negative control serum (Lawman et al., 1984). Figure 2 shows a series of standard antibody-binding curves obtained using serum from *Brucella*-positive, vaccinated, and *Brucella*-negative animals.

It is of interest that protein A does not detect bovine immunoglobulins well and shows a marked preference for immunoglobulins of the $IgG_{\gamma 2}$ subtype (Lawman et al., 1984). This preferential reactivity has been used for the detection of *Brucella*-specific antibodies in vaccinated and infected cattle and may prove to be of value for monitoring *Brucella* infections in cattle (Lawman et al., 1984, 1986).

The general approach described to detect *Brucella* antigens is applicable to any antigen–antibody pair. In developing any new assay, a series of

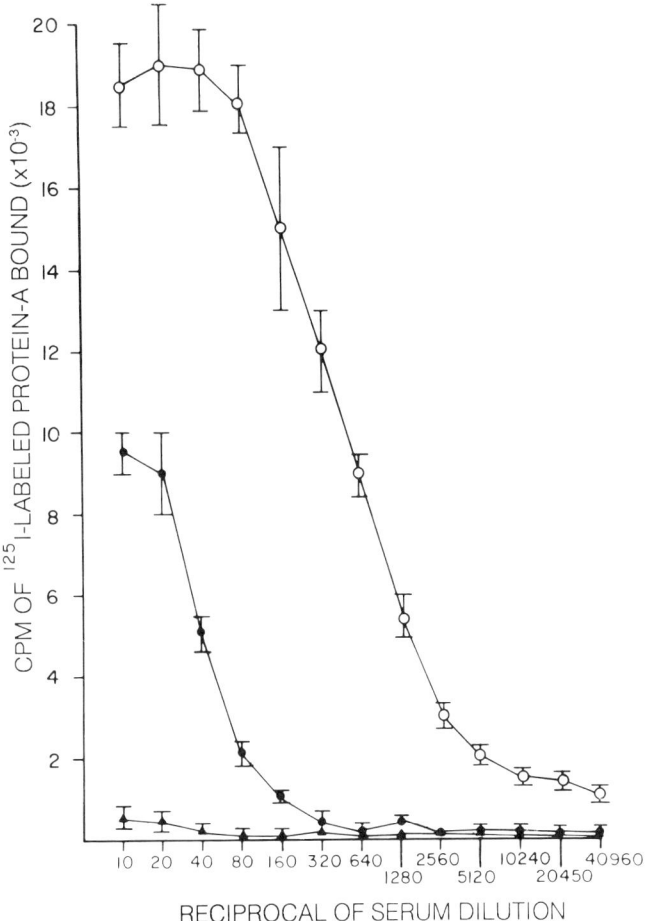

FIGURE 2
Representative standard curves generated from a solid-phase radioimmunoassay to detect anti-*Brucella* specific antibody. Serum from *Brucella*-infected animals (○-○). Serum from *Brucella*-vaccinated animals (●-●). *Brucella*-negative serum control (▲-▲). The error bars represent the mean ± SEM for each of triplicate experimental observations. (Reproduced from Lawman *et al.*, 1986, with permission.)

preliminary experiments is essential to optimize assay conditions, e.g., time, temperature, buffers, blocking agents, etc. If the antigen is already immobilized, e.g., on a cell, stage one of the procedure just described can be eliminated.

III. Detection of Antibodies to Tumor-Associated Antigens

Binding of specific antibodies to tumor cells can be monitored by use of suitably labeled Fc-binding proteins. Specific antibodies bind to their cognate antigen on the cell via $F(ab')_2$ domains, and cell-associated antibodies can then be detected, following washing, by their reactivity with a suitable tracer form of an Fc-binding protein. This can be a radiolabeled derivative, an enzyme-labeled derivative, a gold-labeled derivative, or a fluorescent derivative.

The procedure to detect tumor antigens is similar to that described earlier, except that in this system the antigen is "naturally" immobilized on the cell surface. It is necessary, in optimizing any assay for cell-surface antigens, to have available an appropriate positive serum. When detecting antibodies directed against antigens that are expressed in low concentrations, it is necessary to use a high enough cell number to provide sufficient, immobilized antigen in the assay system. In the preliminary studies, it is also necessary to carry out kinetic studies similar to those described in section II, to ensure that the time and temperature for antibody and tracer binding are adequate. It should be noted that patching and capping of surface antigen–antibody complexes can occur, and that this effect is enhanced by incubation of the cells for prolonged periods at elevated temperatures. These problems can be minimized, either by carrying out the reactions on ice, or by addition of chemicals that interfere with antigen movement on the cell surface, e.g., sodium azide, cytochalasin B, etc. (Unanue *et al.*, 1973; Taylor *et al.*, 1971; Edidin and Weiss, 1974; de Petris, 1974; Boyle *et al.*, 1975). It is also important to include appropriate controls of (1) cells alone or (2) cells incubated with either a similar sublcass of nonimmune antibody of the same isotype and subclass, or serum obtained from the animal before immunization, to quantitate nonspecific or background binding.

The procedure to detect cell-associated antigens is carried out by adding 0.1 ml of dilutions of antigen-positive tumor cells (ranging from 10^6 to 10^8 cells per ml) to an equal volume of differing dilutions of serum, ascites fluid, or antibody-containing supernatants, and incubating for 30–60 min at 37°C. (The optimal time and temperature should be established for each system in preliminary experiments.) Unbound antibodies are removed by adding 2 ml of veronal-buffered saline, pH 7.35, containing Ca^{2+}, Mg^{2+}, and 0.1% gelatin (VBS-gel), pelleting the cells by centrifugation at 2000 × *g* for 5 min and discarding the supernatant fluid containing unbound antibodies and other proteins. This washing procedure is carried out three times. The antibody-coated tumor cells are then incubated with 0.1 ml of ^{125}I-labeled Fc-binding protein (~30,000 counts per minute (cpm)/tube) and incubated for 1 hr at 37°C; then washed twice as described above with 2 ml of veronal-buffered saline containing 0.01 M ethylenediaminetetraaacetic acid (EDTA) and 0.1% gelatin. The washed cell pellet is counted in a gamma counter. Phosphate-buffered saline containing a nonspecific protein source or tissue culture medium can be used as diluent or for washing cells in these assays. The formulations for all buffers are presented in the Appendix.

An example of this procedure applied to the detection of rabbit antibodies to antigens on two guinea pig hepatoma cell lines will be presented in this chapter. This procedure was initially described by Langone *et al.* (1977) and the details of the preparation of antibodies, growth of the hepatoma cell lines etc., can be found in Boyle and Langone (1979). In the experiment described here, 1×10^5 tumor cells were sensitized by incubation with differing concentrations of rabbit antibodies to line-1 or line-10 tumor cells for 30 min at 30°C. Control tubes included (i) antibody incubated in the absence of cells, (ii) cells incubated in the absence of antibody, and (iii) cells incubated with preimmunization serum. After the initial incubation period, unbound antibody and other serum proteins were separated from the tumor cells by washing three times with 2 ml VBS-gel. The cell pellet was then incubated for 1 hr at 30°C with ^{125}I-labeled protein A (~30,000 cpm/sample) in a total volume of 0.2 ml VBS-gel. [These conditions have been shown to be optimal for binding of ^{125}I-labeled protein A to antibody-sensitized tumor cells (Langone *et al.*, 1977).] After washing three times with 2 ml of VBS-gel buffer, the radiolabel associated with the cell pellets was measured in a gamma counter. The results presented in Figure 3 show that antibodies of the IgG isotype specific for line-1 or line-10 cells could be detected. Tumor cells sensitized with IgM antibodies did not bind Protein A (Langone *et al.*, 1977) and no significant binding of radiolabeled tracer was observed, either to the cells themselves or to tumor cells following incubation with normal rabbit serum (Boyle and Langone, 1979).

This approach can also be used with preparations of antibodies of known specificity and titer to determine differences in antigen expression on tumor cells. Studies by Gee *et al.* (1987) have demonstrated that, following selection by treatment with an excess of a mouse monoclonal antibody specific for the common acute lymphoblastic leukemia antigen (cALLa) and complement, cells from a human leukemia cell line (NALM-16) displayed different levels of tumor-associated antigen on their surface. In these studies, the NALM-16 cells were treated with DU-ALL-1 monoclonal antibody (Jones *et al.*, 1982) (kindly provided for that study by Dr.

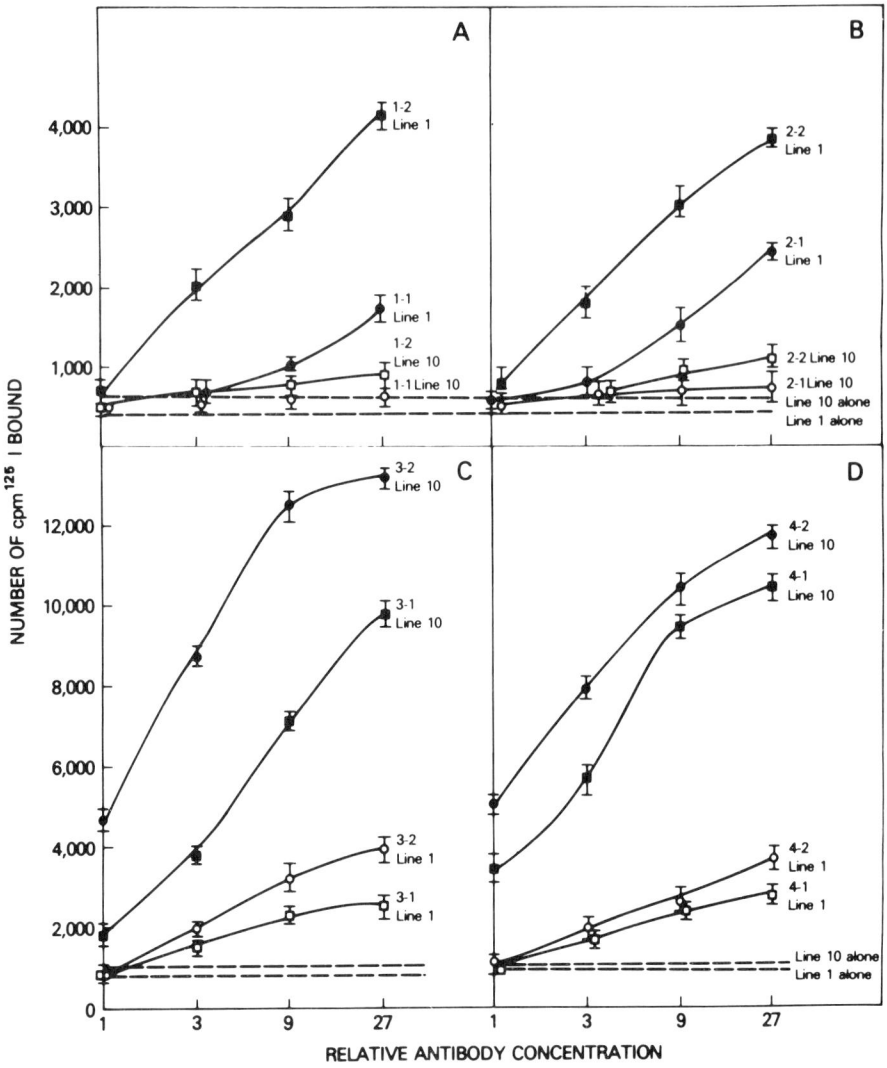

FIGURE 3
Binding of ^{125}I-labeled protein A (~30,000 cpm added) to 10^3 line-1 or line-10 tumor cells sensitized with differing amounts of: Panel (A) Antiserum 1-1 or 1-2 from a rabbit immunized with line 1 tumor cells. Panel (B) Antiserum 2-1 or 2-2 from a rabbit immunized with line-1 tumor cells. Panel (C) Antiserum 3-1 or 3-2 from a rabbit immunized with line-10 tumor cells. Panel (D) Antiserum 4-1 or 4-2 from a rabbit immunized with line-10 tumor cells. A relative concentration of 1 is equivalent to 1:243 dilution of the serum. For details of immunization protocols and tumor cell lines, see Boyle and Langone (1980). (Reproduced from Boyle and Langone, 1980.)

Richard Metzgar of Duke University Medical Center, Durham North Carolina), and excess rabbit complement. Residual viable cells were expanded in culture as described by Gee *et al.* (1987).

The expression of cALLa on the surface of each of the cell populations following antibody–complement treatment was studied by measuring the quantity of monoclonal antibody bound. This was assayed by measuring the binding of ^{125}I-labeled protein A to cells sensitized with different dilutions of the cALLa-specific, protein A-fixing, monoclonal antibody, following the method previously outlined. The results, in Figure 4, demonstrate major differences in the antigen expression among each of the selected populations of leukemic cells. The greatest quantity of antibody, and therefore the greatest level of cALLa expression, was associated with the untreated, parent cell line (Figure 4). Progressively lower quantities of antigen were expressed following each antibody–complement treatment (Figure 4). These results indicate that cALLa expression per cell, as

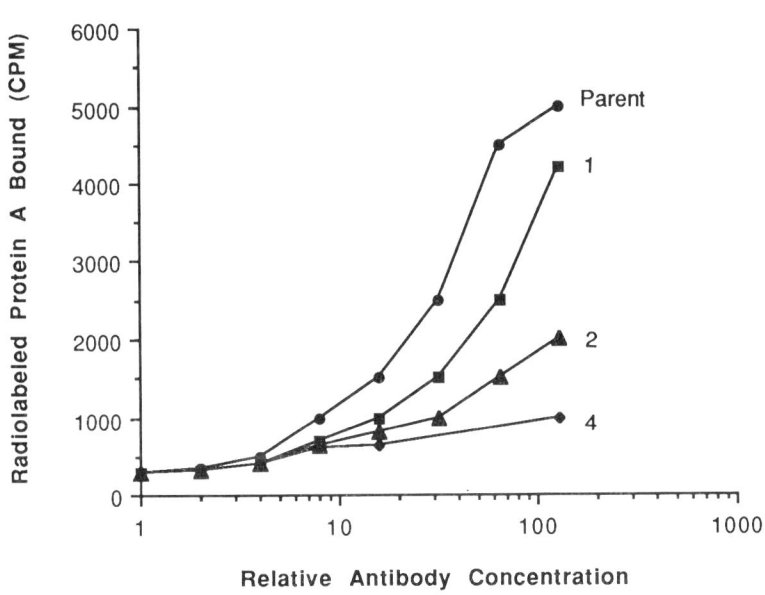

FIGURE 4
Analysis of binding of an anti-cALLa monoclonal antibody to complement-resistant subpopulations of NALM-16 leukemia cells. Binding of DU-ALL-1 monoclonal antibody (MoAb) to the parental line of NALM-16 cells (P) and the complement-resistant selected subpopulations (1, 2, and 4) was measured with the use of ^{125}I-labeled protein A. For precise experimental detail, see Gee *et al.* (1987). (Reproduced from Gee *et al.*, 1987.)

detected by the DU-ALL-1 monoclonal antibody binding, differed significantly between the various derived lines (Gee *et al.*, 1987).

It should be noted that these procedures yield an average value for surface antigen expression within a population. The results do not distinguish between (1) uniform lowered antigen expression on all cells, (2) changes in surface area of the tumor cells, or (3) total loss of antigen expression by a percentage of the cells and unaltered expression by the remainder. The explanation for changes in total antibody binding requires the use of more sophisticated techniques, such as flow cytometry. When these cell populations were analyzed by flow cytometry, there was no marked difference in cell size-related forward light scatter signals observed among the various selected cell populations. The fluorescent intensity then must decrease due to a decrease in the expression of the antigen recognized by the monoclonal antibody, rather than an increase in cell surface area (Gee *et al.*, 1987).

IV. Detection of Rabbit IgM Antibodies to Sheep Erythrocytes

All of the assays for detection of antibodies described thus far in this chapter have been based on the ability to detect antibodies that are reactive with an Fc-binding protein tracer. This limits the procedure to antibodies of species, isotypes, and subclasses for which suitable tracer molecules are available. In this section, we describe a sandwich immunoassay that can be used to detect antibodies of unreactive isotypes. This example describes an assay to quantify rabbit IgM antibodies specific for the Forssman antigen expressed on the surface of sheep erythrocytes (E). This assay uses a second antibody specific for rabbit IgM heavy chains and ^{125}I-labeled protein A as the tracer. The second antibody was prepared in goats, and although fluid-phase goat IgG binds poorly with protein A, we have found that this antibody binds protein A with an enhanced affinity when complexed with its antigen (Boyle and Langone, 1979). The IgM anti-Forssman antibody was isolated as described in Boyle and Langone (1980) and quantified using the C1 fixation and transfer test (Borsos *et al.*, 1968). The quantitation of complement-fixing IgM molecules can be carried out accurately using the complement fixation and transfer test (Borsos *et al.*, 1968; Moyer *et al.*, 1968). In this test, the first component of complement binds to cell-bound IgM under conditions of low ionic strength. The cells are washed in low ionic strength buffer, allowing $\overline{C1}$ associated with cell-bound IgM antibodies to be separated from unbound $\overline{C1}$. The $\overline{C1}$ associated with the antibody-sensitized cells can be dissociated by incubation in a buffer of higher ionic strength and the released $\overline{C1}$ can be quantified on a molecular basis using a standard $\overline{C1}$ titration assay (Rapp and Borsos, 1970). This procedure, developed by Borsos and colleagues has proven to be a very reliable method for the detection of IgM complement-fixing antibodies (Borsos et al., 1968). We have used this $\overline{C1}$ fixation and transfer test to determine the number of $\overline{C1}$-fixing IgM molecules per cell on the various preparations of sheep erythrocytes used in these experiments.

For the experiments described here, sheep erythrocytes were standardized to 10^9/ml (Rapp and Borsos, 1970) and sensitized with specific IgM antibodies, by incubation of an equal volume of erythrocytes with a solution of IgM antibody (containing approximately 200 $\overline{C1}$-fixing IgM molecules/erythrocyte) for 15 min at 37°C (Boyle and Langone, 1979). The antibody-sensitized cells (EAIgM) were washed twice in VBS-gel buffer and resuspended to a concentration of 10^9/ml.

In the initial experiments, differing numbers of EAIgM were incubated with varying dilutions of goat anti-rabbit IgM for 1 hr at 30°C. After this time, the cells were washed twice with 3 ml of VBS-gel and the cell pellet was incubated with 0.1 ml of ^{125}I-labeled protein A (approximately 30,000 cpm/tube) for 1 hr at 30°C. This incubation time was sufficient for maximal binding of ^{125}I-labeled protein A to antibody-sensitized cells (Langone et al., 1977). Differing concentrations of goat anti-IgM were tested for the ability to bind to varying numbers of EAIgM (Figure 5A). When the goat anti-rabbit antibody was diluted 1/10 or 1/20, equivalent binding was observed, which increased as the cell number increased. As expected, at higher dilutions of goat anti-rabbit IgM (1/160), the second antibody reagent became limiting and the number of counts bound did not increase as greater numbers of IgM-sensitized erythrocytes were added (Figure 5A). No significant binding of protein A to EAIgM occurred in the absence of goat anti-rabbit IgM (Boyle and Langone, 1980).

Similar experiments were carried out with sheep erythrocytes sensitized with differing dilutions of IgM anti-Forssman antibodies. Based on the results presented in Figure 5A, these studies were carried out using 10^8 sensitized cells. As shown in Figure 5B, differing levels of IgM can be detected on the surfaces of the sensitized red cells. As expected for IgM antibodies, there was a direct proportion between the number of molecules bound to E and the dilution of IgM used to sensitize the cells (Figure 5C). Hoyer et al. (1968) have measured the absolute number of specific anti-Forssman IgM molecules and the percentage of that IgM that is C-fixing in similar preparations of anti-Forssman antisera. These estimates indicate that approximately 20% of the antigen-specific IgM was of the C-fixing type (Hoyer et al., 1968). Assuming these estimates were valid for this

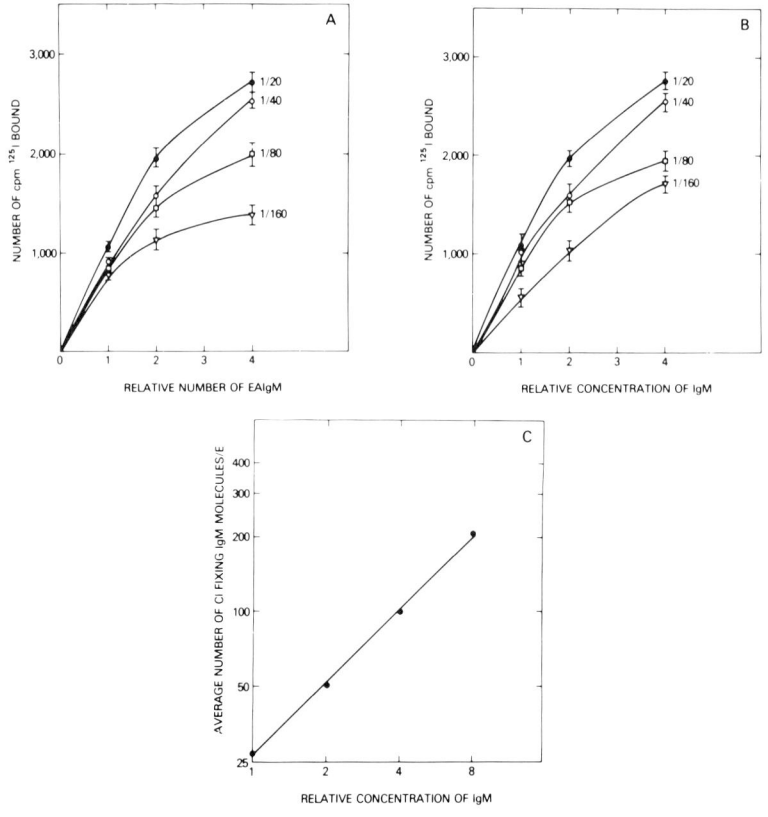

FIGURE 5

Quantitative determination of IgM bound to sheep erythrocytes (E). (A) Binding of ^{125}I-labeled protein A to differing numbers of E sensitized with 200 $C\overline{1}$-fixing IgM molecules/cell, following incubation with varying dilutions of goat anti-rabbit IgM. A relative cell concentration of 1 is equivalent to 2.5×10^7 cells. Approximately 30,000 cpm ^{125}I-labeled protein A were added per tube. (B) Binding of ^{125}I-labeled protein A to 10^8 E sensitized with varying dilutions of IgM following incubation with varying dilutions of goat anti-rabbit IgM. A relative IgM concentration of 1 is equivalent to 50 $C\overline{1}$-fixing IgM molecules/cell. Approximately 30,000 cpm ^{125}I-labeled protein A were added per tube. (C) Binding of $C\overline{1}$ to 10^7 EA sensitized with differing dilutions of IgM anti-Forssman antibody measured by the $C\overline{1}$-fixation and transfer test (Borsos et al., 1968). A relative concentration of 1 is equivalent to 1/80 dilution of the purified IgM antibody. (Reproduced from Boyle and Langone, 1979.)

serum, we calculated that it contained 3×10^{11} C-fixing IgM molecules/ml and 1.5×10^{12} molecules/ml of total IgM. If one further assumes that a direct relationship exists between the ^{125}I-labeled protein A bound and the quantity of IgM bound to the cell, then from the data presented in Figure 5, we can estimate that 1000 cpm bound under the conditions of this experiment are equivalent to approximately 10^{10} C-fixing IgM molecules and approximately 5×10^{10} total IgM antibody molecules. [It should be noted that many normal rabbit sera contain natural antibodies to sheep erythrocytes and other antigens, so it may be necessary to preabsorb the second antibody used if high background levels of nonspecific binding are detected.]

The preceding experiments were carried out in a sequential fashion. The reaction of the second antibody with the antibody-sensitized cells was carried out in the first step. In the second step, complexes of second antibody with antibody-sensitized cells were separated from unbound, second antibody by washing and were then incubated with the tracer. Previous studies have shown that protein A reacts poorly with fluid-phase goat IgG (Langone, 1978). Consequently, we tested whether the assay would yield similar results if the reaction were carried out in a single step, i.e., if goat anti-rabbit IgM and ^{125}I-labeled protein A were present together in the reaction mixture. The results in Figure 6 demonstrate that similar findings were obtained when ^{125}I-labeled protein A and goat anti-rabbit IgM were present together. These findings suggest that goat IgG either only binds protein A when complexed to an appropriate antigen or that its affinity for protein A, once complexed, is markedly enhanced (Boyle and Langone, 1979).

For this procedure to be applicable to detection of IgM in serum, it is necessary first to remove any IgG antibodies that would react directly with the tracer. This can be achieved by preabsorbing the antiserum with a source of the immobilized Fc-binding protein used as the tracer. This approach has been applied successfully to measure IgG and IgM antibodies to tumor cells (Boyle and Langone, 1980). IgG antibodies were measured by direct interaction with the tracer; IgM antibodies were quantified following absorption with immobilized protein A in a sandwich assay using a μ chain-specific antibody and the procedure just described (Boyle and Langone, 1979). Since antibodies of different isotypes may also compete for binding to the same antigen, it may also be important to selectively remove other isotypes of unreactive immunoglobulins or to vary the antigen concentration to ensure that the antibody isotype of interest can be detected and quantified accurately.

The examples described in this section demonstrate how, by use of a suitable second antibody, any unreactive primary antibody can be detected. It is of interest that second antibodies can be used, which have either been prepared in a species of animal whose IgG is reactive directly with the Fc-binding protein tracer or, as in the example just presented, which become reactive only when they are complexed to the specific antigen.

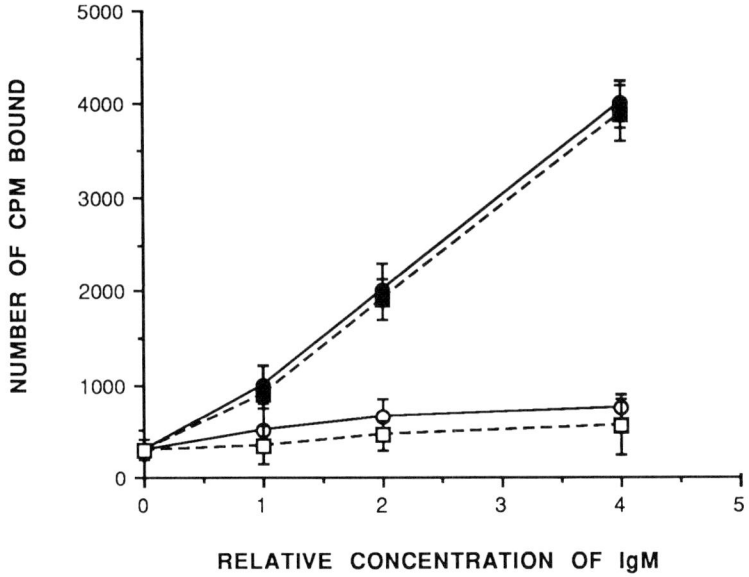

FIGURE 6
Detection of rabbit IgM anti-sheep red cell antibodies in a sandwich assay using goat anti-rabbit IgM and ^{125}I-labeled protein A. This experiment compares the results of studies in which the anti-IgM antibody (1/20) is preincubated with 10^8 IgM-sensitized sheep erythrocytes for 60 min at 30°C and washed prior to addition of ^{125}I-labeled protein A (●--●), with equivalent samples in which the anti-IgM antibody and labeled tracer are present throughout the incubation period (■--■). The corresponding samples in the absence of added goat anti-rabbit IgM are shown by the corresponding *open* symbol. A relative concentration of 1 for IgM is equivalent to 50 C1-fixing molecules/cell. (Reproduced from Boyle and Langone, 1979).

V. Summary

The general procedures outlined in this chapter permit antibodies to either cell surface or soluble antigens to be detected. Antibodies whose Fc regions bind to the Fc-binding protein tracer can be detected directly, while immunoglobulins of unreactive species or isotypes can be detected using an appropriate, reactive, second antibody reagent. The examples provided in this chapter have used an ^{125}I-labeled form of Fc-binding protein as tracer; however Fc-binding proteins can also be labeled with an enzyme, gold particle, fluorescent dye, or biotin tag. An example of this basic procedure for the detection of antibodies to cell surface antigens, utilizing an enzyme-labeled tracer is provided in the previous chapter.

References

Borsos, T., Colten, H. R., Spalter, J. S., Rogentine, R., and Rapp, H. J. (1968). *J. Immunol.* **101,** 392–398.
Boyle, M. D. P., and Langone, J. J. (1979). *J. Natl. Cancer Inst.* **62,** 1537–1544.
Boyle, M. D. P., and Langone, J. J. (1980). *J. Immunol. Methods* **32,** 51–58.
Boyle, M. D. P., Ohanian, S. H., and Borsos, T. (1975). *J. Immunol.* **115,** 473–475.
De Petris, S. (1974). *Nature* (*London*) **250,** 54–56.
Edidin, M., and Weiss, A. (1974). *Proc. Natl. Acad. Sci. U.S.A.* **69,** 2456.
Gee, A. P., Bruce, K. M., van Hilten, J., Siden, E. J., Braylan, R. C., Bauer, P. C., and Boyle, M. D. P. (1987). *J. Natl. Cancer Inst.* **78,** 29–35.
Hoyer, L. W., Borsos, T., Rapp, H. J., and Vannier, W. E. (1968). *J. Exp. Med.* **127,** 589–603.
Jones, N. H., Borowitz, M. J., and Metzgar, R. S. (1982). *Leuk. Res.* **6,** 449–464.
Kaneene, J. J. M., Anderson, R. K., Johnson, D. W., and Muscoplat, C. C. (1978). *Infect. Immun.* **22,** 486–491.
Langone, J. J. (1978). *J. Immunol. Methods* **24,** 269–285.
Langone, J. J., Boyle, M. D. P., and Borsos, T. (1977). *J. Immunol. Methods* **18,** 281–293.
Lawman, M. J. P., Thurmond, M. C., Reis, K. J., Gaunlett, D. R., and Boyle, M. D. P. (1984). *Vet. Immunol. Immunopathol.* **6,** 291–305.
Lawman, M. J. P., Ball, D. R., Hoffman, E. M., Des Jardin, L. E., and Boyle, M. D. P. (1986). *Vet. Microbiol.* **12,** 43–53.
Rapp, H. J., and Borsos, T. (1970). "Molecular Basis of Complement Action." Appleton (Century-Crofts), New York.
Taylor, R. B., Duffus, W. P. H., and de Petris, S. (1971). *Nature* (*London*) *New Biol.* **223,** 225.
Unanue, E. R., Karnovsky, M. J., and Engers, H. D. (1973). *J. Med.* **137,** 675.

CHAPTER **11**

Use of fluorescent-conjugated bacterial immunoglobulin-binding proteins

Stephen N. Sisson

I. Standand Methods

A. Commonly Used Linkers

There are a variety of fluorescent dyes that are used for labeling proteins, mainly antibodies (Coons and Kaplan, 1950). The most popular dye is fluorescein isothiocyanate (FITC), which is a derivative of fluorescein. This is a green fluorescing dye introduced by Riggs *et al.* in 1958, which introduces a linkage to proteins via a thiocarbamide bond.

Another commonly used dye is the rhodamine derivative, tetramethylrhodamine isothiocyanate (TRITC). The rhodamine derivative fluoresces a red to orange color and is valuable in conjunction with fluorescein when counterstaining or double-staining the same sample or preparation. There are two other fluorochromes that have been developed recently and which are useful in double-staining; these are XRITC (5 and 6 carboxyxrhodamine isothiocyanate) and Texas Red. They are useful because their emission spectra are longer in wavelength than the emission spectrum of TRITC.

Another set of fluorescent dyes currently in use are the phycobiliproteins (Oi *et al.*, 1982), which are naturally occurring fluorescent proteins that are found in algae. The main groups of phycobiliproteins are R-phycoerythrin from red algae, allophycocyanin from cyanobacteria, and phycocyanins. These contain alpha, beta, and gamma polypeptide subunits with tetrapyrrole chromophores attached and these chromophores can be excited over a wide range of wavelengths. Another advantage of using the phycoerythrins is that the color does not fade or bleach as quickly as the fluorescein or rhodamine dyes. In some cases this may be very important. Still another advantage is that nonspecific binding, under the same conditions, is generally much lower than with FITC or TRITC. This may be due to the fact that these proteins do not have a highly negative charge, as is the case with the fluoresceins. These phycobiliproteins are also useful in flow cytometry, as shown by Parks and Herzen-berg (1984).

Conjugation of FITC or TRITC to a bacterial immunoglobulin-binding protein, such as protein G, can be accomplished very easily in the laboratory. A good fluorescent/protein (F/P) ratio can be obtained and the separation of free from bound fluorochrome can be achieved by gel chromatography with Sephadex G-25. A frequent problem with protein G and other bacterial immunoglobulin-binding proteins is that they can lose their ability to bind to the Fc portion of the IgG molecule following labeling by certain conjugation methods. One of the ways to overcome this problem is to use a fluorescein- or rhodamine-labeled protein that has a spacer between the protein G and the fluorochrome. A set of fluorescein and rhodamine dyes that contain spacers can be obtained from Research Organics, Inc. (Cleveland, Ohio).

Another method involves the use of a protein G that has been biotinylated (Calbiochem, La Jolla, California) and a streptavidin tracer that has been conjugated to the fluorochrome. It should be noted that streptavidin (from *Streptomyces avidinii*) is preferred over avidin because streptavidin has a higher affinity for biotin and a much lower isoelectric point. Consequently, the background nonspecific binding of streptavidin conjugates is lower then the corresponding avidin tracers.

When conjugating phycoerythrins, a linker that has given good results is GMBS (N-γ-Maleimidobutyryloxy-succinimide ester).

The selectivity of the conjugation can be controlled using different pH conditions that will form reactivity with either the maleimide or the N-hydroxy-succinimide ester with thiol groups or amino groups, respectively, on the protein. GMBS may be obtained from Calbiochem (La Jolla, California).

B. Determination of Fluorescence/Protein Ratios

When preparing and using fluorochromes on protein G and probing for IgG either directly (immobilized IgG as target), or by indirect assay (immobilized antigen to which IgG becomes complexed and then protein G binds to the complex), the F/P ratio is one of the most important parameters that will influence the performance of the fluorescent probes. If the molar ratio of fluorochrome to protein G is low (less than 2), there may be competition by the unconjugated protein G and the intensity of the protein G fluorescence will be low. If the molar ratio is too high (greater than 5), there may be a loss of functional activity of the protein G because of steric hinderance. When rhodamine is the fluorochrome, self-quenching can also be a problem. In the case of rhodamine, it is more difficult to determine the exact F/P ratio because of its absorption spectrum with the peak increase at 515 nm (Goding, 1983).

The problem is reversed with phycoerythrins. In this system, the question becomes how many protein G molecules should be attached to each phycoerythrin molecule. The molecular weight of phycoerythrin is between 240,000 and 260,000, while the molecular weight for protein G is approximately 54,000 for the wild type protein (Boyle and Reis, 1987) and 32,000 (Fahnestock et al., 1986) for the recombinant type. A ratio that works well and gives a very low background is two protein G molecules to one phycoerythrin.

The formula derived by The and Feltkemp (1970) can be was used to determine the F/P ratio for FITC:

$$\text{F/P ratio} = \frac{2.87 \times OD_{495}}{OD_{280} - 0.35 \times OD_{495}}$$

The conjugation procedures using FITC and TRITC are straightforward and well documented (Coons and Kaplan, 1950; Riggs et al., 1958; Parks and Herzen-berg, 1984; Goding, 1983; Wood et al., 1965) and will not be discussed here. The F/P ratio for each of these derivatives can be calculated from the formula above using the optical density (OD) at an appropriate wavelength for the fluorescent label employed.

II. Conjugation Method Using GMBS

The example given is the conjugation of protein G (wild type M_r approximately 54,000) to a phycoerythrin (M_r 240,000, obtained from BioMeda (Foster City, California). GMBS (Calbiochem, La Jolla, California) is a heterobifunctional linker that contains a seven-atom spacer. It contains a maleimide group at one end that will attach to the sulfhydryl group of a cysteine amino acid, and an N-hydroxysuccinimide ester at the other end that will attach to the amino group of a lysine amino acid. This linker can be used to modify protein G without loss of its immunoglobulin-binding activity.

A. Conjugation Protocol

The first step is to attach the GMBS to protein G. This is accomplished by dissolving 5 mg protein G in 0.5 ml 50 mM NaHCO$_3$ buffer, pH 8.5, in a small reaction vial that is protected from light. Dissolve 1.2 mg GMBS in a minimum volume of dimethyl sulfoxide (DMSO). Add the GMBS in small portions at room temperature to the protein G solution while stirring slowly over a period of one hour. When the last portion has been added, stir the reaction for one additional hour. On a G-25 column (~15 ml) (foil-covered), pre-equilibrated with phosphate-buffered saline (PBS), pH 6.0, load the protein G–GMBS mixture, elute the column with the same buffer and collect 1 ml fractions. The protein G–GMBS conjugate will elute in the void volume. This volume will be approximately 4 ml. The free GMBS will be retarded and will elute from the column much later. Monitor the protein G by measurement of the OD$_{280}$ spectrophotometrically. Pool the fractions containing the peak OD$_{280}$.

Make a solution (48 mg/5 ml) of the phycoerythrin (PE) in PBS, pH 6.0. While the phycoerythrin solution is stirring, slowly add the protein G–GMBS dropwise into the vortex of the PE solution. After all of the protein G–GMBS has been added, let the reaction continue to stir overnight, with protection from light.

B. Chromatography

If the reaction has gone to completion, there should be approximately two protein G molecules on every phycoerythrin, but in practice this ratio will not be achieved. A second chromatographic step will have to be performed to separate residual, free phycoerythrin from the protein G-bound PE. The free PE has an M_r of 240,000 and the two protein G–PE mixture has a molecular weight of approximately 340,000. A good gel for this separation is the Sepharose S-300 (Pharmacia, Sweden).

Degas and pre-equilibrate the gel in PBS, pH 7.4, and pour into a 1 × 60 cm column. Since the phycoerythrin is light-sensitive, it is best to wrap the column with foil and keep exposure of the sample to light to a minimum. Apply the sample to the column, elute with PBS, and collect 1 ml fractions. The phycoerythrin is a bright pink color and this property makes it easy to determine when the conjugate is eluting from the column. The protein G-bound PE will elute in the void volume, and the free phycoerythrin will be retarded on the column. The fractions containing PE–protein G conjugate are kept separate at this point. After each fraction has been tested for protein G activity using a suitable assay, high, specific activity fractions can be pooled. Remember to keep the conjugate protected from light throughout the entire process.

C. Functional Assay System

A suitable standard assay system is the AFT^R kit (Behring Diagnostics, Inc., Sommerville, New Jersey), which contains slides with fixed HEP-2 cells and are designed for ANA (anti-nuclear antibodies) detection. The kit provides a positive and a negative control. By the use of the fluorescein-conjugated antibody in the kit, one is able to establish the dilution at which the conjugate provides the best signal to noise ratio. This is dependent both on the intensity of the positive sample and the low background staining of a negative sample.

III. Comparison of Recombinant Protein G to Wild Type Protein G Isolated from *Streptococcus* Cell Membranes

A. Fluorescence/Protein Ratios

Two forms of bacterial Type III Fc-binding protein G are commercially available from Calbiochem (La Jolla, California). One is a wild type protein, isolated from streptococcal cell membranes and has an M_r of approximately 54,000. The other is a recombinant product, which has an M_r of approximately 32,000. Because of the larger molecular weight, it is possible to obtain higher fluorescence/protein (F/P) ratios (up to about 3.5) with the wild type protein when using fluorescein or rhodamine derivatives. With the recombinant form, an F/P ratio of about 1.5 is obtainable. When the fluorescein conjugates are compared side by side in the AFT^R system, the wild type has a working dilution of 1:50 along with good intensity and low background. The recombinant however, even without dilution, is not as intense and the background not as low. Under these conditions, the wild type protein G conjugate also seems to perform much better as a probe for human IgG.

B. Functional Testing

The protein G–fluorochrome conjugates could be useful in a wide variety of analytical systems. They work well in the system described earlier with human IgG, and should also work well as probes for rabbit IgG, goat IgG, or mouse IgG. This is a very versatile probe, which can replace secondary antibodies conjugated to fluorescein in many immunofluorescent assays. If more than one species of IgG is used as a primary antibody in the same laboratory, then the protein G–X–fluorescein may be the probe of choice in these systems.

C. Background and Albumin Binding

Nonspecific binding by a fluorochrome may make it difficult, if not impossible, to read the intended target. It is important to establish an optimal working dilution. This is the dilution that gives a maximum ratio of target signal intensity to background signal intensity. A technique used to reduce background, which works well with the π-electron-rich fluorescein conjugate, is the anionic detergent SDS (sodium dodecyl sulfate). The presence of 0.02% SDS on the slide prior to and during the use of the fluorescein–X–protein G probe improves the signal detection and sensitivity when used at the same working dilution as fluorescein–X–protein G without SDS. If more than 0.02% SDS is used, the solution may wash fixed cells from the slide.

Wild type protein G has a portion at its amino terminus that will bind to human serum albumin. This portion can be advantageous when increasing the F/P ratio of protein G. This is a segment of the molecule where a chromophore may attach and not interfere with IgG Fc-binding properties. There appears to be no interference in the system when using the AFT[R] HEP-2 cells and the human control sera, both positive and negative, which contain high concentrations of albumin. However, there may be systems where the human serum albumin-binding portion of the wild type protein G could cause interference. The addition of a low concentration of human serum albumin to the buffers would minimize this background without influencing the ability of protein G to bind to immunoglobulin.

References

Boyle, M. D. P., and Reis, K. J. (1987). *Biotechnology* **7,** 697.
Coons, A. H., and Kaplan, M. H. (1950). *J. Exp. Med.* **91,** 1.
Fahnestock, S. R. and Fisher, K. E. (1986). *J. Bacteriol.* **167,** 870.
Goding, J. W. (1983). "Monoclonal Antibodies: Principles and Practice." Academic Press, New York.
Oi, V. T., Glazer, A. N., and Stryer, L. J. (1982). *J. Cell Biol.* **93,** 981.
Parks, D. R., and Herzen-berg, L. A. (1984). [19] *In* "Methods in Enzymology" (G. Di Sabato, J. J. Langone, and H. van Vukakis, eds.), Vol. 108. 19
Riggs, J. L., Seiwald, R. J., Burekhalter, J. H., Downes, C. M., and Metcalf, T. G. (1958). *Am. J. Pathol.* **34,** 1081–1098.
The, T. H., and Feltkemp, T. E. W. (1970). *Immunology* **18,** 865–881.
Wood, B. T., Thompson, S. H., and Goldstein, G. (1965). *J. Immunol.* **95,** 225.

CHAPTER 12

Biotinylated IgG-binding proteins—doubly versatile

Laurence J. McIntyre

I. Introduction

The main advantage in using labeled bacterial IgG-binding proteins for the detection of immunoglobulin is the fact that they bind to a variety of different types of immunoglobulin. The use of biotin as the means of labeling the IgG-binding protein extends this versatility to the detection system by permitting the use of a wide range of enzyme-based, fluorescent, or radioactive methods. The biotin/avidin detection system is based on the observations that proteins are easily and gently, covalently labeled with biotin, a small vitamin molecule, and that biotin binds almost irreversibly at up to four sites on avidin, a protein isolated from egg white. Avidin, in turn, can be labeled directly with enzymes, fluorescent molecules, or a radioisotope, or can be detected in its unlabeled form using a biotin-labeled enzyme (Wilchek and Bayer, 1988). In this way, one biotinylated IgG-binding protein can be used to detect a number of different primary antibodies and a number of different avidin labels can be used as reporter molecules. In immunohistochemistry, this versatility has to be balanced against two main drawbacks of the use of IgG-binding proteins. One is that, in certain systems, they are not as sensitive as the corresponding secondary antibody (Hsu *et al.*, 1981a; Lanzillo and Fanburg, 1982) and the second is that binding to endogenous IgG in the tissue sections can lead to high background and masking of positive staining (Hsu *et al.*, 1981a).

The most commonly used biotin/avidin detection system in immunohistochemistry is the Avidin Biotin Complex (ABC) method described by Hsu *et al.* (1981b,c). In this technique, biotinylated molecules are detected by their interaction with a preformed complex of avidin and biotinylated horseradish peroxidase, followed by incubation with a peroxidase substrate. The multivalency of both molecules produces a complex containing numerous enzyme molecules and this leads to the high sensitivity of the ABC method. Many examples of the use of biotinylated IgG-binding proteins in immunohistochemistry have employed the ABC method and biotinylated protein A. In one of the first studies of biotinylated protein A in immunohistochemistry, a detailed comparison was made of the sensitivity of a number of different staining methods on formalin-fixed, paraffin-embedded sections of tonsil, skin, and thyroid tissue using rabbit anti-human IgG as the primary antibody (Hsu et al., 1981a). The lower sensitivity of biotinylated protein A compared to the biotinylated secondary antibody mentioned previously was ascribed to the fact that the biotinylated protein A reacts with the primary antibody at a 1:1 ratio, while the biotinylated secondary antibody reacts with the primary antibody at multiple antigenic sites. Another possibility is that the difference in size between biotinylated protein A and biotinylated secondary antibody permits access of more ABC complexes to the biotin groups in the latter instance. A second use of biotinylated protein A was also described in this study, where an unlabeled, swine anti-rabbit secondary antibody was used, followed by biotinylated protein A and ABC complex. This gave a staining intensity similar to that obtained with biotinylated secondary antibody but with a higher background staining. The authors also found that preincubation of the biotinylated protein A with 10 μg/ml of mouse liver powder for 15 min before use and blocking of the sections with 100 μg/ml mouse liver powder reduced the background staining.

Biotinylated protein A and the ABC technique were also used to localize S-100 protein and carcinoembryonic antigen (CEA) in sections of paraffin-embedded skin using rabbit primary antibodies (Schaumberg-Lever, 1986). They have been used to detect neutral metalloendopeptidase in prostate and kidney (Erdos et al., 1985), growth hormone-releasing factor in hypothalamus (De Gennaro et al., 1986), and ubiquitin in the brain following cerebral ischemia (Magnusson and Wieloch, 1989). Brain and spinal cord were the tissues studied in a series of experiments to localize peptide hormones and structural proteins using biotinylated protein A and the ABC technique (Zang et al., 1985; Xu and Nilaver, 1986; Vandenbark et al., 1986; Friedman et al., 1986; Loftus et al., 1986; Bodnar et al., 1986; Sloviter and Nilaver, 1987). Both vibratome sections and sections of paraffin-embedded tissue were used in these experiments and Triton X-100 was added to the buffers used with the vibratome sections in order to facilitate penetration of the reagents. The primary antisera used were rabbit antibodies to glial fibrillary acidic protein (Zang et al., 1985; Xu and Nilaver, 1986; Vandenbark et al., 1986; Friedman et al., 1986), myelin basic protein (Vandenbark et al., 1986; Friedman et al., 1986), neurofilament protein (Friedman *et al.*, 1986), motilin, growth hormone and prolactin (Loftus *et al.*, 1986), vasopressin (Bodnar *et al.*, 1986), gamma amino butyric acid, somatostatin, vasoactive intestinal polypeptide, and cholecystokinin (Sloviter and Nilaver, 1987). The same immunohistochemical technique was also used in a series of experiments concerned with the proteins involved in vitamin D-dependent calcium metabolism (Zhou *et al.*, 1986; Craviso *et al.*, 1987; Sloviter, 1989; Clemens *et al.*, 1988). Calcium-binding protein was localized in frozen and vibratome sections of bone (Zhou *et al.*, 1986), in cultured kidney cells (Craviso *et al.*, 1987), and along with parvalbumin, in brain tissue (Sloviter, 1989). In most experiments using the ABC technique, the peroxidase substrate used was diaminobenzidine tetrahydrochloride (DAB), but in the study of calcium-binding protein in brain, the use of benzidine dihydrochloride as a substrate revealed a novel localization of the antigen (Sloviter, 1989). Biotinylated protein A and the ABC technique were used to identify the 1,25-dihydroxyvitamin D3 receptor in cultured bone cells, osteogenic sarcoma cells, intestine, liver, and brain tissue (Clemens *et al.*, 1988). One interesting aspect of this experiment was that the primary antibody was a rat monoclonal antibody and it was detected by sequential incubations with biotinylated rabbit anti-rat IgG, biotinylated protein A, and then the ABC complex. In this way, the biotinylated protein A was used to amplify the binding of a biotinylated secondary antibody. Biotinylated protein A and the ABC technique have also been used to overcome nonspecific binding problems with the rabbit peroxidase–antiperoxidase method. Rabbit immunoglobulins bind to particular areas of the pig hypothalamus (Meijer *et al.*, 1986) and therefore, localization of luteinizing hormone-releasing hormone in that tissue was carried out using a swine primary antibody and biotinylated protein A (Meijer *et al.*, 1986).

A very different use of biotinylated IgG-binding proteins in immunohistochemistry is the technique of radioimmunocytochemistry using biotinylated protein A, avidin, and tritiated biotin (Hunt and Mantyh, 1984). Sections of brain tissue were incubated with rabbit antibodies to substance P, enkephalin, pancreatic polypeptide, tyrosine hydroxylase, or somatostatin and the sections were then incubated with biotinylated protein A. The sections were finally incubated with a premixed solution of avidin and tritiated biotin and the radioactivity was localized either by dipping in nuclear emulsion or by exposure to tritium-sensitive film. As a control, some sections were incubated with a conjugate of avidin and horseradish peroxidase instead of the avidin-tritiated biotin complex and the antigen was localized with peroxidase substrate. One advantage of this technique is that the tritium-sensitive film can be analyzed by computer-controlled densitometry. A double-labeling technique was also described in which the first primary antibody is localized using biotinylated protein A and avidin–

peroxidase. After developing the colored precipitate, the section is incubated with unlabeled protein A, fixed again, and then the second primary antibody is applied and detected using biotinylated protein A and the avidin/tritiated biotin complex.

The research just described demonstrates that biotinylated IgG-binding proteins can be used in a wide variety of immunohistochemical staining systems in terms of tissue type, fixation, and embedding techniques. The next section will provide more detailed methodology for the labeling and use of biotinylated IgG-binding proteins in standard immunohistochemical staining and these should provide an adequate basis for use in more specialized situations.

II. Biotinylation of IgG-Binding Protein

Biotinylated protein A can be purchased from a number of manufacturers, particularly those specializing in biotin/avidin reagents. This section will describe the biotinylation of a different IgG-binding protein, where the labeled form of the protein is not so readily available, protein G from *Streptococcus* species (Boyle and Reis, 1987). The method can be easily adapted for the biotinylation of protein A or other IgG-binding proteins. A considerable number of reactive derivatives of the biotin molecule have been prepared (Wilchek and Bayer, 1988) and one of the best for labeling proteins is Biotin (Long Arm) NHS or BNHS, which has the chemical structure: N-hydroxysuccinimidyl 6-(biotinamido) hexanoate. BNHS reacts with amino groups on proteins. This reagent is prepared by dissolving BNHS in N,N-dimethylformamide or dimethyl sulfoxide at 25–50 mg/ml. It may be necessary to warm the solution slightly to completely dissolve the BNHS. The reagent should be made up just prior to use and slightly more than is needed should be prepared to permit accurate dispensing. Protein G is dissolved in 100 mM N-2-hydroxyethyl-piperazine-N'-2-ethanesulfonic acid (HEPES) or sodium bicarbonate buffer, pH 8.5, at a concentration of 2–10 mg/ml. An aliquot of the BNHS reagent, sufficient to give a final ratio of 1 : 10 by weight of BNHS to protein G, is added and incubated at room temperature for 2 hr with occasional stirring. The reaction is stopped by the addition of 10 mg of glycine or 5 μl of ethanolamine per milligram BNHS used. The biotinylated protein is then dialyzed against three changes of at least 2 liters of buffer to remove unreacted or hydrolyzed BNHS. The BNHS can also be removed by gel filtration.

A. Assay for Percentage of Biotinylation

In most cases, about 95% of the protein G molecules will be labeled with biotin by the method just described. To ensure that this is the case, an aliquot of the biotinylated protein G can be taken, after removal of any free biotin derivatives, and passed through a small column of agarose-bound Avidin D. By measuring the amount of protein G passing through the column, the percentage of the biotinylated protein G preparation capable of binding avidin (i.e., percentage of biotinylation) can be determined. This is done by placing a small plug of fine glass wool in a pasteur pipet and adding 2 ml of a 1:1 slurry of agarose–Avidin D. The column is then washed with four to five column volumes of phosphate-buffered saline (PBS) or until the optical density at 280 nm (OD_{280}) of the effluent equals that of PBS. An aliquot of biotinylated protein G, sufficient to give a final OD_{280} of around 0.15, is added to 1 ml of PBS (solution B). An identical aliquot of the biotinylated protein G is loaded onto the column and washed by gravity with 1 ml PBS. The effluent during loading and washing is collected in the same tube (solution A). The OD_{280} of both solution A and solution B is then measured and the percentage of biotinylation is calculated as follows:

$$\text{percentage of biotinylation} = \frac{OD_{280} \text{ solution B} - OD_{280} \text{ solution A}}{OD_{280} \text{ solution B}} \times 100$$

III. Immunohistochemical Staining Using Biotinylated IgG-Binding Proteins

As previously mentioned, the most commonly used immunohistochemical detection system for biotinylated IgG-binding proteins is the ABC method. Because the biotinylated IgG-binding proteins are not as sensitive as the corresponding biotinylated secondary antibodies, better results can be obtained using a more sensitive ABC system, the VECTASTAIN® *Elite* ABC Kit, and this is the method that will be described in this section, using routinely processed, formalin-fixed, paraffin-embedded tissue sections. The VECTASTAIN® *Elite* ABC (Vector Laboratories, Inc. Burlingame, California) reagent should be prepared 30 min before use by adding 2 drops of reagent A to 5 ml of PBS, followed by 2 drops of reagent B to the same solution and mixing immediately. The immunohistochemical staining procedure is as follows:

1. Deparaffinize and hydrate the tissue sections through xylene or other clearing agents and a graded alcohol series.
2. Rinse for 5 min in distilled water.
3. If quenching of endogenous peroxidase activity is required, incubate the sections for 30 min in 0.3% hydrogen peroxide (H_2O_2) in methanol.

4. Wash in PBS for 20 min.
5. Incubate sections for 20 min in blocking solution. Suitable blocking solutions include 2% normal chicken serum in PBS or 1–5 mg/ml crystalline grade bovine serum albumin in PBS. Any normal serum used in blocking solutions should be one with which the IgG-binding protein does not cross-react.
6. Blot excess blocking solution from sections.
7. Incubate sections for 30 min with primary antiserum diluted in blocking solution.
8. Wash slides for 10 min in PBS.
9. Incubate sections for 30 min with biotinylated IgG-binding protein diluted to 5 μg/ml in blocking solution.
10. Wash slides for 10 min in PBS.
11. Incubate sections for 30 min with VECTASTAIN® *Elite* ABC reagent.

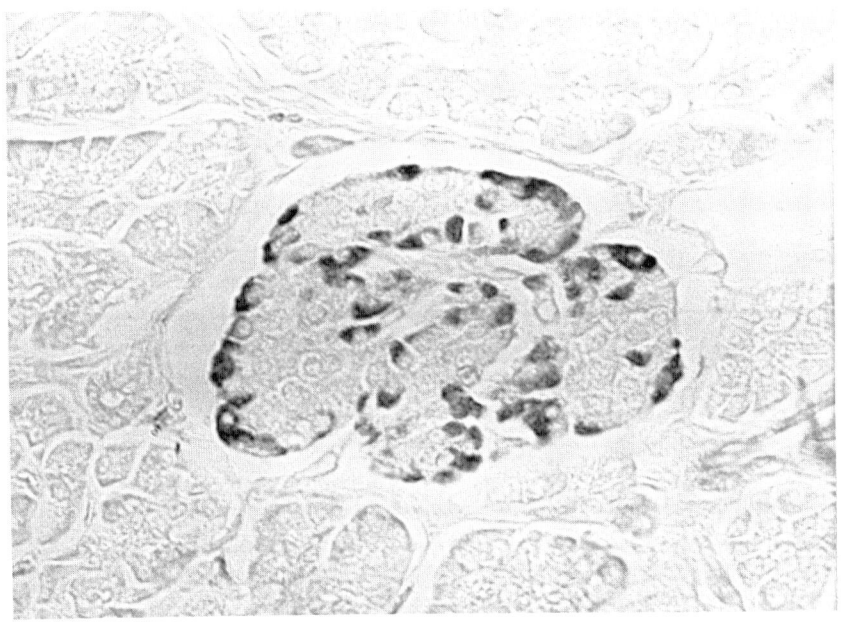

FIGURE 1
Formalin-fixed, paraffin-embedded human pancreas stained with rabbit anti-glucagon and detected with biotinylated protein G, followed by VECTASTAIN® ABC reagent and DAB ($\times$256).

Chapter 12. Biotinylated IgG-Binding Proteins 211

12. Wash slides for 10 min in PBS.
13. Incubate sections for 2–7 min in peroxidase substrate solution, which is prepared by mixing together an equal volume of 0.02% hydrogen peroxide (made in distilled water from a 30% stock) and 0.1% (1 mg/ml) diaminobenzidine tetrahydrochloride (DAB) made in 0.1 M Tris buffer, pH 7.2. The substrate solution should be prepared just prior to use.
14. Wash sections for 5 min in tap water.
15. Counterstain, clean, and mount.

This protocol provides a basis from which many different biotin/avidin immunohistochemical techniques can be derived by further experimentation. Different substrates such as 3-amino-9-ethylcarbazole or DAB/nickel can be used for the peroxidase enzyme. Other enzymes such as alkaline phosphatase or glucose oxidase can be used in the

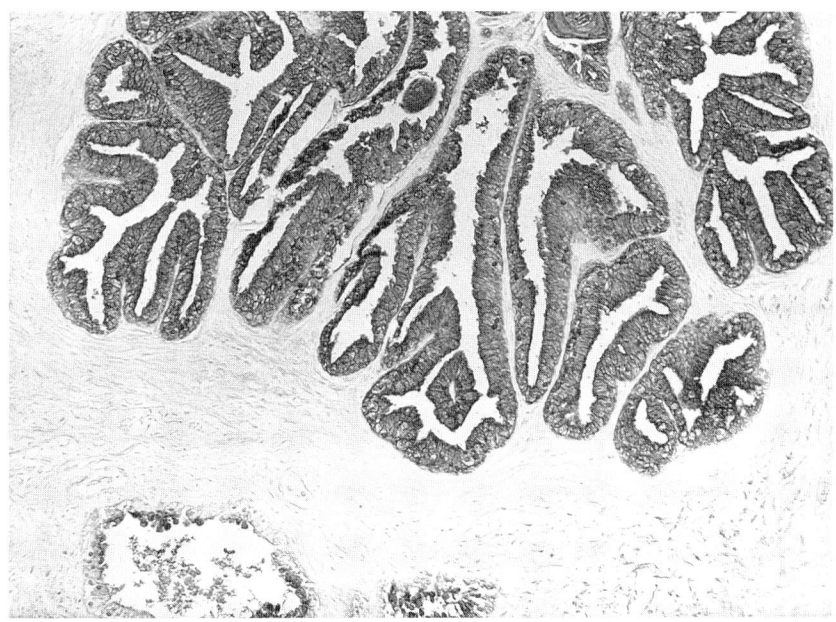

FIGURE 2
Formalin-fixed, paraffin-embedded human prostate tissue stained with rabbit anti-prostate specific antigen, biotinylated protein G, and VECTASTAIN® *Elite* ABC reagent. The peroxidase substrate was DAB (×64).

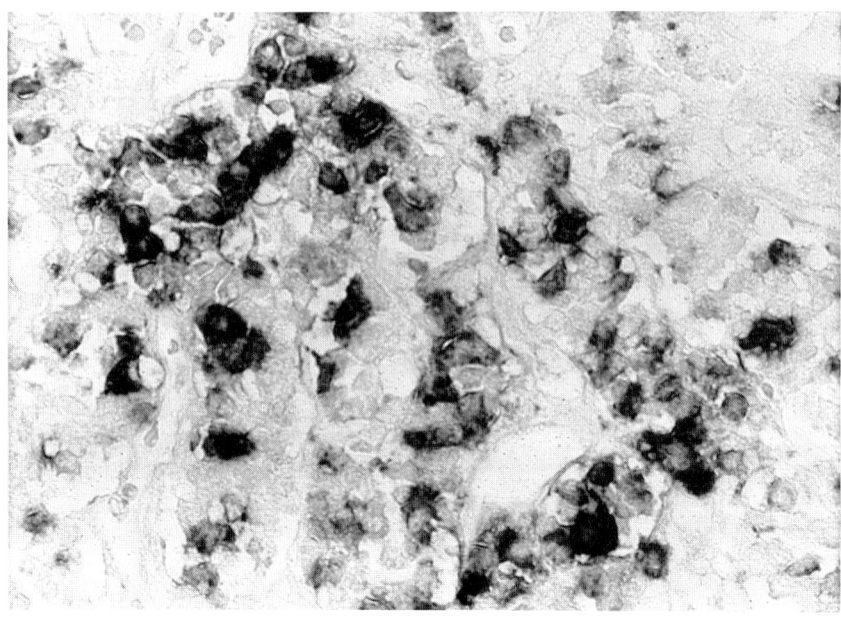

FIGURE 3
Formalin-fixed, paraffin-embedded human pituitary stained with rabbit anti-luteinizing hormone followed by biotinylated protein A and VECTASTAIN® ABC-AP reagent, a preformed complex containing biotinylated alkaline phosphatase. The enzyme was detected using Alkaline Phosphatase Substrate Kit II (×256).

VECTASTAIN® ABC Kit or conjugates of avidin or streptavidin with enzymes can be substituted in the detection step. With avidin–enzyme conjugates, a suitable concentration range would be 1–5 µg/ml. When fluorescent avidin derivatives such as fluorescein–Avidin D, AMCA–Avidin D, or Texas Red–Avidin D are used, a suitable working dilution would be approximately 20 µg/ml. As with all immunohistochemical systems, the optimal reagents, concentrations, and incubation conditions will have to be determined by experimentation in each particular situation. Representative examples of the staining that can be obtained using biotinylated IgG-binding proteins are shown in Figures 1–5.

In addition to being used in immunohistochemical staining techniques, biotinylated IgG-binding proteins have also been utilized in methods that will be covered in greater detail in other chapters. Biotinylated protein A has been used in enzyme immunoassay systems to measure human serum angiotensin-1-converting enzyme (Lanzillo and Fanburg, 1982), antibodies

Chapter 12. Biotinylated IgG-Binding Proteins

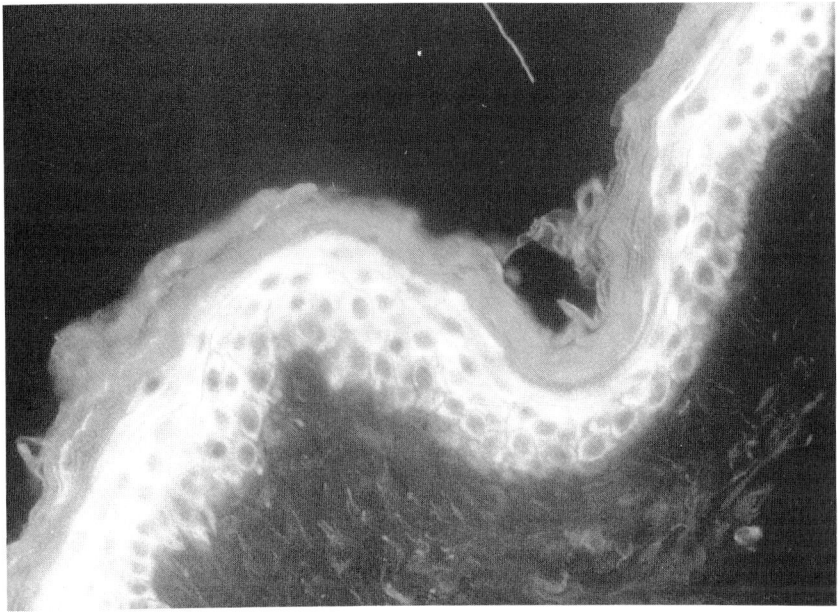

FIGURE 4
Methacarn-fixed, paraffin-embedded human skin stained with rabbit anti-keratin and detected with biotinylated protein A followed by Texas Red–Avidin D (×256).

to Japanese encephalitis virus (Chang *et al.*, 1984), *Taenia solium* cysticerci (Larralde *et al.*, 1986), and herpes simplex virus (Katz *et al.*, 1986). A recently developed assay for hog cholera virus combines enzyme immunoassay and immunohistochemistry by using biotinylated protein A and a horseradish peroxidase–Avidin D conjugate to stain virus-infected cells cultured in microtiter plates (Afshar *et al.*, 1989). Biotinylated protein A has also been use in Western blots of *Taenia solium* cysticerci (Larralde *et al.*, 1986), skeletal myosin (Katayama *et al.*, 1984), alpha-actinin (Mabuchi *et al.*, 1985), and molecular weight marker proteins (Conter *et al.*, 1986). The last example describes a useful technique for accurately locating molecular weight markers on Western blots using antibodies to the marker proteins.

These final examples of the use of biotinylated IgG-binding proteins once more emphasize the double versatility of such reagents, as they can bind to immunoglobulins from a wide variety of species and they can serve as link proteins to a large number of biotin/avidin detection systems.

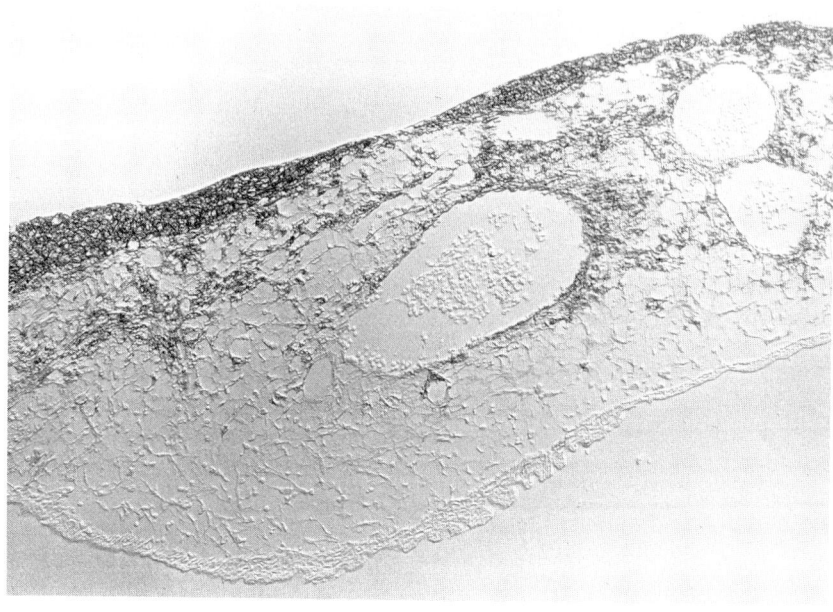

FIGURE 5
Formalin-fixed, paraffin-embedded chorioallantoic membrane infected with vaccinia virus and stained with rabbit anti-vaccinia virus. The primary antibody was detected using biotinylated protein A, VECTASTAIN® *Elite* ABC Reagent, and DAB (×64).

Acknowledgments

I would like to thank all of the scientific staff at Vector Laboratories, Inc. who developed the protocols on which this article is based.

References

Afshar, A., Dulac, G. C., and Bouffard, A. (1989). *J. Virol. Methods* **23,** 253–262.
Bodnar, R. J., Truesdell, L. S., Haldar, J., Aral, I. A., Kordower, J. H., and Nilaver, G. (1986). *Peptides* **7,** 111–117.
Boyle, M. D. P., and Reis, K. J. (1987). *Biotechnology* **5,** 697–703.
Chang, H.-C., Takashima, I., Arikawa, J., and Hashimoto, N. (1984). *J. Virol. Methods* **9,** 143–151.
Clemens, T. L., Garrett, K. P., Zhou, X.-Y., Pike, J. W., Haussler, M. R., and Dempster, D. W. (1988). *Endocrinology* **122,** 1224–1230.
Confer, A. W., Durham, J. A., and Simons, K. R. (1986). *J. Immunol. Methods* **93,** 285–286.
Craviso, G. L., Garrett, K. P., and Clemens, T. L. (1987). *Endocrinology* **120,** 894–902.

De Gennaro, V., Redaelli, M., Locatelli, V., Cella, S. G., Fumagalli, G., Wehrenberg, W. B., and Muller, E. E. (1986). *Neuroendocrinology* **44,** 59–64.
Erdos, E. G., Schulz, W. W., Gafford, J. T., and Defendini, R. (1985). *Lab. Invest.* **52,** 437–447.
Friedman, E., Nilaver, G., Carmel, P., Perlow, M., Spatz, L., and Latov, N. (1986). *Brain Res.* **378,** 142–146.
Hsu, S.-M., and Raine, L. (1981a). *J. Histochem. Cytochem.* **29,** 1349–1353.
Hsu, S.-M., Raine, L., and Fanger, H. (1981b). *Am. J. Clin. Pathol.* **75,** 734–738.
Hsu, S.-M., Raine, L., and Fanger, H. (1981c). *J. Histochem. Cytochem.* **29,** 577–580.
Hunt, S. P., and Mantyh, P. W. (1984). *Brain Res.* **291,** 203–217.
Katayama, E., Wakabayashi, T., Reinach, F., Masaki, T., and Fischman, D. A. (1984). *J. Biochem.* **95,** 721–727.
Katz, D., Hilliard, J. K., Eberle, R., and Lipper, S. L. (1986). *J. Virol. Methods* **14,** 99–109.
Lanzillo, J. J., and Fanburg, B. L. (1982). *Anal. Biochem.* **126,** 156–164.
Larralde, C., Laclette, J. P., Owen, C. S., Madrazo, I., Sandoval, M., Bojalil, R., Sciutto, E., Contreras, L., Arzate, J., Diaz, M. L., Govezensky, T., Montoya, R., and Goodsaid, F. (1986). *Am. J. Trop. Med. Hyg.* **35,** 965–973.
Loftus, C. M., Nilaver, G., Beinfeld, M. C., and Post, K. D. (1986). *Neurosurgery* **19,** 201–204.
Mabuchi, I., Hamaguchi, Y., Kobayashi, T., Hosoya, H., Tsukita, S., and Tsukita, S. (1985). *J. Cell Biol.* **100,** 375–383.
Magnusson, K., and Wieloch, T. (1989). *Neurosci. Lett.* **96,** 264–270.
Meijer, J., Poot, P., Molenaar, G., and Goede, R. (1986). *J. Neurosci. Methods* **17,** 269–274.
Schaumberg-Lever, G. (1986). *Int. J. Dermatol.* **25,** 217–223.
Sloviter, R. S. (1989). *J. Comp. Neurol.* **280,** 183–196.
Sloviter, R. S., and Nilaver, G. (1987). *J. Comp. Neurol.* **256,** 42–60.
Vandenbark, A. A., Nilaver, G., Konat, G., Teal, P., and Offner, H. (1986). *J. Neurosci. Res.* **16,** 643–656.
Wilchek, M. and Bayer, E. A. (1988). *Anal. Biochem.* **171,** 1–32.
Xu, Z. and Nilaver, G. (1986). *Chin. Med. J.* **99,** 708–712.
Zang, X., Nilaver, G., Stein, B. M., Fetell, M. R., and Duffy, P. E. (1985). *J. Neuropathol. Exp. Neurol.* **44,** 486–495.
Zhou, X. Y., Dempster, D. W., Marion, S. L., Pike, J. W., Hausler, M. R., and Clemens, T. L. (1986). *Calcif. Tissue Int.* **38,** 244–247.

CHAPTER **13**

Use of IgG-binding proteins in immunoelectronmicroscopy

Sylvia E. Coleman

I. Introduction

Colloidal gold has been used extensively as a tracer in transmission electronmicroscopy since about 1975, although seventeenth century alchemists were familiar with colloidal gold and preparative methods were described by Faraday in 1857 (Smit and Todd, 1986). Colloidal gold is now widely used for localizing antigenic sites via gold-labeled antibodies and for labeling proteins for detection of receptor sites. The electron opacity and range of sizes in which colloidal gold may be prepared make it particularly useful for ultrastructural studies with the electron microscope. The ability to enhance gold particles and to conjugate them to such useful systems as proteins A and G and biotin–avidin add to their usefulness as structural markers.

II. Preparation of Colloidal Gold

Colloidal gold particles of various sizes are remarkably easy to produce and consistency in size is good. Gold colloids can be made in almost any laboratory. A technique for making gold colloidal particles by reducing tetrachloroauric acid with 1% sodium citrate was introduced by Frens in 1973 and is still widely used. Larger particles of 15–20 nm are the easiest to make and the most consistent in size. Smaller particles of 5 nm are more complicated to produce and require an ultracentrifuge for concentration of the colloid.

Commercial sources of gold colloids are available, but these are considerably more expensive than ones made in the laboratory and the quantity is more limited. There are also commercial sources of many gold conjugates such as antibodies, protein A, and avidin.

A. Glassware and Solutions

Glassware used for the production of colloidal gold should be scrupulously clean including graduate cylinders, beakers, and bottles used for storing distilled water and gold colloids. A good detergent such as F1-70 (Fisher, Pittsburg, Pennsylvania) should be used in about a 2% solution and glassware left soaking at least overnight. It is a good idea to isolate a set of glassware for colloidal gold and leave it soaking in the detergent between uses.

Distilled water used in preparing colloidal gold should be of high quality, at least double-distilled. All distilled water used for colloidal gold should be filtered through a 0.2 μm filter, including the distilled water used for rinsing glassware and for preparation of solutions.

B. Preparative Procedures
1. Preparing 15 nm Gold Particles
a. Start with a 4% solution of gold chloride ($AuCl_4$ or $AuCl_3$). Make up the whole sample at once since gold chloride is very hydroscopic and the 4% solution will last indefinitely.
b. Put the 4% gold chloride solution on ice. Filter 50 ml of double-distilled water through a 0.2 μm filter to rinse the flask, then filter the water to be used in making the gold colloid.
c. Make 10 ml of 1% trisodium citrate and place on ice.
d. Boil 200 ml double-distilled water in a round bottomed flask (be sure this has been soaked in F1-70 and rinsed with filtered, distilled water).
e. When water is boiling, add 0.5 ml of the 4% gold chloride.
f. Immediately add 5 ml of 1% trisodium citrate. If the procedure has worked, the solution will start turning black almost immediately, then purple, and finally bright deep red. (If the solution is blue, the gold has not stabilized. If this happens, discard all the solutions and repeat the procedure with a new source of distilled water.)
g. After the solution turns red, let it boil 1–2 min longer and then cool to room temperature.
h. Adjust the pH of about 50 ml of the colloid to that appropriate for the particular protein to be conjugated. This is usually 0.2–0.3 pH units above the isoelectric point (pI).

Chapter 13. IgG Binding in Immunoelectronmicroscopy

Figure 1 is an electron micrograph of 15 nm colloidal gold particles prepared by this method and shows the uniform size distribution.

2. Preparing 4.0—11.5 nm Gold Particles

A useful method for preparing colloidal gold particles of between approximately 3 and 17 nm has been reported by Slot and Geuze (1985). This method has several advantages over those previously reported: (1) the particle size can be controlled accurately; (2) the sols (colloidal dispersions in liquid) are homodisperse even when the average particle size drops to almost 3 nm; (3) the method is simple and the reagents are much less hazardous than compounds such as white phosphorus, which is used in other procedures for preparation of small colloidal gold.

It is of practical use to have homogeneous preparations of gold particles of several different sizes for use in multiple labeling experiments. The procedure for preparing 4 nm to 11.5 nm gold particles (Table 1) is as follows:

Two solutions are mixed to make 100 ml of a sol:

a. Gold Solution. Add 1 ml of a 1% solution of $HAuCl_4$ to 79 ml distilled water (80 ml total).

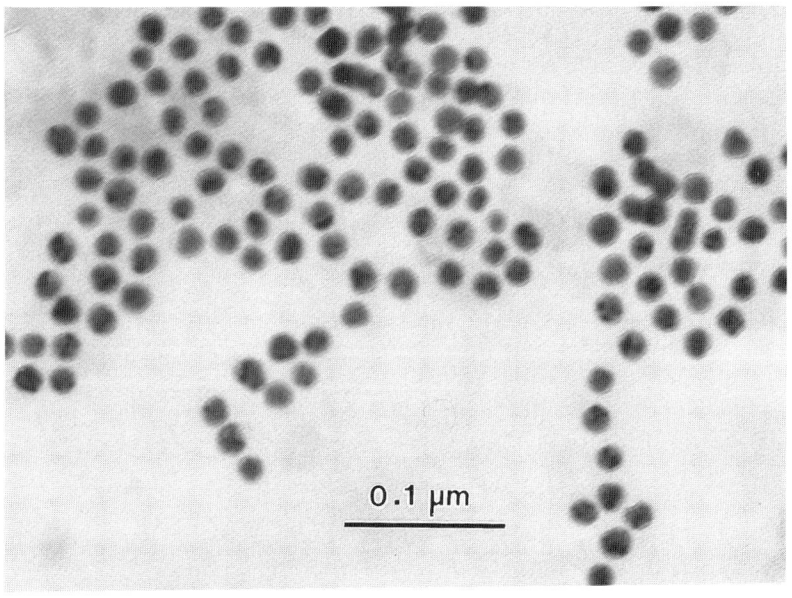

FIGURE 1
Electron micrograph of 15 nm colloidal gold particles prepared by the trisodium citrate method, using gold chloride. The particles are uniform in size ($\times 215,000$).

b. Reducing Mixture. Add 4 ml of 1% trisodium citrate $2H_2O$ to the appropriate solution listed in Table 1 (20 ml final volume) to make each size particle.

Bring both the gold solution and the reducing mixture to 60°C on a hot plate. Quickly add the 20 ml of reducing solution (b) (having added solution 1, 2, 3, or 4 listed in Table 1) to the 80 ml of gold solution (a), while stirring.

The reaction is complete in 1 s for high concentrations of 1% tannic acid, with the time required gradually increasing for lower concentrations, up to about 60 min in the absence of tannic acid.

Heat sols until boiling. When sol formation is finished, it will be evident by the red color.

Establish the average particle diameter and the coefficient of variation by measuring at least 100 particles on negatives of electron micrographs at about 80,000×. Catalase crystals (lattice spacing of ~8.6 nm) are used as calibration standards for exact measurements of particle size.

The tannic acid used in this procedure does not interfere with the binding of proteins to the sols and with most proteins, it does not impair the biological activity. However, to minimize possible interaction between any sensitive proteins and excess tannic acid, the gold–protein complexes may be layered immediately onto a 7% glycerol cushion containing 0.1% bovine serum albumin in phosphate-buffered saline (PBS), pH 7.2. The complexes are then centrifuged in an SW 41 rotor (Beckman Instruments, Palo Alto, California) for 45 min at 41,000 rpm for 5 nm gold or 30 min at 20,000 rpm for 12 nm gold (Slot and Geuze, 1984). The pellet formed is free of tannic acid and also devoid of excess, complexed protein (Slot and Geuze, 1985).

For the removal of aggregates and excess protein, a subsequent gradient centrifugation step is recommended (Slot and Geuze, 1984), by re-

TABLE 1
Method for Preparing 4.0–11.5 nm Colloidal Gold Particles

Average Diameter	Solutions Added[a]
1) 4.0 nm ± 11.7%	2.0 ml 1% tannic acid + 16 ml distilled water (DH_2O) + 2 ml 25 mM K_2CO_3[b]
2) 6.0 nm ± 7.3%	0.5 ml 1% tannic acid + 19.5 ml DH_2O
3) 8.2 nm ± 6.9%	0.125 ml 1% tannic acid + 19.875 ml DH_2O
4) 11.5 nm ± 6.3%	0.03 ml 1% tannic acid + 19.970 ml DH_2O

[a] Solutions added to 4 ml of the reducing mixture (1% trisodium citrate) described in the text (Section IIB,2).
[b] The potassium carbonate is added to solution 1 to compensate for the acidifying effects of the 2 ml of tannic acid, but when 0.5 ml or less is added, this is not necessary.

suspending the pellet and layering it over a 10–30% continuous sucrose or glycerol gradient (volume, 10.5 ml; length, 8 cm) in PBS, pH 7.2. The gradient is then centrifuged in an SW 41 rotor for 45 min at 41,000 rpm for the 5 nm gold or 30 min at 20,000 rpm for 12 nm gold. The nonaggregated complexes are collected from the gradients in one band.

C. Storage of Colloidal Gold

Colloidal gold preparations should be stored at 5–8°C and will remain stable for long periods of time, with 0.02% sodium azide added to maintain sterility. If the preparation turns blue, it should be discarded.

III. Coupling of Proteins to Colloidal Gold

The conjugation of colloidal gold to immunoglobulins and isolated immunoglobulin-binding proteins is useful for the ultrastructural localization of receptor sites and antigens on whole bacteria and on sections of bacteria or other cells.

When proteins interact with gold particles, the number of binding sites for a protein on a particle of given size is inversely proportional to the molecular weight of the protein. These results are compatible with the presence of a monomolecular shell of protein surrounding the gold particle at saturation. From this, the number of molecules able to saturate a gold particle may be predicted with reasonable accuracy, if the average diameter of the gold particle and the molecular weight of the globular protein are known. The affinity will also increase as a function of the molecular weight (de Roe *et al.*, 1987).

For optimal binding of colloidal gold to proteins, the general rule is that the pH should be adjusted to just above the isoelectric point of the protein. However, de Roe *et al.* (1987) have reported from their adsorption experiments performed at the same pH, that affinity is not dependent upon the isoelectric point of the protein. They have further reported that the pH for maximum protein adsorption is not related to the isoelectric point and the dissociation constant is not affected by pH.

Before conjugation to colloidal gold, a protein that is dissolved in a solvent such as phosphate-buffered saline should be dialyzed overnight in a buffer solution not exceeding a 5 mM concentration, and in distilled water if possible.

The procedures for conjugating colloidal gold to immunoglobulins (IgA and IgG), protein A (type I immunoglobulin-binding protein), and protein G (type III immunoglobulin-binding protein) are given in this section.

A. Immunoglobulins IgA and IgG

1. Dialyze the solutions (1 mg/ml) against 2 mM sodium borate (pH 9.0) overnight and centrifuge for 1 hr at 100,000 ×g prior to the coupling step in order to remove aggregates.
2. Determine the appropriate ratio of IgG (M_r of 150,000) or IgA (M_r of 170,000) to colloidal gold (see Section C).
3. Adjust colloidal gold sol to pH 9.0 with 0.2 M K_2CO_3.
4. Make a freshly prepared and filtered 10% solution of 20 M polyethylene glycol (PEG 20). The PEG 20 is in flakes, and the use of a stir bar will help to dissolve it.
5. While stirring, add the immunoglobulin to the colloidal gold in the ratio determined by titration.
6. After stirring for 2–3 min, continue mixing, and add dropwise 0.01 ml of the 10% PEG 20 per milligram of conjugate (100 μl PEG 20 for 10 ml of conjugate).
7. Centrifuge the preparation at 14,000 × g (15–20 nm particles) or 60,000 × g (5 nm particles) for 1 hr.
8. Suspend in an equal volume of Tris-buffered saline (pH 7.5) containing 0.5 mg/ml of 20 M PEG (TBS-PEG 20). Centrifuge at low speed (250 × g for 15–20 nm particles, 4800 × g for 5 nm particles) for 20 min to remove aggregates of gold particles.

Figure 2 is a negative stain of 15 nm colloidal gold particles complexed to IgG. A thin layer of protein can be observed in this electron micrograph taken at high magnification (×400,000).

B. Protein G from Group G Streptococci and Protein A from *Staphylococcus aureus*

For the past 10 years, the type I immunoglobulin-binding protein (protein A, M_r of 42,000, pI 5.6), which is a constituent of the cell wall of *Staphylococcus aureus*, has been widely used for pre-embedding (Romano and Romano, 1977) and postembedding (Roth *et al.*, 1978) ultrastructural localization of a wide variety of antigenic sites. In 1984, a protein known as protein G was isolated from the cell wall of group G streptococcus (Björck and Kronvall, 1984) and a corresponding protein from a group C streptococcus (Reis *et al.*, 1984a,b). This protein is a type III immunoglobulin-binding protein (M_r 47,000, pI < 3.5) and has a high affinity for binding to immunoglobulins from sheep, goats, and cows (Åkerström and Björck, 1986; Åkerström *et al.*, 1985), in contrast to protein A. Reis *et al.* (1984b)

Chapter 13. IgG Binding in Immunoelectronmicroscopy 223

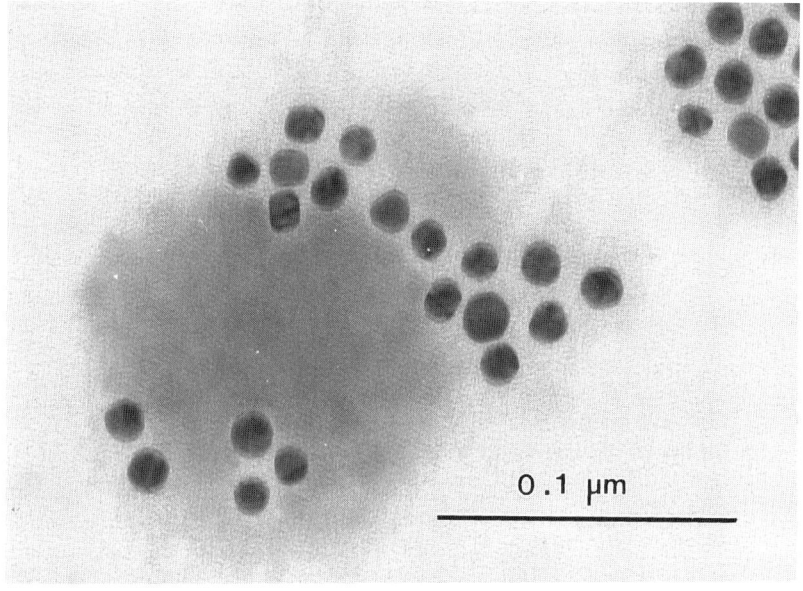

FIGURE 2
Negative stain (2.5% potassium phosphotungstate) of 15 nm colloidal gold after conjugation to IgG. The thin layer of protein surrounding the gold particles can be observed at this high magnification (×400,000).

also compared protein A to a group C type III streptococcal immunoglobulin-binding protein. They demonstrated that it bound more efficiently to goat, sheep, and cow IgG, whereas protein A bound more efficiently to dog IgG, and neither binding protein bound with a high affinity to rat IgG.

In addition, protein G has a high affinity for mouse and rat monoclonal antibodies, with which protein A reacts poorly. Bendayan (1987) recognized it as a tool in immunocytochemistry for high resolution, ultrastructural localization of tissue antigens. In a comparative study of protein A–gold and protein G–gold, Bendayan and Garzon (1988) concluded that because of enhanced reactivity with monoclonal antibodies and broader affinity for polyclonal antibodies, protein G–gold complexes appear to be better and more versatile probes for high resolution immunocytochemistry.

A recent study by Taatjes *et al.* (1987), however, disputed these findings by reporting that no difference was observed in binding to protein G–gold or protein A–gold with a battery of monoclonal antibodies and that protein A–gold reacted well with both sheep and goat IgG molecules.

Protein A–gold complexes are readily available commercially and the procedure for preparing them is similar to that of protein G (Bendayan *et al.*, 1980; Roth *et al.*, 1978). However, according to Romano and Romano (1977), the protein A–colloidal gold complex is dissociated by osmium tetroxide and should not be used when postfixation with osmium is required.

The methods for complexing protein G (type III immunoglobulin-binding protein) and protein A (type I immunoglobulin-binding protein) to colloidal gold are as follows.

1. Adjust the concentration of the protein to 1 mg/ml and dialyze overnight in distilled water, in the cold.
2. Adjust the colloidal gold to pH 4.8–5.4 for protein G and pH 5.8–6.0 for protein A (Bendayan and Garzon, 1988). Note: Many published reports indicate that any pH from 6–7.5 is effective for protein A.
3. Titrate the amount of protein G or protein A to be conjugated to the colloidal gold (whatever particle size desired) as described in section (C).
    Or follow the method of Bendayan and Garzon (1988), who used 14 nm colloidal gold:
    Protein G: mix 0.25 mg of protein, dissolved in 0.2 ml of distilled water, with 10 ml of colloidal gold.
    Protein A: mix 0.3 mg, dissolved in 0.2 ml of distilled water, with 10 ml of colloidal gold
4. Centrifuge for 1 hr at 4°C at:
    14,000 $\times$ g for 15–20 nm gold,
    43,000 $\times$ g for 14 nm gold (Bendayan and Garzon, 1988),
    and, or 60,000 $\times$ g for 5 nm gold
5. After centrifugation, resuspend in 1 ml of 0.01 M PBS, pH 7.2, + 1 mg PEG 20 + 3 mM sodium azide.

C. Titration of the Amount of Colloid to Bind a Protein Sample

Conjugates of gold colloids to proteins must be prepared so that there will be neither excess gold particles nor excess protein in the mixture. To do this, a simple titration is performed.

1. Adjust the pH of the colloidal gold solution to the appropriate pH (as a general rule, this is several tenths of a pH unit above the pI of the protein to be coupled).

For polyclonal antibodies, adjust to pH 9.0. Use 0.2 M K_2CO_3 to raise the pH and acetic, formic, hydrochloric, or phosphoric acid to lower the pH.
2. Prepare ten small test tubes. Pipette 100 μl of distilled water into the last nine tubes, leaving the first tube as an undiluted sample.
3. Pipette 100 μl of protein (1 mg/ml) into the first two tubes. Start serial two-fold dilutions from the second tube. Discard 100 μl from the last tube. Mix between each dilution.
4. Add 0.5 ml of the gold solution to each tube. Mix.
5. Add 0.5 ml of 10% NaCl. Mix and wait several minutes. Any tube containing free, unconjugated gold will turn blue. This can be monitored visually or spectrophotometrically at 420 nm. Placing the tubes in the cold for 30 min will enhance the color difference.
6. Take the last tube that displays a pink color as the endpoint and then add 20% more protein to prepare the desired conjugate.

An example to prepare 10 ml of protein–gold conjugate:

The fifth tube displays the last definite pink color (equivalent to 63 μl of the stock protein solution added). This means 63 μl of this particular protein solution will bind 0.5 ml of the gold colloid. One ml of gold colloid will bind 126 μl of protein and 10 ml will bind 1.3 ml of the stock protein solution.

Consequently, to prepare 10 ml of the protein–gold conjugate, add 20% of 1.3 ml or 1.55 ml of the stock protein solution.

D. Storage of Gold Colloids

Colloidal gold labels should be stored at 4°C where they are stable for long periods of time, many for at least a year. The addition of 3 mM sodium azide will help maintain sterility. The gold colloids can also be frozen at −70°C if resuspended in 20% glycerol.

IV. Use of Gold-Labeling for Localization of Immunoglobulin-Binding Sites and Antigen–Antibody Complexes in Bacteria

Methods are introduced in this section for the direct labeling of binding sites on whole bacteria and on thin sections using gold-labeled immunoglobulins and sandwich procedures for reacting cells with a specific antiserum followed by reaction with gold-labeled protein G.

A. Localization of Immunoglobulin-Binding Molecules on Whole Bacteria

Localization of Fc-binding sites for immunoglobulins on bacterial cells using gold-conjugated Fc fragments was performed using unfixed, whole cells. It was found that the reactivity was much higher on unfixed cells and decreased with the length of fixation time. Where fixation is necessary, use as short a fixation period as possible (5–15 min) with 0.1% glutaraldehyde in 0.1 M cacodylate buffer, pH 7.2. The examples described next focus on studies of the relationship of the β antigen of group B streptococci to the IgA Fc-binding protein associated with these strains. A detailed analysis of the significance of group B streptococci expressing IgA-binding proteins can be found in Coleman *et al.* (1990).

Procedure for localization of IgA-binding sites on whole cells of group B streptococci:

1. The bacteria are grown in broth or on agar plates for 18–24 hr at 37°C and are allowed to settle in the tube or are gently removed from the agar.
2. IgA conjugated to 15 nm gold particles is diluted until just pink and centrifuged 1 min at top speed in a microfuge to remove aggregates.
3. The gold-labeled IgA is mixed with the cells and left for 1 hr at room temperature.
4. The cells are then placed on Formvar-coated grids, allowed to settle, drained, floated on buffer, and then distilled water to wash. The cells can also be fixed for 15 min with 2.5% glutaraldehyde in 0.1 M cacodylate buffer, pH 7.2, after exposure to the gold-labeled immunoglobulin.
5. The grids are then observed with an electron microscope at 80 or 100 kV or by backscatter imaging. A negative stain such as 4% phosphotungstic acid may also be used for obsrving labeling of surface structures such as fimbriae.

Figure 3A is an electron micrograph of whole cells of the group B streptococcus strain SS618c, which has been reacted for 1 hr with a diluted IgA–15 nm colloidal gold conjugate. This is a strain selected for its high reactivity with IgA Fc fragments (Brady & Boyle, 1989). The IgA-binding sites on the surface are visualized by the localization of the 15 nm colloidal gold conjugated to the IgA. Figure 3B is the same preparation observed with backscatter electrons.

B. Procedure for Gold Labeling on Thin Sections

For identification of the structural location of antigens and receptor sites, direct labeling on thin sections of bacteria is a useful technique. Surface-binding sites as well as cytoplasmic sites of antigen secretion can be observed.

Details of the methods used for identifying IgA-binding sites and β antigen in group B streptococci on thin sections are as follows:

1. Fixation and Embedding of Bacteria

a. The bacteria are cultured in broth (Todd-Hewitt or other) for 18–24 hr at 37°C, centrifuged, and fixed for 15 min in 0.1% glutaraldehyde + 4% formaldehyde in 0.1 M cacodylate buffer, pH 7.2.
b. The cells are washed twice in 0.1 M cacodylate buffer, embedded in a small drop of 2% agar and cut with a razor blade or scalpel into 1 mm blocks.
c. The blocks are then dehydrated through 25, 50, 70, 80, 90, and 100% ethanol and embedded in either Lowicryl K4M or LR White resins.

Most of the studies were performed with cells embedded in LR White since the labeling was excellent and LR White does not have the toxic properties of Lowicryl.

2. Localization of IgA- and IgG-Binding Sites on Thin Sections

Thin sections are cut using a microtome equipped with a diamond knife and collected on Formvar-coated, gold grids. It is necessary to use unreactive grids such as gold, nickel, or stainless steel (although the stainless steel grids often have rough edges).

The procedure is as follows:

a. Cut thin sections and pick up on Formvar-coated grids.
b. Float grids on a drop of 1% ovalbumin in PBS for 10 min. Plastic petri dishes are good for this purpose since the surface is hydrophobic and round drops are formed that have good surface tension. Drain the grids but do not dry.

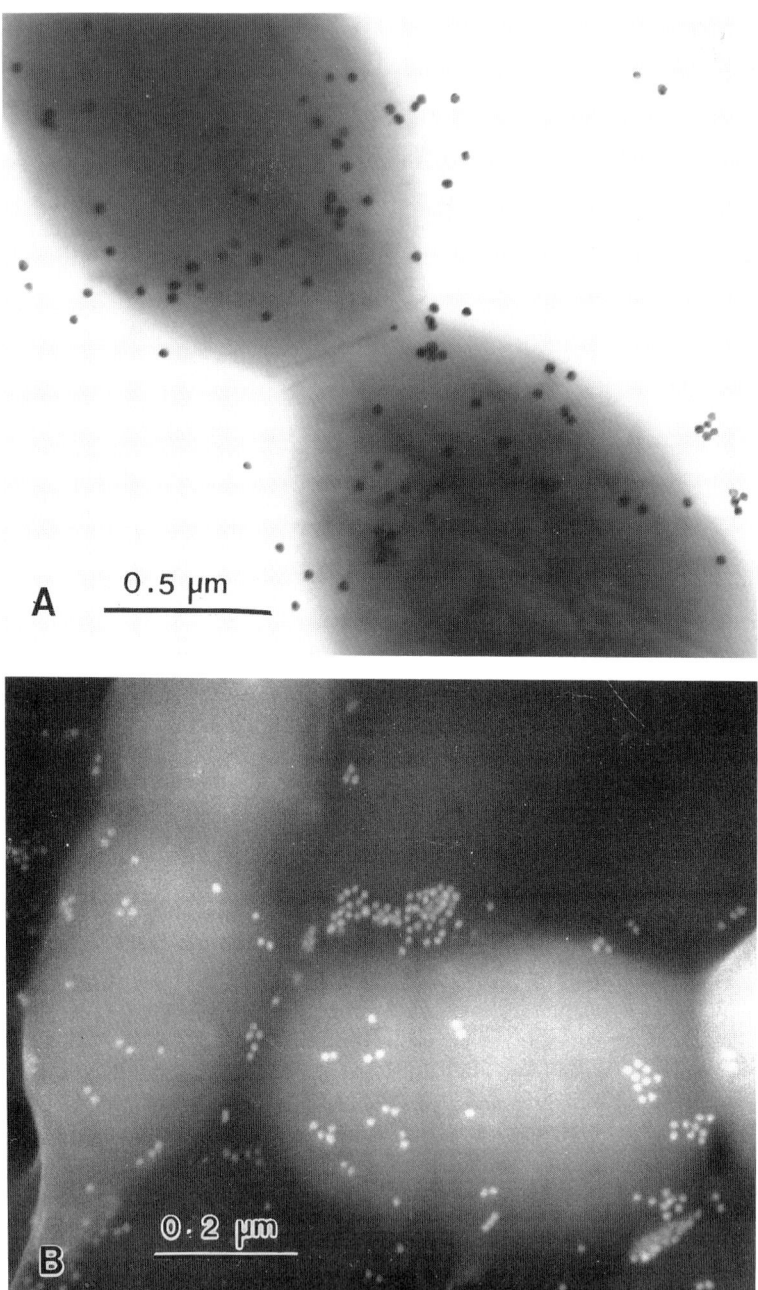

c. Float the grids for 15–60 min on gold-labeled IgA or IgG, which has been diluted until just pink in color (usually 1 : 10).
d. Wash with three changes of PBS over 30 min and then with two changes of distilled water.
e. Observe either without poststaining or after 2 min staining with aqueous 0.5% uranyl acetate. Lead poststaining may be used, depending upon whether it masks the gold particles.

Figure 4A is an electron micrograph of group B streptococcus strain SS618c, which has been reacted with IgA labeled with 15 nm colloidal gold. The surface-binding sites for IgA are marked by the presence of the gold particles.

Figure 4B is group C strain G1400 that binds IgG. Thin sections of the bacteria have been reacted with IgG labeled with 15 nm colloidal gold.

3. Localization of β Antigen of Group B Streptococci Using Anti-β Antiserum and Gold-Labeled Protein G

This is the general "sandwich" method for using an unlabeled, specific antiserum against any antigen, followed by reaction with a gold-labeled immunoglobin-binding protein that will react with the antiserum used. The procedure first calls for reacting the sectioned cells with the antiserum containing specific antibodies of the IgG isotype, washing, and then reacting the sections with a gold-labeled IgG-binding protein.

a. Culture bacteria in broth or on agar. Centrifuge and fix pellet for 15 min with 0.1% glutaraldehyde + 4% formaldehyde in 0.1 M cacodylate buffer, pH 7.2.
b. Embed bacteria in Lowicryl K4M or LR White plastic.
c. Prepare thin sections and place on Formvar-coated grids.
d. Float grids on 1% ovalbumin in PBS for 10 min. Drain grid but do not dry.
e. Float grids for 1 hr on drops of anti-β antiserum (diluted 1 : 500 or higher in PBS) in plastic petri dishes, covered. Float control grids on preimmune serum.
f. Wash with three changes of PBS over 30 min.
g. Dilute 15 nm gold-labeled type III immunoglobulin-binding

FIGURE 3
Electron micrograph of whole cells of group B streptococcus SS618c after exposure for 1 hr to diluted (1 : 10) IgA complexed to 15 nm colloidal gold. (A) Whole cells placed unfixed on a Formvar-coated gold grid and observed at 80 kV (×46,000). (B) The same preparation observed by back-scattered electrons (×95,000).

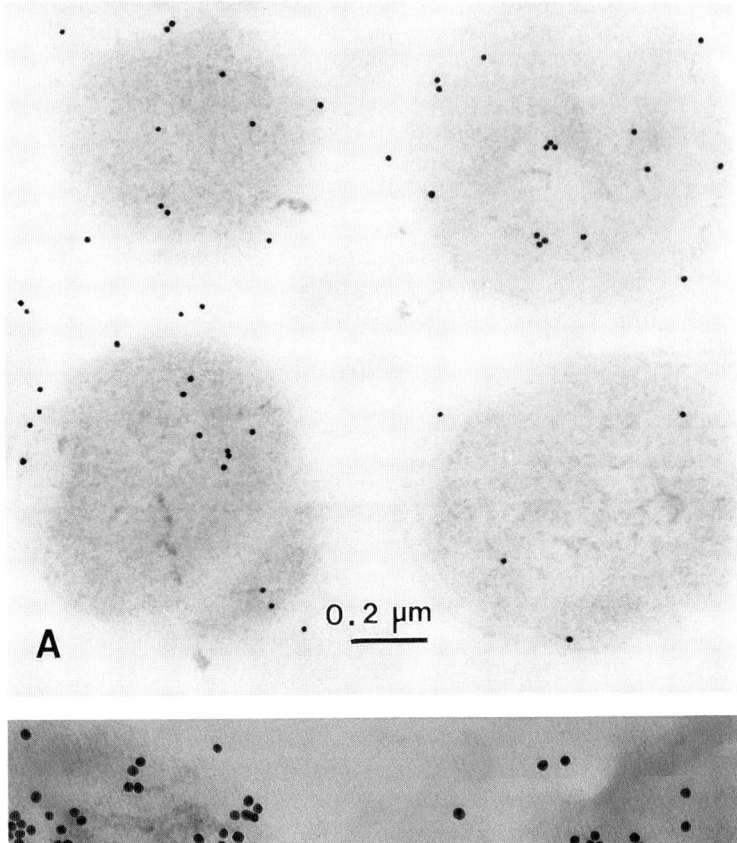
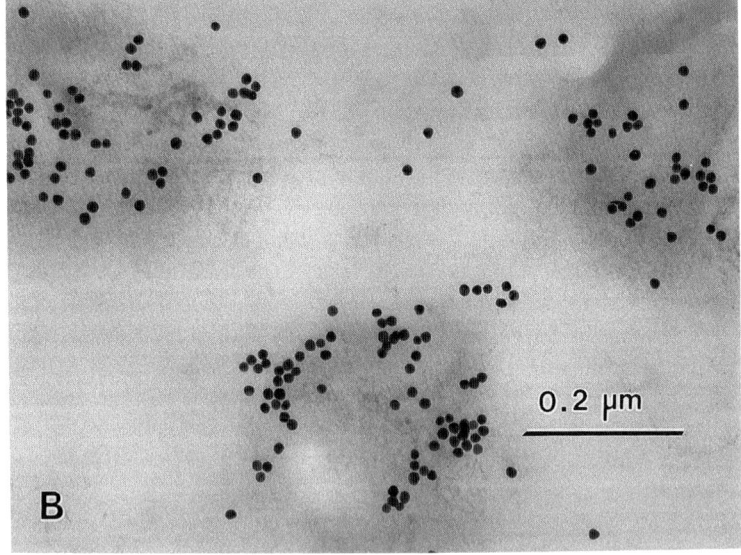

Chapter 13. IgG Binding in Immunoelectronmicroscopy 231

protein (protein G) until just pink (usually 1 : 10) and centrifuge 1–2 min in microfuge to remove aggregates. Incubate grids on gold-labeled protein G for 1 hr (or overnight in the cold).

h. Do not dry grids; wash with two changes of PBS for 15 min each, or with a squirt bottle, and then rinse once with distilled water. (Some investigators fix the grids with 2.5% glutaraldehyde at this point to stabilize the particles, although this does not usually seem necessary).

i. Observe with the electron microscope either without poststaining or after 2 min staining with aqueous 0.5% uranyl acetate. Lead poststaining may be used if contrast permits.

Figure 5A is an electron micrograph of strain HG806 group B streptococcus after exposure of the sections for 1 hr to 1 : 500 dilution of a rabbit anti-β antiserum, followed by incubation for 1 hr with protein G (type III immunoglobulin-binding protein) conjugated to 15 nm colloidal gold and diluted 1 : 10. This strain does not bind IgA to the surface but does secrete β antigen as shown by the gold label in the cytoplasm. The absence of IgA binding is shown in Figure 5B, in which cells of strain HG806 have been incubated with IgA conjugated to 15 nm colloidal gold.

V. Double Labeling Techniques with Different Sizes of Colloidal Gold to Localize Two Different Antigens on Thin Sections

A. Simultaneous Labeling of Sites of IgA Binding and β Antigen in Group B Streptococci

It is possible to localize two different antigenic sites on a thin section by use of proteins conjugated to two differently sized gold particles. In the case of the localization of binding sites for both IgA and β antigen on sections of group B streptococci, the IgA has been labeled with 5 nm gold particles and reacted with one side of the section. Since IgA binding would block the β antigen sites, the localization of β antigen is performed on the back side of the section, which is thick enough to prevent penetration to the other side. For β antigen detection, the section is incubated with anti-β

FIGURE 4
Reaction to gold-labeled immunoglobulins on thin sections. (A) Group B streptococcus strain SS618c reacted 1 hr to IgA labeled with 15 nm colloidal gold (×50,000). (B) Group C streptococcus strain G1400, which possesses binding sites for IgG, incubated for 1 hr with IgG labeled with 15 nm colloidal gold (×105,000).

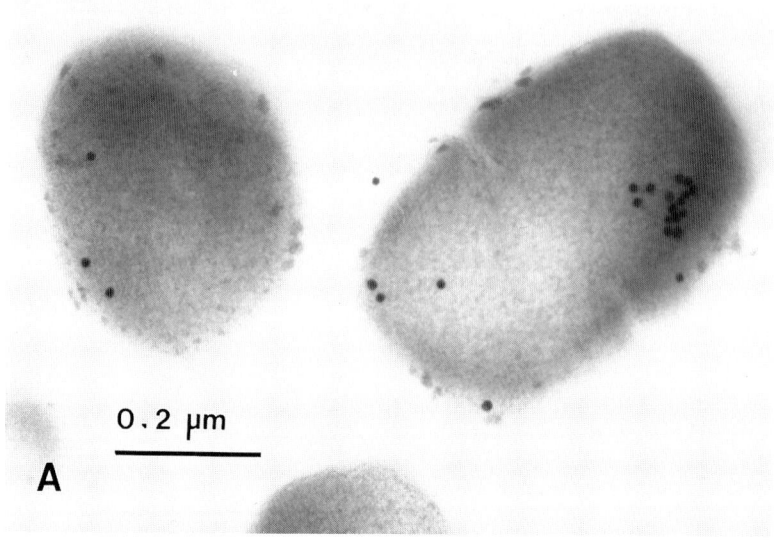

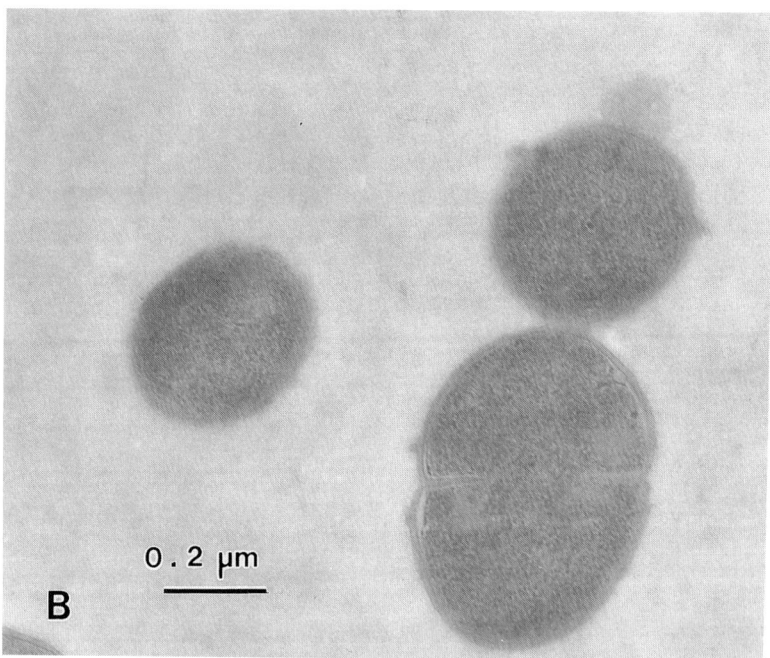

Chapter 13. IgG Binding in Immunoelectronmicroscopy

antiserum, followed by reaction of the anti-β immunoglobulin with 15 nm gold-labeled protein G. The procedure is as follows.

1. The bacteria are cultured in Todd-Hewitt broth for 24 hr at 37°C, pelleted, and fixed for 15 min with 0.1% glutaraldehyde + 4% formaldehyde in 0.1 M cacodylate buffer, pH 7.2. The bacterial sample is then washed twice and embedded in a drop of 2% agar in the same buffer.
2. After cutting the agar-embedded bacteria into 1 mm blocks, they are dehydrated through 25, 50, 70, 80, 90, and 100% ethanol and embedded in LR White resin.
3. Thin sections are prepared and placed on *uncoated gold grids* so that both sides of the sections are accessible.
4. Using plastic petri dishes, carefully float the grids on drops of 1% ovalbumin for 10 min. Drain but do not dry.
5. Float for 1–2 hr on IgA conjugated to 5 nm colloidal gold and diluted until just pink. *Take care to keep the back of the grid dry*.
6. Wash on several drops of PBS and then several drops of distilled water.
7. Drain grid and *carefully turn over*, placing the back side of the section on a drop of 1% ovalbumin for 10 min. Drain but do not dry.
8. Place back side of section on anti-β antiserum diluted 1 : 500 (or as required) for 1 hr.
9. Wash with three changes of PBS over 30 min.
10. Float for 1 hr (or up to overnight in the cold) on a drop of protein G (type III immunoglobulin-binding protein) conjugated to 15 nm gold and diluted until just pink.
11. Wash with two changes of PBS and then two or three changes of distilled water. Dry and observe with the electron microscope, either unstained or stained for 2 min with 0.5% aqueous uranyl acetate.

FIGURE 5
Localization of β antigen in group B streptococcus strain HG806, which does not bind IgA but secretes the β antigen. (A) Thin section exposed for 1 hr to 1 : 500 dilution of rabbit anti-β antiserum followed by incubation for 1 hr with protein G, which has been conjugated to 15 nm colloidal gold ($\times$95,000). (B) Control cells incubated with normal rabbit serum followed by exposure to gold-labeled protein G ($\times$70,000).

Figure 6 is group B streptococcus strain SS618c showing receptor sites for IgA, which has been conjugated to 5 nm particles (small arrow) and localization of the β antigen, which has been reacted with protein G conjugated to 15 nm colloidal gold particles (large arrow).

B. Double-Labeling with Two Different Primary Antibodies by Silver Enhancement of the Colloidal Gold Marker

There are several ways to label two different antigens on the same thin section: (1) use two sizes of gold particles; (2) label on two sides of the same section; (3) label one antigen before embedding and the other afterwards on the section; (4) remove the first antibody or destroy it with formaldehyde vapors; (5) use silver to enhance the size of the gold particles conjugated to one antigen, which distinguishes the first antigen from a second antigen that is conjugated to the same size particle.

The latter method has the advantage of requiring only one size of gold colloid and can be used quite successfully for identifying the loci of two different antigenic sites or two enzyme activities in a bacterium. One note, however, this technique does not seem to work with protein A–gold.

The method described here is essentially that of Bienz *et al.* (1986) with modifications by J. Gokhale (personal communication) who used the method to localize adenosine triphosphatase (ATPase) and methyl-CoM reductase in the methanogenic bacterium *Methanobacterium thermoautotrophicum*.

The silver enhancement procedure is as follows.

1. The bacteria are cultured, fixed, and embedded in Lowicryl K4M or LR White, by standard methods.
2. Thin sections are prepared and picked up on gold (100 mesh), Formvar-coated grids.
3. Developing solution:

    75 mg Microdol X developer

    50 mg anhydrous sodium sulfite

    20 mg sodium thiocyanate

    Dissolve in 10 ml of distilled water. Adjust pH to 6.3. Prepare this solution fresh each time.
4. Preparation of colloidal gold–anti-immunoglobulin conjugate:
    a. Conjugate 10 nm colloidal gold to an anti-immunoglobulin directed against the primary antibodies. Example: if using

Chapter 13. IgG Binding in Immunoelectronmicroscopy

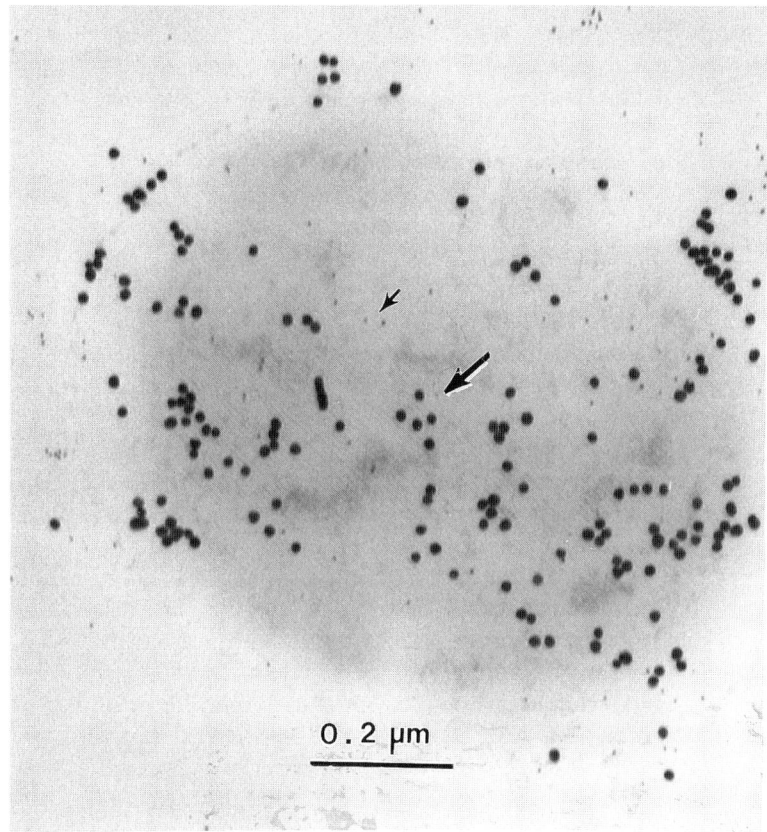

FIGURE 6
Thin section of group B streptococcus strain SS618c, which has been double-labeled by reacting one side of the grid to IgA labeled with 5 nm colloidal gold (small arrow) and reacting the other side with anti-β antiserum followed by protein G conjugated to 15 nm colloidal gold (large arrow) ($\times 95,000$).

        rabbit antibodies, conjugate 10 nm gold to goat anti-rabbit immunoglobulin G (IgG).
- **b.** Dilute 1 : 200 with PBS.
5. Reaction with first antibody
   - **a.** Under a safelight (Ilford filter S902), weigh out Ilford L4 emulsion (gel form) in an empty light-tight container.
   - **b.** Add an appropriate amount of developing solution to give a final concentration of 40 mg of Ilford L4 per ml of developing solution.

c. Stir mixture for 5 min.
d. Using plastic petri dishes, float grids, section side down on 1% ovalbumin for 10 min to block nonspecific sites.
e. Drain but do not dry.
f. Float grids on a 1 : 100 dilution of the first antibody for 60 min at room temperature.
g. Wash briefly in three changes of PBS.
h. Float the grids for 10 min on the 10 nm gold labeled anti-immunoglobulin.
i. Wash with two changes of PBS and wash once in distilled water.
6. Silver enhancement procedure:
   a. Transfer 5–7 ml of the prestirred developer mix into a plastic weighing boat with a magnetic stir bar.
   b. Float gold grids section side down for 20 min on the prestirred developer while stirring slowly (adjust speed so that grids remain on the surface of the solution and do not sink or hit the stir bar).
   The 10 nm particles will be enhanced to about double their original size.
   c. Wash grids with several changes of PBS.
7. Reaction with second antibody
   a. Float the same side (section side) of grid for 60 min on the second antibody. Dilute 1 : 100 in PBS as described.
   b. Wash briefly in three changes of PBS.
   c. Float the grids for 10 min on the 10 nm labeled anti-immunoglobulin.
   d. Wash the grids with several changes of PBS and distilled water.

These particles will label the second antibody and will remain the original 10 nm in size.

Figure 7 illustrates the use of the silver enhancement technique for demonstrating the sites of ATPase (10 nm particles marked with small arrows) and methyl-CoM reductase (enhanced particles marked by large arrows) in the methanogenic bacterium *Methanobacterium thermoautotrophicum*.

VI. Streptavidin/Avidin–Biotin Labeling for Detection of Immunoglobulin-Binding Proteins

A number of years ago, research investigators discovered that feeding large amounts of dried egg white to animals produced a nutritional defi-

Chapter 13. IgG Binding in Immunoelectronmicroscopy   **237**

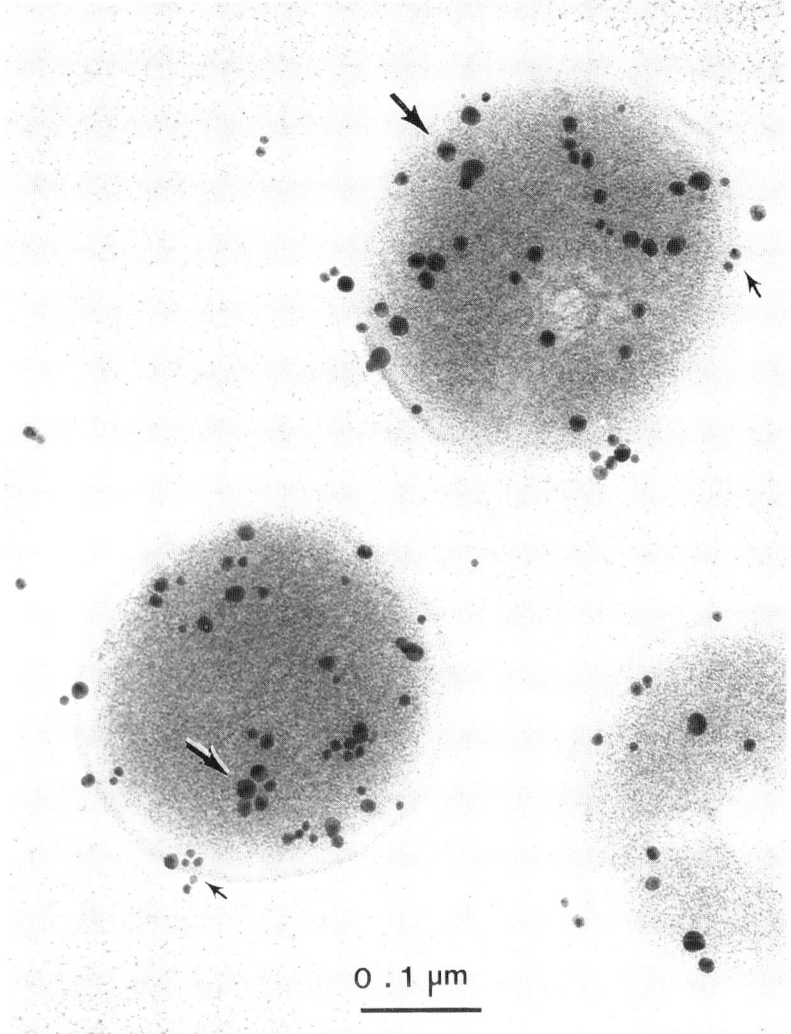

FIGURE 7
The silver enhancement technique used with the methanogenic bacterium *Methanobacterium thermoautotrophicum* to localize the sites of two enzymes. The enzyme ATPase is labeled with 10 nm colloidal gold (small arrows). The large arrows mark the location of methyl-CoM reductase, which is labeled with the larger, enhanced colloidal gold (×160,000). (Courtesy of J. Gokhale, University of Florida, Gainesville, Florida.)

ciency. Eventually, it was discovered that the deficiency was caused by the presence of a protein (M_r 68,000) that was named avidin, which had a high affinity for the vitamin biotin. This affinity is about a million times more powerful than most antigen–antibody reactions, making the bond essentially irreversible. Biotin (vitamin H) is a small molecule (M_r 274) and can be easily conjugated to many proteins without altering biological activity. Only for the last few years has this complex been used widely as a scientific tool to detect, separate, and quantitate minute amounts of biological substances.

The recent discovery of a protein called streptavidin, which is released from cultures of *Streptomyces avidini* has led to the finding that this protein has a number of advantages over avidin. Both proteins are tetramers with subunit molecular weights of about 15,000 and are stable to treatment with urea, guanidine-HCl, and heat.

Streptavidin, because it has a neutral pI and is nonglycosylated, has been found to be a superior reagent for the detection of biotinylated ligands (Chaiet and Wolf, 1964). Applications of the streptavidin/avidin–biotin technique include immunocytochemistry, localization and separation of antigens, affinity chromatography, and immunoassay and hybridization studies (Fuccillo, 1985).

The methods described here are for the conjugation of gold colloids to both streptavidin and egg white avidin as electron-dense markers, which can be reacted with any biotin–protein conjugate desired (antibodies, enzymes, lectins, hormones, immunoglobulin-binding sites, etc.).

The streptavidin/avidin–biotin linkage is a useful alternative to antibody–antigen and protein A– or protein G–IgG interactions because it is formed rapidly and is almost irreversible (Green, 1975; Tolson *et al.*, 1981). This system can also be used with whole cells for surface localization or on thin sections for intracellular localization. Biotinylated protein A or protein G have also been used for immunocytochemistry and these applications are discussed in detail in Chapter 12.

A. Stabilization of Colloidal Gold with Avidin

The procedure for using avidin to stabilize colloidal gold (Geoghegan and Ackerman, 1977; Tolson *et al.*, 1981) is as follows:

1. Prepare a number of tubes containing 1 ml of the gold colloid.
2. Add a range of volumes of 0.1 N NaOH from 10–200 μl to the tubes of gold colloid.
3. Add 10 μl of aqueous avidin (1 mg/ml) to each tube and mix.
4. Add 100 μl of 1% saline to each tube.
5. After 60 min, centrifuge at 200 rpm for 5 min.

Chapter 13. IgG Binding in Immunoelectronmicroscopy

The optimum conditions occur in the tube that requires the minimum amount of NaOH without forming a pellet after centrifugation.

Example: If the tube containing 100 µl of NaOH is the last one without precipitate, then to prepare 10 ml of avidin–gold conjugate:

a. Place 10 ml of gold colloid in a beaker.
b. Add 1 ml of 0.1 N NaOH (10 × 100 µl).
c. Add 100 µl of avidin (1 mg/ml), while rapidly stirring.
d. After several minutes, add 0.5 ml 1% PEG 20 to discourage aggregation.
e. Centrifuge at high speed, 50,000 × g for 3.5 hr (Morris and Saelinger, 1984).
f. Resuspend pellet in 1% PEG 20 in Tris–glycine buffer at pH 11.0 at 278°K (6°C). No loss in ability to bind biotin has been observed over several weeks under these conditions (Tolson *et al.*, 1981).

B. Streptavidin–Gold Labeling for Detection of Immunoglobulin-Binding Proteins

This is the procedure described by Bonnard *et al.* (1984), which is given as follows:

1. All glassware used is siliconized.
2. Prepare 20 ml of gold colloid (2–5 or 10 nm).
3. Add:
   a. 200 µl of 1.0 M NaHCO$_3$
   b. 0.5 ml streptavidin (1 mg/ml) in 1 mM phosphate buffer, pH 7.4
4. Stir for 10 min at room temperature.
5. Add 200 µl of 2% polyethylene glycol (PEG) 6000.
6. Centrifuge:
   a. 2–5 nm gold solutions for 30 min at 11,400 × g (10,000 rpm with a Beckman JA21 rotor);
   b. 10 nm gold solutions for 30 min at 1000 × g (3000 rpm with a Beckman JA21 rotor).
7. Load *supernatant* on top of a 37.5% sucrose cushion in 0.1 M phosphate buffer, pH 7.4, + 0.02% PEG 6000.
8. Centrifuge:
   a. 2–5 nm gold complexes for 30 min at 285,000 × g (40,000 rpm with a Beckman SW40 rotor);
   b. 10 nm gold complexes for 30 min at 138,700 × g (11,000 rpm with a Beckman JA21 rotor).

9. Resuspend the pellet in the same phosphate buffer and add 0.05% sodium azide.
10. Store at 4°C until used.

C. Biotinylation of Proteins for Use with Avidin–Gold

This is the method reported by Bayer *et al.* (1979) for biotinylating ligands in conjunction with avidin–gold colloids:

1. Prepare protein in 1 mg/ml concentration.
2. Add 20 µl of dimethyl formamide containing biotin-N-hydroxysuccinimide ester (Calbiochem, La Jolla, California; 1.4 mg/ml) to 1 ml of protein (5 : 1 molar ratio, 1 : 50 volume ratio).
3. Incubate the reaction mixture at 23°C for 4 hr.
4. Dialyze overnight against 1000 volumes of phosphate-buffered saline (0.15 M NaCl with 0.05 M dibasic sodium phosphate, pH 7.5).
5. Store the biotinylated protein at 4°C until used.

VII. Replica Method with Plasma Polymerization Film by Glow Discharge for Three-Dimensional Demonstration of Colloidal Gold Particles

A. Development of Replica Method

A very useful method for making three-dimensional replicas for the demonstration of the surface distribution of colloidal gold particles has been devised by Tanaka *et al.* (1978). The method uses glow discharge for preparing plasma polymerization films. During development of the plasma polymerization replica method, it was found that the replica membrane formed by the polymerization of ethylene gas in plasma acquired a strong affinity to metal, and the metal particles located beneath the membrane were extracted into the ethylene membrane (Kondo *et al.*, 1983).

When the surface antigens of a cell are labeled with ferritin or gold, the particles are extracted *in situ* from the cell surface into the replica membrane. The particles can be easily observed by transmission electron microscopy on the three-dimensionally polymerized film.

Naphthalene, methane, or ethylene gas may be used to produce a uniform three-dimensional film of 10–50 nm in thickness, which is chemically inert, resistant to heat, and mechanically strong. The plasma polymerization process causes no heat damage to specimens, and being amorphous in texture may give a more accurate image of the specimen with higher resolution (Tanaka *et al.*, 1988).

These workers have published several reports on the application of

Chapter 13. IgG Binding in Immunoelectronmicroscopy 241

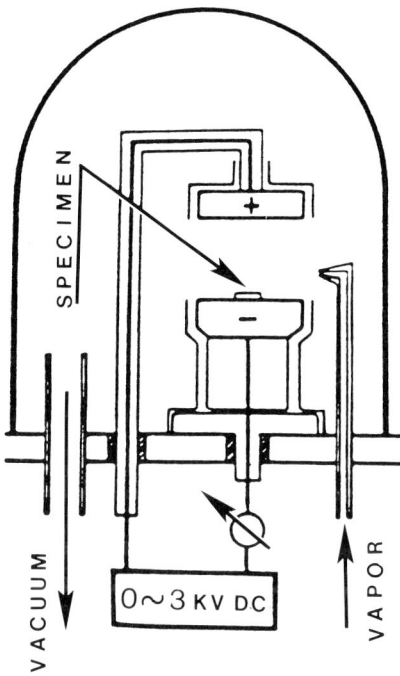

FIGURE 8
Apparatus for the plasma polymerization method (Kondo, 1986), showing the positive electrode above and the negative electrode upon which the specimen is mounted. A hydrocarbon gas (naphthalene, methane, ethylene) is introduced through the vapor tube after evacuation, and an electric current between the electrodes at 1.5–3.0 kV dc, causes a glow discharge field for creating a plasma that polymerizes to form a membrane.

this technique for making surface replicas of biological and inorganic specimens, freeze-fractured tissues, and metal extraction with immunocytochemical markers (Kondo, 1986; Kondo *et al.*, 1982, 1983, 1984, 1986; Tanaka *et al.*, 1988).

B. Technique for Preparation of Replicas by Plasma Polymerization

The method described here is that reported by Kondo (1986) and Tanaka *et al.* (1988). The apparatus for the plasma polymerization replica method consists of a high voltage power supply and a vacuum chamber, as shown in Figure 8. The specimen is placed on a negative electrode stage with the positive electrode above. The procedure is as follows.

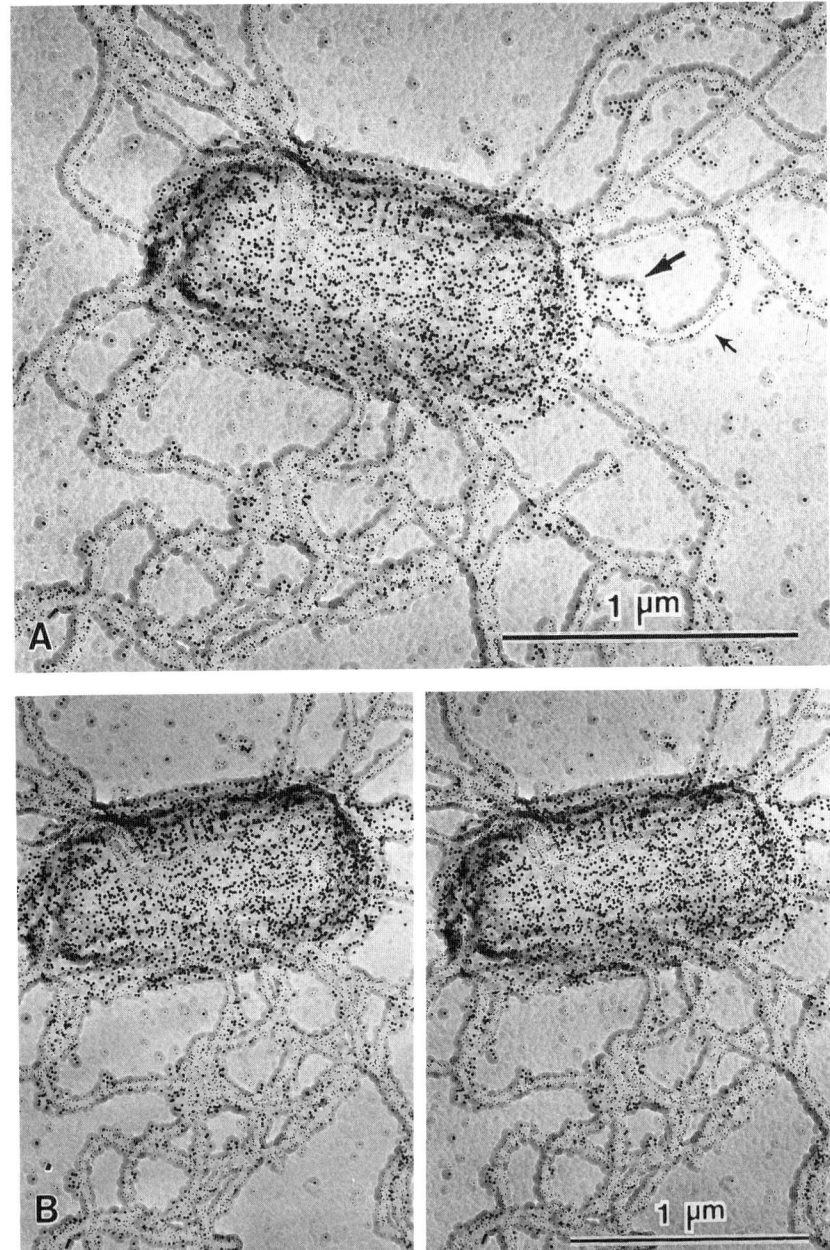

1. Mount the specimen on a collodion film-coated grid or on the flat surface of a block of fractured, crystallized sugar and place the specimen on the negative electrode stage.
2. Evacuate the chamber to 0.05–1.0 Torr and slowly introduce a hydrocarbon gas (naphthalene, methane, ethylene) through the spray tube.
3. When the vacuum reaches 10^{-2} Torr, stop the gas and introduce an electric current between the electrodes at 1.5–3.0 kV dc to cause a glow discharge field for creating a plasma.

The dispersion of the gas is enhanced by the scattering effect of the plasma. The gas covers the whole surface of the specimen with a thin and uniform film, which is immediately polymerized *in situ* by the plasma.

The ionized hydrocarbon molecules diffuse into the surface configurations and are deposited as a three-dimensional, polymerized film of 10–50 nm in thickness.

Figure 9 shows a preparation of *Proteus vulgaris* prepared by this method after double-labeling with rabbit antiflagella factor [H] and protein A–gold, labeled with 5 nm colloidal gold, as well as rabbit anti-somatic antigen factor antibody [0] followed by goat anti-rabbit IgG, conjugated to 10 nm colloidal gold. The cells were fixed with 5% formalin and placed on a collodion-coated grid, treated with the anti-factor [H] antibody followed by protein A, and then postfixed with 2.5% glutaraldehyde and treated with the anti-somatic antigen factor [0] followed by gold-labeled goat anti-rabbit IgG. The grids were placed in the "Plasma nano-replica apparatus" (Ushio Inc., Tokyo, Japan) and the replica film was made with naphthalene gas, polymerized by glow discharge. After the film was produced, the grid was taken from the apparatus, treated with acetone and

---

FIGURE 9

Plasma replica using metal extraction of colloidal gold. (A) Cells of *Proteus vulgaris* fixed with 5% formalin and treated with rabbit anti-flagella serum factor [H] and protein A–gold conjugated to 5 nm colloidal gold, followed by postfixation with 2.5% glutaraldehyde and anti-somatic antigen rabbit serum factor [O] reacted with goat anti-rabbit IgG conjugated to 10 nm colloidal gold. The cells were placed on a grid and a replica film made using a "Plasma nano-replica" apparatus (Ushio Inc., Tokyo, Japan), as described. The 5 nm colloidal gold particles (small arrow) show the location of the flagella factor [H] and the 10 nm particles (large arrow) localize the somatic factor [O] (×40,000). (B) Stereo pair of the same bacterium showing the three-dimensional distribution of the H and O antigens labeled with 5 and 10 nm colloidal gold, respectively (×33,000). (Courtesy of Drs. I. Kondo, M. Yamaguchi, T. Hirano, and A. Tanaka, Taisho Pharmaceutical Company, Ltd., and Jikei University School of Medicine, Tokyo, Japan.)

sodium hypochlorite solution to dissolve both the collodion film and the bacteria, leaving just the replica, which was washed with water, picked up on a grid, and examined in a transmission electron microscope without metal coating or further treatment.

Figure 9A is an electron micrograph at a higher magnification of the replica of *Proteus vulgaris* showing the distribution of flagellar (5 nm gold,

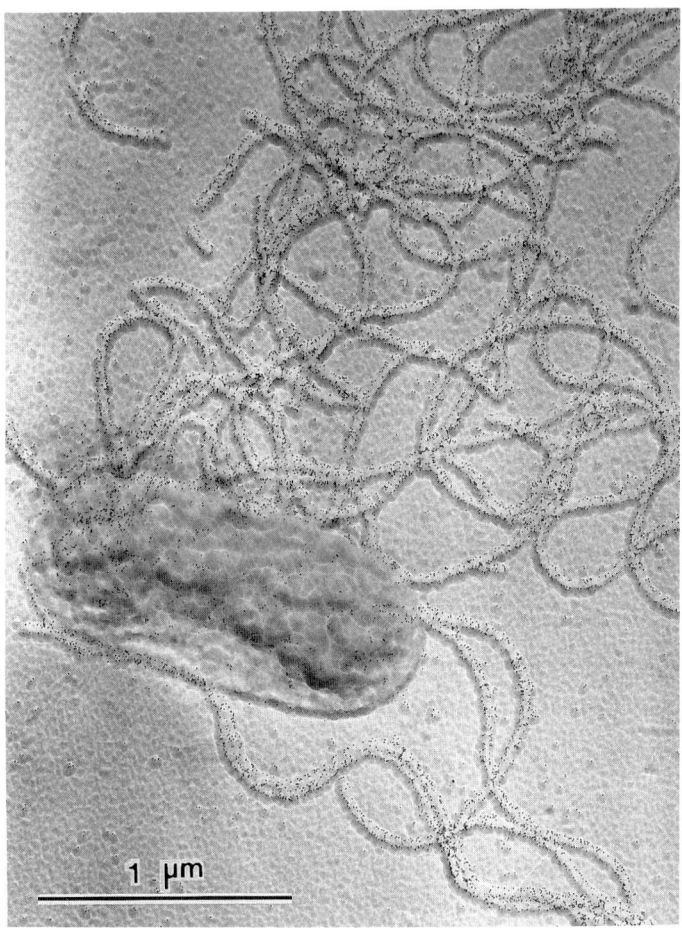

FIGURE 10
Proteus vulgaris fixed with formalin and treated with rabbit serum factor [H] and 5 nm protein A–gold. Replica film was prepared in the same manner as Figure 9 (×35,000). (Courtesy of Drs. I. Kondo and M. Yamaguchi, Taisho Pharmaceutical Company, Ltd., and Jikei University School of Medicine, Tokyo, Japan.)

Chapter 13. IgG Binding in Immunoelectronmicroscopy   **245**

small arrow) and somatic (10 nm gold, large arrow) antigens on the surface. Figure 9B is a stereo pair of the same cell, showing the striking three-dimensional distribution of these antigens as visualized by the deposition of the colloidal gold particles in the plasma membrane.

By contrast, Figure 10 is a cell of *Proteus vulgaris* prepared by the same method but treated only with rabbit serum factor [H] and 5 nm

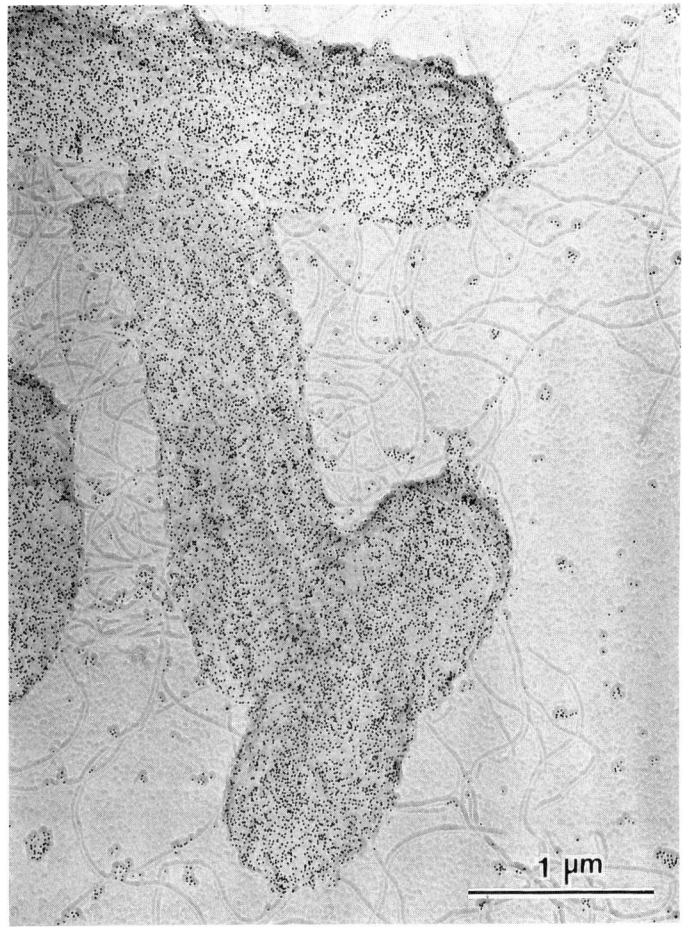

FIGURE 11
Proteus vulgaris fixed with glutaraldehyde and treated with rabbit serum factor [O] and 10 nm gold conjugated to goat anti-rabbit IgG. Replica prepared in the same manner as in Figure 9 (×25,000). (Courtesy of Drs. I. Kondo and M. Yamaguchi, Taisho Pharmaceutical Company, Ltd., and Jikei University School of Medicine, Tokyo, Japan.)

protein A–gold, showing the distribution of 5 nm gold particles on the flagella. Figure 11 shows cells of *Proteus vulgaris* treated with rabbit serum factor [0] and 10 nm gold conjugated to goat anti-rabbit IgG in order to illustrate the distribution of the somatic antigen.

VIII. General Applications of Colloidal Gold Labeling

In research involving biochemical and genetic analyses of microorganisms, an understanding of the spatial orientation of cellular constituents is often important. Cell growth and development and mechanisms of microbial pathogenesis are especially likely to benefit from visualization of the movement and position of cellular components.

Because of the small size of bacteria and other microorganisms, immunocytochemical tools that lend themselves to electron microscopic observation are particularly effective research tools. Methods are advancing steadily, as evidenced by the wide use of colloidal gold techniques. This chapter has detailed a number of techniques useful to studies of immunoglobulin-binding proteins in bacteria and has illustrated that the use of colloidal gold for biochemical and genetic experimentation is straightforward and the methodology generally simpler than that required to obtain the same information by nonultrastructural techniques.

References

Åkerström, B., and Björck, L. (1986). *J. Biol Chem.* **261,** 10240–10247.
Åkerström, B., Brodin, T., Reis, K., and Björck, L. (1985). *J. Immunol.* **135,** 2589–2592.
Bayer, E. A., Skutelsky, E., and Wilchek, M. (1979). *In* "Methods in Enzymology" (D. B. McCormick and L. D. Wright, eds.), Vol. 62, pp. 308–315. Academic Press, New York.
Bendayan, M. (1987). *J. Electron Microsc. Tech.* **6,** 7–13.
Bendayan, M., and Garzon, S. (1988). *J. Histochem. Cytochem.* **36,** 597–607.
Bendayan, M., Roth, J., Perrelet, A., and Orci, L. (1980). *J. Histochem. Cytochem.* **28,** 149–160.
Bienz, K., Egger, D., and Pasamontes, L. (1986). *J. Histochem. Cytochem.* **34,** 1337–1342.
Björck, L., and Kronvall, G. (1984). *J. Immunol.* **133,** 969–974.
Bonnard, C., Papermaster, D. S., and Kraehenbuhl, J.-P. (1984). *In* "Immunolabeling for Electron Microscopy" (J. M. Polak and I. M. Varndell, eds.), pp. 95–111. Elsevier Science Publishing Co., Inc., Amsterdam.
Brady, L. J., and Boyle, M. D. P. (1989). *Infect. Immun.* **57,** 1573–1581.
Chaiet, L., and Wolf, F. J. (1964). *Arch. Biochem. Biophys.* **106,** 1–5.
Coleman, S. E., Brady, L. J., and Boyle, M. D. P. (1990). *Infect. Immun.*, **58,** 332–340.
De Roe, C., Courtoy, P. J., and Baudhuin, P. (1987). *J. Histochem. Cytochem.* **35,** 1191–1198.
Frens, G. (1973). *Natl. Phys. Sci.* **241,** 20–22.

Fuccillo, D. A. (1985). *BioTechniques* **3**, 494–501.
Geoghegan, W. D., and Ackerman, G. A. (1977). *J. Histochem. Cytochem.* **25**, 1187–1200.
Green, N. M. (1975). *Adv. Protein Chem.* **29**, 85–133.
Kondo, I. (1986). *Proc. Int. Congr. Electron Microsc., 11th, Kyoto* 2061–2064.
Kondo, I., Hirano, T., and Tanaka, A. (1982). *Proc. Int. Congr. Electron Microsc., 10th, Hamburg* 33–37.
Kondo, I., Hirano, T., and Tanaka, A. (1983). *Proc. Chin. Jpn. Elecron Microsc. Semin., 2nd, Beijing* 227–232.
Kondo, I., Hirano, T., and Tanaka, A. (1984). *Proc. Eur. Congr. Electron Microsc., 8th, Budapest* **3**, 1593.
Kondo, I., Hirano, T., Yamaguchi, M., and Tanaka, A. (1986). *Proc. Int. Congr. Electron Microsc., 11th, Kyoto* 2305–2306.
Morris, R. E., and Saelinger, C. B. (1984). *J. Histochem. Cytochem.* **32**, 124–128.
Reis, K. J., Ayoub, E. M., and Boyle, M. D. P. (1984a). *J. Immunol.* **132**, 3091–3097.
Reis, K. J., Ayoub, E. M., and Boyle, M. D. P. (1984b). *J. Immunol.* **132**, 3098–3102.
Romano, E. L., and Romano, M. (1977). *Immunochemistry* **14**, 711–715.
Roth, J., Bendayan, M., and Orci, L. (1978). *J. Histochem. Cytochem.* **26**, 1074–1081.
Slot, J. W., and Geuze, H. J. (1984). In "Immunolabeling for Electron Microscopy" (J. M. Polak and I. M. Varndell, eds.), pp. 129–142. Elsevier Publishing Co., Inc., Amsterdam.
Slot, J. W., and Geuze, H. J. (1985). *Eur. J. Cell Biol.* **38**, 87–93.
Smit, J., and Todd, W. J. (1986). In "Ultrastructure Techniques for Microorganisms" (H. C. Aldrich and W. J. Todd, eds.), pp. 469–516. Plenum Press, New York.
Taatjes, D. J., Chen, T.-H., Åkerström, B., Björck, L., Carlemalm, E., and Roth, J. (1987). *Eur. J. Cell Biol.* **45**, 151–159.
Tanaka, A., Sekiguchi, Y., and Kuroda, S. (1978). *J. Electron Microsc.* **27**, 378.
Tanaka, A., Yamaguchi, M., and Hirano, T. (1988). *Proc. Annu. Meet. Electron Microsc. Soc. Am., 46th, Milwaukee* 414–415.
Tolson, N. D., Boothroyd, B., and Hopkins, C. R. (1981). *J. Microsc.* **123**, 215–226.

CHAPTER **14**

The use of bacterial Fc-binding proteins as probes for antigen–antibody complexes immobilized on nitrocellulose membranes

Ervin L. Faulmann

Separation of complexed from noncomplexed reactants is the key step of any immunoassay. Immobilization of soluble antigen or soluble antibody provides a convenient method for separating antigen–antibody complexes from unbound reactants in these assays (Towbin and Gordon, 1979; Gershoni and Palade, 1983; Tsang *et al.*, 1983; Kittler *et al.*, 1984; Bers and Garfin, 1985). This chapter describes procedures to immobilize soluble antigens onto charged membranes and to detect them using specific antibody and a labeled bacterial Fc-binding protein tracer. Bacterial Fc-binding proteins have the advantages of economy, wider species reactivity, higher specific activity, lower background reactivity, and greater batch-to-batch reproducibility when compared to other means of detecting immobilized antigen–antibody complexes (e.g., second antibodies) (Langone, 1982). There are two basic techniques to immobilize soluble antigens onto charged membranes: (1) direct binding of a soluble antigen to a suitable membrane (i.e., dot blot or colony lift) (Hawkes *et al.*, 1982; Koenen *et al.*, 1982; Young and Davis, 1983), and (2) electrophoretic transfer of antigens from a gel matrix onto the charged membrane (Western blot) (Towbin *et al.*, 1979; Burnette, 1981). The examples provided in this chapter are specific assays for soluble protein antigens immobilized onto nitrocellulose membranes using radiolabeled bacterial Fc-binding proteins as tracers; however, other means of visualizing antigen–antibody complexes have been developed using enzyme-labeled (Towbin and Gordon, 1984) or colloidal gold-complexes bacterial Fc-binding proteins (Brada and Roth, 1984; Perides et al., 1986). The procedures involving enzyme-labeled Fc-binding proteins are similar to those using radiolabeled tracers and are also described.

I. Dot Blot Assay

Dot blot procedures involve applying soluble antigen solutions to membranes that nonspecifically bind and immobilize the antigen. Initially, protein solutions were simply dotted onto the membrane and a vacuum was applied to draw the solution through the membrane (Hawkes et al., 1982; Herbink et al., 1982; Jahn et al., 1984). Dot blot suction manifolds are commercially available from a number of suppliers (e.g., Bio-Rad, Richmond, California). These devices contain a series of wells that allow for the application of 96 samples onto a 10 × 16 cm membrane. A slot blot apparatus is also available (e.g., Bio-Rad, Fremond, California) that allows for the application of a small number of samples (typically 48) in well defined slots; the autoradiographs of which are more amenable to quantification by scanning densitometry. Nitrocellulose and other charged membranes have been used with success for immobilizing proteins and other antigens (Renart et al., 1979; Towbin et al., 1979; Burnette, 1981; Gershoni and Palade, 1983; Pluskal et al., 1986; Miribel and Arnaud, 1988). The charged or hydrophobic groups on the membrane form stable complexes with the antigen and the membrane thus becomes a stable matrix of immobilized antigen. Further nonspecific interactions of the membrane can be prevented by the addition of saturating amounts of a blocking agent. The immobilized antigen in turn, can then be probed directly or indirectly with a suitably labeled, fluid-phase reagent, i.e., ligands or specific antibodies. In immunoassays, the amount of antibody associated with the membrane-bound antigen can then be determined by adding radiolabeled bacterial Fc-binding protein and detecting the radioactivity associated with the membrane after washing by autoradiography. The main advantage of the dot blot procedure is that one may screen a large number of samples in a single assay. This procedure is most useful as a qualitative measure of soluble antigen and is able to detect soluble antigen in the nanogram per milliliter (ng/ml) range. The method can be developed into a semi-quantitative procedure; however these approaches are limited by the binding capacity of the membrane and the efficiency of quantifying signals on autoradiographs (Uhl and Newton, 1988).

The basic procedure for carrying out any dot blot procedure follows a sequential protocol (summarized in Figure 1) in which

Chapter 14. Fc-Binding Proteins as Probes on Membranes

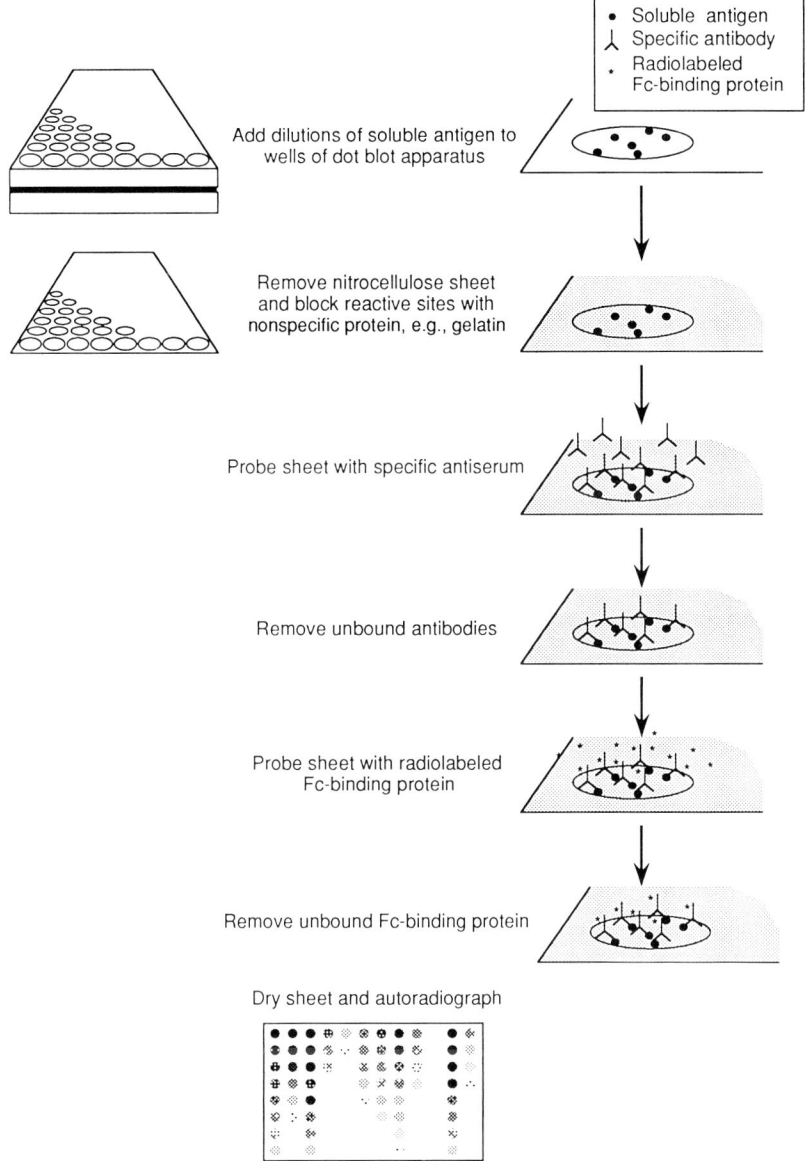

FIGURE 1
Schematic of dot blot assay for soluble antigen using bacterial Fc-binding protein as a tracer.

1) The antigen is immobilized.
2) The unreacted sites on the membrane are blocked.
3) The membrane is probed with specific antibody.
4) Antigen–antibody complexes are probed using a suitable tracer form of bacterial Fc-binding proten.
5) The bound tracer is quantified.

The nitrocellulose blot is washed after each step. The exact experimental procedure for each of these steps and the pitfalls are described in the following section.

A. Initial Experiments in Setting up a Dot Blot Assay

In designing any dot blot assay to detect a specific antigen, preliminary experiments should be carried out to determine the optimal buffer and washing conditions, as well as to optimize concentrations of antiserum and radiolabeled tracer required to obtain the desired sensitivity for the detection of the specific antigen. Initially, the sample buffer must be chosen so that it does not itself affect the binding of proteins to the membrane; the use of acidic buffers is not recommended. Furthermore, samples that contain components that nonspecifically bind either of the probes (immunoglobulin or radiolabeled bacterial Fc-binding proteins) need to be separated from the antigen to avoid high nonspecific backgrounds. Initial experiments used a checkerboard assay of different antigen–antiserum-tracer concentrations are used to determine the sensitivity of the assay and to minimize nonspecific background. This can be performed by adding a constant volume of different dilutions of the antigen solution to parallel rows in a 96-well dot blot apparatus containing a nitrocellulose membrane. The antigen solution is drawn through the membrane by application of a vacuum. The membrane is removed from the apparatus and unreacted sites on the nitrocellulose are blocked by incubation with blocking buffer as will be described later. The membrane is cut into strips and each parallel row can be reacted with a different dilution of antiserum. Following incubation, the strips can be washed and probed with different dilutions of radiolabeled bacterial Fc-binding protein probe (using procedures to be described). The quantity of antigen–antibody complexes associated with each strip is detected by autoradiography. It is recommended that each antigen concentration be immobilized in at least duplicate wells. From this initial experiment it should be possible to determine (1) what concentrations of the antibody and radiolabeled tracer can be used without significant nonspecific background binding, and (2) the sensitivity of the assay (the lowest level of antigen that can be detected in the assay).

B. Immobilizing the Antigen

In the first stage of the assay, the protein or other antigen solution is applied to a membrane so that it forms a dot. The membrane is immersed in phosphate-buffered saline (PBS) or Tris-buffered saline (pH 7.0–8.5) and allowed to equilibrate for 20 min at room temperature. In all of the procedures involving manipulation of charged membranes, gloves should be worn since proteins and oils present on the hands can be detected later in the assay. Aggregates and precipitated material should first be removed from the antigen solution by centrifugation or filtration, and dilutions of the standard antigen solution made in a suitable buffer [i.e., PBS or Tris-buffered saline (pH 7.0–8.5)]. The membrane is then loaded into the apparatus and the samples are added to the wells. The antigens in the solutions are allowed to interact with the membrane for 20 min at room temperature. Vacuum is applied to the apparatus and the samples are drawn through the membrane. The wells are washed twice with 200 μl sample buffer and the membrane is removed from the apparatus.

C. Blocking the Membrane

In the second step of the procedure, sites on the membrane that do not react with antigen are blocked by immersing the membrane into a blocking buffer. The use of an appropriate blocking agent is important in maintaining low background reactivity with either the primary antiserum or radiolabeled bacterial Fc-binding protein. The use of a gelatin solution has been shown to be an effective nonspecific blocking reagent (Jahn *et al.*, 1984; Reis *et al.*, 1985). In our laboratories, a 0.05 M veronal buffer (pH 7.35) containing 0.15 M NaCl, 0.25% gelatin, and 0.25% Tween 20 (referred to as 'blocking buffer') has been very effective for blocking unreacted sites on nitrocellulose membranes. Other researchers use solutions containing bovine serum albumin or nonfat dry milk (Jahn *et al.*, 1984; Koga *et al.*, 1987; Bird *et al.*, 1988; Narendran and Hoffman, 1988; Samuel *et al.*, 1988). Caution must be taken, however, because both of these blocking agents may contain trace quantities of bovine IgG that has the potential of reacting with the radiolabeled bacterial Fc-binding protein. Gelatin-containing buffers, however, should not be used in washing the membrane while it is still within the apparatus because the gelatin from some suppliers will block the pores of the membrane and inhibit the washing process. Ovalbumin (1.0% weight/volume) would also be a suitable nonspecific protein for use in blocking buffers (White and Hoch, 1981). The membrane is washed in 250 ml of blocking buffer for 15 min at room temperature with gentle rocking. The blocking buffer is removed, fresh buffer is added, and the washing process is repeated three more times.

D. Probing the Membrane with Antibody

The third stage in the assay procedure is to probe the immobilized antigen with a suitable dilution of specific antibody. The dilution should be determined from the preliminary studies previously described. As with all immunoassays, the selectivity of the antibody will determine the specificity of the assay.

The antibody probing procedure is carried out in a heat-sealable plastic pouch (Scotch, Minneapolis, Minnesota), which has previously been coated with the blocking buffer. Specific antiserum diluted in blocking buffer (10 ml of diluted antiserum is needed for a 10 × 16 cm nitrocellulose membrane) is added to the pouch (typical hyperimmune antisera can be used at dilutions between 1 : 500 and 1 : 5000), and the mixture is sealed and rotated for 3 hr at room temperature. The membrane is removed from the bag and unbound immunoglobulin is removed by washing four times in blocking buffer as described earlier. Care should be taken to insure that there are no bubbles formed between the membrane and the probing solution that would inhibit effective interaction of the antibody with the antigen.

E. Probing the Membrane with Radiolabeled Fc-Binding Tracer

The fourth stage of the procedure involves the detection of antigen–antibody complexes associated with the membrane. This is achieved by placing the washed membrane in a fresh heat-sealable pouch that has been prewashed with the blocking buffer. Radiolabeled bacterial Fc-binding protein diluted [between 200,000–500,000 counts per minute/milliliter (cpm/ml)] in 10 ml 'washing buffer' (0.1 M EDTA, 1.0 M NaCl, 0.25% gelatin, and 0.25% Tween 20, pH 7.4) is added and the pouch is sealed. The membrane and the probe are then rotated for 3 hr at ambient temperature.

The membrane is removed from the heat-sealable pouch and unbound ^{125}I-labeled bacterial Fc-binding protein is removed by washing four times in 250 ml washing buffer. Other washing buffers containing ovalbumin, etc., can also be used (Gershoni and Palade, 1983). The membrane is allowed to dry, either by air drying or under a heat lamp. *Caution: nitrocellulose can ignite if overheated.*

The preparation of suitable, radiolabeled bacterial Fc-binding protein tracers is described in detail in Chapter 7. As with all procedures involving radioactive tracers, the probing solution and all radioactive washing buffers must be disposed of in an appropriate manner.

F. Autoradiography

The final stage of the procedure is the detection of bound, radioactive tracer and the quantitation of antigen. The dried membrane is wrapped in plastic wrap, loaded along with XAR-5 film into an autoradiographic cassette with intensifying screens, and allowed to develop at $-70°C$ (Laskey and Mills, 1977). At an appropriate time, the film is developed in an X-Omat developer. The time of exposure of the blot to the film will depend on a number of variables, including the number of antigen–antibody complexes present, the affinity of the tracer for the species of antibody used, and the specific activity of the labeled tracer.

Though normally used as a qualitative measure of soluble antigen, there are three methods to quantify the amount of antigenic reactivity of a sample using the dot blot assay. The first is to include a standard antigen dilution series in the assay (e.g., twofold dilutions or less of known concentrations of the pure antigen). The intensity of the signals on the autoradiograph for the unknown samples is then compared with the reactivity of the standards by visual inspection. In this manner, one can "bracket" the relative antigenic reactivity of the unknown by comparison with the standard antigen samples (Kimball *et al.*, 1988; Van Vooren *et al.*, 1988). This method is similar to reporting a hemagglutination titration analysis, however the cutoff between a positive and a negative reaction is not as distinct. Additionally, the sensitivity of the assay is constrained by the dilution scheme; that is, a twofold dilution scheme will only be accurate to $\pm 50\%$ of any dilution.

The second method of quantifying the antigenic reactivity of a sample is to utilize a scanning densitometer that can measure the differential densities of the exposed areas of the autoradiograph (Palfreymen *et al.*, 1988; Uhl and Newton, 1988). Lines of dots are scanned (or whole sheets with some scanners) and the relative density of each dot is determined. Machines equipped with integration capabilities can report numerical values that correlate with the relative intensity of each dot (Palfreymen *et al.*, 1988). Alignment of the light beam of the densitometer through the line of dots is critical because each dot must be scanned across its diameter for reproducible results. Slot blots are preferred for scanning densitometric analysis because alignment of the light beam of the densitometer through the slots of exposed areas of the autoradiograph is more reproducible. A series of dilutions containing a known concentration of antigen should be included on all blots in order to establish a standard curve relating optical density to antigen concentration and to ensure that there is a direct proportionality between the density of the scanned image and the relative concentration of the antigen, i.e., the addition of twofold more antigen yields a peak with twice the area. Common problems in quantifying autoradiographs include overexposure of the X-ray film, yielding dots that are frequently beyond the optical range of the densitometer (Uhl and Newton, 1988), or under-representation of a strong radioactive signal due to coincident radioactive disintegrations that are not reflected in the precipitation of the silver salts in the film emulsion.

The third method for determining the quantity of labeled tracer bound to a dot blot is to cut the dots out of the membrane where the antigen has been immobilized and count them directly in a gamma counter. Yarnall and Boyle (1986) and Yarnall et al. (1986) have used this approach to measure the expression of different receptors on bacteria or as a method for comparing the functional activity of a given Fc-binding protein.

An example of the dot blot procedure to detect β antigen secreted or extracted from a strain of group B streptococcus is presented in the next section (for details of the significance and nomenclature of antigens associated with group B streptococci, see Chapter 9). This example utilizes radiolabeled protein G as the probe. Enzyme-labeled tracers can also be used to detect antigen–antibody complexes immobilized to charged membranes and the general procedures for using enzyme-labeled tracers will also be described.

G. Detection of β Antigen in Culture Supernatants or Extracts of Group B Streptococcus TC795

In this experiment, 100 μl of various dilutions of culture supernatants or extracts of group B streptococcal strain TC795, diluted in phosphate-buffered saline (PBS), pH 7.2, were applied onto a nitrocellulose membrane as previously described. The membrane was washed twice with 200 μl of PBS, removed from the vacuum manifold, blocked using the blocking buffer already described, and probed with a 1 : 1000 dilution of a monospecific rabbit antiserum against the β antigen, diluted in blocking buffer (for details of methods to generate β-specific antibodies, see Chapter 9). Unbound immunoglobulin was then removed by washing the membrane in blocking buffer and the membrane was probed for 3 hr with ^{125}I-labeled protein G (250,000 cpm/ml in blocking buffer). Unbound, radiolabeled probe was washed away using the washing buffer described earlier, the membrane was dried, placed with X-ray film using an intensifying screen at $-70°$C, and the film was finally developed 18 hr later. The results of this procedure are shown in Figure 2.

Chapter 14. Fc-Binding Proteins as Probes on Membranes

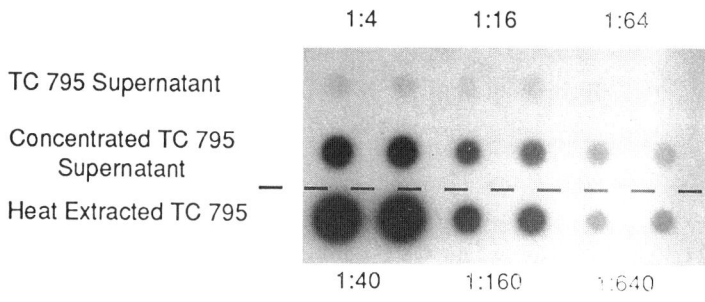

FIGURE 2

Dot blot assay of soluble β antigen from a group B streptococcal strain. Fifty ml of Todd-Hewitt broth was inoculated with strain TC 795 group B streptococcus and grown overnight at 37°C. The culture supernatant was harvested by centrifugation and filtration. An aliquot was removed and the remainder of the culture supernatant was concentrated 20-fold by ultrafiltration (YM30 membrane; Amicon, Danvers, Massachusetts). The bacterial pellet was washed twice in PBS and a 10% solution (wet weight bacteria/volume PBS) was heat-extracted by incubation at 90°C for 10 min. The bacteria were removed from the soluble, extracted material by centrifugation and filtration. The soluble bacterial protein solutions were diluted in PBS and 50 μl samples were added to the wells of the dot blot apparatus. The wells were washed twice with 200 μl of PBS and the nitrocellulose membrane was removed. The membrane was blocked and incubated with a rabbit anti-β monospecific antiserum (diluted 1 : 1000 in 15 ml blocking buffer for a 10 × 16 cm membrane) for 3 hr with rotation. The membrane was washed and probed overnight with ^{125}I-labeled protein G diluted in 15 ml blocking buffer (200,000 cpm/ml). The membrane was washed, air dried, incubated overnight at −70°C with XAR-5 film in a cassette with intensifying screens, and developed.

H. Probing the Membrane with Enzyme-Labeled Bacterial Fc-Binding Tracers

Enzyme-labeled bacterial Fc-binding proteins can be utilized to detect immobilized antigen–antibody complexes (Blake *et al.*, 1984). After the membrane is probed with antibody and washed as described earlier, the membrane is placed in a blocking buffer-coated, heat-sealable, plastic pouch and peroxidase-labeled or alkaline phosphatase-labeled bacterial Fc-binding protein diluted in blocking buffer is added. The sealed bag is rotated at room temperature for a minimum of 3 hr. The membrane is removed from the bag and washed four times in 250 ml Tris-buffered saline with Tween 20 (10 mM Tris-HCl, 150 mM NaCl, 0.05% Tween 20, pH 8.0) as described. The membrane is then washed once in Tris-buffered saline containing Mg^{2+} (10 mM Tris-HCl, 150 mM NaCl, 5 mM MgCl$_2$, pH 8.0). The membrane is blotted dry, immersed in the appropriate substrate solution until it has developed sufficient intensity (usually within 30 min), and then washed twice in H_2O.

Alkaline phosphatase substrate solution:

Combine the following solutions:

25 ml 100 mM Tris-HCl, 100 mM NaCl, 5 mM $MgCl_2$, pH 9.5

0.25 ml p-nitro blue tetrazolium chloride solution (30 mg/ml in 70% dimethylformamide/30% water)

0.25 ml 5-bromo-4-chloro-3-indolylphosphate-toluidine salt solution (15 mg/ml in dimethylformamide)

Substrate solution should be prepared immediately before use. Peroxidase substrate solution:

Add 60 mg 4-chloro-naphthol to 20 ml ice-cold methanol.

Add 60 μl H_2O_2 to 100 ml 20 mM Tris, 0.15 M NaCl, pH 7.5.

Combine the solutions to yield 120 ml of substrate solutions and use immediately.

II. Colony and Plaque Blotting of Antigens Expressed by Bacteria

A number of modifications of the dot blot procedure have been used to detect the presence or production of a given antigen by a bacterial colony. In this procedure, discrete bacterial colonies grown on a replica plate are immobilized on nitrocellulose either by direct adsorption (Koenen *et al.*, 1982) or by electrophoretic transfer (Yarnall *et al.*, 1984). The colonies are then probed directly to detect surface or secreted antigens, or, following lysis in an atmosphere of chloroform, to detect proteins present in the periplasmic space or within the bacteria. The probing procedure is similar to that described earlier for probing the nitrocellulose membranes of a dot blot. Reactive colonies on an autoradiograph can then be aligned with the corresponding colonies on a master plate and used to recover and expand any bacteria containing or expressing a desired antigen. Like all of the procedures involving antigen–antibody complexes immobilized on charged membranes, radiolabeled or enzyme-labeled bacterial Fc-binding proteins can be used as tracer.

With the recent advent of genetic engineering, a number of methods have been developed to monitor the expression of proteins encoded by recombinant DNA in bacteriophage-infected or plasmid-transformed bacterial hosts (Koenen *et al.*, 1982; Young and Davis, 1983). The technique of nonspecifically adsorbing bacterial products from bacteria grown on agar plates onto charged membranes (termed 'colony lifts' or 'plaque lifts' depending on whether the genetically engineered antigen is expressed by a plasmid or during the course of lysis by bacteriophage) and probing these immobilized proteins with specific antibody and radiolabeled bacterial Fc-binding proteins can be used effectively to screen for the production of specific antigens of interest (Koenen *et al.*, 1982; Young and Davis, 1983). Care must be taken to ensure that components in the agar medium and normal host, plasmid, or phage-encoded proteins do not demonstrate nonspecific reactivity in this assay. This activity can be detected by performing lifts and probing membranes from plates of *Escherichia coli* host bacteria transformed with the original plasmid unrecombined vector or infected with wild type phage. In the next section, an example of the use of a colony blot procedure to screen recombinant libraries is presented.

A. Colony or Plaque Lift Procedure

The process is summarized in Figure 3 and is as follows:

1a) Grow the recombinant plasmid-transformed bacterial host on a suitable agar medium overnight at a density of approximately 100–300 colonies per 150 mm diameter plate. If the system is not amenable to the inclusion of antibiotics into the agar medium, replica plates of the overnight plates may be made so that one can work with the colonies without fear of contaminating them during the adsorption process.

1b) For screening recombinant phage, infect a bacterial lawn with sufficient phage to yield 100–300 plaques per 150 mm diameter plate [induction of recombinant proteins using the lambda (λ) phage operator requires the inclusion of isopropyl thiogalactoside (IPTG) into the agar prior to adding the bacteria]. Induce the phage lytic cycle by incubation of the plate for 2 hr at 42°C. Allow the phage plaques to develop for 4–18 hr at 37°C.

2) Carefully place a nitrocellulose filter (i.e., Schleicher & Schuell, Keene, New Hampshire; Bio-Rad, Richmond, California, etc.) on the agar surface so that there are no trapped air bubbles between the agar and the filter. Do not rotate or shift the filter during its application onto the agar

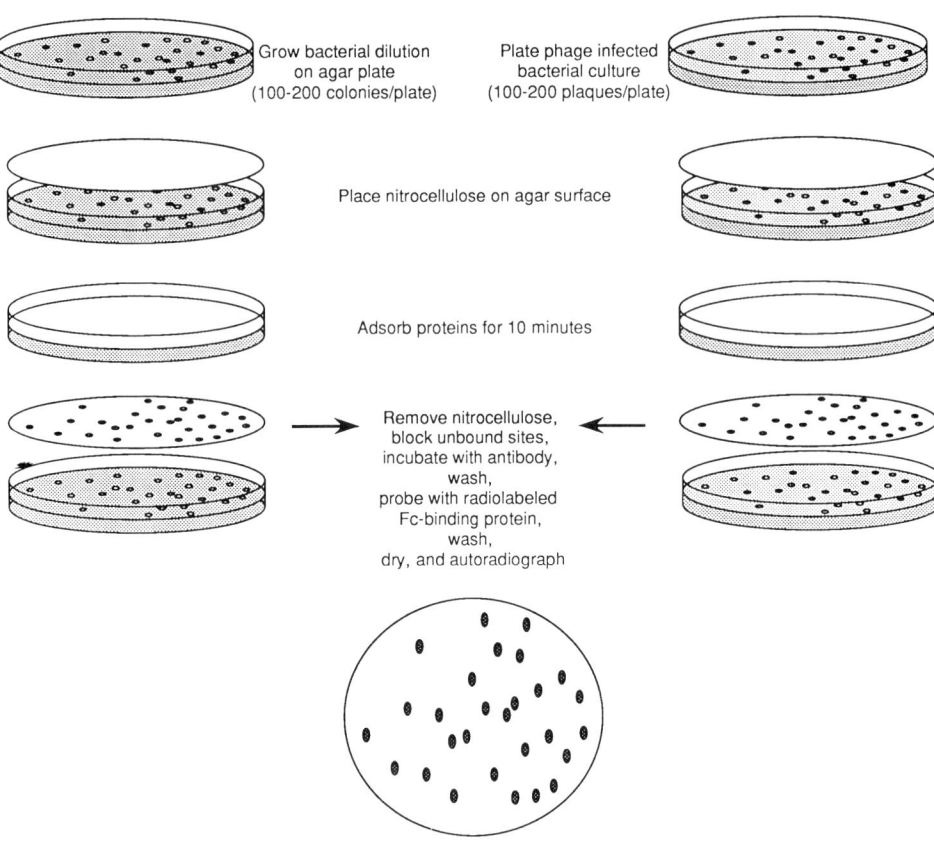

FIGURE 3
Schematic of colony or plaque lift screening for soluble antigen using radiolabeled bacterial Fc-binding protein as a tracer.

surface because significant smearing of the adsorbed proteins will obscure the location of the antigen-producing colony or plaque. Alternatively, the nitrocellulose filter may be placed over the phage-infected lawn and allowed to adsorb proteins during the 4–18 hr incubation at 37°C.

3) Allow the proteins and bacteria to adsorb onto the nitrocellulose for 10 min at room temperature.

4) Mark the membrane to orient it on the plate by making pencil marks on the membrane corresponding to marks on the plate or puncture the membrane and agar at random places with a needle.

5) Carefully remove the membrane with forceps and store the plate at 4°C until the positive colonies or plaques can be selected and subcultured. For bacterial colony lifts, lyse the bacteria by incubation of the nitrocellulose filter in chloroform for 3 min or in a chloroform-saturated atmosphere for 45 min. Allow the chloroform to evaporate at room temperature for 3 min.
6) The membrane is then washed in blocking buffer, probed with specific antibody, washed, probed with radiolabeled bacterial Fc-binding protein, washed, and autoradiographed as described earlier for the dot blot procedure.

This method, using radiolabeled or enzyme-labeled bacterial Fc-binding protein to react with nitrocellulose-immobilized, specific antibody–antigen complexes, provides a rapid screening process that can detect a single recombinant colony or phage plaque expressing the specific antigen, with little background interference. Using this procedure, the expression of a specific antigen by a single colony or phage can be expanded by selecting the colonies or plaques that correspond with exposed areas on the autoradiograph, culturing them, and rescreening the cultures. Care must be taken to align the autoradiograph with the corresponding colony or plaque to ensure selection of the correct recombinant. This process of selection, culturing, and rescreening is repeated until a pure population of recombinant bacteria or phage, all of which express the desired antigen, is produced.

B. Screening of a Recombinant λ Bacteriophage Isolate for the Expression of Streptococcal Plasmin-Binding Protein

An example of the use of the screening procedure just described for the plaque purification of a recombinant phage, which contained a DNA sequence coding for a plasmin receptor expressed by a group A streptococcus (strain 64/14), is shown in Figure 4 (after Lottenberg and Broder, 1990). In this example, the primary mouse antibody specific for the desired antigen displayed poor reactivity with the bacterial Fc-binding probe being used; however, following incubation with a goat anti-mouse IgG secondary antibody, detection by radiolabeled protein G was efficient. Phage from a plaque that had previously been shown to produce the streptococcal plasmin receptor was used to infect a lawn of HB 101 *E. coli* host bacteria. Overnight lysates were adsorbed onto nitrocellulose circles, the nitrocellulose was washed four times in blocking buffer, probed with mouse antiserum specific for the streptococcal plasmin receptor, washed,

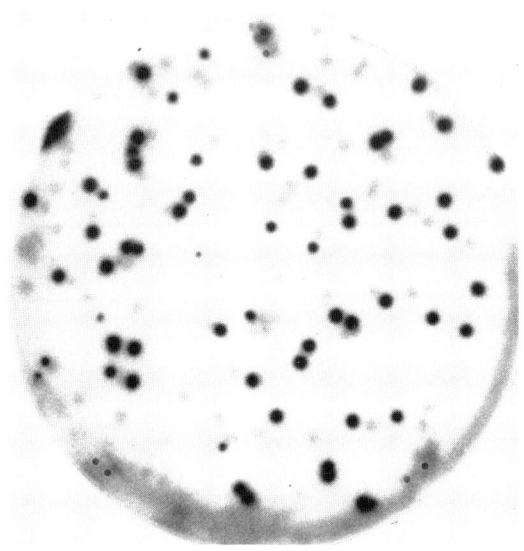

FIGURE 4
A genomic library of group A streptococcal strain 64/14 DNA was generated by mechanical shearing of chromosomal DNA and sizing the DNA into fractions containing 2–7 kilobase (kb) fragments. *Eco*RI linkers were ligated onto the ends of the fragments and they were ligated into the *Eco*RI arms of λ gt11 DNA. The ligated DNA was then packaged into phage heads and used to infect a lawn of HB 101 *E. coli* host bacteria. Positive plaques were screened and plaque-purified by adsorbing expressed proteins onto nitrocellulose circles and probing the membranes as described in the text. The results indicate that the phage preparation is approximately 50% purified (dark plaques denote positive-expressing phage and light plaques are negative).

probed with goat antiserum reactive against mouse IgG, washed, incubated with ^{125}I-labeled protein G, washed, and finally autoradiographed. Positive plaques selected by this procedure were found to express plasmin-binding activity, while other plaques (appearing as faint grey areas in the autoradiograph) failed to express any plasmin-binding potential (R. Lottenberg, personal communication).

III. Western Blot Analysis

The analysis of complex protein solutions by determining their relative migration using sodium dodecyl sulfate polyacrylamide gel electrophoresis (SDS-PAGE) is a widely used technique (Laemmli, 1970). In the last ten years the procedure of transferring the proteins separated by SDS-PAGE onto nitrocellulose or some other suitably charged membrane and then probing the immobilized proteins with specific ligands or antisera (the Western blot procedure) has also gained wide acceptance (Towbin *et al.*, 1979; for review, see Towbin and Gordon, 1984). The use of bacterial Fc-binding proteins as probes for antibody reacting with the separated antigens has expanded the utility of the Western blot procedure for antigenic screening (Burnette, 1981; Howe and Hershey, 1981; Björck and Blomberg, 1987). These reagents are more versatile than the use of secondary antibodies employed in other 'sandwich'-type detection assays because they are highly specific IgG reporting reagents with low nonspecific reactivities that bind with a wide species range of primary antibody (Björck and Blomberg, 1987; Boyle and Reis, 1987).

Soluble proteins are first separated by electrophoresis (in this case SDS-PAGE; however, native gel electrophoresis, isoelectric focusing, etc., can also be used) and then transferred onto nitrocellulose (Van der Sluis *et al.*, 1987; Sittenfeld and Moreno, 1988). The membrane (with proteins adsorbed) is then blocked and reacted with a specific antiserum. Any resulting antigen–antibody complexes are then detected using a radiolabeled or enzyme-labeled bacterial Fc-binding tracer as described previously for the dot blot procedure.

A. General Considerations in Performing Western Blot Assays

The Western blot procedure finds its widest usage as a qualitative assay for the presence of soluble antigen, though with appropriate controls, quantitation of soluble antigen levels in the low microgram range can be achieved (Blake *et al.*, 1984). The major advantage of the Western blotting procedure is the ability to determine a number of characteristics about an antigen, such as its relative molecular weight, homogenicity, pI, etc. (Al-Hussami *et al.*, 1988; Wedege *et al.*, 1988); however, a number of limitations of the procedure should also be considered. Treatment with SDS denatures the protein and the subsequent renaturation of the protein after electrophoretic transfer onto nitrocellulose may not be complete. Consequently, the transferred antigen may differ from the native antigen in the epitopes present. Furthermore, when the SDS gels are electrophoresed under reducing conditions, the reduction of cysteine bonds, together with the denaturation and separation by electrophoresis, will lead to the separation of subunits in proteins containing such structures. This may lead to the loss of antigenic recognition by an antibody prepared to the native protein. As with all procedures involving immobilization of antigens on nitrocellulose, care must be taken to eliminate any components in the sample that could nonspecifically bind to either the primary antibody or to the bacterial Fc-binding protein tracer, since such contaminants can lead to high nonspecific background reactivity.

B. Western Blotting Procedure

The Western blotting procedure is carried out in a sequential fashion as summarized in Figure 5. The initial step is the separation of the antigen sample by SDS-PAGE. The separated proteins are then transferred to nitrocellulose by electroblotting. The nitrocellulose is then reacted with specific antibodies and resulting antigen–antibody complexes are detected using a suitable bacterial Fc-binding protein tracer. The following are examples of procedures for separating protein antigen solutions by SDS-PAGE and transferring the separated molecules to nitrocellulose using a "wet" electroblot apparatus available from a number of commercial sources (i.e., Bio-Rad, Richmond, California; Hoefer, San Francisco, California, etc.).

C. Sodium Dodecyl Sulfate Polyacrylamide Gel Electrophoresis

This procedure follows the published method of Laemmli (1970).

1) All glass plates, spacers, well combs, etc., need to be carefully washed with detergent and water to remove proteins and oils that may inhibit acrylamide polymerization (a final wash in 95% ethanol is suggested).
2) The gel chamber is assembled by placing the spacers between the glass plates, forming a water-tight seal using clamps or tape

Chapter 14. Fc-Binding Proteins as Probes on Membranes

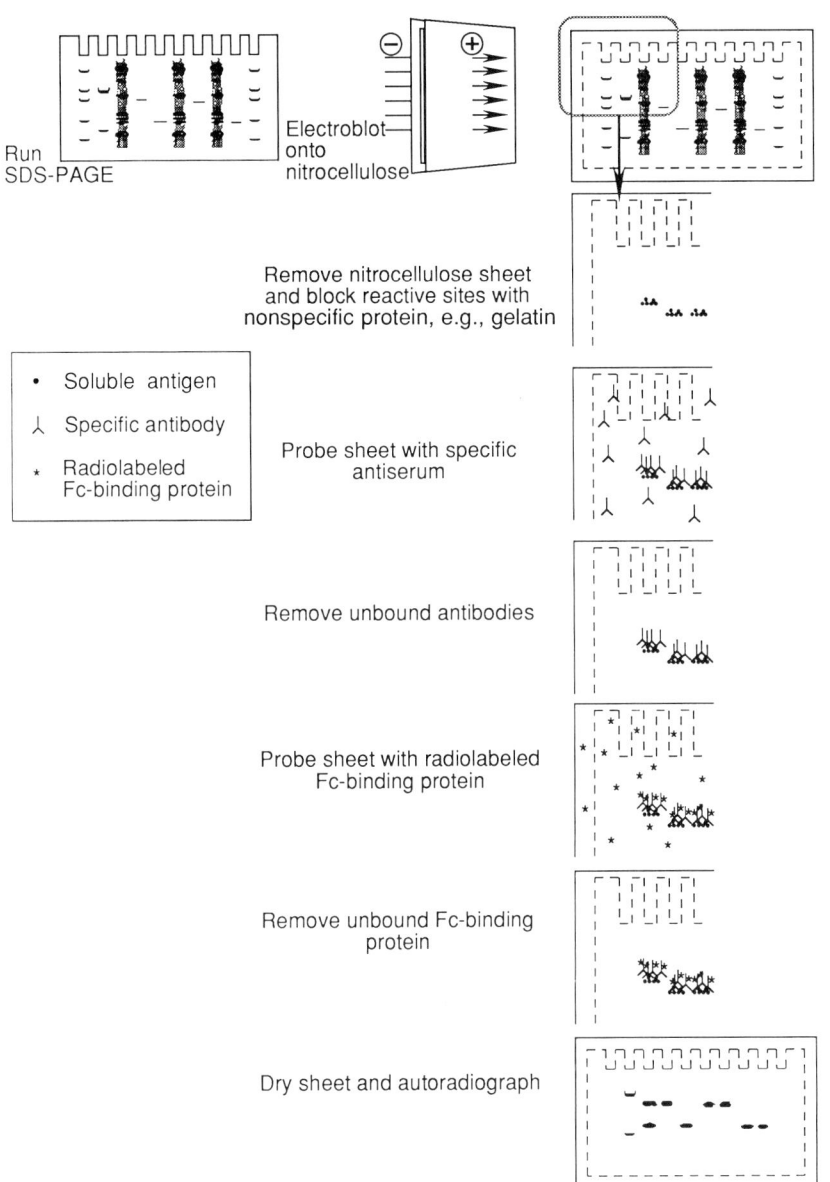

FIGURE 5
Schematic of Western blot assay for soluble antigen using radiolabeled bacterial Fc-binding protein as tracer.

(a light coating of Cell-o-seal on the spacers may prevent leakage). The glass plate assembly is sealed along the bottom edge either by using a commercial gel-casting apparatus or sealing with melted agarose (2% agarose in water) or clay. (Leakage of many commercial casting devices can be avoided by including two layers of Parafilm along the bottom edge of the glass plates.) Water should be added to the gel chamber to test for the presence of leaks.

3) The water is removed from the gel chamber and the separating gel solution containing an acrylamide concentration of between 7.5% and 20% (11.2:1, acrylamide:bis-acrylamide) in 0.375 M Tris (pH 8.8) with 0.1% SDS, 0.05% TEMED (N,N,N',N' tetramethylethylenediamine), and 0.05% ammonium persulfate is poured, overlayered with water, and allowed to polymerize for 1 hr.
Caution: prior to polymerization, acrylamide is a potent neurotoxin with cumulative effects. In preparing stock solutions, avoid breathing powdered acrylamide and take precautions to prevent contact of acrylamide solutions with exposed skin.

4) The water overlay is removed and a stacking gel of 4% acrylamide (11.2:1, acrylamide:bis-acrylamide) in 0.125 M Tris (pH 6.5) with 0.1% SDS, 0.1% TEMED and 0.05% ammonium persulfate is poured with the well comb in place and allowed to polymerize for 1 hr.

5) Samples are diluted 1:2 with sample buffer [0.062 M Tris (pH 6.8), 1.0% glycerol, 0.062% bromphenol blue, 2.0% SDS, and for reduced samples 0.062% 2-mercaptoethanol] and boiled for 1–5 min.

6) The well comb is removed from the gel and the gel, along with the glass plates, is loaded into the electrophoresis apparatus. The upper and lower reservoirs are filled with electrode buffer [190 mM glycine, 25 mM Tris (pH 8.3), and 0.1% SDS].

7) The samples are applied to the wells. It is often convenient to use prestained molecular weight markers to monitor the progress of electrophoresis or the nitrocellulose paper after electroblotting.) Unreduced samples to be electrophoresed should be spaced at least 1.5 cm from samples containing 2-mercaptoethanol or dithiothreitol to prevent the effects of the reducing agent diffusing into the unreduced samples during electrophoresis. Voltage is applied across the gel and typical running times for 160 × 160 × 1.5 mm gels are as follows:

Voltage	Average Running Time
40	20 hr
60	15 hr
200	4 hr

8) Electrophoresis is terminated before the bromphenol blue band runs off the end of the gel, and the gel is removed from the apparatus. At this point, the gel may be cut so portions of the gel can be stained for proteins or carbohydrates, while other portions of the gel can be electroblotted onto nitrocellulose.

D. Electroblotting

1) The gel is immersed in electroblot buffer [190 mM glycine and 25 mM Tris is 60% methanol : 40% water (volume/volume; v/v)] and equilibrated for 20–30 min to remove most of the SDS and to allow the gel matrix to equilibrate in the electrode buffer. (This procedure follows the electroblotting method of Towbin *et al.*, 1979.)
2) The gel is then loaded into a "sandwich" comprised of a pad (Scotchbrite), absorbent paper (Whatman 3MM), a sheet of nitrocellulose, followed by absorbent paper, and another pad (all of which had been saturated in the electrode buffer). Care must be taken to prevent air bubbles between the gel and the nitrocellulose and gloves should be worn to prevent oil and proteins from the hands contaminating the nitrocellulose.
3) The gel "sandwich" is then loaded into the apparatus and should be placed such that the proteins migrating out of the gel in the electric field are directly adsorbed onto the nitrocellulose. In most cases, the SDS coating the proteins imparts a strong, negative charge to the molecules and they are therefore anions in the electroblot buffer, thus the nitrocellulose should be placed between the anode and the gel (electroblotting native gels may require nitrocellulose sheets to be placed on both sides of the gel).
4) Voltage is applied across the gel (using a power supply that can deliver > 200 mA). The voltages and running times for electroblotting vary according to the concentration of the acrylamide in the gel, the molecular weights of the proteins to be eluted from the gel, temperature, and the relative field

strength (which is a function of the distance between the electrodes and the ionic strength of the buffer) but the following are typical findings for electroeluting proteins from a 10% acrylamide gel:

Voltage	Average Running Time
30	14–16 hr
70	3 hr

5) When electroblotting is complete, the gel and nitrocellulose are removed from the apparatus. The efficiency of the electroblotting procedure can be verified by staining the gel to determine if residual proteins are present, or by examining the gel for prestained molecular weight markers, if they are used.

Alternative "semi-dry" blotting devices are also commercially available and facilitate a more rapid transfer of proteins (Bio-Rad, Richmond, California; Hoefer, San Francisco, California, etc.). The manufacturer's recommendations should be followed when using the dry blotting apparatus.

E. Detection of Antigens on Western Blots

The detection of antigen immobilized onto nitrocellulose following electroblotting is carried out as described earlier for the dot blot procedure and an example of this procedure is demonstrated in the following section.

F. Detection of β Antigen in Extracts of Group B Streptococcus TC 795 by Western Blot Analysis

Heat extracts of group B streptococcal strain TC 795 were separated by SDS-PAGE and electroblotted onto nitrocellulose. The protein-binding sites on the membrane were blocked by washing in blocking buffer and the membrane was probed with a monospecific antiserum for the β antigen of group B streptococci (Brady *et al.*, 1988). Unbound immunoglobulin was removed by washing in blocking buffer. The antibodies associated with the separated antigens were visualized by incubation with ^{125}I-labeled protein G, followed by washing and autoradiography (Figure 6). These findings, in agreement with previous studies by Bevanger (1985), Brady and Boyle (1989), Cleat and Timmis (1987), and Russell-Jones *et al.* (1984) demonstrate that the β antigen is expressed by certain group B streptococci as a heterogeneous mixture of proteins with the major molecular form being an ~135,000 dalton protein.

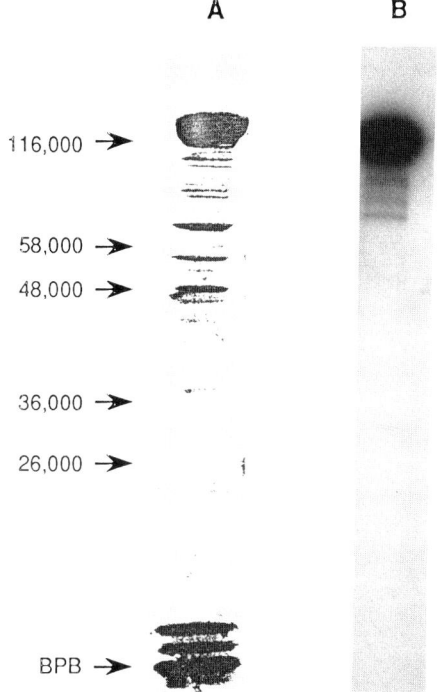

FIGURE 6
SDS-PAGE and Western blot of β antigen extracted from a group B streptococcus strain. Heat-extracted material (25 μl/well added to an equal volume of sample buffer) from strain TC 795 group B streptococcus from Figure 2 was subjected to SDS-PAGE in a 7.5% acrylamide gel. A portion of the gel was stained with Coomassie Blue R-250 (Panel A). The remainder of the gel was electroblotted for 3 hr at 70 V (7 cm electrode separation), blocked with 1% gelatin solution, probed for 3 hr with a monospecific antiserum to the β antigen (diluted 1 : 1000 in blocking buffer), and washed in blocking buffer. The membrane was then probed for 3 hr with ^{125}I-labeled protein G (300,000 cpm/ml in blocking buffer) and washed in washing buffer as described in the text. The membrane was then dried, placed with XAR-5 film for 5 hr at −70°C, and developed (Panel B). (BPB, Bromphenol blue.)

IV. Summary

The methods discussed in this chapter describe a number of examples of the use of radiolabeled bacterial Fc-binding proteins as tracers for antigen–antibody complexes immobilized onto charged membranes. These techniques may be adapted for use with other tracer forms of bacterial Fc-binding proteins, e.g., enzyme-labeled or gold-labeled probes. The dot blot procedure is a rapid method to screen samples for the presence of an antigenic component for which a suitable antiserum is available. The Western blotting procedure combines the techniques that separate molecules by physical characteristics (i.e., molecular size, pI, etc.), before transferring them to a charged membrane and probing them antigenically. These techniques have proven to be of great value for determining heterogeneity in antigen preparations. In general, all the techniques involving the detection of immobilized antigens on charged membranes are analytical but can be made semiquantitative by inclusion of standard antigen preparations combined with densitometry.

Acknowledgments

I would like to thank Drs. M. D. P. Boyle and R. Lottenberg for their contributions of data and expertise, and Dr. R. E. Kris for assistance in editing this manuscript.

References

Al-Hussami, O., Godinot, C., Monier, J. M., Trepo, C., and Monier, J. C. (1988). *J. Immunol. Methods* **113**, 61–73.
Bers, G., and Garfin, D. (1985). *BioTechniques* **3**, 276–288.
Bevanger, L. (1985). *Acta Pathol. Microbiol. Immunol. Scand. B* **93**, 113–119.
Bird, C. R., Gearing, A. H. J., and Thorpe, R. (1988). *J. Immunol. Methods* **106**, 175–179.
Björck, L., and Blomberg, J. (1987). *Eur. J. Clin. Microbiol.* **6**, 428–429.
Blake, M. S., Johnston, K. H., Russell-Jones, G. J., and Gotchlich, E. C. (1984). *Anal. Biochem.* **136**, 175–179.
Boyle, M. D. P., and Reis, K. J. (1987). *Biotechnology* **5**, 697–703.
Brada, D., and Roth, J. (1984). *Anal. Biochem.* **142**, 79–83.
Brady, L. J., and Boyle, M. D. P. (1989). *Infect. Immun.* **57**, 1573–1581.
Brady, L. J., Daphtary, U. D., Ayoub, E. M., and Boyle, M. D. P. (1988). *J. Infect. Dis.* **158**, 965–972.
Burnette, W. N. (1981). *Anal. Biochem.* **112**, 195–203.
Cleat, P. H., and Timmis, K. N. (1987). *Infect. Immun.* **55**, 1151–1155.
Gershoni, J. M., and Palade, G. E. (1983). *Anal. Biochem.* **131**, 1–15.
Hawkes, R., Niday, E., and Gordon, J. (1982). *Anal. Biochem.* **119**, 142–147.
Herbink, P., Van Bussel, F. J., and Warnaar, S. O. (1982). *J. Immunol. Methods* **48**, 293–298.
Howe, J. G., and Hershey, J. W. B. (1981). *J. Biol. Chem.* **256**, 12836–12839.
Jahn, R., Schiebler, W., and Greegard, P. (1984). *Proc. Natl. Acad. Sci. U.S.A.* **81**, 1684–1687.
Kimball, S. R., Rannels, S. L., Elensky, M. B., and Jefferson, L. S. (1988). *J. Immunol. Methods* **106**, 217–223.
Kittler, J. M., Meisler, N. T., Viceps-Madore, D., Cidlowski, J. A., and Thanassi, J. W. (1984). *Anal. Biochem.* **137**, 210–216.
Koenen, M., Rüther, U., and Müller-Hill, B. (1982). *EMBO J.* **1**, 509–512.
Koga, K., Abe, S., Hasimoto, H., and Yamaguchi, M. (1987). *J. Immunol. Methods* **105**, 15–21.

Laemmli, U. K. (1970). *Nature (London)* **227,** 680–685.
Langone, J. J. (1982). *J. Immunol. Methods* **51,** 3–22.
Laskey, R. A., and Mills, A. D. (1977). *FEBS Lett.* **82,** 314–316.
Lottenberg, R., and Broder, C. C. (1990). In preparation.
Miribel, L., and Arnaud, P. (1988). *J. Immunol. Methods* **107,** 253–259.
Narendran, A., and Hoffman, S. A. (1988). *J. Immunol. Methods* **114,** 227–234.
Palfreyman, J. W., Vigrow, A., Button, D., and Glancy, H. (1988). *J. Immunol. Methods* **109,** 199–201.
Perides, G., Plagens, V., and Traub, P. (1986). *Anal. Biochem.* **152,** 94–99.
Pluskal, M. G., Przekop, M. B., and Kavonian, M. R. (1986). *BioTechniques* **4,** 272–283.
Reis, K. J., Ayoub, E. M., and Boyle, M. D. P. (1985). *J. Microbiol. Methods* **4,** 45–58.
Renart, J., Reiser, J., and Stark, G. R. (1979). *Proc. Natl. Acad. Sci. U.S.A.* **81,** 1684–1687.
Russell-Jones, G. J., Gotschlich, E. C., and Blake, M. S. (1984). *J. Exp. Med.* **160,** 1467–1475.
Samuel, D., Pall, R. J., and Abuknesha, R. A. (1988). *J. Immunol. Methods* **107,** 217–224.
Sittenfeld, A., and Moreno, E. (1988). *J. Immunol. Methods* **106,** 175–179.
Towbin, H., and Gordon, J. (1984). *J. Immunol. Methods* **72,** 313–340.
Towbin, H., Staehelin, T., and Gordon, J. (1979). *Proc. Natl. Acad. Sci. U.S.A.* **76,** 4350–4354.
Tsang, V. C. W., Peralta, J. M., and Simons, A. R. (1983). *In* "Methods in Enzymology" (J. J. Langone and H. Van Vunakis, eds.), Vol. 92, pp. 377–391. Academic Press, New York.
Uhl, J., and Newton, R. C. (1988). *J. Immunol. Methods* **110,** 79–84.
Van der Sluis, P. J., Pool, C. W., and Sluiter, A. A. (1987). *J. Immunol. Methods* **104,** 65–71.
Van Vooren, J. P., Turner, M., Yernault, J. C., DeBruyn, J., Burton, E., Legros, F., and Farber, C. M. (1988). *J. Immunol. Methods* **113,** 45–49.
Wedege, E., Bryn, K., and Froholm, L. O. (1988). *J. Immunol. Methods* **113,** 51–59.
White, P. J., and Hoch, S. O. (1981). *Biochem. Biophys. Res. Commun.* **102,** 365–371.
Yarnall, M., and Boyle, M. D. P. (1986). *J. Immunol.* **136,** 2670–2673.
Yarnall, M., Reis, K. J., Ayoub, E. M., and Boyle, M. D. P. (1984). *J. Microbiol. Methods* **3,** 83–93.
Yarnall, M., Ayoub, E. M., and Boyle, M. D. P. (1986). *J. Gen. Microbiol.* **132,** 2049–2052.
Young, R. A., and Davis, R. W. (1983). *Proc. Natl. Acad. Sci. U.S.A.* **80,** 1194–1198.

CHAPTER 15

Application of bacteria expressing immunoglobulin-binding proteins to immunoprecipitation reactions

Michael D. P. Boyle
Ervin L. Faulmann

I. Introduction

The use of immobilized bacterial immunoglobulin-binding proteins to remove IgG or immune complexes containing IgG from solution are among the most widespread applications for this family of functional proteins. A suitably fixed form of a bacteria expressing an IgG-binding protein represents the most economical and convenient form of the immobilized IgG-binding protein reagent. The use of bacterial immunosorbents has the advantage that the binding protein does not need to be isolated and conditions for immobilizing the proteins in a functionally active form do not need to be established. Consequently, procedures using intact bacteria expressing a new or different type of IgG-binding protein represent the easiest way to establish the potential for these reagents. Bacteria, however, express receptors for other serum proteins, e.g., plasmin-binding proteins (Lottenberg *et al.*, 1987), albumin receptors (Wiedback *et al.*, 1983), Clq receptors (Yarnall *et al.*, 1986), etc., and consequently will remove not only immunoglobulin via the Fc region but may remove other serum proteins. Furthermore, many sera contain naturally occurring antibodies that may bind to bacteria via specific antigenic recognition domains in the $F(ab')_2$ region. Despite these limitations, bacterial-bound IgG-binding proteins have proven to be of value for a variety of different procedures.

The next three chapters describe the use of immunoglobulin-binding proteins attached to bacterial cell walls for a number of immunological applications. In this chapter, the focus is directed toward the use of bacterial-bound immunoglobulin-binding proteins for immunoprecipitation reactions. These procedures were among the earliest applications described for protein A and are still in wide use today despite the availability of more completely characterized sources of immobilized protein A reagents. The uses and limitations of bacteria expressing immunoglobulin-binding proteins as immunosorbents for immunoprecipitation and selective depletion of IgG antibodies are described in detail.

II. General Background

All of the procedures using immunoglobulin-binding proteins bound to bacteria are based on the premise that the bacteria can bind free antibody or antigen–antibody complexes with a high affinity via regions of the immunoglobulin molecule not involved in its antigen recognition properties.

In systems using intact bacteria as the immunosorbent, binding of proteins other than antibodies can occur. Consequently, this approach is of limited value as a purification procedure. However, if either a specific antibody and/or a labeled form of antigen is available, this procedure can be used successfully for analytical applications. There are four basic types of applications that will be described in this chapter.

1) The use of bacterial-bound IgG-binding proteins to analyze labeled antigens,
2) The use of bacterial-bound IgG-binding proteins in place of second antibodies for radioimmunoassay,
3) The use of bacterial-bound IgG-binding proteins for detection of specific antibodies, and
4) Depletion of IgG from serum to facilitate measurement of isotypes of antibodies other than IgG.

Before discussing the practical applications of bacterial-bound immunoglobulin-binding proteins as immunosorbents, a general review of the preparation of reagents, selection of conditions, etc., will be presented. As with the majority of practical applications utilizing bacterial immunoglobulin-binding proteins, most studies have been carried out with protein

A, or in this case, formalin-fixed *Staphylococcus aureus* Cowan I bacteria. More recently, applications using heat-killed protein G-positive streptococci have emerged and it is likely that, because of the ease of generating these bacterial reagents, many of the other types of bacterial immunoglobulin-binding proteins will find their first application in the types of assay systems described here.

III. Preparation of Bacterial Immunosorbent Reagents

A. Protein A-Positive *Staphylococcus aureus*

In the pioneering studies using *Staphylococcus aureus* Cowan I as a source of immobilized protein A (Jonsson and Kronvall, 1974; Kessler, 1975, 1976; Goding, 1978), investigators carried out a series of experiments to identify the best way to treat *Staphylococcus aureus* Cowan I to obtain a bacterial immunosorbent expressing a stable, high level of protein A. The parameters that were considered included, (1) the optimal growth and media conditions for culturing the bacteria, (2) the optimal method for killing the bacteria and fixing the cell membrane to maximize their IgG-binding capacity, and (3) stability of IgG-binding activity on fixed bacteria. All of these parameters have been carefully established for protein A-bearing *Staphylococcus aureus* (Jonsson and Kronvall, 1974; Kessler, 1981). These conditions have been published by Kessler (1981), and the major findings are summarized here.

1. Growth of Bacteria

Staphylococcus aureus Cowan I (ATCC #12598) is grown in enriched medium with aeration overnight (stationary phase). The bacteria are harvested by centrifugation and resuspended in 0.15 M phosphate-buffered saline, pH 7.3, containing 0.02% NaN_3 (PBS-azide) at 10% wet weight/volume concentration.

2. Fixation of Bacteria

Formaldehyde is added to a 10% wet weight/volume suspension of bacteria in PBS-azide to yield a final concentration of 1.5% and stirred slowly on a magnetic stirrer for 1.5–2 hr at ambient temperature. The bacteria are pelleted by centrifugation and washed twice with PBS-azide. The washed pellet is resuspended at a concentration of 10% and heated rapidly at 80°C for 5 min. This heating step was reported by Jonsson and Kronvall (1974) to yield a more stable immunoglobulin-binding reagent. Other methods of immobilization of protein A have been reported, including treatment with glutaraldehyde or trichloroacetic acid (Lindmark, *et al.*,

1982; Shantz, 1983). Most commercial sources of protein A-bearing immunosorbents use the formalin fixation procedure, which has proven satisfactory and leads to relatively few bacterial aggregates.

B. Protein G-Positive Streptococci

The applications for which protein A bound to *Staphylococcus aureus* have proven successful could be extended to a wider range of immunoglobulin species if a corresponding protein G-positive streptococcal isolate could be prepared. In our laboratory, we have used a similar approach to that just described to prepare a protein G-positive bacterial immunosorbent. For these studies, we used a protein G-positive, group G streptococcal isolate, G1400, that displayed the greatest IgG-binding capacity of any type III IgG-binding protein-positive strain studied in our laboratory (von Mering and Boyle, 1986). A variety of culture conditions were compared and maximal binding of IgG was observed with bacteria that had been grown as overnight, stationary cultures at 37°C in Todd-Hewitt broth. The bacteria were harvested from overnight cultures, pelleted by centrifugation, and washed twice with PBS-azide. The washed bacterial pellet was resuspended at a concentration of 10% wet weight/volume and then treated with a number of fixatives including glutaraldehyde and formaldehyde, followed by washing and heat-killing at 85°C for ten min. In our studies, we found that the heat-killed organisms retained their ability to bind IgG, while those bacteria treated with glutaraldehyde or formaldehyde displayed decreased IgG-binding capability.

C. IgG-Binding Capacity of Bacterial Immunosorbents

The IgG-binding capacity of different batches of bacteria has been found to vary. This may be due to differences in the expression of binding proteins as a function of the growth or fixation conditions. For example, many bacteria produce proteases that become active as the pH of the culture medium falls, which can lead to digestion of IgG-binding proteins (Elliott and Dole, 1947; Liu and Elliott, 1965; Schalén *et al.*, 1982). Batch-to-batch variation of the amount of surface IgG-binding proteins on the immunosorbent is not highly critical since in most assays the binding proteins are added in gross excess. It is, however, important for reproducible experimental protocols to standardize any new batch of bacterial immunosorbent as a record for future reference, in order to be able to study the stability of the reagent. There are a variety of simple methods to determine the IgG-binding capacity of any lot of bacterial immunosorbent.

In general, 1 ml of a 10% suspension of bacteria is pelleted by centrifugation and washed twice in PBS-azide. The resulting bacterial pellet is then resuspended in 1 ml of a 10 mg/ml solution of any species of IgG diluted in PBS-azide. The bacteria are resuspended in the immunoglobulin solution and rotated, end over end, for 1 hr at room temperature. The bacteria are removed by centrifugation and the quantity of IgG remaining in the supernatant is compared to a similar sample of IgG not incubated with bacteria. An estimate of IgG levels can be carried out using commercially available, radial immunodiffusion plates (Kalstead Laboratories, Austin, Texas), by radioimmunoassay (Langone *et al.*, 1977), or by enzyme-linked immunosorbent assay (Reis *et al.*, 1988a). The binding capacity can also be determined by calculating depletion of a radiolabeled or fluorescent-labeled IgG molecule from a standard IgG stock solution. It is customary to express the binding capacity of bacterial immunosorbents as milligram per milliliter (mg/ml) of IgG removed by 1 ml of a 10% bacterial suspension. Bacterial immunosorbents should be calibrated for each species of immunoglobulin that the investigator intends to immunoprecipitate with the reagent. In particular, the reactivity of any bacterial immunosorbent with a monoclonal antibody must be determined on an antibody by antibody basis.

D. Storage and Stability

The shelf-life of bacterial immunosorbents is found to vary with the bacterial source, the fixation procedure, and the method of storage. The most extensive data on stability of bacterial immunosorbents have been reported for formalin-fixed *Staphylococcus aureus* Cowan I. Most investigators have reported that the IgG-binding capacity of formalin-fixed *Staphylococcus aureus* remains greater than 80% for over one year at 4°C (Kessler, 1981). However, it is generally agreed that stability can be prolonged by freezing the bacteria at $-20°$ or $-70°C$ (Shantz, 1983; Ivarie and Jones, 1979). Repeated freezing and thawing of bacterial immunosorbents significantly increases clumping. Consequently, it is recommended that bacterial immunosorbents are stored frozen as aliquots and discarded after use. Some vendors offer lyophilized bacterial immunosorbent stocks, which should be used within a few weeks of reconstitution (Shantz, 1983).

It is important to wash any form of stored *Staphylococcus aureus* Cowan I strain before use in any procedure. We have found that the bacteria lose protein A from their surfaces over time and the presence of fluid-phase protein A in the reaction mixture significantly reduces the efficiency of the bacteria as solid-phase immunosorbents.

Our experience with protein G-positive bacteria is more limited. We have stored aliquots of heat-killed bacteria for over two years at $-70°C$

without loss of IgG-binding capacity. Bacteria stored in PBS-azide at 4°C are stable for at least 12 months. Increased clumping of heat-killed protein G-positive bacteria has also been noted on repeated freezing and thawing. In general, protein G seems to be more firmly associated with the streptococcal cell wall than protein A is with the staphylococcal cell wall; however, it is recommended that all bacterial immunosorbent preparations be washed prior to use.

E. Commercial Source of Bacterial Immunoglobulins

At the present time there are many suppliers of protein A-positive bacterial immunosorbents suitable for use in the immunoprecipitation applications described in this chapter. Recently, protein G-positive bacterial immunosorbents and bacterial immunosorbents expressing other types of immunoglobulin-binding activities have become commercially available. For a detailed listing of suppliers, see Linscott (1989).

F. Selection of Appropriate Bacterial Immunosorbent for Use with a Monoclonal or Polyclonal Antibody

One of the major problems with studies involving immunoprecipitation of antibodies by bacterial Fc-binding protein-positive bacteria is the perception that any antibody of a given species and subclass will react in a predictable way with a bacterial IgG-binding protein. While it is possible to predict which species and subclasses of IgG would most probably react with protein A or protein G (see Tables 3 and 4 of Chapter 1), many investigators have noted differences in the reactivities of mouse and rat monoclonal antibodies of the same subclass with protein A or protein G (see Reis *et al.*, 1988b; Chapters 16 and 17). Indeed, the best example of selective binding is that observed between human IgG_3 and staphylococcal protein A. The majority of human IgG_3 antibody does not bind with protein A, however, IgG_3 antibodies of the s^+t^+ allotype are found to react. This reactivity can be shown to be due to a single amino acid substitution at position 435 of the heavy chain. A histidine residue at this position facilitates IgG binding, while an arginine residue at this site does not lead to a significant degree of reactivity with IgG_3 (Haake *et al.*, 1982).

It is, therefore, strongly recommended that some preliminary studies be carried out to determine that the antibody of interest will bind to the bacterial immunosorbent selected. This can be carried out in a straightforward manner by incubating the immunosorbent with the antibody source for one hour at room temperature. Unbound antibodies are removed by pelleting the bacteria by centrifugation and washing twice with PBS-azide. The bacterial pellet is then boiled for 5 min in SDS-PAGE sample buffer containing β-mercaptoethanol [0.062 M Tris (pH 6.8), 1.0% glycerol, 0.062% bromphenol blue, 2.0% SDS, and 0.062% β-mercaptoethanol] (Laemmli, 1970). Solubilized proteins are then separated on an SDS-polyacrylamide gel and protein eluted from the bacterial immunosorbent can be visualized following staining with Coomassie Brilliant Blue. The presence of heavy and light chains can be identified by comparison with reduced immunoglobulin standards included on the same gel. An example of this procedure is shown in Figure 1. In this experiment a formalin-fixed *Staphylococcus aureus* Cowan I immunosorbent and a heat-killed type VI-positive *Streptococcus zooepidemicus* strain were compared for reactivity with a mouse IgE monoclonal antibody and five rat monoclonal antibodies (three rat IgMs, one rat IgG_{2b}, and one rat IgG_1). The results shown in Figure 1 indicate a number of interesting findings and underscore the differences that can exist between monoclonal antibodies of the same isotype. Of the three IgM antibodies tested, one bound to the type VI immunosorbent (Lane 5) and not the protein A immunosorbent (Lane 4); one bound to the protein A immunosorbent (Lane 6) and not the type VI immunosorbent (Lane 7); and one antibody failed to bind either immunosorbent (data not shown). The type VI immunosorbent showed reactivity with the IgG_{2b} antibody (Lane 11) and a mouse IgE antibody (Lane 15) but was unreactive with a rat IgG_1 antibody (Lane 9). Analysis of the interaction of the type VI immunosorbents with polyclonal rat immunoglobulins demonstrated reactivity with rat IgM, IgG_1, and IgG_{2b} (Reis *et al.*, 1988b).

These findings underscore the potential difficulties in predicting reactivity of a monoclonal antibody with a bacterial immunosorbent or any immobilized form of bacterial IgG-binding protein. As discussed in Chapters 16 and 17, the interaction of monoclonal antibodies with bacterial immunoglobulin-binding proteins can be influenced by the ionic strength and pH of the reaction mixture. For example, the interaction of the type VI immunosorbent with polyclonal rat IgG is more efficient at pH 5.0 than at pH 7.0 (Figure 2).

IV. Practical Applications Using Bacterial Immunosorbents

Four types of practical applications using bacterial immunosorbents are described in this section.

A. Use of Bacterial Immunoglobulin-Binding Proteins to Analyze Labeled Antigens

Immunological techniques have been used extensively for the analysis of cell surface antigens. Kessler (1975, 1976) has demonstrated the value of

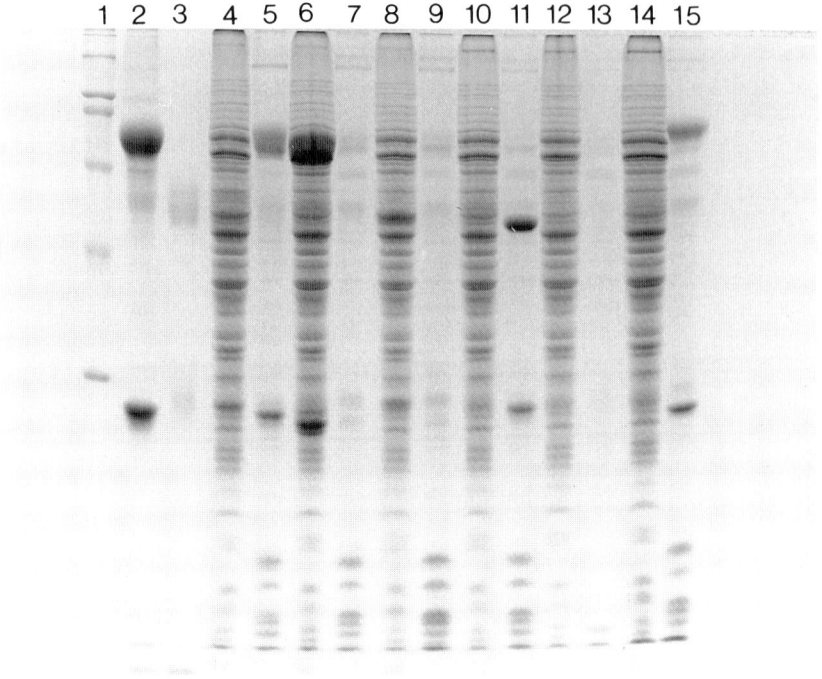

FIGURE 1
Monoclonal antibodies bound to *Staphylococcus aureus* or *Streptococcus zooepidemicus* strain RSS-212. Lane 1, Sigma high molecular weight markers. Lane 2, MOPC 104E murine IgM. Lane 3, murine hybridoma SP39 IgG; even-numbered lanes 4–14, *Staphylococcus aureus* Cowan I; odd-numbered lanes 5–15, *Streptococcus zooepidemicus* strain RSS-212. Lanes 4 and 5, B23.1 IgM rat monoclonal antibody to a mast cell determinant (Katz et al., 1983). Lanes 6 and 7, RA3-EA1 (IgM) rat anti-murine B220 antigen (Coffman and Weisman, 1981). Lanes 8 and 9, Bet 1 (IgG$_1$) rat anti-murine IgM (Kung et al., 1981). Lanes 10 and 11, 14.8 (IgG$_{2b}$) rat anti-murine B220 (Kincade et al., 1981). Lanes 12 and 13, control supernatant. Lanes 14 and 15, IgE murine monoclonal anti-TNP antibody (Rudolph et al., 1981). (Reproduced from Reis et al., 1988b, with permission.)

using immobilized protein A on *Staphylococcus aureus* Cowan I for isolating and characterizing antigens from cells. In these assays, the cellular antigens are labeled either biosynthetically with a radioactive amino acid or posttranslationally using lactoperoxidase and ^{125}I-labeled sodium iodide (for details of labeling cellular proteins biosynthetically or labeling proteins with ^{125}I, see the excellent review by Kessler, 1981). The solu-

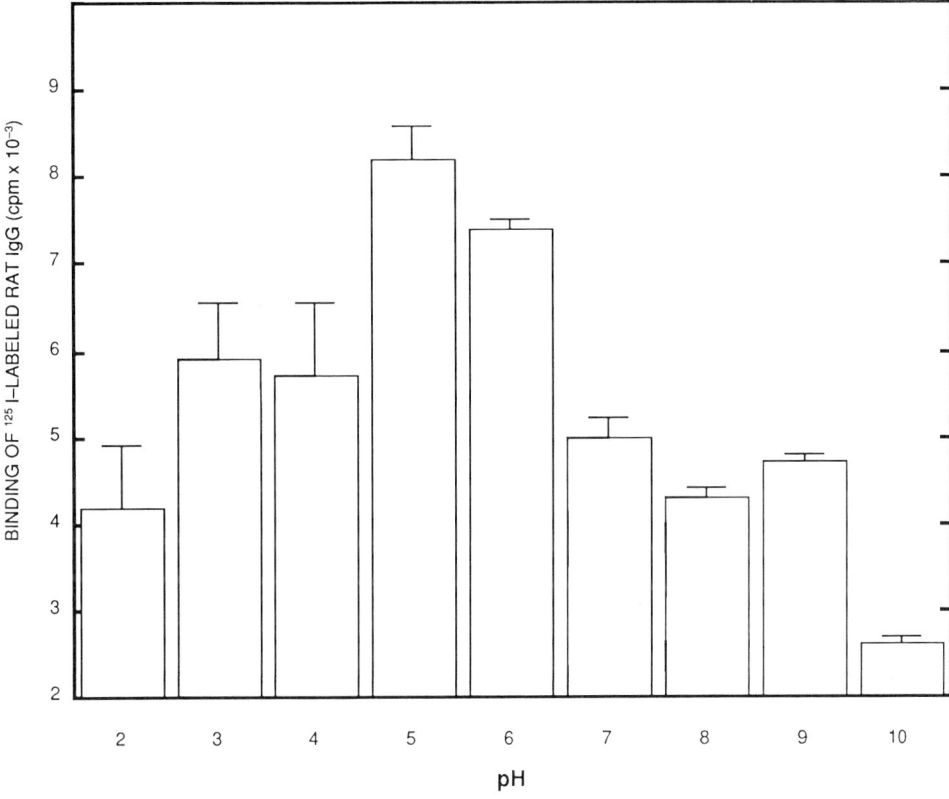

FIGURE 2
Binding of ^{125}I-labeled polyclonal rat IgG to *Streptococcus zooepidemicus* strain RSS-212 as a function of pH. (Reproduced from Reis *et al.*, 1988b, with permission.)

bilized, radiolabeled antigens are reacted with a specific antibody and the resulting immune complexes are recovered by addition of excess protein A-positive *Staphylococcus aureus* immunosorbent and subsequent centrifugation. The labeled antigens can then be extracted from the bacterial pellet by treatment with a variety of ionic or nonionic detergents, high salt, or chaotrophic agents (MacSween and Eastwood, 1977, 1981; Kessler, 1981). The antigens solubilized from the bacteria can then be analyzed by SDS gel electrophoresis followed by autoradiography.

The experimental protocol for studying cell surface antigens was originally developed by Kessler for the analysis of lymphocyte surface antigens (Kessler, 1975). These studies defined a number of the critical parameters necessary for this approach to be applicable to analysis of any antigen. First, labeling conditions must be established to ensure that the specific activity of the antigen is sufficiently high to be detected at the end of the precipitation procedure. Secondly, a suitable, monospecific antibody that recognizes the desired antigen is essential, and finally, the immunosorbent should bind the antibody with a high affinity. The basic procedure is summarized in Figure 3.

In these studies the labeled antigen-containing extract should be preincubated with an aliquot of the bacterial immunosorbent for 30 min at room temperature to remove any directly reactive constituents (Barber and Delovitch, 1978). The bacteria are pelleted and the bacterial-free supernatant recovered. An excess of specific antibody is added to the labeled antigen in the supernatant and incubated for 30 min at 37°C. At this time an excess of the immunosorbent is added to this mixture, mixed, and incubated for 15 min at 37°C to facilitate binding of antigen–antibody complexes to the immunosorbent. The bacteria are pelleted by centrifugation and washed three times with PBS-azide. This can be conveniently carried out in 1.5 ml polypropylene centrifuge tubes, using a microcentrifuge. Care must be taken, however, to limit the speed and duration of the centrifugation in order to minimize the "packing" of the bacterial pellet which inhibits effective resuspension of the immunosorbent and increases nonspecific trapping of proteins. Nonspecific binding of proteins to the bacterial immunosorbent can be minimized by the addition of a low amount of non-ionic detergent (e.g., 0.02% Tween 20) to the wash buffer. A variety of comparative studies have been performed by MacSween and Eastwood (1977) to determine optimal methods for eluting the labeled antigens from the bacterial pellet. The eluted samples can then be analyzed under reducing or nonreducing conditions with any of a variety of different one- and two-dimensional gel electrophoresis systems (Laemmli, 1970; O'Farrell, 1975).

These approaches have been extended to studies of a wide variety of antigens extracted from cell surfaces, secreted by cells or bacteria, or produced in *in vitro* translation systems (Hall *et al.*, 1979; Graves, 1981; Thompson *et al.*, 1978; Shapiro and Young, 1986; Scharfstein *et al.*, 1979; Shuman *et al.*, 1980). The majority of these applications have utilized a protein A-positive, formalin-fixed, *Staphylococcus aureus* Cowan I strain as the immunosorbent. More recently, a number of similar applications have been described using immobilized protein G as the immunoprecipitating agent (Tobin *et al.*, 1989; Barton, 1989).

In all of these assays, it is essential to carry out preliminary studies to establish optimal conditions for each stage of the assay. A control sample in which a nonimmune or irrelevant antibody is substituted for the specific

Chapter 15. Immunoprecipitation Reactions

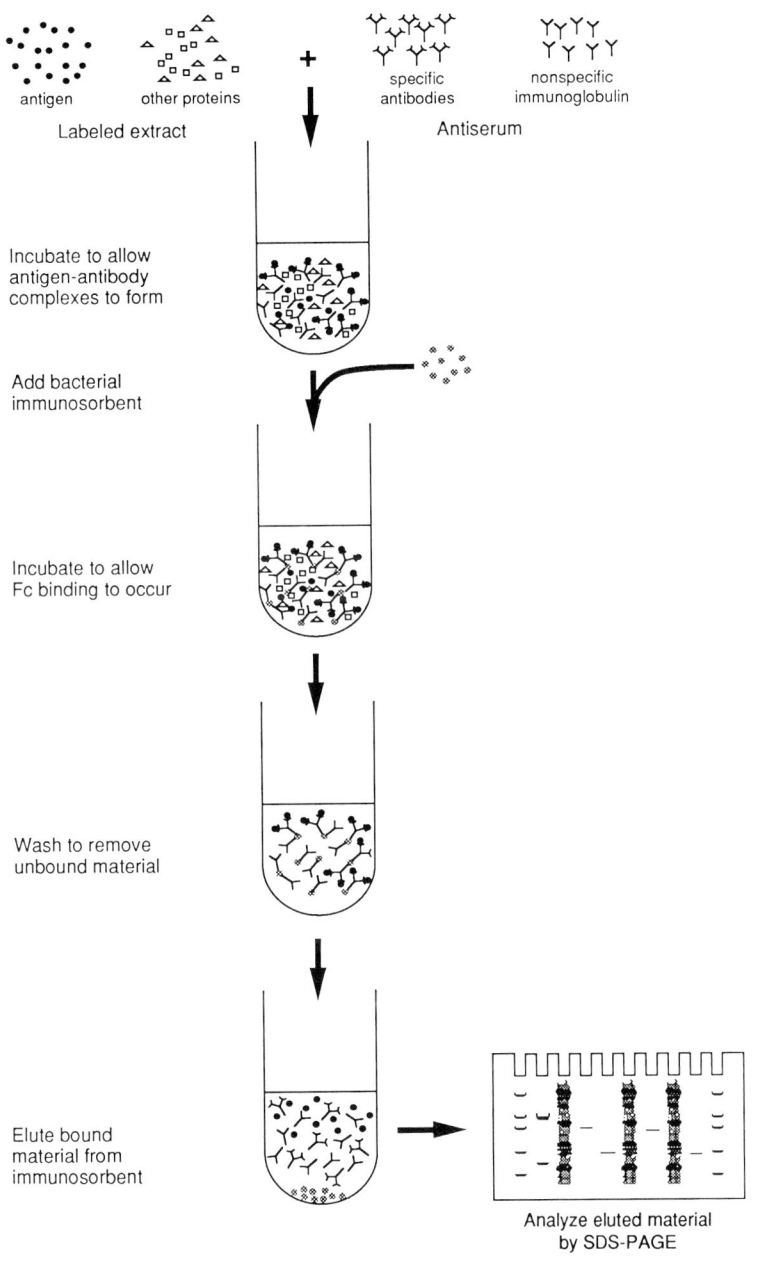

FIGURE 3
Schematic representation of the selective immunoprecipitation procedure to analyze labeled antigens.

antibody should be included in each assay. Some investigators substitute the so-called protein A-negative *Staphylococcus aureus* Wood 46 strain and the specific antibody as the negative control. It should be noted that the Wood strain is not devoid of protein A but expresses the IgG-binding protein at a much lower level than is expressed on the Cowan I strain (Boyle, 1990; Fehrer *et al.*, 1988).

If the nonspecific binding of labeled proteins is found to be unacceptably high, the procedure can be modified utilizing a two-stage immunoprecipitation procedure. The basic immunoprecipitation procedure is performed, and the antigens and antibodies are eluted from the bacterial immunosorbent in a small volume of the eluting agent [e.g., 30 μl 1% SDS (w/v)] for 10 min at ambient temperature. Bacteria are separated from the eluted material by centrifugation, diluted at least 1 : 20 with wash buffer, added to a pellet of fresh bacterial immunosorbent, and the adsorption and elution process is repeated. This procedure results in a much lower, nonspecific background signal (John and Firestone, 1986; Platt *et al.*, 1986).

B. The Use of Bacterial-Bound IgG-Binding Proteins in Place of Second Antibody for Radioimmunoassays

The use of a second antibody to precipitate antigen–antibody complexes in radioimmunoassays was widely used in the 1970s. In this procedure it was necessary to optimize concentrations of primary and secondary antibodies to ensure equivalence and maximal precipitation. While these procedures worked well for separating free, labeled antigen from antibody-complexed antigen, optimizing conditions and reagents for use in this assay was tedious and time consuming. In 1974, Jonsson and Kronvall described a radioimmunoassay for α-fetoprotein in human serum using a specific primary rabbit antibody to α-fetoprotein and formalin-fixed *Staphylococcus aureus* Cowan I (used in place of a second antibody) to separate antigen–antibody complexes from free antigen. These studies demonstrated the practicality of using a bacterial immunosorbent for separation of reactants in radioimmunoassays. This method was found to be as sensitive for the detection of the α-fetoprotein as the classical second antibody precipitation technique, while having many practical advantages. These advantages include the following.

1) The stability of the immunoprecipitating reagent and its lot-to-lot reproducibility
2) The ease of separating free antigen from antigen–antibody complexes
3) The efficiency of precipitation by the bacterial immunosorbent

was independent of the physicochemical composition of the antigen–antibody complexes
4) The lower levels of nonspecific precipitation of labeled antigen observed in the presence of an unrelated antibody

Furthermore, the use of a bacterial immunosorbent was also superior to the use of chemical precipitating agents in that it was applicable to systems in which differential precipitation conditions for antigen and antigen–antibody complexes could not be established.

A variety of different radioimmunoassays utilizing formalin-fixed *Staphylococcus aureus* Cowan I have been described (for review see Kessler, 1981; Mitchell *et al.*, 1980; Shantz, 1983). These applications have not all been limited to the use of primary antibodies that react directly with protein A. Ruch and Knight (1980) described a radioimmunoassay for human α-fetoprotein that used a primary antibody prepared in goats. Goat immunoglobulins display a low affinity for protein A and consequently these investigators used as the immunosorbent a formalin-fixed *Staphylococcus aureus* preparation that had been precoated with rabbit anti-goat IgG. This selective immunosorbent proved to be an efficient immunoprecipitating reagent when compared with the use of the same rabbit anti-goat IgG antibody as a second antibody reagent for direct precipitation. With the availability of bacterial immunosorbents expressing protein G, some of the direct assays are now applicable to specific antibodies from a wider range of species. For a detailed review of the use of protein A immunosorbents in place of second antibodies in immunoassays, see reviews by Shantz, 1983; Goding, 1978; Kessler, 1981; Langone, 1982.

C. The Use of Bacterial-Bound IgG-Binding Proteins for Detection of Specific Antibodies

Bacterial immunosorbents have been used in a modification of the procedure just described to detect antibodies. In this procedure, a source of labeled antigen is mixed with a sample of serum suspected of containing antibodies to that antigen. An excess of bacterial immunosorbent is added. The reaction mixture is mixed by end-over-end rotation and incubated for 30 min at room temperature. The bacteria are pelleted by centrifugation, washed twice with PBS-azide containing 0.1% gelatin and 0.02% Tween 20, and the antigen associated with the resulting bacterial pellet is quantified by counting radioactivity in an appropriate counter. Control tubes to which a known negative serum has been added should be included in each assay. Using this approach, it is possible to detect specific antibodies of an isotype and subclass that is reactive with the immunoglobulin-binding protein on the bacterial absorbent. This approach has been used to measure a variety of autoantibodies in human serum (Tindall et al., 1981; Oliver et al., 1982), as well as an assortment of other antigens (for review see Shantz, 1983). This basic procedure has also been used in a number of laboratories as a procedure for screening supernatants from myeloma–spleen cell fusions to detect the presence of specific monoclonal antibodies.

D. Use of Bacterial Immunosorbents to Deplete Serum of IgG Antibodies

Measurement of IgM antibodies to bacterial or viral antigens is of practical value for detection of exposure to certain pathogens. In studies of infected newborns, it is difficult to distinguish between antibodies derived by placental transfer from the mother and those synthesized by the baby. Only antibodies of the IgG isotype cross the placenta; consequently, any antibodies of the IgM isotype can be attributed to synthesis by the baby. It is frequently difficult in specific radioimmunoassays or enzyme-linked immunoassays to detect IgM antibodies in the presence of large quantities of IgG antibodies with a similar specificity. To facilitate this procedure, serum can be depleted of IgG antibodies by absorption with an immobilized form of bacterial IgG-binding protein prior to measurement of the presence of specific antibodies of other isotypes. This procedure has been used to detect IgM antibodies to a number of bacterial and viral antigens (Ankerst et al., 1974; Rasmussen et al., 1982; Kawano and Minamishima, 1987; Joassin and Reginster, 1986; Kobayashi et al., 1986).

We have used protein A–Sepharose in a similar fashion to remove IgG from rabbit serum, providing an IgM antibody preparation suitable for use in complement assays (Boyle and Langone, 1980). We have also removed IgG from serum in order to determine IgE levels in human serum using a sandwich assay, in which ^{125}I-labeled protein A was used as tracer (Langone et al., 1979). These procedures were successful since there was no significant loss of either the anti-sheep red cell IgM antibody or the human IgE during the IgG depletion step. Grangeot-Kerus et al. (1982) carried out a critical study on the value and limitations of formalin-fixed *Staphylococcal aureus* Cowan I for use in separating IgG and IgM. They reported a number of limitations to this procedure, including loss of certain populations of IgM antibodies and variation from sera to sera in the efficiency of IgG depletion. Although all of these factors should be taken into account, the use of bacterial immunosorbents in depleting samples of IgG is much more economical in time and labor than the use of physicochemical separation procedures. Some of the problems of binding to antibodies of isotopes other than IgG can be minimized by using bacterial absorbents expressing protein G. In this regard it is of interest to note that the ability of wild type protein G to bind to human serum albumin does not affect the efficiency of binding of all four IgG subclasses from human serum (Faulmann *et al.*, 1989).

V. Summary

Bacterial immunosorbents are an economical source of immobilized IgG-binding proteins that can be used for a variety of applications involving selective precipitation of soluble antigen–antibody complexes. These approaches include (1) selective precipitation of labeled antigens from complex mixtures using a specific antibody, (2) precipitation of antigen–antibody complexes in radioimmunoassays, (3) detection of specific antibodies, and (4) depletion of IgG from samples to facilitate measurement of antibodies of other isotypes. Other applications utilizing bacterial-bound immunoglobulin-binding proteins are described in the following two chapters.

Acknowledgments

We would like to thank Drs. Kathy Reis and Ed Siden for carrying out the experiments presented in Figures 1 and 2, and *Biotechniques* for permission to reproduce the data.

References

Ankerst, J. (1974). *J. Infect. Dis.* **130,** 268–273.
Barber, B. H., and Delovitch, T. (1978). *J. Immunol.* **122,** 320–325.
Barton, D. (1989). Ph.D. dissertation, Department of Microbiology, Medical College of Ohio.
Boyle, M. D. P. (1990). *In* "Bacterial Immunoglobulin-Binding Proteins" (M. D. P. Boyle, (ed.), Vol. 1, pp. 17–28. Academic Press, San Diego.
Boyle, M. D. P., and Langone, J. J. (1980). *J. Immunol. Methods* **32,** 51–58.
Coffman, R. L., and Weisman, I. L. (1981). *Nature (London)* **289,** 681–683.
Elliott, S. D., and Dole, V. P. (1947). *J. Exp. Med.* **895,** 305–310.
Faulmann, E. L., Otten, R. A., Barrett, D. J., and Boyle, M. D. P. (1989). *J. Immunol. Methods* **123,** 269–281.
Fehrer, S. L., Boyle, M. D. P., and Halliwell, R. E. W. (1988). *Am. J. Vet. Res.* **49,** 697–701.
Goding, J. W. (1978). *J. Immunol. Methods* **20,** 241–253.
Grangeot-Kerus, L., Leburn, L., Briantais, M. J., and Pillot, J. (1982). *J. Immunol. Methods* **51,** 183–195.
Graves, M. C. (1981). *J. Virol.* **38,** 224–239.

Haake, D. A., Franklin, E. C., and Frangione, B. (1982). *J. Immunol.* **129,** 190–192.
Hall, W. W., Lamb, R. A., and Choppin, P. W. (1979). *Proc. Natl. Acad. Sci. U.S.A.* **76,** 2047–2051.
Ivarie, R. D., and Jones, P. P. (1979). *Anal. Biochem.* **97,** 24–35.
Joassin, L., and Reginster, M. (1986). *J. Clin. Microbiol.* **23,** 576–581.
John, N. J., and Firestone, G. L. (1986). *Biotechniques* **4,** 404–406.
Jonsson, S., and Kronvall, G. (1974). *Eur. J. Immunol.* **4,** 29–33.
Katz, H. R., LeBlanc, P. A., and Russell, S. (1983). *Proc. Natl. Acad. Sci. U.S.A.* **80,** 5916–5918.
Kawano, K., and Minamishima, Y. (1987). *Arch. Virol.* **95,** 41–52.
Kessler, S. W. (1975). *J. Immunol.* **115,** 1617–1624.
Kessler, S. W. (1976). *J. Immunol.* **117,** 1482–1490.
Kessler, S. W. (1981). *In* "Methods in Enzymology" (J. J. Langone and H. Van Vunakis, eds.), Vol. 73, pp. 442–459. Academic Press, New York.
Kincade, P. W., Lee, G., Watanabe, T., Sun, I., and Scheid, M. P. (1981). *J. Immunol.* **127,** 2262–2268.
Kobayashi, N., Suzuki, M., Nakagawa, T., and Matumoto, M. (1986). *J. Clin. Microbiol.* **23,** 1143–1145.
Kung, J. T., Sharrow, S. O., Sieckmann, D. G., Lieberman, R., and Paul, W. E. (1981). *J. Immunol.* **127,** 873–876.
Laemmli, U. K. (1970). *Nature (London)* **227,** 680–685.
Langone, J. J. (1982). *Adv. Immunol.* **32,** 158–252.
Langone, J. J., Boyle, M. D. P., and Borsos, T. (1977). *J. Immunol. Methods* **28,** 281–293.
Langone, J. J., Boyle, M. D. P., and Borsos, T. (1979). *Anal. Biochem.* **93,** 207–215.
Lindmark R., Birriel C., and Sjöquist, J. (1981). *Scand J. Immunol. (1981).* **14,** 409–420.
Liu T. Y., Elliot S. D. (1965). *J. Biol. Chem.* **240,** 1138–1144.
Linscott D. (1989). "Linscott's Directory of Immunological and Biological Reagents," fifth Ed. Mill Valley, California.
Lottenberg, R., Broder, C. C., and Boyle, M. D. P. (1987). *Infect. Immun.* **55,** 1914–1918.
MacSween, J. M., and Eastwood, S. L. (1977). *J. Immunol. Methods* **23,** 259–267.
MacSween, J. M., and Eastwood, S. L. (1981). *In* "Methods in Enzymology" (J. J. Langone and H. Van Vunakin, eds.), Vol. 73, pp. 459–471. Academic Press, New York.
Mitchell, M. L., McKenna, J. J., and McIver, J. (1980). *Clin. Chem.* **26,** 1140–1142.
O'Farrell, P. H. (1975). *J. Biol. Chem.* **250,** 4007–4021.
Oliver, J. R., Hakendorf, P., Zeegen, P., and Ross, W. (1982). *Clin. Chem.* **28,** 121–123.
Platt, E. J., Karlsen, K., Lopez-Valdivieso, A., Cook, P. W., and Firestone, G. L. (1986). *Anal. Biochem.* **156,** 126–135.
Rasmussen, L., Kelsall, D., Nelson, R., Carney, W., Hirsch, M., Winston, D., Preiksaitis, J., and Merigan, T. C. (1982). *J. Infect. Dis.* **145,** 191–199.
Reis, K. J., von Mering, G. O., Karis, M. A., Faulmann, E. L., Lottenberg, R., and Boyle, M. D. P. (1988a). *J. Immunol. Methods* **107,** 273–280.
Reis, K. J., Siden, E. J., and Boyle, M. D. P. (1988b). *Biotechniques* **6,** 131–136.
Ruch, F. E., Jr., and Knight, G. J. (1980). *Clin. Chem.* **26,** 1133–1136.
Rudolph, A. K., Burrows, P. D., and Wabl, M. R. (1981). *Eur. J. Immunol.* **11,** 527–529.
Schalén, C., Svensson, M.-L., and Christensen, P. (1982). *Acta Pathol. Microbiol. Scand. Sect. B* **90,** 237–351.
Scharfstein, J., Correa, E. B., Gallo, G. R., and Nussenzweig, V. (1979). *J. Clin Invest.* **63,** 437–442.
Shantz, E. M. (1983). "Immunological Applications of Fixed Protein A-Bearing *Staphylococcus aureus* Cells." Calbiochem Corp., San Diego.

Shapiro, S. Z., and Young, J. R. (1986). *J. Biol. Chem.* **256,** 1495–1498.
Shuman, H. A., Silhavy, T. J., and Beckwith, J. R. (1980). *J. Biol. Chem.* **255,** 168–174.
Thompson, D. M. P., Rauch, J. E., Weatherhead, J. C., Friedlanger, P., O'Connor, R., Grosser, N., Shuster, J., and Gold, P. (1978). *Br. J. Cancer* **37,** 753–775.
Tindall, R. S. A., Kent, M., and Wells, L. (1981). *J. Immunol. Methods* **45,** 1–14.
Tobin, G. J., Young, D. C., and Flanegan, J. B. (1989). *Cell* **59,** 511–519.
Von Mering, G., and Boyle, M. D. P. (1986). *Mol. Immunol.* **23,** 811–821.
Wiedback, K., Havlicek, J., and Kronvall, G. (1983). *Acta Pathol. Microbiol. Immunol. Scand. Sect. B* **91,** 373–382.
Yarnall, M., Ayoub, E. M., and Boyle, M. D. P. (1986). *J. Gen. Microbiol.* **132,** 2049–2052.

CHAPTER **16**

Use of bacteria expressing immunoglobulin-binding proteins in coagglutination assays

Kathleen J. Reis
Michael J. P. Lawman
Michael D. P. Boyle

I. Introduction

The coagglutination assay is widely used for the rapid identification of a variety of bacteria. The assay is based on the ability of IgG antibodies to bind via their Fc region to protein A on a *Staphylococcus aureus* strain or other suitable bacteria expressing Fc-binding proteins, resulting in an immobilized antibody that can be used as a typing reagent. Since the IgG antibodies bind to the bacterial Fc-binding protein via the Fc portion of the molecule, the antigen-combining sites remain functional. When the antibody-coated staphylococci are mixed with bacteria carrying the corresponding antigen, coagglutination occurs. The basic procedure is outlined in Figure 1.

The coagglutination procedure is similar in basic principle to hemagglutination assays (Rose *et al.*, 1986). The procedure is adaptable to the detection of antigens on cell surfaces, as well as antibodies and antigens in solution. As would be predicted from the schematic representation in Figure 1, this technique requires either a polyvalent or immobilized antigen, or an immobilized hapten. However, haptens could be detected by inhibition of coagglutination while not themselves being capable of mediating an agglutination reaction. Coagglutination reactions have become popular for rapid detection of the presence of antigens, particularly those on the surface of bacteria. The assays are rapid, easy to perform, and are

Reagents

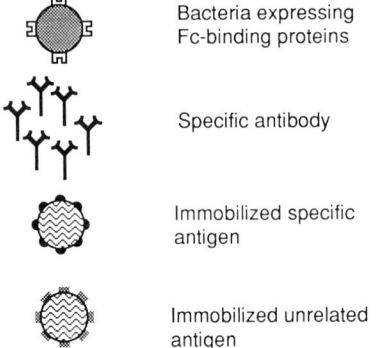

Bacteria expressing Fc-binding proteins

Specific antibody

Immobilized specific antigen

Immobilized unrelated antigen

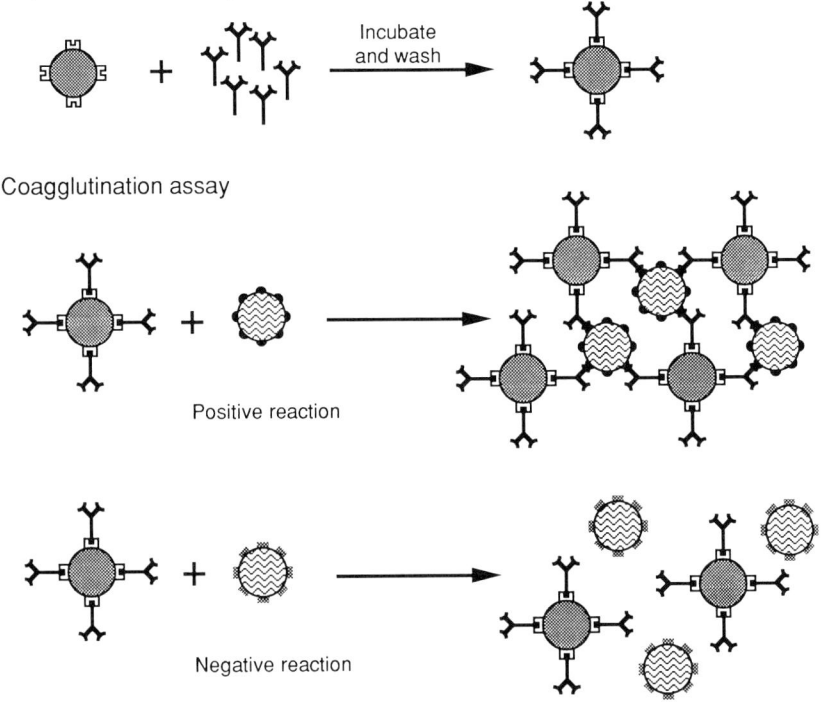

FIGURE 1
Schematic representation of a coagglutination assay to detect immobilized antigens.

economical in their requirements for specific antibodies. In addition to detecting bacterial antigens, coagglutination assays have been used for the detection of specific antibodies. Examples of each of these applications are presented in this chapter. In each case, a series of preliminary experiments are required to establish the optimal conditions for a particular assay. These will vary from system to system depending on such factors as the titer and affinity of the antibody, distribution of antigen, buffer conditions, etc. One example of how an assay was developed has been included as a guide to the general considerations that are involved in developing a coagglutination assay.

II. Detection of Cell-Bound Antigens

The coagglutination method was developed by Kronvall and was first used to type pneumococci, using protein A-positive staphylococci coated with antibodies to pneumococcal capsular antigens (Kronvall, 1972). Eighty-nine pneumococcal strains, representing thirteen different types were typed by this method and the results were in complete agreement with the more time-consuming Neufeld capsule-swelling method (Kronvall, 1972). The advantages of the coagglutination assay for pneumococcal typing were that, (1) 1–2 colonies could be lifted directly from the growth plate for typing; (2) the reaction was easy to read; (3) in most cases agglutination occurred within seconds; (4) less typing sera was used compared to capsular swelling techniques; (5) the staphylococcal typing reagent was stable for months when stored at 4°C.

A series of reports followed soon thereafter, using the coagglutination technique to identify streptococci (Christensen *et al.*, 1973; Leland *et al.*, 1978), mycobacteria (Juhlin and Winblad, 1973), *Neisseria gonorrhoeae* (Danielsson and Kronvall, 1974), *Neisseria meningitidis* (Olcén *et al.*, 1975; Svenungsson and Lindberg, 1978, 1979), and *Haemophilus influenzae* type b (Suksanong and Dajani, 1977). In addition to identifying bacterial isolates in slide agglutination assays, antibody-sensitized staphylococci have been used to group beta-hemolytic streptococci (Edwards and Larson, 1974) and *Neisseria meningitidis* (Zimmerman and Smith, 1978) directly on blood agar plates. Similar strategies have been used to identify *Salmonella* and *Shigella* using antibodies of appropriate specificity immobilized on *Staphylococcus aureus* (Edwards and Hilderbrand, 1976; Svenungsson and Lindberg, 1979), and more recently for the diagnosis of amoebiasis (Parijka *et al.*, 1989).

A coagglutination test was first introduced commercially in 1975 by Pharmacia ENI Diagnostics Inc. (Fairfield, New Jersey) for the identification of streptococci. The Phadebact® coagglutination test utilized rabbit antibodies to streptococcal carbohydrate antigens coated on nonviable *Staphylococcus aureus*. The Phadebact® *Streptococcus* Test, based on the coagglutination technique, allows definitive identification of streptococcal groups A, B, C, D, F, and G using a simple and rapid slide technique. In this coagglutination assay, antibodies specific for each streptococcal group-specific carbohydrate are bound to protein A on the surface of nonviable staphylococci. When a sample containing streptococci belonging to one of these groups is mixed with bacteria coated with an antibody that recognizes specific antigens on the surface of the streptococci, agglutination of the test bacteria and the antibody-coated bacteria will occur. A coagglutination lattice is formed that is visible to the naked eye. In the commercial kit, the staphylococci have been dyed with methylene blue to enhance detection of the agglutination reaction. Similar kits for the identification of *Neisseria gonorrhoeae*, *Haemophilus influenzae*, and pneumococci have been subsequently introduced. The assays allow identification of bacteria directly from agar plates or from broth cultures. Like the original studies of Kronvall (1972), these assays are accurate, rapid, and easy to perform.

III. Detection of Specific Antibody

We have used a similar approach to detect IgG antibodies to *Brucella* antigens in the serum of cattle. A serum sample from a cow suspected of having antibodies to *Brucella* is mixed with a standard suspension of heat-killed bacteria expressing protein G. (For details of preparation and standardization of bacteria as immunosorbents, see Chapter 2.) The protein G-expressing strain, G1400, was chosen for this application because of its stronger reactivity with bovine IgG compared to that of protein A (Wallner *et al.*, 1987). In the first stage of the reaction, IgG antibodies in the cattle serum were immobilized to the bacteria via their Fc regions. Unbound antibodies and other serum proteins were removed by pelleting the bacteria by centrifugation and washing three times with 0.01 M trisodium ethylenediaminetetraacetate containing 0.1% gelatin and 0.1% Tween 20 (EDTA-gel) (for exact information of all buffers, see Appendix). The bacterial pellet was resuspended in 0.1 ml of this buffer and a drop of the suspension was mixed with a drop of a standardized preparation of a soluble *Brucella* antigen on a glass microscope slide or waxed card. The reagents are mixed using a wooden applicator stick. The slide is rocked gently from side to side for about a minute and then observed for agglutination. For ease of reading, the *Brucella* antigen preparation was prestained with a blue dye. The general protocol is outlined in Figure 2. The presence of specific *Brucella* antibodies is demonstrated by agglutination

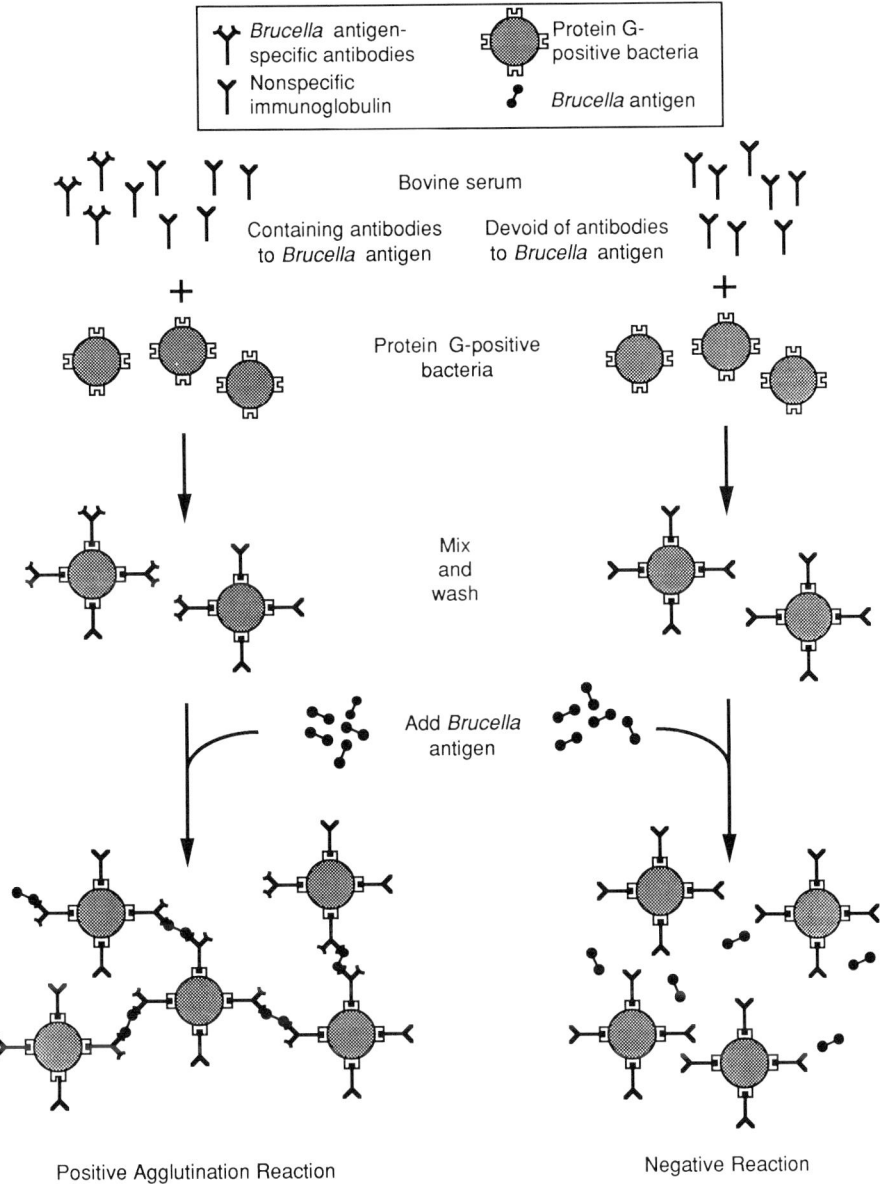

FIGURE 2
Coagglutination assay to detect specific antibodies to *Brucella* antigens.

Appropriate positive and negative controls should be included in each assay, as shown in Figure 2. As with all immunoassays, it is necessary to first carry out a series of preliminary checkerboard titrations to optimize the assay for sensitivity and specificity. This agglutination assay is semi-quantitative and can be used to distinguish serum containing high levels of specific antibodies from those devoid of antibody or from those in which antibodies are present at low levels (Lawman, unpublished observations).

It is advisable when using this approach to monitor antibodies to infectious agents, to include serum samples collected at different times since false negative results may be obtained by testing serum from infected animals early in the disease course. The advantage of this type of assay is that it is easy to perform, rapid, and economical. Measurement of *Brucella*-reactive antibodies has been shown to be of value for identification of infected cattle (Lawman *et al.*, 1984, 1986), and the coagglutination assay described above may prove to be of value as a simple field test.

IV. Procedure for Establishing a Coagglutination Assay to Measure a Polyvalent Soluble Antigen

Any coagglutination assay that can be used to measure a cell-bound, i.e., immobilized, antigen can be adapted as an assay to measure the corresponding soluble, polyvalent antigen. Direct agglutination of protein A-positive *Staphylococcus aureus* strains coated with specific antibodies has been used to detect soluble meningococcal antiens in cerebrospinal fluid (Olcén *et al.*, 1985), soluble *Haemophilus influenzae* type b antigens in cerebrospinal fluid, serum and urine (Suksanong and Dajani, 1977), diphtheria toxin (Sophianou and Bonifas, 1978), and heat labile enterotoxin of *Escherichia coli* (Brill *et al.*, 1979). All of these assays are based on a similar principle, namely, that the presence of the specific soluble antigen facilitates the formation of a lattice of specific antibody-coated bacteria via crosslinking of specific $F(ab')_2$ regions on antibodies immobilized to bacteria via their Fc region.

This approach is generally applicable to detection of any antigen for which a corresponding specific antibody is available. An illustration of this general procedure to the detection of equine IgG will now be presented. In this example, anti-equine IgG is immobilized onto heat-killed, formalin-fixed *Staphylococcus aureus* and the ability of different dilutions of horse serum to cause agglutination is measured.

In the initial preliminary experiments, conditions for coating *Staphylococcus aureus* Cowan I with the specific antibody were determined. For these studies, a 10% formalin-fixed preparation of *Staphylococcus aureus*

Cowan I was prepared according to the method of Kessler (1975). The bacteria were colored by addition of 25 µl of Coomassie Blue dye to 1 ml of a 10% suspension of the bacteria. The mixture was incubated for 10 min at 37°C and then washed three times to remove unbound dye.

The antibody used for this application was a commercial rabbit antiserum to equine IgG heavy and light chains (Jackson Immuno Research Laboratories, West Grove, Pennsylvania). Equal volumes of the 10% solution of bacteria and dilutions of the antiserum were mixed on an end-over-end rotator for 1 hr at ambient temperature. At the end of this incubation time, the bacteria were washed twice with phosphate-buffered saline containing 0.02% sodium azide, (PBS-azide), and any unreactive protein A molecules on the bacteria were blocked by addition of 1% normal rabbit serum. The washed, antibody-coated bacteria were resuspended as 10% suspensions and their ability to agglutinate in the presence of differing dilutions of equine IgG was determined in checkerboard titrations.

For this test a drop of each antibody-coated bacterial preparation was compared for its ability to agglutinate in the presence of different concentrations of antigen (equine IgG). Sensitizing conditions that would agglutinate in the presence of an equal volume of a solution containing approximately 100 µg/ml of equine IgG were chosen. In this example, this was achieved using bacteria that had been coated by preincubation of 1 ml of a 10% solution of *Staphylococcus aureus* with an equal volume of a 1:40 dilution of the antiserum. The coated bacteria were stored at 4°C in the presence of 0.1% sodium azide and maintained their selective, reactive properties for at least two months.

Using the coating conditions established in the preliminary experiments, the assay was applied to detecting IgG in various horse serum samples. Doubling dilutions of horse serum were prepared in PBS-azide. A drop of each dilution was mixed with a drop of the immobilized, bacteria-specific antibody reagent on a glass slide and mixed using an applicator stick. The slide was rocked gently back and fourth and scored for agglutination after 15–30 seconds. All samples resulted in agglutination over a range of dilutions. The minimal dilution required to cause agglutination correlated to the level of IgG in the serum previously determined by radioimmunoassay. Foal samples obtained prior to suckling (n = 8), containing low levels of IgG (0.01–0.1 mg/ml), resulted in agglutination using undiluted serum. Sera (n = 9) containing intermediate levels of IgG (2–8 mg/ml) had to be diluted greater than 1:16. Sera (n = 17) containing normal levels of IgG (> 8 mg/ml) had to be diluted 1:64 or greater. A prozone effect was observed in the presence of high levels of antigen. Consequently, this type of assay should be carried out over a wide range of dilutions to ensure that the failure to agglutinate is due to the absence of antigen rather than to the presence of a gross excess. While the results obtained by this procedure correlated well with the values obtained by classical radioimmunoassay techniques, the coagglutination assay is only semiquantitative and is only of value for distinguishing high from intermediate and low levels of antigen.

V. Summary

The agglutination assays described in this chapter demonstrate the general principle of immobilizing specific antibodies via the Fc region to bacteria expressing Fc-binding proteins and the ability to agglutinate such antibody-coated bacteria in the presence of the corresponding antigen. The procedure can be used to measure specific antibodies or cell-bound and soluble polyvalent antigens and has many practical applications for rapid diagnostic procedures. These assays are not as sensitive or quantitative as many of the other procedures described in this volume, but have the advantages of being rapid, economical, and amenable to being performed without requiring sophisticated equipment.

References

Brill, B. M., Wasilauskas, B. L., and Richardson, S. H. (1979). *J. Clin. Microbiol.* **9,** 49–55.
Christensen, P., Kahlmeter, G., Jonsson, S., and Kronvall, G. (1973). *Infect. Immun.* **7,** 881–885.
Danielsson, D., and Kronvall, G. (1974). *Appl. Microbiol.* **27,** 368–374.
Edwards, E. A., and Hilderbrand, R. L. (1976). *J. Clin. Microbiol.* **3,** 339–343.
Edwards, E. A., and Larson, G. L. (1974). *Appl. Microbiol.* **28,** 972–976.
Juhlin, I., and Winblad, S. (1973). *Acta Pathol. Microbiol. Scand. Sect. B* **81,** 179–180.
Kessler, S. W. (1975). *J. Immunol.* 115; 1617–1624.
Kronvall, G. (1972). *J. Med. Microbiol.* **6,** 187–190.
Lawman, M. J. P., Thurmond, M. C., Reis, K. J., Gauntlett, D. R., and Boyle, M. D. P. (1984). *Vet. Immunol. Immunopathol.* **6,** 291–305.
Lawman, M. J. P., Ball, D. R., Hoffman, E. M., Des Jardin, L. E., and Boyle, M. D. P. (1986). *Vet. Microbiol.* **12,** 43–53.
Leland, D. S., Lachapelle, R. C., and Wlodarski, F. M. (1978). *J. Clin. Microbiol.* **7,** 323–326.
Olcén, P., Danielsson, D., and Kjellander, J. (1975). *Acta Pathol. Microbiol. Scand. Sect. B* **83,** 387–396.
Parijka, S. C., Kasinathan, S., and Rao, R. S. (1989). *J. Microbiol. Methods* **10,** 53–57.
Rose, N. R., Friedman, H., and Fahey, J. C. (1986). "Manual of Clinical Laboratory Immunology," 3rd Ed. A.S.M. Press, Washington, D.C.
Sophianou, D., and Bonifas, V. (1978). *Ann. Microbiol.* **129,** 323–327.
Suksanong, M., and Dajani, A. S. (1977). *J. Clin. Microbiol.* **5,** 81–85.
Svenungsson, B., and Lindberg, A. A. (1978). *Acta Pathol. Microbiol. Scand. Sect. B* **86,** 283–290.

Svenungsson, B., and Lindberg, A. A. (1979). *Acta Pathol. Microbiol. Scand. Sect. B* **87,** 29–36.
Wallner, W. A., Lawman, M. J. P., and Boyle, M. D. P. (1987). *Appl. Microbiol. Biotechnol.* **27,** 168–173.
Zimmerman, S. E., and Smith, J. W. (1978). *J. Clin. Microbiol.* **7,** 470–473.

CHAPTER **17**

Utilization of whole bacteria expressing IgG-binding proteins to detect cell surface antigens

Edward J. Siden

I. Introduction

Large microscopic particles, such as red blood cells or acrylamide beads, have been used to detect the binding of antibodies to mammalian cell surface differentiation antigens (Parish *et al.*, 1974; Ammann *et al.*, 1977). Binding of antibodies to these reagents must be accomplished by the covalent attachment of the antibody or "sandwich" of antibodies to the particle. In the methods to be described here, antibodies bound to whole bacteria expressing immunoglobulin-binding proteins are used as a probe for specific mammalian differentiation antigens. The major advantages of this type of assay, which was first described by Uchanska-Ziegler *et al.* (1982) include the convenience of direct antibody binding without chemical modification of the bacteria or antibody, the increased avidity of the antigen–antibody reaction resulting from monoclonal antibodies adsorbed all over the bacteria, and the simplicity of analyzing the resulting cell–bacteria complexes by light microscopy.

Particular strains of bacteria can also be chosen for their unique immunoglobulin-binding specificities. We have used both *Staphylococcus aureus* Cowan I strain and *Streptococcus zooepidemicus* strain S-212 for assays of expression of murine cell surface proteins. Many of these antigens are defined by rat monoclonal antibodies, which as a rule bind poorly to the *Staphylococcus* strain. The *Streptococcus* strain was specifically selected for its binding to rat immunoglobulins (Reis *et al.*, 1988). The species and isotype specificities of antibody binding to various bacterial strains are discussed in Chapter 1 and may be used to determine whether direct adsorption of a particular antibody could occur. It should be noted however, that binding of a particular isotype or species of monoclonal antibody is not always predictable and must be confirmed by an independent assay such as polyacrylamide gel electrophoresis (Reis *et al.*, 1988).

Alternatively, binding of all monoclonal antibodies of a particular species to the bacteria can be facilitated using a polyvalent, xenogeneic, anti-immunoglobulin second antibody preparation. The resulting anti-Ig-coated or directly reactive bacteria can be incubated in crude hybridoma-conditioned medium to prepare a reagent to detect mammalian cell surface proteins. The bacterial reagent and cells are incubated together in small tubes or in microtiter dishes. The cells are separated from unbound bacteria and prepared for analysis by cytocentrifugation and histological staining. Rosettes formed by the hybridoma-coated bacteria are finally detected by light microscopy.

II. Reagents and Equipment

A 10% suspension of *S. aureus,* Cowan strain (Calbiochem 50761 or equivalent) or *S. zooepidemicus* strain S-212 (Calbiochem 341384)

Dulbecco's Phosphate-buffered Saline (PBS), pH 7.25 (5 liters):
1. Sodium phosphate, monobasic (Na_2HPO_4)   7.18 g
2. Potassium phosphate, dibasic (KH_2PO_4)   1.25 g
3. Sodium chloride (NaCl)   50.00 g
4. Potassium chloride (KCl)   1.25 g

Antiserum: Rabbit anti-rat IgG, (ICN Biomedicals, Inc., Costa Mesa, California, 65-160)

BFAM Buffer:
1. Balanced salt solution (BSS)
   Dissolve components for solutions #1 and #2. Adjust each to 1 liter. Add equal amounts of each and dilute to a ten-fold volume of each stock. The pH should be maintained between 7.2 and 7.4. Filter sterilize through a 0.2 μ filter.
   a) Solution #1 (10x)

Dextrose	10.00 g
KH_2PO_4	0.60 g
$Na_2HPO_4 \cdot 7H_2O$	4.83 g
0.5% phenol red solution	20 ml

Chapter 17. Detection of Cell-Surface Antigens

b) Solution #2 (10x)

$CaCl_2 \cdot 2H_2O$	1.86 g
KCl	4.00 g
NaCl	80.00 g
$MgCl_2$	1.04 g
$MgSO_4 \cdot 7H_2O$	2.00 g

2. Fetal bovine serum: heat inactivate at 56°C for 30 min. Add to 1.0% final concentration.
3. Sodium azide to 0.1% weight/weight (w/w)
4. 2-mercaptoethanol to 50 μM

Hydridoma cell cultures: always pair specific with isotype-matched, nonspecific antibodies.

Cytocentrifuge spin solution:
1. BFAM buffer   5 ml
2. Fetal bovine serum   5 ml

Wright's–Giemsa Stain:
1. Stain
   a) Wright's stain   300 mg
   b) Giemsa stain   30 mg

   Grind powder in methanol, adjust to 100 ml.

2. Buffer solution (1 liter), pH 6.6:
   a) Na_2HPO_4 3.8 g
   b) KH_2PO_4 5.47 g

Clay-Adams "Nutator" Rocker

Microfuge (20,000 rpm)

Superspeed centrifuge (20,000 rpm)

Cytocentrifuge

Vortex mixer

Plate mixer (Dynatech, Arlington, Virginia)

96-well, U-bottom PVC microtiter dish

0.2 μ membrane filter

Slides, coverslips

1.5 ml microfuge tubes

12 × 75 mm tubes

III. Preparation of Antibodies

Rat hybridoma culture supernatants (100–400 ml) are prepared by culturing the hybridoma cells to stationary phase, resulting in a decline in cell viability to approximately 10–30%. Spent medium is centrifuged at 10,000 × g in a Beckman JA-14 rotor to remove cell debris, filtered through a 0.22 μ Nalgene filter, and stored after the addition of sodium size to 0.02%. IgM hybridoma supernatants have been stored for as long as one year at 4°C without significant loss of antibody activity, IgM- and IgG-containing hybridoma supernatants are also reportedly stable when stored at −20°C (Underwood and Bean, 1985).

Polyvalent anti-immunoglobulin is initially reconstituted from lyophilized stocks, dissolved by gentle suspension, and cleared by centrifugation in a microfuge for 5 min at 20,000 × g. The specific antibody concentration was standardized by analyzing the absorbance at 280 nm (A_{280}) of the solution and assuming an extinction coefficient of 1.4 per milligram for the total IgG fraction. This solution has been stored in aliquots at 4°C for one year without significant loss of activity.

IV. Preparation of Anti-Immunoglobulin-Coated Bacteria

Heat-killed, 10% (w/w) suspensions of *S. aureus* and *S. zooepidemicus* may either be purchased from a commercial supplier or grown from seed stocks using the method of Kessler (1981). Precautions against contamination by these live, pathogenic microorganisms must be observed.

All bacterial centrifugations are performed in 1.5 ml microcentrifuge tubes spun for 1 min at 10,000 × g. Fc-binding protein-bearing bacteria are washed once in BSS + 0.1% azide before incubation with anti-immunoglobulin. The washed bacterial cell suspension is incubated in 100 μg/ml of species-specific, polyvalent anti-Ig that is reactive with the specific isotype of the hybridome to be added at later steps. After 30 min at room temperature, the bacteria are washed twice with BFAM. The coated bacteria can be stored at 4°C for at least one week and should be rewashed twice before subsequent use.

V. Preparation of Hybridoma Antibody-Coated Bacteria

Anti-immunoglobulin-coated bacteria are saturated with monoclonal antibody either by incubation in crude, high titer, tissue culture supernatants or a dilute solution of purified antibody. Fifty microliters of anti-Ig-coated bacteria is usually incubated with 5 μg of primary antibody or 1 ml of hybridoma-conditioned medium.

Binding is performed overnight at 4°C in a rocker or roller and the unbound hybridoma antibodies are washed away by three successive washed in BFAM. After the last wash, the bacterial cells are resuspended as a 2.5% suspension (w/w) in BFAM. They can be used immediately or can be stored, rewashed, and used for a number of weeks.

The extent of antibody binding to the bacteria can be analyzed by SDS gel electrophoresis of proteins solubilized from the bacteria (Reis *et al.*, 1988).

VI. Binding Assay

The binding reactions are carried out in vessels appropriate to the number of samples being assayed, Less than six samples are usually prepared using 1.5 ml microfuge tubes. Larger numbers are analyzed using microtiter dish methodology. The same conditions are used for both.

With the microtiter dish assay, the cells to be screened are washed in BFAM buffer at 4°C twice by centrifugation for 2 min at 100 $\times$ g. They are then resuspended in BFAM at 10^6 cells/ml. Aliquots (100 μl) are dispensed into U-bottom microtiter wells (or microfuge tubes) and the cells are pelleted by centrifugation at 4°C for 2 min at 100 $\times$ g. Supernatant can be removed simultaneously from all wells by crisply "flicking" the dish's contents into the sink. The dish is kept upside down and blotted briefly by tapping on paper towels. All cell pellets are loosened before resuspension by vibrating the drained multiwell dish for 5 s with a vortex mixer or plate mixer.

Hybridoma-coated bacteria (2.5%, 20 μl) are added to the loosened, mammalian cell pellets. The reactants are mixed by tapping the dish or tube and incubated on ice for 30 min. After incubation, the volume of the wells is brought to 100 μl with BFAM. The unbound bacteria are washed away by alternately washing the cells in BFAM and spinning the resus-

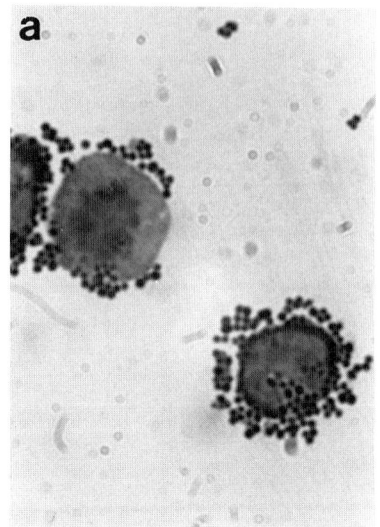 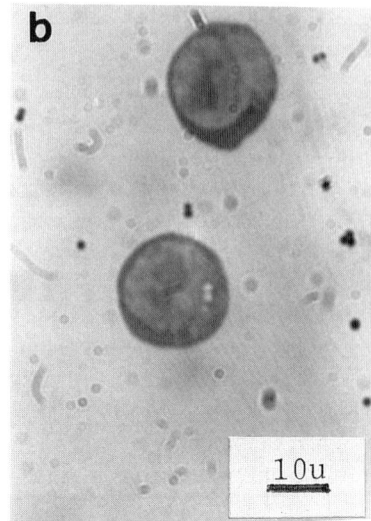

FIGURE 1
B220 differentiation antigen detection on the murine pre-B cell line FLE1-11. Rat IgM anti-B220 (a) or IgM anti-TNP (b) were adsorbed to anti-rat Immunoglobulin-coated *S. aureus*. The bacterial complexes were used to stain the cells and photographed using a Leitz orthopian microscope (Wright's–Glemsa stain, ×848).

pended cells (100 μl) through a layer of fetal bovine serum (75 μl). The wells can be examined with an inverted microscope to assess the efficiency of the washing process. Typically, four to six washes are common and lead to final cytocentrifuge preparations with clean backgrounds (Figure 1).

To deposit the bacteria-stained cells on a microscope slide and determine the fraction of antibody-reactive cells, 100 μl of a serum-containing spin solution is first placed deep into the cytocentrifuge bucket, followed by an aliquot of approximately 3×10^4 washed cell–bacteria complexes. The cytocentrifuge is brought rapidly to 1000 rpm then to 800 rpm for 5 min. When centrifugation is complete, the slides are air dried, fixed 1 min in dry methanol, then stained with a histological stain.

VII. Staining and Quantitation

We have obtained excellent results with May–Grunwald Giemsa stain, but use a Wright's–Giemsa stain to avoid extensive use of volatile, organic solvents. We dip the fixed slides in the methanolic stain for 2 min, briefly drain the excess stain, and dip in two sequential baths of Wright's buffer for 2 min each. The slides are finally dipped in water, air dried, and coverslipped using permount.

To examine a slide, a zone of dispersed cells is located using 100-fold magnification, then examined at 400–600 power. Cells binding five or more bacterial cells are considered arbitrarily positive and reproducible data can be generated by counting as few as 200 cells of a stained, continuous cell line.

VIII. Variations on the Theme

Important advantages of these bacterial tools can also be exploited for other purposes. The multivalency has allowed high avidity interactions to facilitate cell fractionation procedures (Randall, 1983). Whole Fc-binding protein-expressing bacteria adhere to petri dishes and can be used as solid-phase adsorbents.

The simple, visual analysis of the binding of the round Fc-binding protein-positive bacteria to the cells can be exploited in assays using a second, morphologically distinct bacterial strain. We have prepared rod-shaped *Escherichia coli* as a probe for mammalian Fc receptors by attaching the trinstrophenyl hapten (TNP) to the bacteria, then coating these with monoclonal, anti-hapten antibodies of IgE or other isotypes (Siden and Siegel, 1986). The high valency of Fc regions enables reliable quantitation of these receptors.

Finally, to automate the analysis of bacterial binding, we have started to directly label the bacterial–hybridoma complexes with fluorescein. These complexes can then be detected and more accurately quantitated using a cytofluorograph.

IX. Comments

As with any sensitive assay, the ratio of signal to noise must be high to generate good data. High levels of residual, free bacteria are a common cause of unreadable cytocentrifuge preparations. Observing the correct centrifuge speed during the final washes and monitoring contamination with free bacteria will facilitate good slides. Isotype-matched or other nonspecific globulin fractions should be used as negative controls for specific binding. These values can be subtracted from specific antibody binding to correct for either nonspecific binding to sticky cell surfaces or inadequate washing.

Because dead cells have pronounced nonspecific binding properties and lack well-defined cell borders and proper staining characteristics, these cells should not be counted. Using this strategy and the criterion of greater than five bound bacteria for positive scoring, we generate data that have routinely been confirmed by other methods such as northern blotting or immunoprecipitation.

For experiments using limiting amounts of cells, such as examining cells from colonies growing *in vitro*, poly-L-lysine-coated slides increase the recovery of cells onto each slide. Clean slides are coated in 100 μg per ml for 30 min, then washed for 15 min in running H_2O.

Acknowledgments

Thanks to Lydia Lopez for skillful preparation of this manuscript and Ram Roth for preparation of the photomicrograph samples in Figure 1.

References

Amman, A. J., Borg, D., Kondo, L., and Wara, D. W. (1977). *J. Immunol. Methods* **17**, 365–371.
Kessler, S. W. (1981). *In* "Methods in Enzymology" (J. J. Langone and H. van Vunakis, eds.), Vol. 73, pp. 442–459. Academic Press, New York.
Parish, C. R., Kirov, S. M., Bowern, N., and Bladen, R. V. (1974). *Eur. J. Immunol.* **4**, 808–815.
Randall, R. E. (1983). *J. Immunol. Methods* **60**, 147–165.
Reis, K. J., Siden, E. J., and Boyle, M. D. P. (1988). *Biotechniques* **6**, 130–136.
Siden, E., and Siegel, M. (1986). *J. Immunol. Methods* **87**, 252–255.
Uchanska-Ziegler, B., Wernet, P. W., and Ziegler, A. (1982). *Br. J. Haematol.* **52**, 155–160.
Underwood, P. A., and Bean, P. A. (1985). *J. Immunol. Methods* **85**, 1989–197.

CHAPTER **18**

Use of immobilized protein A to purify immunoglobulins

Larry Schwartz

I. Introduction

Immunoglobulins are widely used for a variety of applications in therapeutics, diagnostics, and research. They are used in the treatment of immune diseases and in highly selective, diagnostic procedures (immunoprecipitation, immunodiffusion, immunoelectrophoresis, radioimmunoassays [RIA], enzyme-linked immunosorbent assays [ELISA], etc.) to detect and quantitate the presence of "antigens." Immunoglobulins are also used to purify specific antigens or anti-antibodies by affinity chromatography, a technique which exploits biospecific interactions between molecules.

Immunoglobulins (antibodies) are an extremely heterogeneous class of glycoproteins, which have defined similarities but which also exhibit unique differences in chemical, physical, and biological properties from each other. They are among the most hydrophobic molecules found in serum. Isotypic, allotypic, and idiotypic variations of immunoglobulins give rise to their tremendous heterogeneity. There are potentially hundreds of thousands of different antibodies, each having a unique biospecificity. Purification of a specific antibody is thus not a trivial matter.

Early techniques used to purify immunoglobulins included paper and zone electrophoresis, and ethanol and ammonium sulfate precipitation. In the 1960s, ion-exchange chromatographic procedures were introduced.

Researchers were first able to isolate monospecific antibodies for amino acid sequencing by using sera from patients suffering from a multiple myeloma. The purified immunoglobulin fraction contained high levels of one specific antibody.

In the early 1960s, it was discovered that tumors produced by malignant antibody-secreting cells could be induced in mice by injection of mineral oil into the peritoneal cavity (Potter and Boyce, 1962; Merwin and Redmon, 1963). This technique has been widely used to produce thousands of well characterized mouse myelomas.

Normal B lymphocyte cells could not be cultured to produce antibodies. In 1975, Kohler and Milstein developed a revolutionary technique to fuse myeloma cells with spleen cells from immunized mice (cell hybridization). The fusion product, when injected into mice, was capable of forming tumors (hybridomas) that produced large quantities of highly specific antibodies. Through this technique, it was possible to produce continuous cell lines secreting large quantities of "monoclonal antibody" (antibody with a specificity against a single antigenic site).

Hybridoma cell lines are grown both in culture and in ascites fluid. There are specific differences between using cell culture and intraperitoneal injection into mice. The concentration of antibody found in mouse ascites fluid (2–5 ml/mouse) is in the range of 1–15 mg/ml, while it is only about 5–50 μg/ml in culture fluid. While much higher levels of antibody are found in ascites, so are other proteins and more importantly, host immunoglobulins, which can make the job of purification more difficult.

These new techniques allow production of antibodies of unique specificity. However in all cases, the serum or culture fluid must be collected and purified to obtain the antibodies. Several separation techniques are used to purify immunoglobulins including electrophoresis, precipitation, and liquid chromatography.

Electrophoresis, a high-resolution technique, is most commonly used as an analytical tool to check for purity and specificity. Isoelectric focusing has been used preparatively.

Ethanol precipitation (Cohn fractionation, Cohn *et al.*, 1946) is used by plasma fractionators for purifying large quantities of immunoglobulin G (IgG). It does not work well for small samples and induces polymerization. Precipitation with ammonium sulfate is used either as a one-step procedure or as a preliminary step in a purification scheme. Ammonium sulfate precipitation generally results in a two- to threefold purification with approximately 90% recovery of immunoglobulin. Adjusting conditions to improve the purification factor results in a decrease in recovery. Other techniques such as ethylene glycol and isoelectric precipitation are less commonly used.

Liquid chromatographic techniques are the most widely used methods. Included are ion exchange (anion and cation), gel filtration (size exclusion), hydrophobic interaction, hydroxyapatite, and affinity chromatography.

Immunoglobulins are very heterogeneous. Within a class such as IgG, different antibodies are very similar in molecular size and weight but may differ substantially in charge. Isoelectric points range between 5 and 8 (Carlsson *et al.*, 1985) and are typically higher than most other proteins present. These charge differences make ion exchange chromatography (IEC), an excellent purification technique to use.

Anion exchange is most commonly used. A sample is loaded onto the column under conditions where most proteins bind. The column is then eluted with a shallow salt gradient (step or continuous). Immunoglobulins of the IgG subclass typically elute first, free of most proteins but normally contaminated with a small amount of transferrin and albumin. The more acidic the immunoglobulin, the greater the tendency for contamination with other proteins. Antibodies of the IgM class coelute with more acidic proteins, such as albumin.

Cation exchange is an excellent technique, provided the antibody is stable under mildly acidic conditions, which is usually the case. A strong cation exchanger is used so that it is fully charged at the working pH. A sample is applied under acidic conditions in which the immunoglobulins bind but most other proteins, including albumin, do not. Less chromatographic medium is required for the same size sample than is required with anion exchange because there is less total protein binding.

With ion exchange, conditions need to be optimized for each immunoglobulin. Serum IgG and polyclonal antibodies may elute over a broad pH range with varying contamination. Resolution can be improved by using high-performance, ion-exchange media. However, in all cases the immunoglobulins will still be contaminated with other proteins. If a higher degree of purity is required, the antibody of interest can be further purified, normally by gel filtration. This is a simple and very mild technique. It is commonly used to remove the albumin and transferrin left after ion exchange or to separate IgG from IgM.

Hydrophobic interaction chromatography (HIC) is one of the newer techniques used to purify monoclonal antibodies. Samples are loaded onto a column equilibrated in high salt, e.g. 0.8–1.7 M ammonium sulfate (below concentration required to cause precipitation). Elution is achieved by using a decreasing salt gradient. Elution patterns from a hydrophobic column are similar to cation exchange, with the immunoglobulins eluting last.

Hydroxyapatite (HA) chromatography may also be used. A sample is applied to the column in phosphate buffer at a neutral pH and elution is achieved by using an increasing phosphate salt gradient. The elution pattern is similar to HIC and cation exchange. Hydroxyapatite is a mild technique and can have an advantage over the other techniques when purifying a very labile antibody. Like HIC, resolution is influenced by variations in sample load, flow rate, and temperature, much more so than cation exchange. In all three techniques, resolution and elution position are dependent on the specific antibody being purified.

Affinity chromatography is the technique that is likely to give the highest resolution in a single chromatographic step. A ligand (antigen or anti-antibody) having a biospecificity for the antibody to be purified, is immobilized by covalently coupling it to an insoluble matrix. If a sample containing antibody to the ligand is applied to the column, only that specific antibody will bind strongly. If the ligand is an antigen, it is possible that there may be several different antibodies that will bind, each directed against a different antigenic determinant. Nonspecifically-bound material is washed off with excess buffer. The bound antibody is eluted by lowering the pH to 3.0. If the binding affinity is too high, it is possible that the antibody will not be released from the column. It is also possible that loss of activity can occur from the harsh elution conditions.

The most common purification procedure for immunoglobulins is affinity chromatography on protein A immobilized on agarose (Sepharose® CL-4B). Protein A will bind to most but not all subclasses of immunoglobulin G from human, as well as most other mammals. It will also bind to some IgM, IgA, and IgE. The bound immunoglobulin is eluted from the column by lowering the pH. It is also possible to selectively elute specific immunoglobulin subclasses by decreasing the pH in steps. This procedure will be discussed later in detail.

The high specificity of protein A for immunoglobulins makes it extremely useful for purifying monoclonal antibodies. One affinity medium and set of buffers can be used to purify a tremendous number of different immunoglobulins, in contrast to an immunoaffinity column, which will only purify a single antibody. Protein A will not bind all immunoglobulins from any species. Therefore one must first confirm binding between a specific immunoglobulin and protein A before proceeding. Protein A affinity gels are commercially available, whereas an immunoaffinity column requires purification and immobilization of the ligand, a reasonably tedious task. The interaction between protein A and an immunoglobulin appears to be weaker than that between an antigen and an immunoglobulin. Consequently, less harsh conditions can be used to elute the antibody from a protein A column with greater change of recovering active material.

Hjelm *et al.* (1972) first reported the use of Protein A Sepharose as an immunosorbent for the isolation of human immunoglobulins. IgG from guinea pig was isolated on Protein A Sepharose 4B by Grov (1973). Hjelm (1975) showed that human IgG_3 could be purified from immunoglobulin isolated on a DEAE anion exchange column by using Protein A

Sepharose 4B to remove the other IgG subclasses. It was also shown that some IgA bound to protein A and copurified with the IgG.

This procedure was confirmed by Skvaril (1976), who also demonstrated that a minor portion of IgG_3 always bound to Protein A Sepharose CL-4B at neutral pH and eluted with the other three subclasses at acidic pH. Goding (1976) reported the use of Protein A Sepharose as a simple one step procedure for preparation of rabbit IgG from whole serum, removal of undigested IgG after pepsin treatment, and concentration of dilute solutions of IgG. Several investigators [Ey et al. (1978), MacKenzie et al. (1978a), Chalon et al. (1979), and Watanabe et al. (1981)] have published procedures for isolating the major IgG subclasses of mouse or Protein A Sepharose by elution using discrete pH changes. Seppälä et al. (1981) further demonstrated that the elution characteristics on mouse IgG depended on the haplotype of the donors. Duhamel et al. (1979) reported a method to subfractionate human IgG subclasses on Protein A Sepharose. There are numerous reports showing selective binding and isolation of IgG subclasses from different mammalian species, as well as binding of some IgA, IgE, and IgM. Table 1 summarizes methods for the isolation of immunoglobulin classes and subclasses on Protein A Sepharose. A summary of many of these methods is presented in a review article by Langone (1982).

Protein A binds to the Fc region of immunoglobulin. The protein A molecule is a single polypeptide (M 42,000), highly extended, and asymmetric. It is comprised of five domains; four are highly homologous and are Fc-binding whereas the fifth, C-terminal domain is not (Leatherbarrow and Dwerk, 1983). The protein A binding site is formed by the unique, longitudinal interaction of the CH_2 and CH_3 domains of IgG (Deisenhofer et al., 1978, 1981) and involves tyrosine residues of the Fc region. Binding involves ionic, electrostatic, and hydrophobic interactions and is dominated by interactions between aromatic residues (Bywater et al., 1983). The strength of this interaction is dependent on the specific class, subclass, and species of the immunoglobulin, as is obvious from the extensive list of classes and subclasses that bind protein A and the various methods employed to elute the antibody.

II. Overview of Purification Procedure

The affinity chromatography procedure, using immobilized protein A can be very simple if a commercially prepared adsorbent is used. Protein A Sepharose CL-4B (Pharmacia LKB, Piscataway New Jersey) is the most commonly used and cited material. Adsorbent can be prepared in the

TABLE 1
Summary of Reported Methods for the Purification of Immunoglobulins on Protein A–Sepharose[a]

Species	Class/Subclass	Start pH	Elution pH	Elution Buffer	Comments	References
Human	Whole IgG	7.0	3.0	0.1 M glycine-HCl	Contaminated with IgA and IgM.	Hjelm et al. (1972)
Human	Whole IgG IgM, IgA	7.35	4.0 2.5	applied in 0.025 M phosphate. 0.1 M citric acid–sodium citrate	Less IgM and IgA than at pH 2.5; 40% of bound IgM, 32% IgA, 6% IgG.	Vidal and Conde (1980)
Human	IgG_3 IgG_2 IgG_1 (IgG_2, IgG_4)	7.0	7.0 4.7 4.3	0.2 M phosphate/ 0.1 M citric acid, pH gradient elution; pH 7.0 to 2.2	IgG_2 90–95% pure; 60% total IgG_2, 90% IgG_1, 6% IgG_2, 40% total IgG_2.	Duhamel et al. (1979)
Human	IgG_3	7.0	7.0	0.1 M phosphate	IgG from IEC[b], IgG_3 in void volume.	Hjelm (1975);
Human	IgM	7.5	2.5	0.1 M glycine-HCl	Void fraction from G-200 on proAS[b]; Different levels of IgM from four samples.	Balint et al. (1981)
Human	IgA_1, IgA_2, IgG_3 IgA_1, IgA_2, IgG_1, IgG_2, IgG_4	7.4	7.4 3.0	PBS 0.1 M glycine-HCl	70% of IgA does not bind, 30% binds; Unbound IgA passed through second time still does not bind.	Van Kamp (1979)

Species	Ig class			Buffer	Notes	Reference
Mouse	IgM, IgA, IgE	8.0	8.0	0.14 M phosphate	Purity > 90%, yield 90–100%, except IgG$_{2b}$, 60%; Optional wash step at pH 5.5; Fractions neutralized with 1 M Tris.	Ey et al. (1978)
	IgG$_1$		6.0	0.1 M citrate		
	IgG$_{2a}$		4.5	0.1 M citrate		
	IgG$_{2b}$		3.5	0.1 M citrate		
Mouse	IgG$_1$	8.0	6	0.1 M phosphate;	Step gradient (0.5 pH units/step); Fractions neutralized with 1 M Tris, pH 9.0; Elution characteristics of IgG$_{2a}$ are dependent on allotype.	Seppälä et al. (1981)
	IgG$_{2a}$ (allotypes a,j)		5.0	0.1 M citrate/citric acid		
	IgG$_{2a}$ (allotype b), IgG$_3$		4.5			
	IgG$_{2b}$		3.0–5.0			
Mouse	IgG$_1$	8.0	6.6–5.8	0.1 M phosphate	Continuous gradient (nonlinear); Fractions neutralized with 1 M Tris, pH 8.5; Partial separation of IgG$_{2a}$, IgG$_b$ and IgG$_3$.	Seppälä et al. (1981)
	IgG$_{2a}$		4.8–4.5			
	IgG$_{2b}$		4.4–4.0	0.1 M citrate		
	IgG$_3$		4.7–4.4			
Mouse	IgG$_1$	7.4		0.5 M NaSCN[a]		MacKenzie et al. (1978a)
	IgG$_{2a}$ and IgG$_{2b}$			1.5–2.0 M NaSCN		
Mouse	IgM	7.4	7.4	3 M NaSCN	Only one of five IgM samples bound.	Mackenzie et al. (1978b)

(continued)

TABLE 1 (Continued)

Species	Class/Subclass	Start pH	Elution pH	Elution Buffer	Comments	References
					these conditions.	
Rat	IgG$_{2a}$ IgG$_{2b}$ and IgG$_1$ IgG$_1$	8.0	8.0 8.0 7.0	0.14 M sodium phosphate	Elution with step gradient pH 8.0, 7.0, 6.0, 5.0, 4.0; Better if sample applied at pH 9.0.	Rosseaux et al. (1981)
Rat	IgG$_1$ IgG$_{2c}$ IgG$_{2a}$ IgG$_{2b}$		8.0 7.0	0.05 M NaSCN 1.0 M NaSCN 5 mM phosphate 0.14 M phosphate	Effluent onto DEAE cellulose column; 15 mM PO$_4$[h] fractions off DEAE cellulose.	Nilsson et al. (1982)
Rabbit	IgG	7.4	3.0	0.1 M glycine–HCl or 0.58% HAc containing 0.15 M NaCl	Yield: 5–6 mg/ml serum.	Goding (1976) Miller and Stone (1978)

(continued)

Goat	IgG$_1$	9.1	9.1	0.1 M phosphate	IgG$_1$ elutes in second peak, free of most contaminants.	Delacroix and Vaerman (1979)
	IgG$_2$		5.9			
Goat	IgG$_1$	7.1	6.5–6.9	0.2 M phosphate/ 0.1 M citric acid, pH gradient from pH 7.1 to 2.2	Weak interaction between goat IgG and protein A.	Duhamel et al. (1980)
	IgG$_2$		5.6–6.0			
Guinea pig	IgG$_1$ and IgG$_2$	9.0	4.5	0.1 M phosphate (pH step gradient)	60% elutes at pH 4.5, 40% at pH 3.2; Rechromatography elutes a single peak at the specific pH for each.	Ricardo et al. (1981)
	IgG$_1$ and IgG$_2$		3.2			
Guinea pig	IgG$_1$ (IgG$_2$)	7.3	4.7	0.02 M phosphate/ .01 M citrate pH gradient from 7.3 to 2.1	Five-chamber gradient maker used to generate a smooth pH gradient.	Martin (1982b)
	IgG$_2$		4.3			
Pig	IgG (IgA, IgM)	7.6	3.0	0.1 M glycine–HCl, applied in 0.01 M phosphate, pH 7.6	20–25 mg/ml porcine IgG binds to protein A–Sepharose.	Milon et al. (1978)
Syrian hampster	IgG$_2$	8.0	5.9	0.2 N acetate/acetic acid gradient from pH 7.5–3.0		Coe et al. (1981)
	IgG$_1$		5.3			
Syrian hampster	IgM	8.0	8.0	0.1 M phosphate 0.1 M sodium citrate/citric acid	Free of any IgG; Suggests IgG$_2$ is heterogeneous.	Escribano et al. (1982)
	IgG$_2$		6.5			
	IgG$_2$		6.0			
	IgG$_1$		5.0			

(continued)

TABLE 1 (*Continued*)

Species	Class/Subclass	Start pH	Elution pH	Elution Buffer	Comments	References
Dog	IgG, IgM, IgA IgG, IgM, IgA	7.2	7.2 2.5	PBS 0.1 M glycine-HCl	Neutralized with 0.5 M Tris.	Goudswaard *et al.* (1978)
Dog	IgG, IgM IgM IgG	8.0 8.0	8.0 8.0	0.58% HAc, 0.15 M NaCl 0.05 M THAM, 0.15 M NaCl	Applied in 0.5 M THAM[c] 0.1 M NaCl GF[i] on Sepharose CL-6B, first peak; Second peak off GF column.	Warr and Hart (1979)
Dog	IgM	7.5	2.5	0.1 M glycine-HCl	>80% yield of IgM from G-200 Peak; IgM first purified on Sx[f] G-200 pH 3.0; pH adjusted to 7.5 with 2.5 M NaOH	Balint *et al.* (1981)
Rhesus monkey	IgG$_I$ IgG$_{II}$ IgG$_{III}$	7.3	5.0–4.72 5.1–4.65 4.6–4.25	0.1 M citrate/0.2 M phosphate	Did not bind DEAE IEX[g] in .01 M PO4[g]; Eluted off DEAE IEX[f] before ProAS[b] purified fractions were obtained.	Martin (1982a)
Cow	IgG$_1$ IgG$_2$, IgG$_1$	7.2	7.2 2.5	PBS 0.1 M glycine–HCl	Neutralized with 0.5 M THAM[e].	Goudswaard *et al.* (1978)

Species	Ig class	pH	Buffer	Notes	Reference
Sheep	IgG$_1$	7.2	PBS		Goudswaard et al. (1978)
	IgG$_2$	2.5	0.1 M glycine–HCl	Neutralized with 0.5 M THAM^e.	
Horse	IgG$_{a+b}$, IgG$_c$, IgG(T)	7.2	PBS		Goudswaard et al. (1978)
	IgG$_{a+b}$, IgG$_c$, IgG(T)	2.5	0.1 M glycine–HCl	Neutralized with 0.5 M THAM^e.	

^{a} Copyright 1990, Pharmacia LKB Biotechnology Inc., Piscataway, New Jersey. This table is an expansion of one prepared by Langone (1982).
^{b} IEC: Ion exchange chromatography
^{c} ProAS: Protein A–Sepharose
^{d} NaSCN: Sodium thiocyanate
^{e} THAM: Tris(hydroxymethyl)aminomethane
^{f} Sx: Sephadex
^{g} IEX: Ion exchange column
^{h} PO4: phosphate buffer
^{i} GF: Gel filtration

laboratory, but it will add extra work and considerable variability to the results.

The main points to consider in performing an affinity chromatography purification procedure include:

Choice of ligand:
  protein A source
  purity

Choice of a matrix:
  dextran, agarose, synthetic resin, etc.
  standard versus high performance media

Immobilization procedure:
  activation method CnBr, epoxy, tresyl, etc.
  ligand density
  homemade versus commercial media

Determination of available binding capacity

Column preparation
  size
  sample load (capacity)
  equilibration procedure
  flow rates
  prevention of microbial contamination

Sample preparation: serum or ascites versus cell culture, desalting, dialysis, centrifugation, dilution, buffer exchange, precipitation, etc.

Sample application

Elution procedures

Fraction collection and detection
  neutralization after acid eluton

Column reequilibration, reuse, and storage

Limitations of method

Each of these points will be discussed. General methods for purification of IgG from mouse and human will then be outlined.

III. Choice of Ligand

It is important to choose a ligand that is as pure and as highly specific as possible.

Protein A can be obtained from different strains of *Staphylococcus aureus*. Much of the early work used protein A from Cowan I strain. This protein A is covalently bound to the cell wall and is isolated by digestion with lysostaphin followed by ion exchange and gel filtration on DEAE Sephadex® A-50 and Sephadex G-100 (Sjöquist *et al.*, 1972) or affinity chromatography on IgG–Sepharose.

Most methicillin-resistant strains of *Staphylococcus aureus* lack or only excrete protein A. Strain A676 produces high levels of protein A which can be purified by affinity chromatography on IgG–Sepharose 4B (Lindmark *et al.*, 1977). It is this type of strain that is used to produce the protein A commercially supplied by Pharmacia LKB. Recombinant protein A is also available commercially.

The physiochemical and immunochemical properties of protein A from strain A676 and Cowan I are very similar. There are however, differences in their amino acid composition (Lindmark *et al.*, 1977). Protein A from strain A676 is a true extracellular protein and as such, contains no contamination cell wall fragments, as is the case with protein A from Cowan I. Enzymatic digestion and harsh extraction conditions are not used in the production of protein A from A676 and this results in a pure, homogeneous product.

IV. Choice of Matrix

The best matrix for affinity chromatography exhibits macroporosity, a high degree of stability, low nonspecific adsorption, and a large number of accessible sites for ligand attachment. Beaded agarose is the most widely accepted matrix for this purpose. The first reported use was by Grov in 1973, who used Sepharose 4B (4% agarose from Pharmacia). Crosslinked agarose (Sepharose CL–4B) is the preferred matrix as this material is more stable to the harsh elution conditions (low pH) required to elute immunoglobulin from the column. Beaded agarose of higher concentrations (>4%) is less porous, especially after activation, which causes internal crosslinking and a possible reduction in the available binding capacity for immunoglobulin. Lower concentrations (<4%) result in a softer matrix, which has poorer stability and flow characteristics. A new gel, Sepharose 4 Fast Flow has recently been presented as a good matrix for preparative applications (Tranell *et al.*, 1988).

Several different high-performance matrices have been used to immobilize protein A. Superose® 12 is a 12% beaded agarose available from Pharmacia LKB (Uppsala, Sweden). It has a particle diameter of 13 ± 2 μm compared to an average particle size of 100 μm for Sepharose. Silica

300 A (10 μm) is available commercially from Pierce Chemical Co. (Rockford, Illinois). A disadvantage of silica is that it begins to dissolve above pH 8.0 and alkaline solutions can not be used. Bio-Rad Laboratories (Richmond California), uses protein A coupled to a 40–60 μm, hydrophilic polymer.

For most applications, Sepharose CL-4B is sufficient and in many cases better to use than high-performance media. It can be activated to give a high-binding capacity. It can be run fast, especially when packed in short columns. It is much less expensive to use and doesn't require any elaborate equipment to run. On the other hand, the efficiency of a Sepharose column is lower than that of a high-performance column, resulting in a greater dilution of the eluting material. Binding is more efficient at high flow rates in a high-performance column. The bottom line is that high-performance columns are better if many small samples need to be run, as in a clinical application. But for most other applications, a protein A Sepharose CL-4B or 4 Fast Flow column is the best choice.

V. Immobilization Procedure

The three major methods of attachment of protein A to a matrix are cyanogen bromide, tresyl, and epoxide activation. Cyanogen bromide activation is the most common method of immobilization of protein A to agarose (Porath *et al.*, 1967). Activation by cyanogen bromide results in the formation of cyanate esters, which react with nucleophiles (primary and secondary amines). This method results in a relatively stable attachment of the protein through an isourea linkage and also causes internal crosslinking of the agarose chains, which increases the stability of the matrix.

Tresyl activation is another procedure that has been used. The reaction of tresyl chloride with the hydroxyl groups of agarose results in sulfonate esters, which in turn react with nucleophiles. The bonds that are formed are more stable to hydrolysis than those formed by cyanogen bromide activation, especially under alkaline conditions (Nilsson and Mosbach, 1984). However, no crosslinking of the matrix occurs.

Epoxide activation with bis oxirane results in a stable alkylamine linkage with primary amines and introduces a spacer arm between the matrix and the ligand (protein A). It also causes crosslinking of the agarose chains, increasing the stability of the matrix (Sundberg and Porath, 1974). Ligand density is normally lower with epoxide coupling than with cyanogen bromide or tresyl.

Other coupling procedures (carbodiimide, N-hydroxysuccinimide, etc.) are also used. Cyanogen bromide activation is, by far, the dominant method.

There has been much discussion about the stability of the isourea linkage formed in cyanogen bromide activation. In fact, this bond is quite stable under the acidic conditions used with protein A. The long history and wide acceptance of this method is in itself proof of its usefulness. There is some leakage of protein A from columns. It is therefore important to wash the column well before use. It has been found that some protein A that leaks is coupled to fragments of agarose, indicating breakage of either the glycosidic linkages or hydrogen bonds holding gel fragments together, rather than the isourea linkages.

The question that really needs to be addressed is whether to make the protein A affinity gel or to use commercially available media. The predominant advantage of preparing it is lower cost. This may be true if fairly large amounts of affinity medium is prepared (> 100 ml), but usually not for only a few milliliters. However, if the real cost of making the media is taken into account—the labor cost, quality control (QC) cost (if any QC is actually done), and wasted material cost—it probably is not cost effective. If a gel is needed with a different degree of substitution than is commercially supplied, the coupling must be performed in the laboratory. Preactivated affinity media are also commercially available for this purpose. The major advantages to commercially supplied materials are defined specifications (coupling capacity) and reproducibility. Even experts at coupling procedures have difficulty making reproducible batches.

VI. Available Binding Capacity

The available binding capacity is a measure of how much immunoglobulin will adhere to a defined volume of the affinity medium under specified conditions. It is related to the amount of protein A coupled per milliliter of Sepharose, the source of protein A, the immunoglobulin class, subclass, or allotype, and the buffer system used.

Ligand density (amount of protein A coupled to a defined volume of affinity media) is a very important variable. It affects the reproducibility of experiments and also recovery. Binding capacity does not increase proportionally with ligand density. At high ligand density, binding capacity and recovery may be reduced due to multiple binding, nonspecific interactions, and steric effects. Typically, a ligand density of about 2 mg of protein A per ml of gel is used. This gives a binding capacity of about 20–25 mg of human IgG/ml, but only 6 mg/ml for mouse. This value differs for various animal species. Protein A Sepharose 4 Fast Flow, with a ligand density of 6 mg/ml has a binding capacity of about 35 mg/ml for human IgG (Tranell *et al.*, 1988).

A comprehensive binding capacity table of protein A Sepharose for immunoglobulin from different animal species does not exist. Many papers refer to work by Kronvall (1973), who compared the IgG-binding capacity of protein A for animal and human sera. These data can be misleading since they were based on the total IgG reactivity of equal volumes of sera. A survey of methods shows that protein A binding is subclass- and subtype-specific. Consequently, the binding capacity for a specific antibody, subclass, or allotype representing only a small part of the total IgG may be high even though the total IgG-binding capacity for that species has been reported to be weak.

One example of this is rat IgG. Work reported by Rousseaux *et al.* (1981) has shown that IgG_{2c} binds to protein A, as does about 60% of the IgG_1. The remaining IgG_1, IgG_{2a}, and IgG_{2b} (~70% of the total IgG) does not. These results help explain the low-binding capacity previously reported for rat IgG. Use of a high salt, high pH buffer to equilibrate the column and load the sample could improve the binding of rat IgG_1 as has been shown to be the case with mouse.

VII. Column Preparation

The first step in preparing the column is to determine the sample volume, the concentration of immunoglobulin in the sample, and the binding capacity of the affinity column. From this information, the size of the column needed can be calculated. Normally, a column that has at least twice the capacity needed to assure complete binding is prepared. If the amount of immunoglobulin in the sample approaches the total capacity of the column, small changes in contact time and flow rate will affect the results and less than the maximal amount of immunoglobulin will be bound. For 5 ml of sample containing 10 mg of IgG/ml and a gel with a binding capacity of 20 mg/ml, a column containing about 5 ml of gel is needed for a sample.

Next, choose a column that will accomodate the gel and leave sufficient volume for the sample, or a column where the gel is retained between two bed supports and can be connected to a sample application device. Almost any type of chromatography column can be used, from a pasteur pipette with a glass wool support to a plastic syringe barrel with a fritted plastic disc to the best commercial columns. Column dimensions should be chosen so that the bed height is 1–5 cm. Longer columns result in increased separation times. For 5 ml of protein A Sepharose CL-4B, a column with a diameter of 1.6 cm will give a bed height of 2.5 cm. If an open column is used, it must be at least 5 cm in length to accomodate the volume of gel and excess buffer. One advantage of affinity chromatography is that column design has little effect on results unless gradient elution is used.

Measure out the volume of settled gel required and dilute it with an equal volume of start buffer (freeze-dried medium must first be rehydrated and washed according to the manufacturer's instructions). Wash the column out and make sure no air is trapped in the support material and that buffer freely flows through the column. Next, stir the medium with a glass rod and pour it down the column wall, being careful not to trap air bubbles. Allow buffer to run from the column but be careful not to let the column run dry. It is best to pass through at least ten column volumes of start buffer to be sure that the column is completely equilibrated.

If an open column is used, then hydrostatic pressure determines the flow rate. As the level of buffer in the column drops, so does the flow rate. In closed systems where a pump is used, the flow rate can be accurately controlled. The type of separation medium and the affinity binding constant influence the maximum flow rate to use. Different flow rates can be used for sample application, elution, and reequilibration within one procedure. Higher flow rates may be used with high-performance medium because the smaller particle diameters allow faster solute equilibration and give less dilution. However, if the binding is weak under the conditions used, not all of the immunoglobulin may be pulled out of solution at high flow rates.

Once a column has been prepared, it is necessary to prevent bacterial contamination. This is accomplished by adding a suitable bacteriostatic agent to the buffer. This agent can easily be removed by washing the column with several volumes of buffer, free of the bacteriostatic agent, prior to use. The bacteriostatic agent need not be removed if its presence does not interfere with further work. Suitable agents that can be used include

ethanol, 20%

sodium azide, 0.02–0.04%

thimerosal, 0.02%

chlorhexidine digluconate 0.002%.

Ethanol is recommended as it is readily available, safe to use, and can be disposed of with ease. A bacteriostatic agent is not necessary if the column is used frequently. However, in this case it is important to use freshly prepared and filtered buffers.

After use, the column should be cleaned and stored below 8°C (not frozen) in buffer at neutral pH containing a bacteriostatic agent.

VIII. Sample Preparation

Proper sample preparation assures that the immunoglobulin will bind to the column and increases the useful life of the affinity column. The pH of the sample should be adjusted to the same pH as the loading buffer. The sample should be free of cell debris and other insoluble substances. Filtration through a 0.02–0.45 micron filter will remove any particulates. Centrifugation (10,000 × g, 20 min) is also useful for removing insoluble material but is not as thorough as filtration since it is dependent on the relative density of the particles to the medium. It is critical that samples are filtered if high-performance columns are used. These columns are easily blocked by particulates.

Ascites fluid and serum require more careful sample preparation than culture fluid. Normally, filtration and pH adjustment are all that is required with culture fluid. Protein concentration is low and the immunoglobulin is concentrated on the protein A column. If serum supplemented culture fluid is used, check for the presence of immunoglobulin in the serum which could ultimately interfere. If found, it can be removed either by passing the serum through or batch adsorbing it to protein A Sepharose before adding it to the culture fluid.

Ascites fluid and serum should be diluted with starting buffer at least two-fold to reduce the viscosity and adjust the pH. They contain high protein levels, hydrophobic substances, (lipids, membrane proteins, coagulation factors) nucleic acids, and additives such as pristine, which can effect column performance. It may be helpful to remove these substances before applying the sample to the affinity column. Gel filtration, dialysis, and precipitation techniques are commonly used. Starting buffer conditions should be chosen carefully because some antibodies (IgM, mouse IgG_{2b}, and IgG_3) exhibit euglobulin properties and may precipitate at low ionic strength.

Gel filtration (desalting) on Sephadex® G-25 is a simple procedure. The column bed volume should be 4–5 times the volume of sample. Desalting removes low molecular weight substances (<1000 daltons), leaves the sample in the desired starting buffer (pH and salt), and also tends to adsorb strongly hydrophobic substances like lipids. The procedure is fast, taking about 15 min. It dilutes the sample about 1.5–2-fold, which is recommended before application onto the protein A column to reduce the viscosity. The desalting column can be cleaned and reused or discarded. Prepacked, disposable columns are commercially available for this purpose.

Dialysis leaves the sample in a correct starting condition and is nondiluting. It reduces or changes the salt concentration more gradually than desalting, which may be better for some immunoglobulins, reducing the chance of precipitation. However, it is time consuming, somewhat tedious, and there is a risk that the dialysis bag will leak or rupture, causing loss of sample.

Ammonium sulfate precipitation is a useful method that gets rid of about 50% (by weight) of contaminating proteins in serum or ascites fluid. Care should be taken as some monoclonals are denatured by this technique (Burchiel, 1986; McGregor et al., 1983). This method is time consuming and normally not necessary as a cleanup step prior to affinity chromatography.

Lipoproteins can be removed if desired, by precipitation with dextran sulfate (van Dalen et al., 1967), polyvinylpyrrolidone (Burstein, 1957), or caprylic acid treatment (Russo et al., 1983). Caprylic acid precipitates about 50% of the contaminating proteins leaving the IgG in solution. Nucleic acids can be removed by precipitation with protamine sulfate (Scopes, 1982).

Degassing the sample prior to application can help prevent air bubbles from forming and distorting the UV elution profile, a very annoying problem which usually starts just as the protein peak begins to elute.

IX. Sample Application

Once the sample has been prepared, it can be applied directly onto the column. Flow rate, pH, and ionic strength are the major factors to consider. Sample volume is relatively unimportant if the total immunoglobulin content has been calculated and does not exceed 80% of the binding capacity of the column.

The pH of the starting buffer depends on the application. Once the pH has been determined, the sample pH should be adjusted to assure that most of the immunoglobulin will bind.

Flow rate should not be so fast that all the immunoglobulin does not have sufficient time to bind. The flow rate to use depends on the sample and buffer composition. Linear flow rates from 10–100 cm/hr can be used on Protein A Sepharose CL-4B and even higher on Sepharose 4 Fast Flow and high-performance columns. If time is important, try using the higher flow rate and test the eluant for immunoglobulin. If none is found, the flow rate is acceptable. If found, cut the flow rate in half and try again. (First determine that the immunoglobulin found will bind at all.) If immunoglobulin is still found in the eluant at 10 cm/hr, check the pH. For large-scale or repetitive applications, one may want to calculate the column binding capacity over a range of flow rates.

Binding of IgG to protein A can be influenced by the ionic strength of the buffer. Immunoglobulins are more hydrophobic than most other serum proteins. Consequently, altering the ionic strength can affect the relative binding of IgG to hydrophobic regions on protein A to a greater extent than for most other proteins. However the risk of contamination with other proteins is increased (Ohlson et al., 1988).

X. Elution Procedures

Elution from the protein A column is normally achieved by lowering the pH of the buffer. The specific procedure depends on the species, the type of sample (serum IgG, monoclonal, polyclonal), and the goal of the procedure (to isolate all immunoglobulin or a specific subclass). Most immunoglobulin can be eluted by dropping the pH to 3.0 with a phosphate/citrate or citric acid buffer. This procedure is sufficient for serum IgG when complete recovery is desired. However, the low pH may denature some immunoglobulin. For some monoclonals and specific subclasses, it is possible to elute at a higher pH. Elution can also be achieved by decreasing the pH in discrete steps or by a continuous gradient. Step elution is the most common procedure. There are numerous references for isolating immunoglobulins and subclasses from different species, as mentioend earlier.

For mouse ascites fluid, a starting buffer of 0.2 M sodium phosphate/ 0.15 M sodium chloride, pH 8, will bind a high percentage of the IgG. Elution is achieved with 100 mM citric acid titrated with NaOH to pH 6.0 for IgG_1, pH 5.0 for IgG_{2a}, and pH 4.0 for IgG_{2b} and IgG_3

Mouse IgG_1 binds weaker to protein A than other mouse immunoglobulin subclasses. Using the described starting buffer, a specific IgG_1 may or may not bind. It is possible to improve binding by increasing the ionic strength and enhancing hydrophobic interactions.

Protein G is another bacterial receptor protein which also binds IgG. It has been reported to bind tighter to mouse and many other species of IgG than protein A. While it may bind more IgG for specific species (i.e., rat), it is not clear whether it binds significantly more mouse IgG (specifically IgG_1) than protein A. Elution from a Protein G affinity column requires lowering the pH below 3.0 for all IgGs. Applications of protein G affinity purifications of IgG are reviewed in Chapter 20.

Other methods to elute immunoglobulins from protein A columns have been reported. Chaotropic ions (Kristiansen, 1974) have been used, but again these are rather harsh conditions. Bywater *et al.* (1978, 1983) have reported that solutions of glycyl-tyrosine, L-tryptophan, and glycyl-L-histidine at pH 7.0 are mild and reasonably effective eluting agents for IgG. This work showed that some IgG eluted but it was not determined if this IgG was subclass-specific. Morgan *et al.* (1978) have reported an electrophoretic method for removal of immunoglobulins from Protein A Sepharose CL-4B. These last two methods are mild and could prove to be useful in specific cases, but pH elution is still by far the most accepted method.

XI. Collection and Detection Methods

Since elution is affected by discrete pH changes, it is possible to collect all of the material eluting between pH changes into a single test tube. No fraction collector or detector is required. However, use of a fraction collector, a detector, and a recording device can improve the collection procedure by reducing dilution and documenting results. A flow-through UV monitor set at an absorbance of 280 nm is normally used. The monitor lets you see when no more material is eluting and the next buffer can be applied. Collection of fractions can be started as soon as material begins to elute and stopped when the absorbance peak returns to the base line. In this way, both the void volume and the volume eluted after the peak has eluted are not collected. Peak material may be collected in a single tube or in several smaller fractions. A small volume of a ten-fold concentrated buffer at neutral pH can be put into the bottom of the collection tubes to raise the pH of the sample as it elutes and reduce the chance of denaturation from low pH.

XII. Column Reequilibration, Reuse, and Storage

After the immunoglobulin has eluted, the column is washed with several volumes of buffer at pH 3.0 to remove any remaining bound material. It is then reequilibrated by passing through ten column volumes of start buffer. You should test the pH of the effluent to be sure it is the same as that being applied. At this point the column is ready for application of the next sample.

When finished, the column should be stored in 20% ethanol in the cold (4–8°C). Care should be taken to prevent bacterial contamination. If necessary, Protein A Sepharose CL-4B can be sterilized by treatment with 70% ethanol for 17 hr at 22°C.

A useful column life depends on several factors:

1. the number of cycles it has gone through,
2. the extremes of pH and temperature to which it has been exposed and for how long,
3. the type of sample (ascites or culture fluid); whether it contains proteolytic enzymes that can digest protein A and exposure time,
4. method of sample pretreatment, and
5. the age of the medium and its storage conditions.

With proper sample pretreatment and following standard procedures, several months of column use can be expected. The time for column replacement can be determined by measuring the capacity of the medium periodically.

XIII. Limitations of Method

Protein A binds selectively to several classes and subclasses of immunoglobulins from human, mouse, and many other mammalian species. it does not bind to all and the degree and tightness of binding varies between species, classes, and subclasses. It is important to first determine whether the immunoglobulin to be purified binds to protein A and the conditions under which this binding takes place. If it doesn't bind, protein G may work. In general, if the IgG binds to both protein A and G, protein A is usually the better choice since the IgG can be eluted under less harsh conditions. Protein G columns require using acid elution at a pH between 2 and 3.

Protein A does not bind to most human IgG_3. Therefore, serum IgG purified on protein A will contain little IgG_3. The same is true for other species that show selective subclass binding. If all of the immunoglobulin needs to be recovered from these species, another method must be used, such as ion exchange, ammonium sulfate precipitation, or Protein G affinity chromatography.

Since protein A binds some IgA, IgE, and IgM, as well as IgG, it is possible that purified IgG will be contaminated with these other immunoglobulins. If the final use requires their removal, other purification steps will be required. IgM can be removed by gel filtration on Sephacryl® S-300HR. IgA can possibly be removed by ion-exchange. Protein G only bind IgG.

Monoclonal antibodies from ascites fluid will be contaminated with host immunoglobulins. Partial purification of the monoclonal from host can be achieved by high-performance ion-exchange, or hydrophobic interaction chromatography.

Monoclonal antibodies exhibit substantial microheterogeneity resulting from differential gene expression, posttranscriptional and posttranslational modifications, variations in glycosylation, aggregation, proteolytic degredation, etc. Many, but not necessarily all of the variants will be copurified by protein A affinity chromatography, precipitation, or conventional chromatographic methods. They can be further subfractionated using high-performance cation exchange (Mono S) chromatography or isoelectric focusing. Keep in mind that a technique like protein A affinity chromatography may selectively enrich or eliminate specific variants. Use of anion exchange is less selective and may give an IgG preparation which is more representative of the total IgG population. You should consider using one or more of the high performance techniques (cation exchange, Isoelectric focusing, etc.) to characterize the monoclonals you work with.

Protein A can leach from the column and elute with the immunoglobulin. Although the level of leakage is extremely small, it may be a concern, especially if the immunoglobulin will be used as a therapeutic agent. It is important that the protein A affinity column be thoroughly washed prior to use to remove any free protein A. It is possible to test for protein A leakage by using a sensitive ELISA method such as reported by Olsvik and Berdal (1981) or Dertzbaugh *et al.* (1985).

The most important point to remember is that there is no single method or set of conditions that is optimal for the purification of all immunoglobulins. A researcher should always confirm that a method works on a small scale before applying all of the sample. Keeping in mind the parameters that have been discussed, it should be possible to modify or design a method that meets the specific needs of the investigator. Also keep in mind that protein A affinity chromatography is not always the best technique for purification of immunoglobulins. There are other selective techniques such as ion exchange, hydrophobic and protein G affinity chromatography. Each one has specific benefits and limitations.

The following methods may be used for the purification of human and mouse IgG from serum, ascites, and culture fluids.

XIV. General Methods Using Protein A Sepharose CL-4B and Protein A Sepharose 4 Fast Flow for Mouse and Human IgG Purification

A. Mouse IgG: Monoclonal, or Polyclonal

1. Materials

Protein A Sepharose CL-4B or Protein A Sepharose 4 Fast Flow (Pharmacia LKB, Piscataway, New Jersey)

Buffer A: 0.2 M Na_2HPO_4, 0.1 M NaCl, pH 8.0

Buffer B: 0.1 M citric acid/NaOH, pH 6.0

Buffer C: 0.1 M citric acid/NaOH, pH 5.0

Buffer D: 0.1 M citric acid/NaOH, pH 4.0

Buffer E: 0.1 M citric acid/NaOH, pH 3.0

Buffer F: 0.5 M Na_2HPO_4, 0.5 M NaCl, pH 8.0

Buffer G: 1.0 M Tris HCl, pH 8.0

2. Equipment

Column C10/10 with one or two adaptors AC10 (Pharmacia, LKB) will hold up to 7 ml Protein A Sepharose CL-4B (use or for up to 25 mg bound IgG). Column size depends on the volume of sample and the concentration of IgG.

Flow through UV monitor, 280 nm (UV-1)

Potentiometric recorder (REC 2)

Sample application valve (LV-3)

Solvent selection valve (LV-3)

Peristaltic pump (P-1)

Fraction collector (FRAC-100) with flow diversion valve (PSV-100)

The components of a liquid chromatography system for affinity chromatography can be seen in Figure 1.

3. Method

Prepare the protein A Sepharose CL-4B according to manufacturer's directions. Suspend the gel in buffer A and pack the required volume into the column (approximately 1.0 ml of gel for each 0.5 ml of ascites fluid, 2 ml of serum, or 100 ml of culture fluid). (Actual binding capacity should be

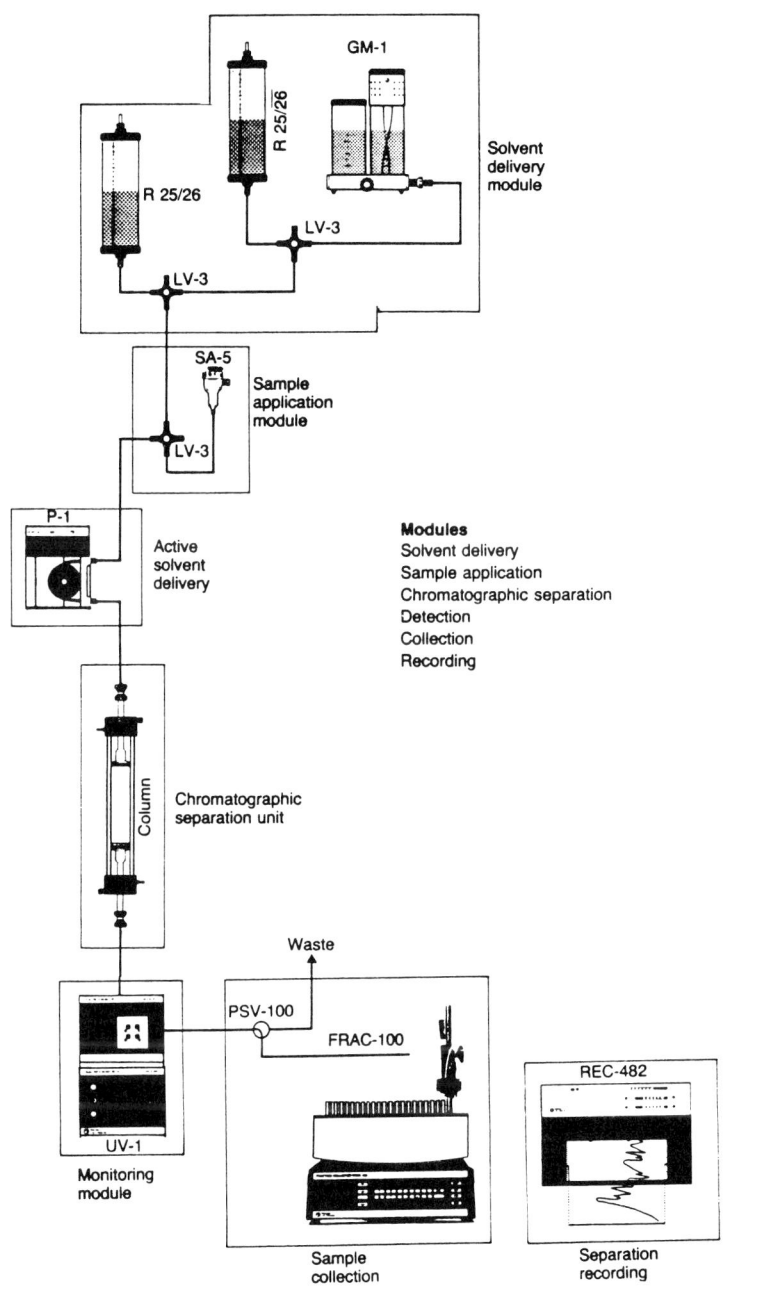

FIGURE 1
Components of a liquid chromatography system for affinity chromatographs. (Copyright 1990, Pharmacia LKB Biotechnology, Inc., Piscataway, New Jersey)

determined for the specific sample. Sample load should not exceed 50% of capacity for highest recovery.) Insert the adaptor into the column and adjust it down to the surface of the gel.

a. Ascites Fluid or Serum. Equilibrate the column with five bed volumes of buffer A. Use a linear flow rate of up to 1 cm/min. (Volumetric flow rate = linear flow rate × cross-sectional area of column.)

Dilute the sample with an equal volume of buffer F and put it through a 0.45 μm filter. Alternatively, buffer exchange the sample on a column of Sephadex G-25 Medium equilibrated in Buffer A. For sample volumes up to 2.5 ml, PD-10 prepacked, disposable columns (Pharmacia LKB) may be used.

Apply the sample to the column and follow it with more buffer A. Monitor the effluent for protein. (Choose an absorbance range which gives at least 50% full-scale response when protein elutes). When the absorbance value returns to the base line, switch to the first elution buffer. IgG subclasses can be selectively eluted from the column as follows:

Buffer B, pH 6.0 elutes IgG_1.

Buffer C, pH 5.0 elutes IgG_{2a}.

Buffer D, pH 4.0 elutes IgG_{2b} and IgG_3.

For whole serum, start elution with buffer B. Turn the fraction collector on when the monitor signal indicates material is starting to elute from the column and begin collecting the IgG_1. When the absorbance returns to near the base line, stop collecting, but continue with buffer B until the absorbance returns to base line. Switch to buffer C to elute the IgG_{2a} following the same procedure. After the IgG_{2a} has eluted, the procedure is repeated with buffer D to elute the IgG_{2b} and IgG_3 (Figure 2). Antibodies eluting below pH 5.0 should be rapidly neutralized to prevent denaturation. This is accomplished by adding 1.0 M Tris-HCl (buffer G) (a volumn equal to 10% of the fraction size) to the tubes in the fraction collector prior to collection.

Wash the column with 5–10 bed volumes of buffer E and then 5–10 bed volumes of buffer A to regenrate the column. The pH of the effluent should be checked to make sure that it is the same as the equilibrating buffer prior to applying the next sample.

Monoclonal antibodies can be applied to the column in Buffer A and

Chapter 18. Use of Protein A to Purify Immunoglobulins

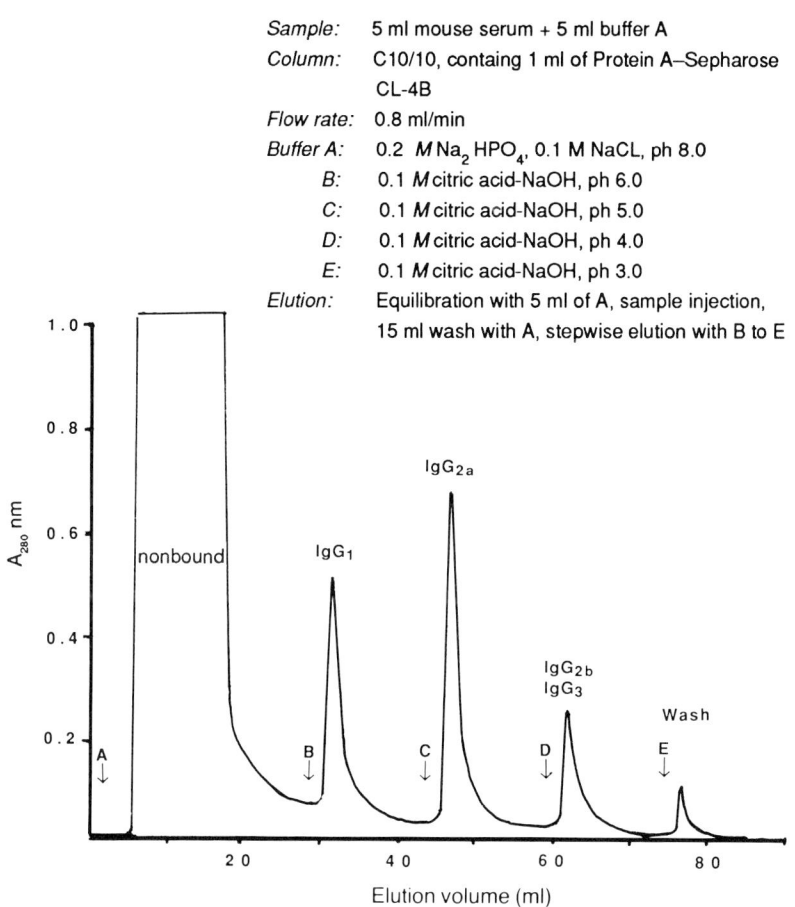

FIGURE 2
Representative chromatographic profile of IgG subclasses from mouse serum using stepwise elution. The column was eluted in four steps, as indicated by the arrows.

eluted using only the specific buffer for its subclass. Once the monoclonal has eluted, follow the wash and equilibration steps.

b. Cell Culture: IgG_{2a}, IgG_{2b}, IgG_3. Equilibrate the column with five bed volumes of 10 mM phosphate buffer, pH 8.0. Use a linear flow rate of up to 1 cm/min.

Centrifuge the supernatant to remove cells and debris (10,000 × g, 20–30 min) or alternatively, use a tangential flow cassette ultrafiltration system with a 0.3 μ Omega series membrane (Pharmacia LKB) to harvest the culture fluid. Adjust the pH of the culture fluid to 8.0 with dropwise addition of 1.0 M NaOH and then pass it through a 0.45 μ filter. Apply the sample to the column and follow it with at least one column volume of equilibration buffer.

Choose the appropriate elution buffer for the monoclonal subclass being purified. Apply the elution buffer. Turn the fraction collector on when the monitor signal indicates material is starting to elute from the column and begin collecting. When the absorbance returns to near base line, stop collecting and divert the effluent to waste. Antibodies eluting below pH 5.0 should be rapidly neutralized to prevent denaturation. To do this, add a volume of 1.0 M Tris-HCl, equal to 10% of the fraction size, to the tubes in the fraction collector prior to collecting.

Wash the column with 5–10 bed volumes of buffer E and then 5–10 volumes of equilibration buffer. Check that the pH of the effluent matches the pH of the equilibrating buffer prior to application of the next sample.

Monoclonal antibodies of subclass IgG_1 from cell culture are best purified by other methods because the large sample volumes and weak binding of IgG_1 to protein A often gives poor recovery and reproducibility. Purification by cation exchange on S Sepharose Fast Flow in an acetate buffer at pH 5.0 is recommended. The purified IgG_1 fraction can be desalted and/or further purified on the protein A column if required, using the method for ascites samples.

Ammonium sulfate precipitation is not a good choice because of the large volumes. The culture fluid should first be ultrafiltered using a tangential flow cassette system with a 0.3 μ Omega series membrane. It can then be concentrated by ultrafiltration on a 10,000k cutoff Omega membrane. The immunoglobulin can then be purified on a Protein A–Sepharose column using the method for ascites samples.

B. Human IgG: Serum or Cell Culture
1. Materials
Protein A Sepharose CL-4B or Protein A Sepharose 4 Fast Flow

Buffer A: 0.2 M Na_2HPO_4, pH 7.0 adjusted with 0.1 M citric acid

Buffer B: 0.1 M glycine-HCl, pH 4.0

Buffer C: 0.1 M glycine-HCl, pH 3.0

Buffer D: 1.0 M Tris-HCl, pH 8.0

2. Equipment
Same as for mouse IgG.

3. Method

Prepare the Protein A Sepharose CL-4B according to manufacturer's directions. Suspend the gel in buffer A and pack the required volume into the column (approximately 1.0 ml of gel for each ml of serum). Adjust the adaptor down to the surface of the gel.

Equilibrate the column with five bed volumes of buffer A. Use a linear flow rate of up to 1 cm/min.

For serum, dilute the sample with an equal volume of buffer A and put it through a 0.45 μ filter. Alternatively, desalt the sample on a column of Sephadex G-25 (medium). For sample volumes up to 2.5 ml, prepacked, disposable columns (Pharmacia LKB) may be used.

For culture fluid, centrifuge the supernatant to remove cells and debris (10,000 $\times$ g, 20–30 min). Alternatively, use a tangential cassette ultrafiltration system with a 0.3 μ Omega series membrane (Pharmacia LKB) to filter the culture fluid. Adjust the pH to 7.0 by dropwise addition of 1.0 M NaOH or HCl while stirring and then pass it through a 0.45 μ filter.

Apply the sample to the column and follow it with more buffer A.

Monitor the effluent for protein. When the absorbance value returns to base line, switch to the eluting buffer. Buffer B will elute the IgG containing reduced levels of IgM and IgA (Vidal and Conde, 1980). Buffer C will elute the entire immunoglobulin fraction. The acid-eluted immunoglobulins should be neutralized to prevent denaturation. This is accomplished by adding 1.0 M Tris-HCl, pH 8.0 (buffer D) at a volume equal to 10% of the fraction size, to the tubes in the fraction collector prior to collection.

Turn the fraction collector on when the monitor signal indicates that material is starting to elute from the column and begin collecting the immunoglobulin. When the absorbance returns to near the base line, stop collecting. If buffer B was used for elution, switch to buffer C to wash the column of any remaining material. This material can be collected if desired, as it will contain an appreciable amount of IgM and IgA.

When the monitor signal indicates no additional material is being eluted, switch to buffer A and equilibrate the column with at least five bed volumes. Check that the pH of the eluent matches the equilibrating buffer prior to applying the next sample.

References

Balint, Jr., J. P., Ikeda, Y., Nagai, T., and Terman, D. S. (1981). *Immunol. Commun.* **10,** 533–540.

Burchiel, S. (1986). "Methods in Enzymology" (J. J. Langone and H. van Avunakis, eds.), Vol. 121, pp. 596–615.
Burstein, M. C. R. (1957). *Acad. Sci.* **244,** 3189–3191.
Bywater, R. (1978). *Chromatogr. Synth. Biol. Polym.* **29,** 237–240.
Bywater, R., Eriksson, G., and Ottosson, T. (1983). *J. Immunol. Methods* **64,** 1–6.
Carlsson, M., Hedin, A., Inganäs, M., Harfast, B., and Blomberg, F. (1985). *J. Immunol. Methods* **79,** 89–98.
Chalon, M., Milne, R., and Vaerman, J.-P. (1979). *Scand. J. Immunol.* **9,** 359–364.
Coe, J. E., P. R. Coe and M. J. Ross. (1981). *Molec. Immunol.* **18,** 1007.
Cohn, E. J., Strong, L. E., Hughes, W. L., Mulford, D. J., Ashworth, J. N., Melin, M., and Taylor, H. L. (1946). *J. Amer. Chem. Soc.* **68,** 459.
Deisenhofer, J. (1981). *Biochemistry* **20,** 2361–2370.
Deisenhofer, J., Jones, T. A., Sjödahl, J., and Sjöquist, J. (1978). *Hoppe-Seylers Z. Physiol. Chem.* **359,** 975–985.
Delacroix, M., Fluckinger, M., and Lebherz, III, W. (1985). *J. Immunol. Methods* **83,** 169–177.
Duhamel, R., Schur, P., Brendel, K., and Meezan, E. (1979). *J. Immunol. Methods* **31,** 211–217.
Duhamel, R., Meezan, E., and Brendel, K. (1980). *Mol. Immunol.* **17,** 29–36.
Escribano, M. J., Haddada, H., and de Vaux Saint Cyr, Ch. (1982). *J. Immunol. Methods* **52,** 63–72.
Ey, P. L., Prowse, S. J., and Jenkin, C. R. (1978). *Immunochemistry* **15,** 429–436.
Fredriksson, U.-B., Fägerstam, L. G., Cole, A. W. G., and Lundgren, T. (1986). *Int. Congr. Immunol. 6th, Toronto, July* 6–11.
Goding, J. W. (1976). *J. Immunol. Methods* **13,** 215–226.
Goding, J. W. (1978). *J. Immunol. Methods* **20,** 241–253.
Goudswaard, J., van der Donk, J. A., Noordzig, A., van Dam, R. H., and Vaerman, J.-P. (1978). *Scand. J. Immunol.* **8,** 21–28.
Grov, A. (1973). *Acta Pathol. Microbiol. Scand. Sect. A* **236,** 77–83.
Hjelm, H., K. Hjelm and J. Sjöquist. (1972). *FEBS Lett.* **28,** 73.
Hjelm, H. (1975). *Scand. J. Immunol.* **4,** 633–640.
Hjelm, H., and Sjöquist, J. (1975). *Scand. J. Immunol.* **4** (Suppl. 3), 51–57.
Kohler, G., and Milstein, C. (1975). *Nature* (*London*) **256,** 495–497.
Kristiansen, T. (1974). *Biochim. Biophys. Acta* **263,** 567.
Kronvall, G. (1973). *J. Immunol* **111,** 1401–1406.
Langone, J. (1982). *J. Immunol. Methods* **55,** 277–296.
Leatherbarrow R. J., Dwerk, R. A. (1983). *FEBS Lett.* **164,** 2.
Lindmark, R., Movitz, J., and Sjöquist, J. (1977). *Eur. J. Biochem.* **74,** 623–628.
McGregor, J. L., Brochier, J., Wild, F., Follea, G., Trzeciak, M.-C., James, E., Dechavanne, M., McGregor, L., and Clemetson, K. J. (1983). *Eur. J. Biochem.* **131,** 427–436.
MacKenzie, M., Warner, N., and Mitchell, G. (1978a). *J. Immunol.* **120,** 1493–1496.
MacKenzie, M., Gutman, G., and Warner, N. (1978b). *Scand. J. Immunol.* **7,** 367–370.
Manil, L., Motté, P., Pernas, P., Troalen, F., Bohuon, C., and Bellet, D. (1986). *J. Immunol. Methods* **90,** 25–37.
Martin, L. N. (1982a). *J. Immunol. Methods* **50,** 319–329.
Martin, L. N. (1982b). *J. Immunol. Methods* **52,** 205–212.
Merwin, R. M., and Redmon, L. W. (1963). *J. Natl. Cancer Inst.* **31,** 997–1017.
Miller, T. J. and H. O. Stone. (1978). *J. Immunol. Methods* **24,** 111.
Milon, A., Houdayer, M., and Metzger, J. (1978). *Dev. Comp. Immunol.* **2,** 699–709.

Chapter 18. Use of Protein A to Purify Immunoglobulins

Morgan, M. R. A., Johnson, P. M., and Dean, P. D. G. (1978). *J. Immunol. Methods* **23,** 381–387.
Nilsson, K., and Mosbach, K. (1984). *In* "Methods in Enzymology" (W. B. Jakoby, ed.), Vol. 104, pp. 56–69. Academic Press, New York.
Nilsson, R., Myher, E., Kronvall, G., and Sjögren, H. O. (1982). *Mol. Immunol.* **19,** 119–126.
Olsvik, O., and Berdal B. P. (1981). *Acta Pathol. Microbiol. Scand. Sect. B* **89,** 289–290.
Ohlson, S., Nilsson, R., Niss, U., Kjellberg, B., and Freiburghaus, C. (1988). *J. Immunol. Methods* **114,** 231–235.
Porath, J., Axén, R., and Ernbach, S. (1967). *Nature (London)* **215,** 1491–1492.
Potter, M., and Boyce, C. R. (1962). *Nature (London)* **193,** 1086–1087.
Ricardo, Jr., M. J., Trouy, R. L., and Grimm, D. T. (1981). *J. Immunol.* **127,** 946–951.
Rousseaux, J., Picque, M. T., Bazin, H., and Biserte, G. (1981). *Mol. Immunol.* **18,** 639–645.
Russo, C., Callegaro, L., Lanza, E., and Ferrone, S. (1983). *J. Immunol. Methods* **65,** 269–271.
Scopes, R. (1982). "Protein Purification: Principles and Practice." Springer-Verlag, New York.
Seppälä, I., Sarvas, H., Peterfy, F., and Mäkelä, O. (1981). *Scand. J. Immunol.* **14,** 337–344.
Sjöquist, J., Meloun, B., and Hjelm, H. (1972). *Eur. J. Biochem.* **29,** 572–578.
Skvaril, F. (1976). *Immunochemistry* **13,** 871–872.
Sundberg, L., and Porath, J. (1974). *J. Chromatogr.* **90,** 87–89.
Tranell, C., Westerlund, K., Magnusson, B., Johansson, H., Mellåker, H., and Svensson, R. (1988). *Int. Symp. HPLC Proteins, Peptides Polynucleotides, 8th, Copenhagen, Oct. 31–Nov 2.*
van Dalen, A., Seijen, H. G., and Gruber, M. (1967). *Biochim. Biophys. Acta* **147,** 421–426.
van Kamp, G. J. (1979). *J. Immunol. Methods* **27,** 301–305.
Vidal, M. A., and Conde, F. P. (1980). *J. Immunol. Methods* **35,** 169–172.
Warr, G. W., and Hart, I. R. (1979). *Am. J. Vet. Res.* **40,** 922–926.
Watanabe, M., Ishii, T., and Nariuchi, H. (1981). *Jpn. J. Exp. Med.* **51,** 65–70.

CHAPTER **19**

Purification and quantitation of monoclonal antibodies by affinity chromatography with immobilized protein A

Susan M. Scott
Hector Juarez-Salinas

I. Purification of IgG$_1$ Monoclonal Antibodies

Due to its affinity for the Fc portion of IgG, *Staphylococcus aureus* protein A has been extensively used in the purification of immunoglobulin molecules (for review see Langone, 1982). However, its application in the purification of monoclonal antibodies was curtailed by the low affinity of protein A for mouse antibodies belonging to the IgG$_1$ subclass. This fact is of considerable importance, since a good portion of the monoclonal antibodies currently available belong to the IgG$_1$ subclass. Even before the discovery of monoclonal antibodies, Kronvall *et al.* (1970) and Grey *et al.* (1971) observed that mouse IgG$_1$ polyclonal antibodies did not bind to protein A. Later, Goding (1976) showed that mouse IgG$_1$ was only retarded when chromatographed on a protein A column. Using slightly alkaline (pH 8.1) buffer conditions, Ey *et al.* (1978) showed that mouse IgG$_1$ was retained on a protein A column. However, the IgG$_1$–protein A capacity observed was too low to be of practical use. The weak binding of mouse IgG$_1$ to protein A was also observed by other investigators (Mackenzie *et al.*, 1979; Chalon *et al.*, 1979; Bywater *et al.*, 1983). The inability of protein A to effectively bind mouse IgG$_1$ has been overcome by the discovery of binding buffer solutions that dramatically increase the capacity of protein A for mouse IgG_1 (Affi-Gel® Protein A, 1984; Juarez-Salinas et al., 1986a; Juarez-Salinas and Ott, 1987). This binding buffer solution has been commercially available from Bio-Rad Laboratories under the trade name of MAPS® buffers since 1984. Over the years, these buffer solutions have found wide application in the isolation of monoclonal antibodies and are now routinely used in this endeavor. The effectiveness of the MAPS binding buffer is best assessed by comparing the performance of protein A chromatography using both a published protocol (Bigbee et al., 1983) and using the MAPS process (Figure 1). Three different IgG_1, one IgG_{2a}, and one IgG_{2b} monoclonal antibodies were purified on protein A columns using either the MAPS buffer or phosphate-buffered saline (PBS), pH 8.2, as binding buffer. It is apparent that the use of the MAPS method produces a several-fold increase in the yield of purified IgG_1 monoclonal antibodies when compared with the yield obtained using PBS as binding buffer. It is also apparent that the yield of IgG_{2b} monoclonal antibodies is also improved by the MAPS process, while the yield of IgG_{2a} antibodies was the same under both conditions.

Figure 2 shows that the monoclonal antibodies purified using the MAPS process are electrophoretically pure. Lane 1 shows the sodium dodecyl sulfate polyacrylamide gel electrophoresis (SDS-PAGE) (Laem-

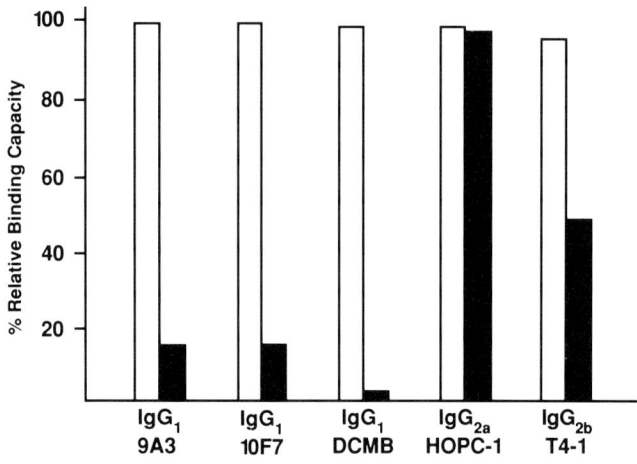

FIGURE 1
Comparison of the relative binding efficiencies of IgG_1, IgG_{2a}, and IgG_{2b} murine monoclonal antibodies to Affi-Gel–protein A (Bio-Rad Laboratories) following the MAPS method (open bars) and a published method (solid bars). Mouse ascites, containing 5 mg of murine monoclonal antibody, were chromatographed in a 1 ml column of Affi-Gel–protein A. (Reproduced from Juarez-Salinas et al., 1986a, with permission.)

Chapter 19. Protein A Monoclonal Antibody Purification

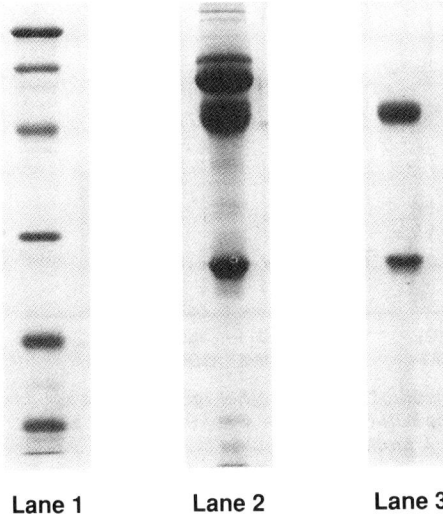

FIGURE 2
Reducing SDS-PAGE of IgG$_1$-containing mouse ascites before and after Affi-Gel–protein A MAPS chromatography. Lane 1, Bio-Rad low molecular weight (LMW) standards; Lane 2, IgG$_1$-containing mouse ascites; Lane 3, Affi-Gel–protein A MAPS-purified IgG$_1$. (Reproduced from Juarez-Salinas *et al.*, 1986a, with permission.)

mli, 1970) profile of low molecular weight protein standards (Bio-Rad Laboratories). Lane 2 shows the SDS-PAGE profile of mouse ascites containing an IgG$_1$ monoclonal antibody before purification; the light (25,000 M_r) and heavy (50,000 M_r) immunoglobulin chains and other contaminant bands (albumin and transferrin) are apparent. Lane 3 shows the SDS-PAGE profile of the protein A-purified IgG pattern; only the light and heavy immunoglobulin chains are present. Thus, the use of the MAPS process increases the protein A capacity without infringing on the quality of purification expected from protein A chromatography.

II. Purification of IgM Monoclonal Antibodies

As in the case of mouse IgG$_1$, IgM binds weakly, if at all, to protein A (Ey *et al.*, 1978; Seppala *et al.*, 1981; Lindmark *et al.*, 1983). Thus, the binding capacity of protein A for mouse IgM was considered to be too low to have practical applications in the purification of mouse IgM monoclonal antibodies. Data obtained in our laboratories indicate that some IgM monoclonal antibodies can be effectively purified by protein A chromatography

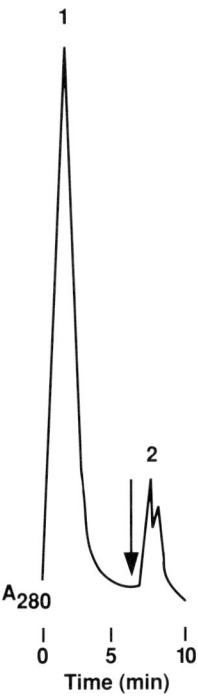

FIGURE 3
Affi-Prep–protein A MAPS (Bio-Rad Laboratories) of mouse ascites containing an IgM monoclonal antibody. Mouse ascites (0.5 ml), containing 4 mg of an IgM monoclonal antibody, were diluted 1:1 with Affi-Prep–protein A MAPS binding buffer and injected into a MAPS preparative HPLC system (Bio-Rad Laboratories) equipped with a 30 × 4.6 mm Affi-Prep–protein A cartridge. Unbound proteins were eluted with binding buffer (peak 1). Immunoglobulins were eluted with Affi-Prep–protein A elution buffer at the time indicated by the arrow (peak 2). Flow rate was 0.5 ml/min. Absorbance was monitored at 180 nm. (Reproduced from Juarez-Salinas *et al.*, 1987, with permission.)

when using the MAPS buffers (Juarez-Salinas *et al.*, 1987). Figure 3 shows the purification of an IgM monoclonal antibody using the MAPS method in a high-performance system. The effect of the MAPS process in increasing the protein A–IgM capacity has been confirmed by Mariani *et al.* (1989a,b). These investigators succeeded in purifying two IgM monoclonal antibodies using protein A in conjunction with the MAPS buffer system, achieving yields greater than 80%.

Chapter 19. Protein A Monoclonal Antibody Purification

III. Quantitation of Monoclonal Antibodies

The availability of the MAPS process has also made it possible to use protein A chromatography for the quantitative determination of monoclonal antibodies (Crowley and Walters, 1982; Hammen *et al.*, 1988). Recently, Duffy *et al.* (1989) were able to generate a linear standard curve by chromatographing increasing amounts of an IgG_1 monoclonal antibody using an Affi-Prep® protein A high-performance cartridge in conjunction with the MAPS buffers. The standard curve was then used to determine the concentration of monoclonal antibodies in unknown samples. Figure 4 shows the chromatographic patterns obtained with different IgG_1 concentrations. The area under the eluted peak was then plotted against concentration to obtain the standard curve, as shown in Figure 5.

This technique proved to be faster and more accurate than enzyme-linked immunosorbent assays (ELISA). The amount of antibody quantitated by ELISA is usually overstated, since this method detects free light

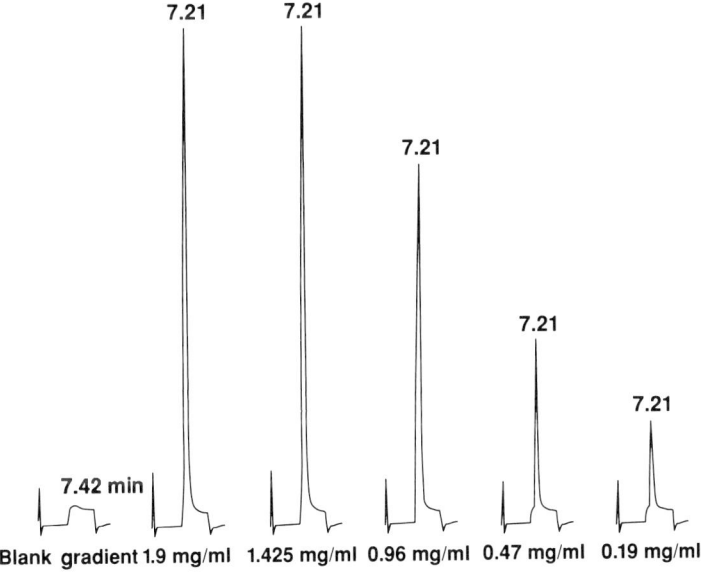

FIGURE 4
Affi-Prep–protein A (30 × 4.6 mm HPLC cartridge) chromatograms of various amounts of purified IgG_1. The peak heights are directly proportional to the injected amounts of IgG_1. The small peak at the left of each trace is the injection spike. The retention time (in min) is given for each peak. (Reproduced from Duffy *et al.*, 1989, with permission.)

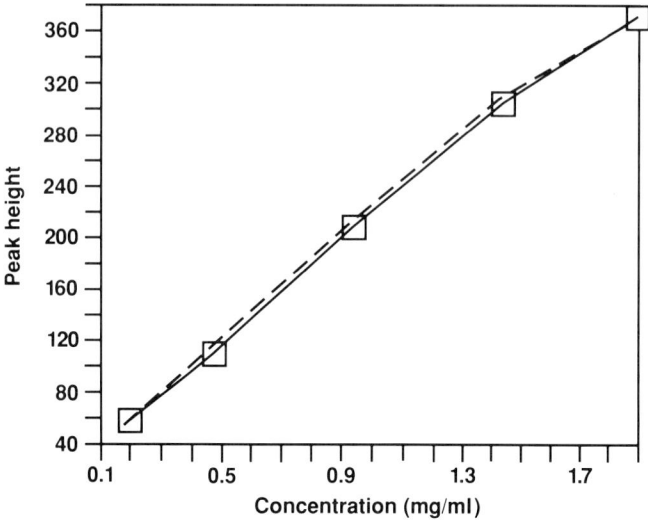

FIGURE 5
Standard curve generated from data obtained by injecting known amounts of purified IgG_1 into an Affi-Prep–protein A HPLC cartridge (see Figure 4). Standards were run in both PBS (---) and 5% fetal bovine serum (—). The correlation coefficients (r^2) for the two curves are similar ($r^2 = 0.998$ for PBS; $r^2 = 0.996$ for 5% fetal bovine serum); the interference from serum components is apparently minimal (Reproduced from Duffy *et al.*, 1989, with permission.)

chains as well as the intact antibody, while protein A chromatography detects only the intact antibody. With the use of currently available high-performance liquid chromatography (HPLC) systems and automatic sample injectors, the method can be automated for the operator-free analysis of many samples per day. Other investigators have shown that extremely low amounts of antibody (0.25–250 μg) can be quantitated by protein A high-performance chromatography when binding and elution buffers with a low absorbance at 280 and 220 nm are used (Compton *et al.*, 1989).

IV. Purification of Injectable-Grade Monoclonal Antibodies

A. Resistance of Protein A to Treatment with 1 *N* NaOH

Many monoclonal antibodies have been developed for therapeutic applications. Often, these applications require that the purification of the antibody be performed under pyrogen-free conditions. One of the preferred methods for achieving these conditions is the treatment of the chromatographic supports with 1 N NaOH (Berglof et al., 1988). Recently, Bio-Rad Laboratories introduced a new polymer-based protein A support that complies with this requirement (Bio-Radiations 70, 1988) Affi-Prep–protein A support. Figure 6, panel A, shows the IgG_1 protein A chromatographic pattern under maximal binding conditions. In panel B, the same experiment was performed after the column was subjected to four chromatographic cycles. Each cycle included a wash with 30 ml (60 bed volumes) of 1 N NaOH. At the end of the four chromatographic cycles, the cartridge was washed with 240 bed volumes of 1 N NaOH. It can be observed that the chromatographic pattern was not changed by the NaOH treatment,

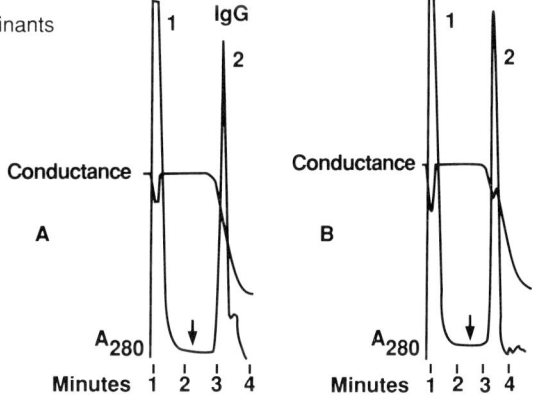

FIGURE 6
Panels A and B show the Affi-Prep–protein A (30 × 4.6 mm) pattern of mouse ascites containing an IgG_1 monoclonal antibody before and after four washing cycles with 1 N NaOH. Each washing cycle consisted of 15 ml of water, 30 ml of 1 N NaOH, 15 ml of Affi-Prep–protein A MAPS binding buffer. At the end of each 1 N NaOH washing cycle, chromatography of 0.8 ml of mouse ascites was performed under the same conditions used before the cartridge was washed with 1 N NaOH. Mouse ascites (0.8 ml) were diluted 1:1 with Affi-Prep–protein A MAPS binding buffer before application. Flow rate was 0.5 ml/min. After sample application, the cartridge was washed with MAPS binding buffer until the base line was stabilized. Elution was started at the time indicated by the arrow using Affi-Prep–protein A MAPS elution buffer (Reproduced from Bio-Radiations 70, 1988, with permission.)

indicating that the protein A capacity is not affected by these conditions. The ability of Affi-Prep–protein A to withstand this treatment removes an important obstacle for the use of protein A chromatography in the purification of injectable-grade monoclonal antibodies.

B. The Role of Protein A Chromatography in Multistep Purification Protocols

Regardless of the method used, the purification of injectable-grade monoclonal antibodies usually requires a multistep procedure. Several current publications dealing with this issue use protein A chromatography in combination with other chromatographic steps such as ion-exchange chromatography (Duffy *et al.*, 1989; Bio-Radiations 70, 1988) or hydroxylapatite chromatography (Juarez-Salinas *et al.*, 1984, 1986b; Stanker *et al.*, 1985; Mariani *et al.*, 1989a; Zola and Neoh, 1989).

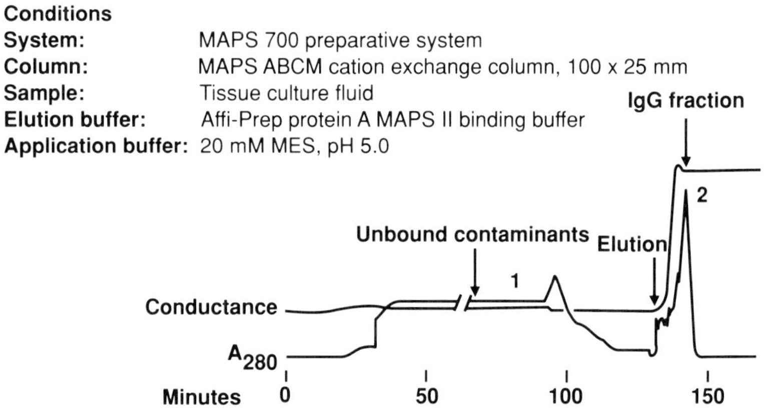

Conditions
System: MAPS 700 preparative system
Column: MAPS ABCM cation exchange column, 100 x 25 mm
Sample: Tissue culture fluid
Elution buffer: Affi-Prep protein A MAPS II binding buffer
Application buffer: 20 mM MES, pH 5.0

FIGURE 7
Tissue culture fluid (250 ml) containing a mouse IgG_1 monoclonal antibody was titrated to pH 5.0 with 1 M 2-(N-morpholino) ethanesulfonic acid (MES) buffer, pH 3.5. The sample was then diluted 1:1 with deionized water and prepared for chromatography by filtration through a 0.2 μm filter. The sample was then chromatographed in a 1 N NaOH-sanitized, MAPS preparative system equipped with a 100 × 25 mm preparative MAPS ABCM column, previously equilibrated with 20 mM MES buffer, pH 5.0 (application buffer). Sample application flow rate was 4 ml/min. The absorbance at 280 nm (A_{280}) was monitored at 0.16 AUFS (Absorbance Units Full Scale). After sample application, the column was washed with application buffer until the A_{280} approached zero. The bound material containing the monoclonal antibody was eluted at the time indicated by the arrow with Affi-Prep–protein A MAPS binding buffer. A_{280} was monitored at 1.28 AUFS during elution. (Reproduced from Bio-Radiations 70, 1988, with permission.)

A typical purification of 350 mg of an IgG_1 monoclonal antibody from culture medium using high-performance, cation-exchange chromatography (MAPS ABCM high-performance preparative column, Bio-Rad Laboratories), followed by protein A chromatography on an Affi-Prep–protein A, preparative, high-performance column is presented in Figures 7 and 8, respectively. Since the concentration of monoclonal antibodies in culture medium is usually extremely low, the first step with cation-exchange chromatography is used to achieve concentration and partial purification. Another advantage of this step is that it efficiently removes phenol red, DNA, and most of the unbound endotoxin contaminants. Although most antibodies will require acidic binding conditions (pH 5–6), some will bind

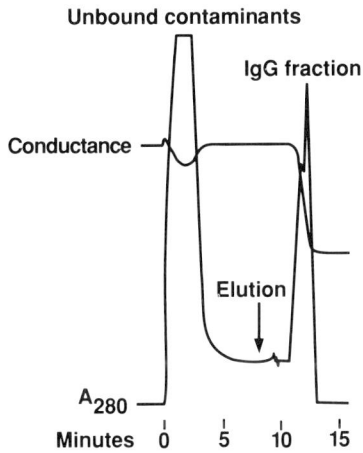

FIGURE 8
The material eluted form the MAPS ABCM column (Figure 7) was chromatographed in a sanitized MAPS preparative system equipped with a 100 × 25 mm, preparative Affi-Prep–protein A column. Sample application flow rate was 4 ml/min. The A_{280} was monitored at 1.28 AUFS. After sample application, the column was washed with Affi-Prep–protein A MAPS binding buffer until the base line was stabilized. The IgG was then eluted with Affi-Prep–protein A MAPS elution buffer. (Reproduced from Bio-Radiations 70, 1988, with permission.)

well at neutral pH. The antibody is then eluted with MAPS binding buffer, taking advantage of the high salt, high pH conditions of this buffer. The partially purified antibody is then directly applied to the protein A column to achieve complete purification (Figure 8).

The culture medium used for hybridoma growth frequently needs to be supplemented with fetal calf serum. This serum usually contains variable amounts of bovine IgG. The separation of monoclonal antibodies from bovine IgG has been successfully achieved by the combination of protein A and hydroxylapatite chromatography (Juarez-Salinas et al., 1986a). Figure 9 shows the hydroxylapatite (Bio-Gel® high performance hydroxylapatite (HPHT), Bio-Rad Laboratories) chromatographic pattern of a protein A-purified IgG containing a human monoclonal antibody and bovine serum IgG. The bulk of the bovine IgG elutes as a broad peak (peak 1), preceeding the elution of the monoclonal antibody, which is seen as the narrower peak (peak 2). The identity of the peaks was confirmed by performing an activity assay on each of the peaks (data not shown). Thus, most of the bovine IgG was separated from the monoclonal antibody.

The combination of protein A and hydroxylapatite chromatography has also proven useful in the purification of light and heavy chain monoclo-

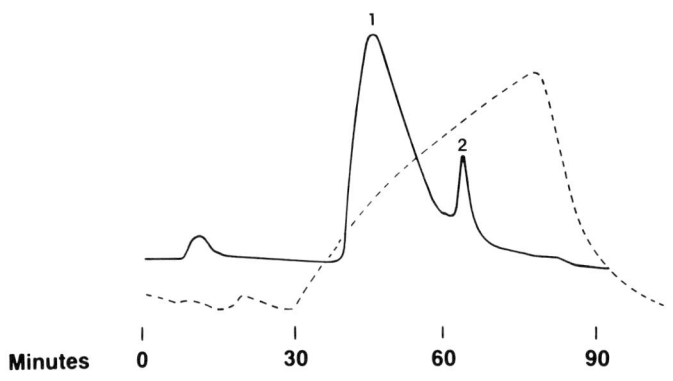

FIGURE 9
HPHT profile of Protein A-purified fetal calf serum supplemented (10%) tissue culture medium containing a human IgG monoclonal antibody. Peak 1 represents the fetal calf serum IgG; peak 2 is the monoclonal antibody. After Protein A purification, the sample was extensively dialyzed against 10 mM sodium phosphate, pH 6.8, and injected into a Bio-Gel HPHT column (7.8 × 100 mm analytical column and a 7.8 × 30 mm guard column; Bio-Rad). After sample application, the column was washed with 10 ml of buffer A (10 mM sodium phosphate, pH 6.8). IgG was eluted with 30 min gradient from buffer A to buffer B (300 mM sodium phosphate, pH 6.8). Flow rate was 1 ml/min. (———) A_{280}; (----) conductivity.

nal antibody variants. These situations arise when the myeloma cell line used to generate the hybridoma is a light-chain producer or when two hybridomas are fused to produce a quadroma or tetradoma cell line.

Figure 10 shows the hydroxylapatite chromatography of a protein A-purified monoclonal antibody preparation derived from a hybridoma cell line that produced two different light chains (Juarez-Salinas et al., 1984, 1986b, 1987). Three peaks were separated; peak 1 was inactive and contained two inactive light chains; peak 2 showed moderate activity and was a hybrid with one of the antibody arms containing the active light chain and the other arm the inactive light chain; peak 3 was the most active and both arms contained the correct light chain.

Quadroma cell lines are generated with the purpose of producing bispecific monoclonal antibodies. With 2 different heavy and light chains in the same cell, 16 different combinations are possible if random chain

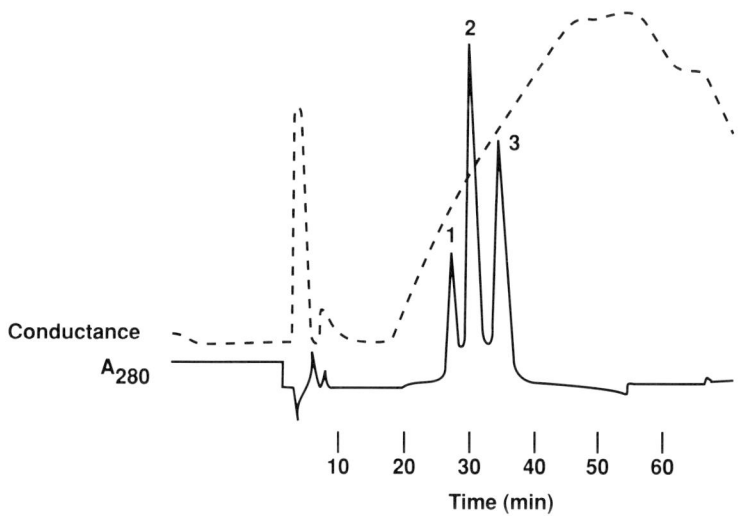

FIGURE 10
High-performance hydroxylapatite (HPHT) chromatography of protein A-purified IgG_1 (H-1) monoclonal antibody. Protein A-purified IgG was dialyzed against 10 mM sodium phosphate buffer, pH 6.8 (buffer A). Two milliliters of dialysate containing 2 mg pure H-1 IgG was filtered through a 0.22 μm membrane filter prior to chromatography. HPHT chromatography was performed in a MAPS preparative system equipped with a Bio-Gel HPHT column set (7.8 × 100 mm analytical column and a 7.8 × 30 mm guard column, Bio-Rad Laboratories). After sample application, the column was washed with a 30 min gradient from 10 mM sodium phosphate, pH 6.8, to 300 mM sodium phosphate, pH 6.8 (buffer B). Flow rate was 1 ml/min. (———) Absorbance at 280 nm; (----) conductance. (Reproduced from Juarez-Salinas et al., 1986b, with permission.)

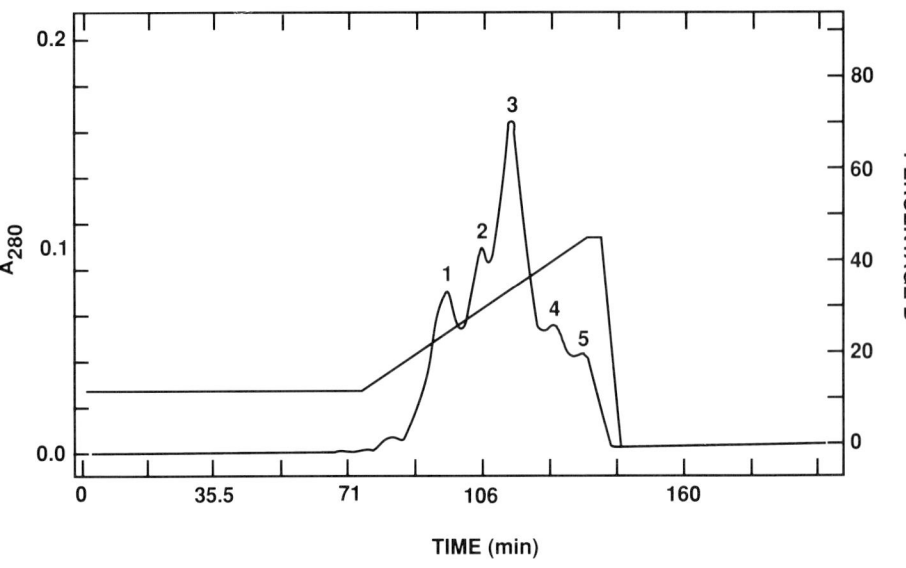

FIGURE 11
High-performance hydroxylapatite (HPHT) chromatography of bispecific monoclonal antibody AB8.28 × Ep2 after affinity chromatography purification on an Affi-Prep–protein A column. Peak 3 contains the active bispecific antibody, while peaks 1 and 5 contain the two parental antibodies. Peaks 2 and 4 represent different inactive rearrangements of the parental heavy and light chains. Chromatographic conditions were as in Figure 9. (Reproduced from Mariani et al., 1989, with permission.)

association is assumed (Suresh et al., 1986). Only a fraction of the total number of species will have the required bispecificity. Figure 11 shows the hydroxylapatite chromatography of protein A-purified quadroma IgG (Mariani et al., 1989). Five peaks are apparent; peak 3 contained the active bispecific antibody, while the others represented different inactive arrangements of the parental heavy and light antibody chains.

V. Conclusions

Due to the availability of optimized buffer solutions (MAPS buffers) to increase the affinity of protein A for the mouse IgG_1 subclass, the purification of monoclonal antibodies by affinity chromatography with protein A is now a well established procedure. A growing body of information indicates that the MAPS buffers also promote the binding of mouse IgM monoclonal antibodies to protein A. The ability of protein A to withstand treatment with 1 N NaOH without losing its activity increases the attraction of protein A for use as an alternate procedure in the purification of monoclonal antibodies under sanitized conditions. Finally, protein A chromatography is carving a permanent niche in the multistep protocols designed for the purification of injectable-grade monoclonal antibodies. Particularly noteworthy is the combination of protein A and hydroxylapatite chromatography to separate active monoclonal antibodies from inactive light and heavy chain variants and bovine IgG.

Acknowledgments

We would like to acknowledge Dr. Ann Stevens, Bio-Rad Laboratories, for her critical review of this manuscript.

References

Affi-Gel Protein A (1984). Technical Bulletin. Bio-Rad Laboratories, Richmond, California 94806.
Bigbee, W. L., Vanderlaan, M., Fong, S. S. N., and Jensen, R. H. (1983). *Mol. Immunol.* **20,** 1353–1359.
Bio-Radiations 70 (1988). Bio-Rad Laboratories, Richmond, California.
Bywater, R., Erikson, G.-B., and Attosoon, T. *et al.* (1983) *J. Immunol. Methods* **64,** 1–6.
Cassone, A., Torosantucci, A., Boccanera, M., Cianfriglia, M., and Mariani, M. (1988). *J. Med. Microbiol.* **27,** 233–238.
Chalon, M. P., Milne, R. W., and Vaerman, J. P. (1979). *Scand. J. Immunol.* **9,** 359–364.
Compton, B. J., Lewis, M., Whigham, F., Gerald, J. S., and Countryman, G. E. (1989). *Anal. Chem.* **61,** 1314–1317.
Crowley, S. C., and Walters, R. R. (1982). *J. Chromatogr.* **266,** 157–163.
Duffy, S. A., Moellering, B. J., Prior, G. M., Doyle, K. R., and Prior, C. P. (1989). *BioPharmacology* 35–47.
Ey, P. L., Prowse, S. J., and Jenkin, C. R. (1978). *Immunochemistry* **15,** 429–436.
Goding, J. S. (1976). *Aust. Soc. Immunol. Proc.* p. 15 (Abstr.).
Grey, H. M., Hirst, J. W., and Cohn, M. (1971). *J. Exp. Med.* **133,** 289–304.
Hammen, R. F., Pang, D., Remington, K., Thompson, H., Judd, R. D., and Szuba, J. (1988). *J. Biochromatogr.* **3,** 54–61.
Juarez-Salinas, H., and Ott, G. S. (1987). United States Patent No. 4,704,366.
Juarez-Salinas, H., Engelhorn, S., Lowry, M. A., Bigbee, W. L., and Stanker, L. H. (1984). *Biotechniques* **2,** 164–169.
Juarez-Salinas, H., Bigbee, W. L., LaMotte, G. B., III, and Ott, G. S. (1986a). *Am. Biotech. Lab.* **March/April.**
Juarez-Salinas, H., Ott, G. S., Chen, J. C., Brooks, T. L., and Stanker, L. H. (1986b). *In* "Methods in Enzymology" (J. J. Langone and H. van Vunakis, eds.), Vol. 121, pp. 615–622. Academic Press, Orlando, Florida.
Juarez-Salinas, H., Brooks, T. L., Ott, G. S., Peters, R. E., and Stanker, L. (1987). *In*

"Commercial Production of Monoclonal Antibodies" (S. S. Seaver, ed.), Vol. 12, pp. 217–245. Dekker, New York.
Kronvall, G., Grey, H. M., and Williams, Jr., R. C. (1970). *J. Immunol.* **105,** 1116–1130.
Laemmli, U. K. (1970). *Nature (London)* **227,** 680–685.
Langone, J. J. (1982). *J. Immunol. Methods* **55,** 277–296.
Lindmark, R., Thoren-Tolling, K., and Sjöquist, S. (1983). *J. Immunol. Methods* **62,** 1–13.
Mackenzie, M. P., Warner, N. L., and Mitchell, G. F. (1979). *J. Immunol.* **120,** 1493–1496.
Malavasi, F., De Monte, L. B., Nistico, R., Tecce, P., Dellabona, P., Reyna, A., Natali, P. G., and Mariani, M. (1988). *Eur. Immunol. Meet. Satellite Symp. Immunol. Biotechnol., 9th,* in press.
Mariani, M., Cianfriglia, M., and Cassone, A. (1989a). *Immunol. Today* **10,** 115–116.
Mariani, M., Bonelli, F., Tarditi, L., Calogero, R., Camagna, M., Spranzi, E., Seccamani, E., Deleide, G., and Scassellati, G. A. (1989b). *BioChromatography* **4,** 149–155.
Seppala, I., Sarvas, H., Peterfy, F., and Makela, O. (1981). *Scand. J. Immunol.* **14,** 335–342.
Stanker, L. H., Vanderlaan, M., and Juarez-Salinas, H. (1985). *J. Immunol. Methods* **76,** 157–169.
Zola, H., and Neoh, S.-H. (1989). *BioTechniques* 781–808.

CHAPTER **20**

Use of immobilized protein G to isolate IgG

Barbara Webb Walker

I. Introduction

The two bacterial IgG-binding proteins, protein G, a cell wall component from strains of *Streptococcus,* and protein A, a cell wall component of *Staphylococcus aureus* strains, have both been used as affinity ligands for purifying mammalian immunoglobulins from serum, mouse ascites fluid, and hybridoma tissue culture medium. Protein A was the first bacterial immunoglobulin-binding protein identified and isolated (Forsgren and Sjöquist, 1967). It has subsequently been used as a general purpose immunochemical reagent, not only for affinity chromatography, but also for immunoprecipitation and antibody localization in immunoassays such as enzyme-linked immunosorbent assays (ELISA) and Western blots (Goding, 1978; Langone, 1982). As researchers have used protein A, they have identified a number of limitations in its IgG-binding properties. For example, its affinity for immunoglobulins from goats and sheep, two animals that are often used for preparing large quantities of specific antibodies, is so low and subclass specific that it is not a useful reagent for binding IgG from these species (Åkerström *et al.*, 1985; Björck and Kronvall, 1984). It has also been shown that protein A binds poorly to the mouse subclass IgG_1 and to all subclasses of rat IgG (Åkerström *et al.*, 1985; Ohlson *et al.*, 1988). The binding of mouse IgG_1 can be improved by the use of high ionic strength alkaline buffers, but it has been suggested that these buffers increase the risk of nonspecific, hydrophobic adsorption. This leads to a lower degree of purity for the isolated immunoglobulin (Ohlson *et al.*, 1988).

While the majority of monoclonal antibodies that have been described are from mouse hybridomas, rat hybridomas have been reported to have certain advantageous characteristics (Clark *et al.*, 1983; Campbell, 1984). For example, the reversion rate of parental cell lines to nonsecreting lines is lower for rat hybridomas than it is for mouse hybridomas. Rats are also larger and therefore yield larger quantities of ascites per animal. The low affinity of protein A for most rat monoclonals, which makes it an unsuitable reagent for purification of these antibodies, has been cited as a disadvantage of the rat hybridoma system. However, the availability of immobilized protein G, which does bind rat subclasses, should easily overcome any difficulties in purifying rat monoclonals.

The streptococcal IgG-binding protein, referred to as protein G was isolated in 1984 (Reis *et al.*, 1984; Björck and Kronvall, 1984) and the gene was cloned and expressed in *Escherichia coli* shortly thereafter (Fahnestock *et al.*, 1986; Guss *et al.*, 1986; Björck and Blomberg, 1987). Like protein A, protein G binds to antibodies by a mechanism that does not involve the antigen-binding site of IgG. However the binding spectrum of protein G differs from that of protein A in several important respects. Protein G only binds to IgG subclasses, while protein A crossreacts with some IgM, IgA, and IgE antibodies. Protein G also binds well to polyclonal antibodies from goats, sheep, horses, and cattle, as well as mouse and rat monoclonals (Åkerström *et al.*, 1985; Åkerström and Björck, 1986). Protein G and protein A perform equally well in applications that involve IgG from human and rabbit IgGs, making protein G an excellent, general purpose affinity ligand for binding mammalian IgG.

The purification of proteins by affinity chromatography is based on the ability of a specific ligand to interact with its respective binding substance, in this case a protein. The ligand must be chemically immobilized on a support matrix in such a way that the specific binding affinity of the ligand for its binding substrate is retained. Complex mixtures of proteins containing the interacting protein are applied to the immobilized ligand under conditions that allow maximum interaction of the protein with the ligand. After any noninteracting proteins are washed from the matrix, the interacting protein is eluted by adjusting the washing conditions so that the affinity of the ligand for the bound protein is decreased. Two types of affinity chromatography have been used to purify immunoglobulins: (i) specific affinity, in which the ligand is an antigen and the interacting protein is an antibody that recognizes the antigen, and (ii) general affinity, in which the ligand is an IgG-binding protein such as protein G and the interacting protein is an immunoglobulin. Specific affinity chromatography yields a purified preparation of immunoglobulins that recognize only a specific antigen, whereas general affinity yields all of the IgG immunoglobulins in a particular preparation. General affinity chromatography is often the only method available when the antigen to which a particular antibody binds is unavailable in pure form or is available only in small quantities.

II. Determination of Optimal Conditions for Protein G Affinity Chromatography

Recombinant protein G variants, immobilized on a variety of support matrices including agarose, silica, and membranes, are available from several commercial sources. The choice of affinity resin depends on the particular application, as well as on the particular equipment and experimental preferences of the researcher. If the researcher has access to a high-performance liquid chromatography (HPLC) system, he may choose to use protein G immobilized on silica and packed into stainless steel columns. Excellent results can also be obtained with protein G immobilized on agarose, packed in a disposable column, and run with gravity flow.

Regardless of the type of chromatography system used, several variables should be considered when setting up a particular chromatographic procedure to insure that optimal recoveries, as well as high levels of purity are achieved. These include the source of the IgG and the concentration of the IgG in the sample. The maximal binding capacities of protein G agarose vary considerably for different animal species. For example, a 1 ml column of GammaBind®G agarose will bind 20 mg of human IgG, but only 7 mg of mouse polyclonal IgG. The concentration of IgG in sera of different animal species varies considerably, and animal-to-animal variations can be significant as well. Therefore, it is useful to determine the amount of IgG in a particular sample by chromatographing a small sample of the serum, ascites fluid, or tissue culture medium on an analytical GammaBind®G column.

When establishing protocols, it is important to understand the method used by a particular vendor to determine the binding capacity of the particular protein G matrix used. For example, Genex (Gaithersburg, Maryland) determines the maximal binding capacity of its products using conditions where the antibody is applied in at least two-fold excess over the concentration of protein G available for binding.

In setting up an efficient purification procedure, it is necessary to determine the breakthrough binding capacity of the protein G matrix being used with the sample to be purified. The breakthrough binding capacity is defined as the amount of IgG that is bound when the amount of antibody appearing in the column effluent reaches a given level, typically 10–20% of the amount in the starting sample. In the final protocol, the amount of antibody loaded onto the column should not exceed this binding capacity, to insure that the column is not overloaded and a significant fraction of the antibody lost. For GammaBind®G agarose, this can vary between 25 to 70% of the maximal binding capacity, depending upon both the binding affinity of protein G for the particular antibody being purified and the flow rate used to load the sample. Severely underloading the column matrix can result in precious antibody samples being lost on the column due to the antibodies being irreversibly adsorbed to the matrix or being diluted so that they are not detectable.

Another important variable to consider is the flow rate at which the sample is loaded onto the column. Even though the experimental conditions used when loading do not allow a true equilibrium to be reached, the amount of protein G antibody complexes formed is dependent on the local concentration of the two reactants, as well as on the association and dissociation rates of the binding reaction. Since one of the reactants is immobilized, it is important to consider the time that the interacting protein is actually resident in the column matrix when determining flow rates. If the antibody to be purified is extremely valuable, and only small quantities are available, it is best to use a small column and load at a slow flow rate. In other situations, where the time for processing is important, such as in an industrial process, using faster flow rates may be preferable even though some of the antibody may remain in the flow-through. This flow-through can always be passed through the column again so that the antibody is recovered in a second pass. It should also be kept in mind that flow rates are most accurately expressed as volume per cross-sectional area per hour. This allows direct conversion of the chromatographic conditions as the size of the column is increased or decreased, in order to accommodate the quantity of antibody that is to be isolated.

A. Sample Preparation

Some serum and ascites samples contain significant amounts of lipids that can clog columns and cloud samples. In some cases the lipid can be removed easily by centrifuging the sample at 12,000 rpm for 20 min in a Sorvall SS-34 rotor or the equivalent. The lipid will form a visible layer on top of the sample, allowing the sample to be carefully pipetted from under the lipid. Neoh *et al.* (1986) have described a method for delipidating ascites fluid using silicon dioxide powder, which can be used with serum samples as well. The sample can also be passed through a gel filtration column such that the IgG elutes in the void volume. Alternatively, the lipid can be removed by extraction with organic solvents such as 1,1,2-trichloro-trifluoroethane, which is sold under the tradename of Lipi-Free™ (Genex Corporation, Gaitherburg, Maryland) or with butanol and ether, as described by Hardy (1986). Following the lipid removal step, the sample should be diluted 1:1 with loading buffer, then filtered through a low protein-binding, 0.45 μm membrane to remove any small particulate matter. Regardless of the type of column and matrix used, careful sample preparation will both extend the life of the column and help avoid clogging.

III. Examples of Affinity Chromatography Using Protein G Agarose

Materials and Methods: Whole goat serum was purchased from Pel Freeze (Rogers, Arkansas). Lyophilized mouse ascites fluid was purchased from Organon Tekhnika Corporation (Durham, North Carolina). The mouse hybridoma cell line DA4-4 (No. HB57) was obtained from the American Type Culture Collection (ATCC) in Rockville, Maryland and grown in RPMI 1640 medium containing 10% fetal calf serum (Whittaker Bioproducts, Walkersville, Maryland), according to ATCC recommended procedures. The DA4-4 cells were weaned to medium containing 0.5% fetal calf serum and 1% Nutridoma (Boehringer Mannheim, Indianapolis, Indiana), according to the manufacturer's instructions.

GammaBind®G agarose, GammaBind®G Plus agarose (Genex Corporation, Gaithersburg, Maryland), or Protein A Fast Flow Agarose (Pharmacia, Piscataway, New Jersey) were packed into glass columns with medium pressure fittings so that they could be used on a Waters HPLC system (Bedford, Massachusetts) or on the Genex System 100 affinity chromatography system. Samples were loaded onto protein G columns in PBS, 10 mM sodium phosphate, 150 mM sodium chloride at pH 7.0, or in 100 mM sodium acetate, 100 mM sodium chloride, pH 5.0. The column was washed with the loading buffer until the absorbance of the effluent at 280 nm returned to background. Antibodies were eluted with 0.5 M acetic acid adjusted to pH 3.0 with ammonium hydroxide. The solution containing the eluted IgG was neutralized immediately by adding 0.4–0.5 volumes of 1.0 M Tris base to the antibody fractions. The addition of Tris was monitored using pH indicator sticks (EM Sciences, Cherry Hill, New Jersey), to ensure that the pH was adjusted to between 5.5 and 7.0. The antibody was dialyzed or concentrated, as needed. The protein G–agarose column was cleaned with 1.0 M acetic acid to remove any remaining protein before a new sample was loaded.

A. Isolation of IgG from Goat Serum

Goat serum was centrifuged at 12,000 × g for 20 min to clarify and remove the lipids. The serum was diluted 1:1 with either PBS, pH 7.0, for the sample loaded on GammaBind®G agarose or 100 mM sodium phosphate, pH 7.0, for the sample loaded on Protein A Sepharose Fast Flow, immediately before it was applied to the column. The buffer conditions used were those suggested by the respective manufacturers. Scans at 280 nm, showing the purification of IgG from 0.25 ml of diluted serum on 0.5 ml columns of each matrix, are shown in Figure 1 (A, B). The protein G column bound 3.8 mg of IgG from the goat serum, while the protein A

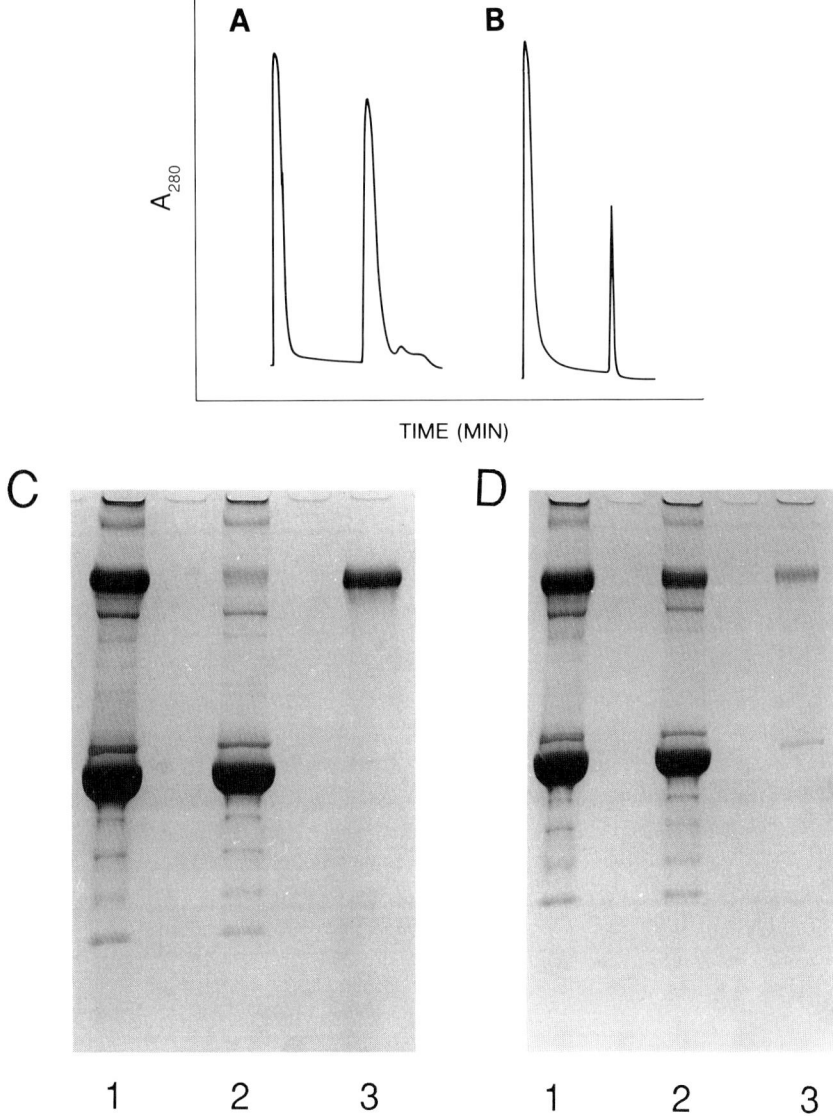

FIGURE 1
Comparison of the purification of goat IgG on GammaBind®G and protein A Fast Flow agarose. Goat serum (250 μl), diluted 1:1 with sample buffer, was chromatographed on a 0.5 ml column of either GammaBind®G agarose or protein A–agarose Fast Flow at a flow rate of 0.5 ml per minute. (A) Trace of the A_{280} scan of the GammaBind®G column chromatography. (B) trace of the A_{280} scan of the protein A Fast Flow column. The scale of the tracings is 0 to 1.5 A_{280} units. Nonreducing SDS–PAGE (polyacrylamide gel electrophoresis) of the proteins in the sample loaded onto the column (lane 1), the flow-through sample (lane 2), and the pH 3.0 eluted sample (lane 3) from the GammaBind®G agarose column (C) and the protein A–agarose column (D).

column bound only 0.41 mg. The proteins in both the load flow-through and the eluted fractions were analyzed on 8–16% nonreducing sodium dodecyl sulfate (SDS) polyacrylamide gels (Novex, Encinitas, California). These results, shown in Figure 1 (C, D) clearly demonstrate that protein G binds significantly more goat IgG in a single chromatographic step. Similar results are obtained when using GammaBind®G to purify IgG from sheep, horse, and bovine sera.

B. Isolation of DA4-4, a Mouse IgG$_1$, from Hybridoma Tissue Culture Medium

An example of the isolation of a mouse monoclonal antibody from hybridoma tissue culture supernatant is shown in Figure 2. DA4-4, an IgG$_1$ mouse monoclonal to human IgM (Maruyama *et al.*, 1985), was grown in RPMI 1640 according to the procedures suggested by the ATCC. The hybridoma supernatant was adjusted to pH 5.0 with 3.5 M acetic acid, then filtered through a 0.45 μm filter to remove the fine precipitate that had formed. The supernatant was supplemented with 50 ml of 100 mM sodium acetate, 100 mM sodium chloride at pH 5.0, before it was loaded onto a column of GammaBind®G Plus agarose (gel bed dimensions 10 × 15 mm) at a flow rate of 1.0 ml/hr. The chromatography was done using the standard method program of the Genex System 100, a dedicated affinity chromatography system. Five milligrams of IgG were recovered from 144 ml of undiluted hybridoma supernatant in a final volume of 20 ml, which represents a seven-fold increase in concentration of the IgG compared to the hybridoma supernatant. The fetal calf serum used in the culture medium was determined to contain 81 μg of IgG per ml of serum by chromatographing 1 ml of the serum on GammaBind®G agarose. Since the medium contained 0.5% fetal calf serum, the purified monoclonal antibody contained no more than 1.3% fetal bovine IgG.

C. Comparison of the Purification of MOPC 21, a Mouse IgG$_1$ Monoclonal Antibody, when Loaded at pH 7.0 and at pH 5.0

Results at Genex have shown that the maximal binding capacity of GammaBind®G for certain mouse monoclonals is increased if the sample is loaded at pH 5.0 instead of pH 7.0. This result was predicted by the binding studies of Åkerström and Björck (1986), which showed that the binding of nonrecombinant protein G is dependent on pH. A comparison of the chromatography of the mouse monoclonal MOPC 21 on GammaBind®G agarose when loading the sample in PBS, pH 7.0, or in 100 mM sodium

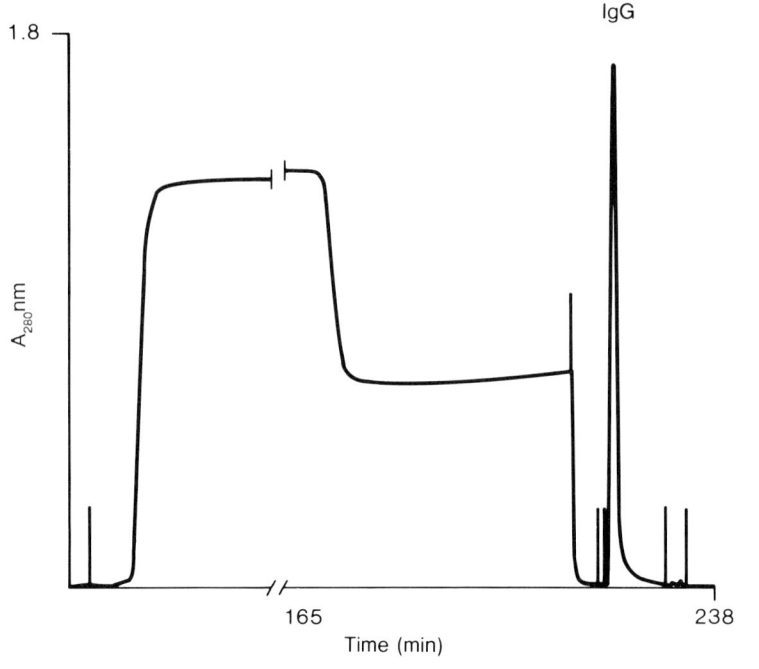

FIGURE 2
Isolation of DA4-4 mouse IgG_1 monoclonal antibody from hybridoma tissue culture supernatant. The tissue culture supernatant was adjusted to pH 5.0 with 3.5 M acetic acid, filtered through a 0.45 μm membrane and supplemented with 50 ml of 100 mM sodium acetate, 100 mM sodium chloride before it was loaded onto a GammaBind®G Plus agarose column (bed dimension 10 × 15 mm, flow rate 1 ml/min). (The last 50 ml loaded was diluted 1:1 with loading buffer, which halved the absorbance of the flow-through material.) Above, trace of the A_{280} scan.

acetate, 100 mM sodium chloride, pH 5.0, is shown in Figure 3. Not only is the amount of recovered MOPC 21 increased by 35% when the sample is loaded at pH 5.0, the elution of IgG is retarded for 1.7 min, suggesting that the binding is stronger at the lower pH. It should be noted that lowering the pH of ascites fluid and tissue culture supernatant can result in the formation of a fine precipitate, which must be removed before the sample is loaded on the column. Results with several different monoclonals have suggested that binding can be increased by adjusting the pH of the sample to 5 before it is applied to the column. Lowering the pH does not significantly effect the binding capacity of Protein G for human, rabbit, or goat IgG.

Chapter 20. IgG Purification Using Protein G

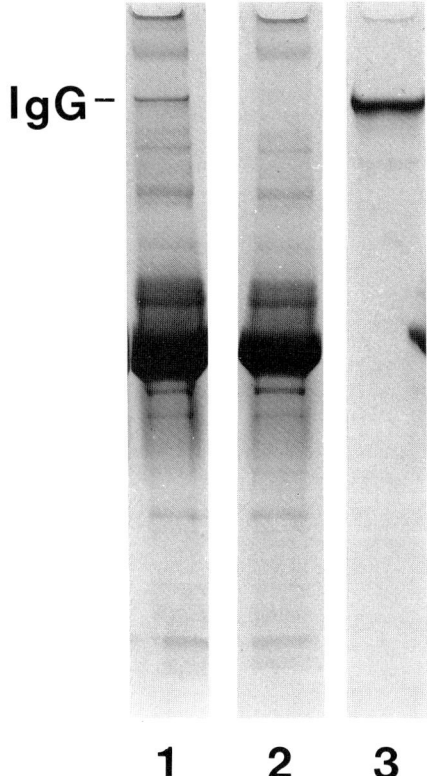

FIGURE 2 *Continued*
Nonreducing SDS–PAGE of the proteins in the supernatant (lane 1), in the flow-through fractions (lane 2), and the eluted IgG (lane 3).

IV. Use of Protein G Agarose to Make an Antigen-Binding Column

Since the binding of protein G to IgG does not interfere with its antigen-binding site, it is possible to use protein G immobilized on agarose as the starting matrix for producing antigen-binding columns, using the methods described by Schneider *et al.* (1982) for Protein A agarose. These methods have been used to make an antibody column for isolating lysozyme using the mouse monoclonal HyHEL-5, an anti-hen egg white lysozyme antibody. Three milligrams of purified HyHEL-5, at a concentration of 1.0 mg/ml, were mixed with 1.0 ml of GammaBind®G agarose, which had

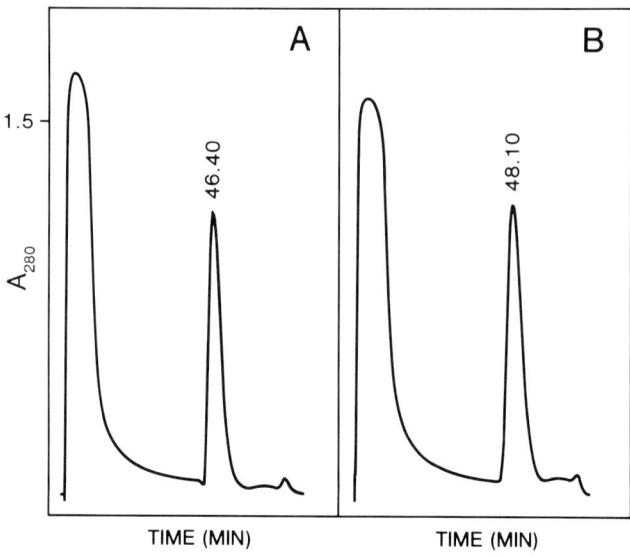

FIGURE 3
Isolation of MOPC 21 IgG$_1$ from mouse ascites fluid. (A) 1 ml of ascites was diluted with PBS, pH 7.0, and loaded onto a 1.0 ml GammaBind®G agarose column at a flow rate of 0.5 ml per minute. (B) 1 ml of ascites diluted 1:1 with 100 mM sodium acetate, 100 mM sodium chloride, pH 5.0, and chromatographed on a 1.0 ml column of GammaBind®G Plus using the same conditions as in the experiment shown in (A), except that the loading/washing buffer was 100 mM sodium acetate, 100 mM sodium chloride, pH 5.0. The time at which the peak of IgG was eluted is indicated for both experiments.

been extensively washed with PBS. The resulting slurry was incubated at room temperature for 1 hr with occasional mixing to allow the binding reaction to go to completion. The agarose beads were washed with PBS to remove any unbound antibody, then washed once with 10 ml of 0.2 M triethanolamine at pH 8.5. The crosslinking solution, which contained 10 mg/ml of dimethylpimelimidate in 0.2 M triethanolamine, was made just before use and the pH adjusted to 8.5. The agarose beads with bound antibody were incubated with the crosslinker for 30 min at room temperature, with occasional mixing. The agarose beads were collected by briefly centrifuging the slurry and carefully removing the supernatant. The beads were then suspended in 0.2 M ethanolamine at pH 8.0, and incubated at room temperature to stop the reaction. After a final wash in ten volumes of PBS, the beads were ready to be packed into a column and used.

The HyHEL-5 affinity column was used to purify lysozyme from hen

Chapter 20. IgG Purification Using Protein G

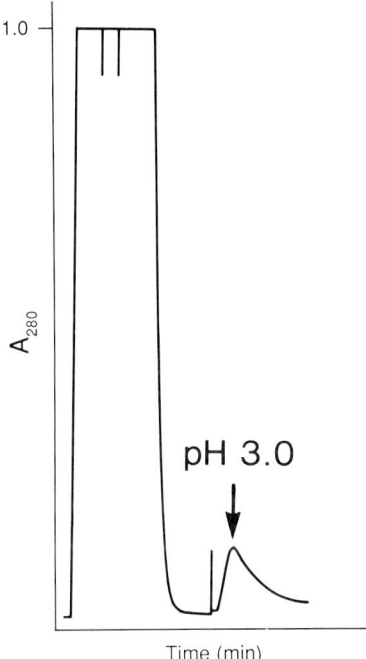

FIGURE 4A
Isolation of hen egg white lysozyme on a GammaBind®G agarose antigen affinity column. Four ml of hen egg white, diluted 1:10 with PBS loading buffer was chromatographed on a column containing HyHEL-5 monoclonal antibody crosslinked to protein G agarose. Above, trace of the scan at A_{280}.

egg white. The egg white was diluted 1:10 with PBS, and the mixture vigorously shaken to break up the viscous egg white. Four milliliters of the diluted egg white was applied to a 1.0 ml column of the HyHEL-5 antibody agarose at a flow rate of 0.5 ml/min. The column was washed with PBS until the absorbance at 280 nm returned to background, and the lysozyme was eluted with 0.5 M acetic acid at pH 3.0. The profile of the absorbance scan at 280 nm is shown in Figure 4A and SDS polyacrylamide gels of the proteins in the column load, flow-through, and eluted peaks are shown in Figure 4B. The eluted fraction contained 110 μg of purified lysozyme.

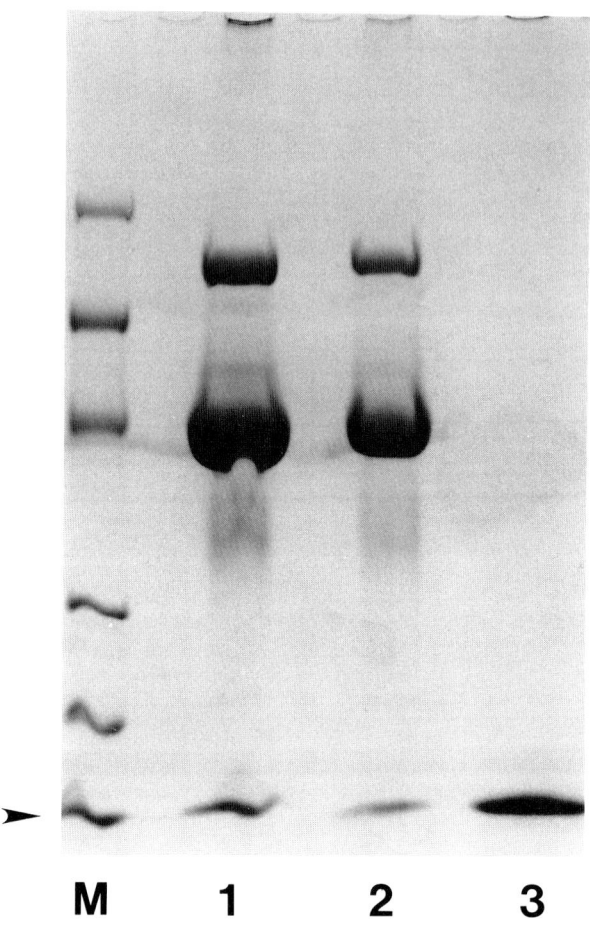

FIGURE 4B *Continued*
Reducing SDS–PAGE of the proteins in the loaded sample (lane 1), the flow-through fraction (lane 2), and the eluted fraction (lane 3). M, molecular weight markers; phosphorylase B, 97,400; bovine serum albumin, 66,200; oval bumin, 45,000; carbonic anhydrase, 31,000; soybean trypsin inhibitor, 21,500; egg white lysozyme, 14,400.

V. Summary

Protein G immobilized on a solid support such as GammaBind®G agarose provides a convenient and efficient matrix for purifying IgG. The procedures for purification are straightforward and can be easily adapted to different experimental systems. The three examples of IgG purification described here provide guidelines for carrying out similar protocols with any IgG isolated from serum, ascites fluid, or hybridoma supernatants. GammaBind®G agarose also provides an excellent beginning matrix for preparing antigen purification columns, since the interaction between protein G and IgG does not interfere with the antigen-binding site of the antibody. In addition, the purification of the IgG can be coupled with the crosslinking reaction in one protocol, eliminating the need for first purifying the antibody.

Acknowledgments

I thank Dr. Kathy Reis for allowing me to use the data in Figure 2 and for helpful discussions and suggestions. I also thank Dr. Jeffrey McGuire for helpful discussions and suggestions and his support while I prepared the manuscript.

References

Åkerström, B., and Björck, L. (1986). *J. Biol. Chem.* **261,** 10240–10247.
Åkerström, B., Brodin, T., Reis, K., and Björck, L. (1985). *J. Immunol.* **135,** 2589–2592.
Björck, L., and Blomberg, J. (1987). *Eur. J. Clin. Microbiol.* **6,** 428–429.
Björck L., and Kronvall, G. (1984). *J. Immunol.* **133,** 969–974.
Campbell, A. (1984). "Monoclonal Antibody Technology: The Production and Characterization of Rodent and Human Hybridomas," pp. 66–67. Elsevier, Amsterdam.
Clark, M., Coffold, S., Hale, G., and Waldman, H. (1983). *Immunol. Today* **4,** 100–101.
Fahnestock, S. R., Alexander, P., Nagle, J., and Filpula, D. (1986). *J. Bacteriol.* **167,** 870–880.
Forsgren, A., and Sjöquist, J. (1966). *J. Immunol.* **97,** 822–827.
Goding, J. W. (1978). *J. Immunol. Methods* **20,** 241–253.
Guss, B., Eliasson, M., Olsson, A., Uhlén, M., Frej, A.-K., Jornvall, H., Flock, J.-I., and Lindberg, M. (1986). *EMBO J.* **5,** 1567–1575.
Hardy, R. (1986). In "Handbook of Experimental Immunology, Vol. 1: Immunochemistry" (D. M. Weir, ed.), pp. 13.1–13.13. Blackwell, Oxford.
Langone, J. J. (1982). *J. Immunol. Methods* **55,** 277–296.
Maruyama, S., Kubagawa, H., and Cooper, M. D. (1985). *J. Immunol.* **135,** 192–199.
Neoh, S. H., Gordon, C., Potter, A., and Zola, H. (1986). *J. Immunol. Methods* **91,** 231–235.
Ohlson, S., Nilsson, R., Niss, U., Kjellberg, B., and Freiburghaus, C. (1988). *J. Immunol. Methods* **114,** 175–180.
Reis, K. J., Ayoub, E. M., and Boyle, M. D. P. (1984). *J. Immunol.* **132,** 3091–3097.
Schneider, C., Newman, R. A., Sutherland, D. R., Asser, U., and Greaves M. F. (1982). *J. Biol. Chem.* **257,** 10766–10769.

CHAPTER **21**

Bacterial immunoglobulin-binding proteins and complement

Michael D. P. Boyle

I. Introduction

The complement system consists of at least 20 serum proteins and regulators that interact in a precise sequence, resulting in the generation of a variety of complement split products and the lysis of an appropriate target (Müller-Eberhard, 1975; Mayer, 1978; Boyle and Borsos, 1980; Frank, 1985). Complement activation can occur by two different pathways, summarized in Figure 1. The classical pathway is initiated by binding of the first component of complement to an antigen–antibody complex. The alternate pathway differs from the classical pathway both in the initial reactants and in the manner in which the cascade starts. Following activation of C1, the classical pathway follows a sequential cascade in which C4, C2, C3, C5, C6, C7, C8, and C9 participate in that order (Müller-Eberhard, 1975; Mayer, 1978; Boyle and Borsos, 1980; Frank, 1985). Unlike the classical pathway, the alternate pathway does not have an absolute requirement for antibody, but is continuously operational in serum (Fearon and Austen, 1975a,b). Spontaneous hydrolysis of zymogen C3 to C3b occurs at a low rate in serum, and as shown in Figure 1, this reactant is the first component necessary for alternate pathway activity. If C3b can bind to a suitable surface, then in combination with activated factor B, a C3bBb complex can be generated. This acts as a C3 convertase and facilitates the cascade of reactions associated with the alternate pathway (Fearon, 1978). Normally, this alternate pathway C3 convertase is closely regulated by factors H and I, and the pathway is not triggered. However, when a suitable surface or chemical structure is present in the reaction mixture,

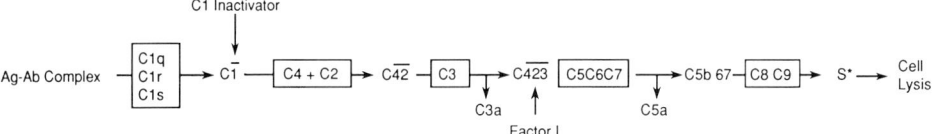

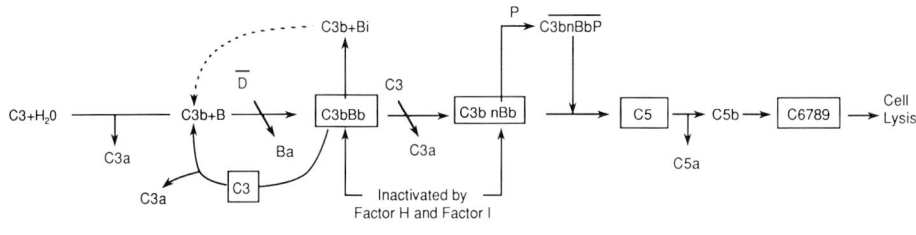

FIGURE 1
Schematic representation of the classical and alternate complement pathway cascade reactions.

the alternate pathway C3 convertase can escape regulation, and the entire pathway becomes operational. In addition to differences between the methods of initiation of the classical and alternate cascades, these pathways differ in their requirements for divalent cations. The classical pathway requires the presence of both Ca^{2+} and Mg^{2+}, while the alternate pathway requires only Mg^{2+}. Consequently, the pathways can be distinguished by comparing their activities in buffers containing Mg^{2+} and Ca^{2+} to their activities in a system containing Mg^{2+} alone. For a comprehensive review of the complement system, see reviews by Müller-Eberhard (1975), Ruddy et al. (1972), and Frank (1985).

One of the most striking features of the bacterial IgG-binding proteins is that they all bind to an identical (or very similar) site on the C_H2–C_H3 interface of the Fc region of the IgG molecule (Wright et al., 1977; Nardella et al., 1986; Woof and Burton, 1990; Schröeder et al., 1987). This site is close to the site at which the C1q subunit of the first component of the classical complement pathway binds. It is therefore not surprising that bacterial IgG-binding proteins can influence the binding of C1q to antibody–antigen complexes (Langone et al., 1978a,b; Laky et al., 1985). In addition, by virtue of their valence, bacterial immunoglobulin-binding proteins can form complexes with IgG that can directly activate the classical complement pathway in serum, in the absence of any specific antigen (Langone et al., 1978a,b).

A number of groups have studied the complement activation potential of soluble protein A and protein A bound to *Staphylococcus aureus* (Sjöquist and Stalenheim, 1969; Kronvall and Gewurz, 1970; Stalenheim *et al.*, 1973; Langone *et al.*, 1978a,b, 1984). The results of these studies have demonstrated effects ranging from inhibition to enhancement of complement activation (for a detailed review, see Boyle, 1990). In general, it has been found that the ability of bacterial IgG-binding proteins to activate complement requires the following:

1. the presence of nonimmune IgG
2. a critical ratio of IgG to bacterial IgG-binding proteins
3. the IgG-binding protein must be at least bivalent
4. the presence of Ca^{2+} and Mg^{2+}

Each of these characteristics should be considered when designing appropriate experiments.

Complement activation can be measured by a variety of functional and antigenic methods. In this chapter, basic methods are described for measuring the ability of bacterial immunoglobulin-binding proteins to activate either the classical or alternate complement pathways, in the presence or absence of IgG.

II. Measurement of Functional Complement Activity

The majority of information on the molecular basis of complement action has been derived from analysis of the ability of antibody-sensitized targets to be lysed on addition of complement (Rapp and Borsos, 1970; Mayer, 1978). This analysis has led, not only to an understanding of the components involved in the reaction and the order in which they participate, but also to a detailed understanding of the chemistry and biochemistry of each reaction step (Müller-Eberhard, 1975; Boyle and Borsos, 1980; Frank, 1985; Mayer, 1978).

Measurement of total, functional, serum complement activity is achieved by measuring the ability of dilutions of a serum sample to mediate lysis of a suitable target. For quantitation of classical pathway activity, sheep erythrocytes sensitized with rabbit anti-sheep red cell antibodies of the IgM isotype have proven to be optimal (Rapp and Borsos, 1970). For detection of alternate pathway activity, erythrocytes have also proven to be the optimal target (Minta and Gee, 1983). The susceptibility of a target cell to the alternate pathway is dependent on certain surface characteristics, e.g., presence of a suitable site for binding of C3b (enabling this bound complement split product to escape regulation by factors H and I). The content of sialic acid on an erythrocyte surface is critical in this regard (Fearon, 1978). Chicken or rabbit erythrocytes can be lysed directly by action of alternate pathway proteins present in human serum (Platts-Mills and Ishizaka, 1974; Polhill *et al.,* 1978; Minta and Gee, 1983). By contrast, sheep erythrocytes are resistant to these activities. Treatment of sheep erythrocytes with neuraminidase (Fearon, 1978) or coating the surface with an appropriate bacterial lipopolysaccharide can render these cells sensitive to lysis via the alternate pathway (Houle and Hoffman, 1984). The choice of erythrocytes as targets for functional complement assays is based on the ability to quantify cell lysis by measuring release of hemoglobin. Erythrocytes also display other characteristics, which make them technically easy to work with, e.g., they do not divide, they pellet well on centrifugation, and they bear suitable membrane antigens to which appropriate IgM antibodies can be prepared.

In addition to lysis of appropriate targets, complement activation can be monitored by the generation of split products (Figure 1). These include C3a, C4a, and C5a, which are released as byproducts of activation of the classical complement pathway, or Ba, C3a, and C5a, produced as a consequence of activity in the alternate pathway. These split products are low molecular weight proteins that have been shown to mediate a variety of biological functions and are generally termed anaphylatoxins (Hugli, 1978, 1979, 1981; Hugli and Müller-Eberhard, 1978; Chenoweth and Hugli, 1980). They are regulated by a series of serum inhibitors that function by removing a key C-terminal arginine residue (Hugli, 1979). Consequently, the split products that are present in serum following complement activation may be a mixture of the physiologically active split product and its biologically less active des-arg form. Detection of either form of the split product by specific antibodies can, however, be used as an accurate reflection of complement activation (Chenoweth and Hugli, 1980; Satoh *et al.,* 1983).

Procedures for measuring total hemolytic complement activity (CH_{50}) of either the classical or alternate pathway, or for quantifying split products, are described in the next section.

III. Detection of Classical Pathway Complement Activity

The detection of classical complement pathway activity (CH_{50}) utilizes a system in which dilutions of the complement source are mixed with antibody-sensitized sheep erythrocytes and the degree of red cell lysis determined spectrophotometrically at the reaction endpoint. This reaction is dependent on a number of factors, including the ionic strength, pH, metal ion content of the buffers, volume of the reaction mixture, temperature, and time (for detailed analysis of these factors, see Rapp and Borsos, 1970). The procedure described here for measurement of classical pathway activity is based on the use of commercially available reagents. Anyone interested in producing their own reagents should consult Gee (1983) for the appropriate protocols.

A. Reagents

Sheep erythrocytes (Pel freez, Rodgers, Arkansas)

IgM anti-sheep red cell antibody (Cordis Corporation, Miami, Florida)

Source of serum complement (A variety of commercial sources of guinea pig and rabbit serum complement are available. Lyophilized serum samples are not recommended for use in complement assays.)

Veronal-buffered saline (VBS)-gel-Ca^{2+}-Mg^{2+} buffer (for exact formulation, see Appendix)

Ethylenediaminetetraacetic acid (EDTA)-gel buffer (for exact formulation, see Appendix)

It is vital in all assays of complement activity that buffers be free of endotoxin.

B. Procedure
1. *Standardization of Sheep Erythrocytes*

Sheep erythrocytes are normally supplied as a suspension in Alsever's solution. It is first necessary to wash the cells and to resuspend them in the appropriate buffer (VBS-gel-Ca^{2+}-Mg^{2+}). This is achieved by removing an appropriate volume of the red cell suspension and centrifuging at 1000 × g for 5 min. The supernatant and any buffy coat should be discarded and the cells resuspended in EDTA-gel buffer. This buffer chelates Ca^{2+} and Mg^{2+} and will destroy any $\overline{C1}$ that may be bound to the erythrocytes. The red cells should be incubated in this buffer for 10 min at 37°C and then washed twice with VBS-gel-Ca^{2+}-Mg^{2+}. At this time, the supernatant should be colorless, i.e., free of any released hemoglobin. If hemoglobin is present in the cell-free supernatant, a third wash should be included. If even a faint color persists in the supernatant at this time, the cells should be discarded.

2. Standardization of Sheep Erythrocyte Concentration

Sheep erythrocytes display a remarkably constant level of hemoglobin. Consequently, by completely lysing an aliquot of cells and determining spectrophotometrically the quantity of hemoglobin released, the absolute number of erythrocytes in the preparation can be determined. An aliquot of the red cell suspension is diluted 1:50 in distilled water and mixed well. This will result in rapid and complete osmotic lysis and release of all the hemoglobin from the cells. The absorbance of the solution is measured at a wavelength of 541 nm in a 1.0 cm path length cuvette. This absorbance can be related to the cell number by simple proportion, given that 10^9 sheep erythrocytes, diluted 1:50 in H_2O will have an absorbance at 541 nm of 0.21.

3. Sensitization of Sheep Erythrocytes with Antibody

Red cells are sensitized with IgM anti-red cell antibodies by mixing equal volumes of sheep erythrocytes (E) at 10^9/ml, with an appropriate dilution of IgM anti-sheep red cell antibody. Polyclonal rabbit IgM antibodies (Rapp and Borsos, 1970), or monoclonal mouse IgM anti-red cell antibodies are suitable for this purpose (Faulmann and Boyle, 1987). It is important to use IgM antibodies for sensitization, since certain problems have been observed when antibodies of the IgG isotype are used (Rapp and Borsos, 1970). The optimal concentration of antibody needs to be determined empirically for each IgM antibody preparation. A dilution of IgM that results in an average of 100–200 $\overline{C1}$-fixing IgM molecules/red cell is ideal. This implies that on addition of excess complement, 100% of the cells can be lysed, without problems resulting from direct agglutination of erythrocytes. If the manufacturer does not indicate a titer for the antibody preparation, preliminary experiments must be performed in which

1. 0.1 ml of E (10^9/ml) is mixed with 0.1 ml of two-fold dilutions of antibody and incubated for 10 min at 37°C.
2. A dilution of excess guinea pig complement (1.3 ml) is added directly to the antibody-sensitized cells. The tubes are mixed and then incubated for 1 hr at 37°C.
3. The reaction mixture is centrifuged to pellet any unlysed cells.
4. The OD_{541} is read in a spectrophotometer and the minimal dilution of antibody that causes 100% lysis in the presence of excess complement is determined.

Note: a control of buffer and complement alone must be included to ensure lysis is antibody dependent, as well as an aliquot of cells diluted in water to determine 100% lysis. In this assay each tube should contain a constant final reaction volume of 1.5 ml. From a preliminary experiment of this type, a suitable concentration of IgM antibody to sensitize the cells can be determined. The sensitizing antibody concentration should be twice that of the lowest dilution, yielding 100% lysis in such a preliminary experiment.

To sensitize the red cells, mix an appropriate volume of E (10^9/ml) with an equal volume of the IgM antibody preparation for 10 min at 37°C. The preparation is washed twice with VBS-gel-Mg^{2+}-Ca^{2+} buffer, resuspended in that buffer, and the cell concentration standardized to 10^9/ml as described earlier. If cell lysis is observed during the sensitization step, this may indicate the presence of complement in the IgM antibody preparation. If this occurs, the sensitization step should be carried out in EDTA-gel buffer, and an additional washing step in VBS-gel-Mg^{2+}-Ca^{2+} should be included. Any preparation in which agglutination of the sensitized red cells is observed should be discarded.

4. Measurement of Complement Activity

Whole complement activity is measured in CH_{50} units. This unit is defined as the reciprocal of the dilution of serum which, when 1 ml is added under defined conditions, produces 50% lysis of optimally sensitized erythrocytes. This is a relative value and will depend on the precise system used to measure red cell lysis, e.g., cell number, reaction volume, etc. These values cannot be compared from laboratory to laboratory and consequently, each experiment must have its own internal control.

5. Procedure

The functional complement assay described here is carried out using 10^8 optimally antibody-sensitized sheep erythrocytes (EA) in a total reaction volume of 1.5 ml. The diluent throughout is VBS-gel-Ca^{2+}-Mg^{2+} and the reaction is allowed to proceed to endpoint. We have found in kinetic studies that any time over 45 min at 37°C is adequate to reach endpoint for lysis of EA under the experimental conditions next described.

The functional activity of the entire classical pathway (C1–C9) is measured in this assay. This is a complicated series of reactions in which no single complement protein is rate limiting. The relationship between the concentration of complement added and the extent of lysis is therefore complex and yields a sigmoid curve of high slope when the percentage of red cell lysis versus complement concentration is plotted (Figure 2). Over a two-fold range of complement concentrations, lysis of optimally sensitized sheep erythrocytes can vary from 100% to less than 10%. Consequently, a narrow concentration range of complement dilutions must be employed in these assays. Preliminary experiments should be conducted to obtain the minimal dilution of the complement source, which, when 1.4 ml is added to 0.1 ml of optimally sensitized EA (10^9/ml), results in lysis of 100% of the erythrocytes at endpoint, under the assay conditions used. For most sources of human serum, this dilution will be about 1:200 to 1:300, and for guinea pig serum about 1:300 to 1:400, using the conditions described. Once this has been established, it is convenient to start with the dilution and add varying volumes of that dilution of the complement source to the antibody-sensitized red cells, as shown in Table 1.

Occasionally, when a heavily hemolyzed serum is used as the complement source, a significant contribution to the absorbance detected in the experimental tubes is due to the presence of this reagent. If this is the case, it is necessary to make an appropriate correction to the observed absorbance values of each experimental tube.

The reactants shown in Table 1 are added in the order shown to 12×75 mm glass test tubes on ice. Once all the reactants have been added, the tubes are mixed thoroughly on a vortex mixer and transferred to a 37°C shaking water bath. The tubes are incubated for 1–2 hr at 37°C (endpoint). Unlysed cells are pelleted by centrifugation at $1000 \times g$ for 5 min; and the quantity of hemoglobin release is determined by reading the absorbance at 541 nm of the supernatant fraction.

TABLE 1
Titration of Classical Complement Pathway

Tube #	1[a]	2	3	4	5	6	7	8[b]	9[c]	10[d]
EA[e] 10^9/ml (ml added)	0.1	0.1	0.1	0.1	0.1	0.1	0.1	0.1	0.1	—
Volume of VBS[f]-gel-Ca^{2+}-Mg^{2+} buffer (ml)	—	0.2	0.4	0.6	0.8	1.0	1.2	1.4	—	0.1
Volume of C[g] diluted 1/300 (ml)	1.4	1.2	1.0	0.8	0.6	0.4	0.2	—	—	1.4
Volume of water (ml)	—	—	—	—	—	—	—	—	1.4	—
Total reaction volume (ml)	1.5	1.5	1.5	1.5	1.5	1.5	1.5	1.5	1.5	1.5

[a] Tubes 1–7 are the experimental samples.
[b] Tube 8 is a measure of the spontaneous or background release of hemoglobin from erythrocytes.
[c] Tube 9 is a measure of the total release of hemoglobin (or 100% lysis).
[d] Tube 10 is a control for any color contributed by the complement source itself.
[e] EA: Antibody-sensitized sheep erythrocytes.
[f] VBS: Veronal-buffered saline.
[g] C: Complement.

The fraction of cells lysed (y) in each tube is calculated as follows:

$$y = \frac{OD_{541} \text{ experimental} - OD_{541} \text{ control}}{OD_{541} \text{ total lysis}}$$

OD_{541} experimental is that measured in each tube (i.e., 1–7). OD_{541} control is the sum of the absorbance in tube 9 plus the absorbance contributed by the color of the complement source (complement color). The complement color control is determined from the OD_{541} value of tube 10 as follows. For tube 1 it will be the same as the OD_{541} value of tube 10, for tube 2 it would be $(\frac{1.2}{1.4}) \times OD_{541}$ value of tube 10, for tube 3 it would be $(\frac{1.0}{1.4}) \times OD_{541}$ value of tube 10, etc.

From these data, it is then possible to generate a graph of the fraction of cells lysed (y) vs. the complement dilution (Figure 2A). It is difficult from the data plotted in this form to obtain an accurate estimate of the CH_{50} value, i.e., the exact dilution of the complement source that will result in exactly 50% lysis of the antibody-sensitized erythrocytes. Consequently, it is conventional to transform the sigmoid curve shown in Figure

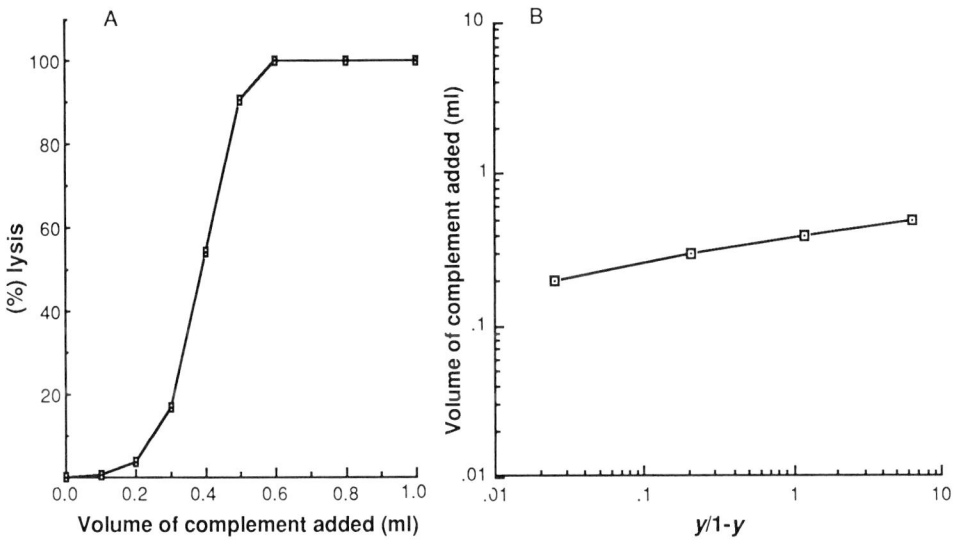

FIGURE 2
Hemolysis of antibody-sensitized sheep erythrocytes by human complement. Plot of hemolysis versus volume of complement added (A). (B) The von Krogh transformation of the data to enable accurate determination of the CH_{50}. For precise details, see text.

2A to a linear form by use of the von Krogh transformation (Figure 2B). The von Krogh equation is used for this purpose:

$$\log x = \frac{1}{n}\left[\log\left(\frac{y}{1-y}\right)\right] + \log k$$

In this equation, (x) represents the volume of complement added, (y) is the degree of hemolysis, and (n) and (k) are constants.

By plotting the term $(\frac{y}{1-y})$ on the abscissa and the volume of complement (x) on the ordinate of a log–log plot, this equation yields a straight line of the form $y = mx + c$. When $y = 0.5$ or 50% of the cells are lysed, the value of $(\frac{y}{1-y}) = 1$. Consequently, the volume of complement required to lyse 50% of the cells can then be determined from the log–log plot when $(\frac{y}{1-y}) = 1$. This can then be used to determine accurately the CH_{50} of the serum sample being studied. If all of the experimental conditions have been fulfilled, the slope of the graph $(\frac{1}{n})$ plotted in this fashion should be $0.2 \pm 10\%$ (Gee, 1983).

IV. Measurement of the Functional Activity of the Alternate Complement Pathway

The functional activity of the alternate pathway can be determined using a suitable erythrocyte target and buffer system, in an analogous way to that just described in detail for the classical pathway. The target used to measure alternate pathway lysis can be chicken erythrocytes, rabbit erythrocytes, neuraminidase-treated sheep erythrocytes, or sheep erythrocytes coated with a suitable source of lipopolysaccharide (Fearon, 1978; Minta and Gee, 1983; Houle and Hoffman, 1984). For convenience, we use rabbit erythrocytes, which are readily available in most research laboratories. The alternate pathway does not require Ca^{2+}, and its activity is measured in an ethyleneglycol-bis-N,N'-tetraacetic acid (EGTA)-Mg^{2+} buffer. This buffer does not facilitate complement activity mediated by the classical pathway. The protocol for detection of the alternate pathway CH_{50} is summarized in Table 2.

In general, the CH_{50} values for the alternate pathway are lower than for the classical pathway and most human serum samples should be diluted in the range of 1:50–1:100 to determine alternate pathway activity. As noted earlier, the precise conditions of the assay system can influence the results, and it is therefore necessary to carry out some preliminary studies to determine optimal conditions for each complement source to be tested.

TABLE 2[a]
Titration of Alternate Pathway Complement Activity

Tube #	1[b]	2	3	4	5	6	7	8[c]	9[d]	10[e]
Rabbit E[f] 10^9/ml	0.1	0.1	0.1	0.1	0.1	0.1	0.1	0.1	0.1	—
Volume of EGTA-gel-Mg^+ buffer (ml)	—	0.2	0.4	0.6	0.8	1.0	1.2	1.4	—	0.1
Volume of C[g] diluted 1/50	1.4	1.2	1.0	0.8	0.6	0.4	0.2	—	—	1.4
Volume of water (ml)	—	—	—	—	—	—	—	—	1.4	—
Total reaction volume (ml)	1.5	1.5	1.5	1.5	1.5	1.5	1.5	1.5	1.5	1.5

[a] This protocol is identical to the protocol in Table 1 for determining classical pathway CH_{50} values, except in the choice of target (rabbit erythrocytes vs. antibody-sensitized sheep erythrocytes), and in the buffer system (EGTA-gel-Mg^{2+} versus VBS-gel-Mg^{2+}-Ca^{2+}).
[b] Tubes 1–7 are the experimental samples.
[c] Tube 8 is a measure of the spontaneous or background release of hemoglobin from erythrocytes.
[d] Tube 9 is a measure of the total release of hemoglobin (or 100% lysis).
[e] Tube 10 is a control for any color contributed by the complement source.
[f] E: Erythrocytes.
[g] C: Complement.

V. Application of Functional Complement Titrations to Measurement of Activity of Immunoglobulin-Binding Proteins

The methods described earlier enable standardization of complement sources and detection of complement activity. Activation of complement, detected by reduction of the CH_{50} value, has been observed in human and guinea pig serum samples following preincubation with *Staphylococcus aureus* expressing protein A, free protein A, or a streptococcal type III Fc-binding protein (protein G) (Langone *et al.*, 1978a,b; Kronvall and Gewurz, 1970; Sjöquist and Stalenheim, 1969; Stalenheim *et al.*, 1973; Boyle *et al.*, 1988). These findings indicate that the bacterial immunoglobulin-binding proteins have the ability to mediate activation of complement. Distinction between the classical and alternate pathways can be made by carrying out the reactions in buffer containing Ca^{2+} + Mg^{2+} or Mg^{2+} alone. In our studies of the complement activating potential of staphylococcal protein A, we could not detect any alternate pathway activation when protein A was added to guinea pig serum (Langone *et al.*, 1978a,b). In similar studies, consumption of guinea pig or human complement activity via the classical pathway could be demonstrated (Langone *et al.*, 1978a,b).

In a series of studies, in which different concentrations of a type III Fc-binding protein isolated from a group C streptococcus or staphylococcal protein A were incubated with a dilution of human serum, the functional activity of the classical complement pathway activity was consumed (Figure 3). In these studies, protein G (FcRc) or protein A was added to a dilution of human complement for 30 min at 37°C, 0.1 ml of optimally sensitized sheep red cells (EA) was added, and the extent of lysis determined at endpoint. The results in Figure 3 show that minimum lysis of sheep erythrocytes (and hence maximum complement consumption) occurred at a concentration of approximately 30 µg of protein A or of protein G added to the reaction mixture. This value corresponded, in the reaction mixture, to a ratio of approximately one bacterial IgG-binding molecule to two IgG molecules (present in the serum used as the complement source). Addition of purified IgG to the reaction could displace the minimum of the lysis curves to the right. These findings underscored a number of key points. First, bacterial IgG-binding protein-mediated classical complement pathway activation was dependent on the presence of IgG. Second, activation of complement occurred only over a narrow range of bacterial immunoglobulin-binding protein concentrations. The importance of the composition of different complexes between IgG and immunoglobulin-binding proteins, to their complement activating potential are further discussed in this chapter. When these experiments were carried out using agammaglobulinemic serum, no complement activation was detected (Boyle *et al.*, 1988). However, addition of normal levels of human IgG (10 mg/ml) to the agammaglobulinemic serum resulted in a similar profile to that observed for the normal serum. In these studies, there was no evidence that bacterial IgG-binding proteins could facilitate alternate pathway activity (Boyle *et al.*, 1988).

VI. Measurement of the Generation of Complement Split Products

The previous example, of measuring complement activating potential, was based on the use of functional assays to determine complement lytic activity. In this section, procedures based on antigenic recognition of complement-split products are described. These assays measure the presence of the complement-split products C4a, C3a, or C5a in a serum sample. These products are recognized antigenically by use of specific antibodies that bind both to the biologically active split product and to the des-arg form of the molecule (Chenoweth and Hugli, 1980; Hugli, 1981; Gorski, 1981).

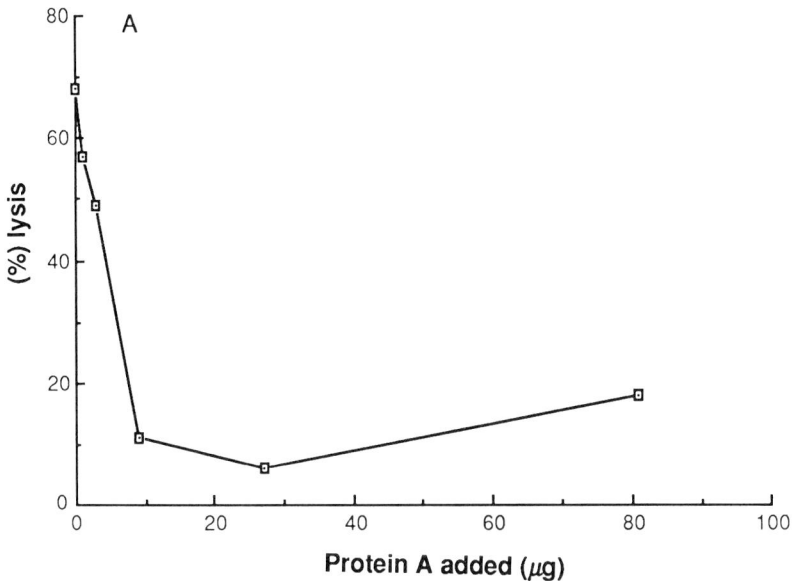
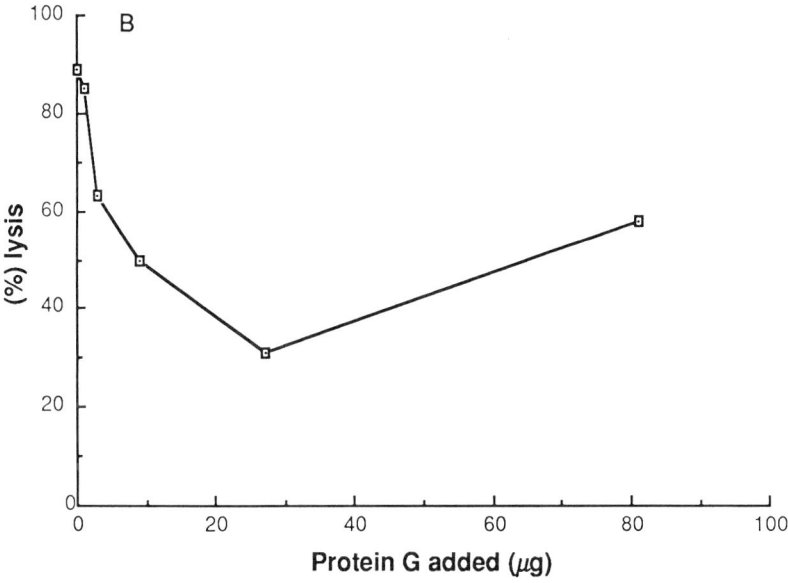

FIGURE 3
Lysis of antibody-sensitized sheep erythrocytes by human serum complement, following preincubation for 30 min at 37°C with different concentrations of protein A (A) or protein G (B). Hemolysis was determined by measuring the quantity of hemoglobin released following incubation of the antibody-sensitized red cells with the complement source for 60 min at 37°C. For precise experimental details, see text.

Measurements of C4a, C3a, or C5a follow a similar protocol. Each assay is based on the availability of specific antibodies to each complement split product and the corresponding radiolabeled ligand. Competition between labeled and unlabeled antigens enables the quantitation of each complement split product in unknown samples. The assay is carried out in three stages (Figure 4). In the first stage, the appropriate complement-split product is separated from the zymogen complement protein by selective precipitation. C3a, C4a, and C5a are similarly sized peptides (approximately 10,000 daltons) and can be readily separated from their respective zymogens by use of a salting out technique employing $(NH_4)_2SO_4$ (ammonium sulfate) or polyethylene glycol (Gorski, 1981; Chenoweth and Hugli, 1980). The split products remain in solution and the zymogen is completely separated from the split form of the component. That is an essential step in the sample preparation for the assay since many of the epitopes present on the split product will be represented on the zymogen. Radioimmunoassay kits for the quantitation of C4a, C3a, and C5a have been developed by the Upjohn Company following the general procedures of Satoh *et al.* (1983) and Chenoweth and Hugli (1980). These kits can be obtained from the Amersham Corporation (Chicago, Illinois), and detect the respective complement split products in the high nanogram to low microgram range. The general procedure for these assays is detailed in this section.

A. Reagents

The radioimmunoassay kits for C4a, C3a, and C5a supplied by Amersham contain all of the necessary reagents including the following:

1. Selective precipitating solution to separate zymogen complement components from split products (step 1 of Figure 4)
2. Labeled split product (^{125}I-labeled C4a, C3a, or C5a)
3. Selective anti-complement split product antibody
4. Unlabeled complement split product standards (C4a, C3a, or C5a)
5. Buffer
   These reagents are needed for the competitive-binding phase of the reaction (Figure 4, step 2).
6. A suitable second antibody to facilitate immunoprecipitation of the antigen–antibody complexes formed (Figure 4, stage 3). This reagent does not precipitate the labeled antigen, (i.e., ^{125}I-labeled C4a, C3a, or C5a) and is used to separate antibody-bound antigen from unbound antigen. [Alternative methods of

Stage 1
Separation of C4 split products from zymogen C4

Sample containing zymogen C4, C4a, and C4a, and C4a des-arg

Separation by selective precipitation

| Zymogen C4 | C4a and C4a des-arg |
| in pellet | in supernatant |

Stage 2
Measurement of split product in the supernatant
Competition phase of the radioimmunoassay

Max binding

^{125}I-labeled C4a des-arg + Ab (antibody specific for C4a des-arg) ⇌ ^{125}I-labeled C4a des-arg–Ab

Sample

C4a or C4a des-arg in sample + ^{125}I-labeled C4a des-arg + Ab ⇌ ^{125}I-labeled C4a des-arg–Ab + C4a des-arg–Ab

Background

Buffer + ^{125}I-labeled C4a des-arg ⇌ ^{125}I-labeled C4a des-arg–Ab

Stage 3
Separation of labeled tracer in antigen–antibody complexes from free tracer

A) Staphylococcal protein A or protein G on beads or fixed to bacteria

or

B) Precipitate with $(NH_4)_2SO_4$, polyethylene glycol, or equivalent,

or

C) Precipitate with a suitable second anitbody to anti-C4a des-arg primary antibody.

FIGURE 4
Schematic outline of the general radioimmunoassay procedure for measuring complement split products. The procedure is for the measurement of C4a and antigenically related split products. The procedures used to measure C3a or C5a are identical, with the substitution of an appropriate, labeled tracer and specific anti-complement split product antibody.

separating complexed antigen from free antigen have been used, including precipitation of the antibody by binding to protein A on the surface of formalin-fixed *Staphylococcus aureus* Cowan strain bacteria (Chenoweth and Hugli, 1980).]

B. Procedure

The samples to be assayed for the presence of complement split products should be first diluted with 0.1 M ethylenediaminetetraacetic acid (EDTA), pH 7.35, to a final concentration of 0.01 M EDTA. This will result in the inactivation of any further split product generation during the assay procedure. An aliquot (0.5 ml) of this sample should then be mixed with 0.5 ml of the precipitating solution, followed by centrifugation at 10,000 × g for 10 min. [Alternative methods for separating C3a and C5a from their zymogens by acidification and centrifugation have also been described (Chenoweth and Hugli, 1980).]

The complement split products are recovered in the fluid phase separated from the zymogen proteins present in the pellet. The supernatant is recovered and a dilution series in duplicate is prepared for the competitive binding stage of the assay (Figure 4, stage 2).

Each competitive-binding immunoassay should include a series of known standard concentrations of the split product being measured. A set of control tubes to determine maximal binding of labeled antigen in the absence of any unlabeled competitor and a set of control tubes to determine the nonspecific background precipitation of the labeled antigen by the second antibody reagent should also be included. The basic assay protocol is carried out as shown in Table 3.

Protocol:

    Incubate reactants shown in Table 3 for 1 hr at room temperature.
        ↓
    Add 50 µl of second antibody to each tube.
        ↓
    Mix well and incubate for 1 hr at 37°C.
        ↓
    Add 2 ml of phosphate-buffered saline.
        ↓
    Centrifuge 2000 × g for 10 min.
        ↓
    Discard supernatant and count pellet in a gamma counter.

TABLE 3
Measurement of Anaphylatoxins by Competitive Binding Radioimmunoassay[a]

	Controls		Standards					Sample #1				Sample #2, etc.			
	1,2[b]	3,4[c]	5,6[d]	7,8[d]	9,10[d]	11,12[d]	13,14[d]	15,16[e]	17,18[e]	19,20[e]	21,22[e]	23,24[f]	25,26[f]	27,28[f]	29,30[f]
Buffer	150	100	—	50	75	87.5	93.75	0	50	75	87.5	0	50	75	87.5
Sample 1			100					100				100			
Complement split product standard (μg/ml)	—	—	—		25	12.5	6.25	—	—	—	—	—	—	—	—
[125]I-labeled antigen	50	50	50	50	50	50	50	50	50	50	50	50	50	50	50
Specific anti-split product antibody	—	50	50	50	50	50	50	50	50	50	50	50	50	50	50

[a] All values in this table are in μl.
[b] Tubes 1 and 2, which determine the nonspecific background binding.
[c] Tubes 3 and 4, which determine the maximal binding.
[d] Tubes 5–14, which provide the data to generate a standard inhibition curve.
[e] Tubes 15–22, which enable the level of split product present in sample 1 to be determined.
[f] Tubes 23–30, which enable the level of split product present in sample 2 to be determined, etc.

Using the data in Table 3, a standard curve is generated by calculating the percentage of labeled antigen bound/free antigen (B/Bo). The results are graphed on log–logit graph paper with the concentration of the complement split product standard on the log axis and the percentage of inhibition on the logit axis. The counts bound for each sample are determined by averaging the counts bound in duplicate tubes and subtracting average nonspecific binding in tubes 1 and 2. Maximal binding is determined from the average number of counts in tubes 3 and 4 versus the average nonspecific binding in tubes 1 and 2. The concentration of split product in any unknown sample can then be determined from the B/Bo ratio for that sample by interpolation of the standard curve and following appropriate corrections for sample dilutions. In our laboratory, we have found the commercial kits to be extremely reliable and reproducible. Values in the high nanogram to low microgram range can be obtained.

The sensitivity of the radioimmunoassay for C4a, C3a, and C5a requires that extreme care must be taken in preparing buffers and other reagents used in preparing samples for these assays. Low levels of endotoxins can activate the alternate complement pathway and generate split products. Similarly, certain types of surfaces (e.g., dialysis tubing) or particles (e.g., Sepharose beads) are all capable of facilitating alternate complement pathway activity and the generation of split products (Chenoweth *et al.*, 1981; Craddock *et al.*, 1980; Langone *et al.*, 1984; Nakanishi *et al.*, 1985). Further, any serum containing immune complexes may also lead to the activation of complement and high levels of split product being detected in control samples of serum incubated in the absence of addition of any other reagent. In general, we have rarely found detectable levels of any of the anaphylatoxins in control samples containing only serum. This usually occurs only when contaminated buffers have been used. Any experiment in which a control serum sample shows greater than 10% of the maximum level of split product activation measured following complete activation of the sample should be repeated. It is also advisable to include a positive control in each experiment to measure the maximal, achievable conversion of split products for the serum sample being used. This can be achieved by addition of an excess of immune complexes for classical pathway activation or by use of suitable polysaccharides, e.g., zymosan, for the alternate pathway potential.

VII. Measurement of Complement Split Products Generated as a Consequence of Complement Activation Mediated by Bacterial Immunoglobulin-Binding Proteins

Langone *et al.* (1984) have used commercial radioimmunoassay kits to determine generation of C3a, C4a, and C5a in serum-incubated, with fluid-phase staphylococcal protein A, protein A associated with intact *Staphylococcus aureus* organisms, or protein A immobilized on Sepharose. In these studies, the authors found that quantitative conversion of C3 to C3a, C4 to C4a, and 40% of the potential C5 to C5a conversion occurred in serum incubated with fluid-phase or immobilized protein A. The maximal generation of split products occurred when ratios of protein A to IgG resulted in maximal precipitation of IgG. This finding once again underscores the importance of the nature of complexes formed between IgG and bacterial IgG-binding proteins with respect to their complement activating potential. Complement split products were also found when protein A–Sepharose, Sepharose alone, or the protein A-poor Wood *Staphylococcus aureus* strain were incubated with human serum (Langone *et al.*, 1984). These observations demonstrate that there are many potential compounds that facilitate complement activation and consequently, carefully controlled experiments are required before attributing the effects on the complement system to a single functional molecule like a bacterial IgG-binding protein.

VIII. Studies of Binding of the First Component of Complement

Many bacterial IgG-binding proteins react with a site on the C_H2–C_H3 interface of the Fc region of IgG (Woof and Burton, 1990). This is also the site on antigen–antibody complexes that binds to the first component of complement (Laky *et al.*, 1985). There has, therefore, been considerable interest in studying the effect of bacterial-binding proteins on the interaction of $\overline{C1}$ with cell-bound antigen–antibody complexes (Langone *et al.*, 1978a,b; Wright *et al.*, 1977; Laky *et al.*, 1985). This can be achieved by monitoring the functional activity of $\overline{C1}$ by use of radioactive C1q, the subunit of the C1 molecule responsible for binding to antigen–antibody complexes.

In a series of studies, we have compared the ability of protein A to inhibit binding of guinea pig $\overline{C1}$ to sheep erythrocytes sensitized with rabbit anti-sheep red cell antibodies of the IgG isotype. In these experiments, sheep erythrocytes (E) were sensitized with sufficient IgG to ensure complete hemolysis if excess guinea pig complement was added (Langone *et al.*, 1977). We demonstrated that protein A inhibited $\overline{C1}$ binding in a concentration-dependent fashion, and at the highest level of protein A tested, $\overline{C1}$ fixation was inhibited by 42% (Langone *et al.*, 1978b).

We also found that $\overline{C1}$ bound to sheep erythrocytes sensitized with rabbit anti-sheep red cell antibodies of the IgG isotype (EAIgG) inhibits the binding of protein A to erythrocytes sensitized with high concentrations of IgG anti-Forssman antibody. These findings highlight the differences in binding of $\overline{C1}$ and protein A to IgG. Protein A binds to each IgG molecule bound to an erythrocyte. Consequently, there is a direct proportion between ^{125}I-labeled protein A-binding and IgG antibody concentration (Langone et al., 1978a,b; Boyle and Langone, 1978). By contrast, $\overline{C1}$ will only bind when two IgG molecules are in close proximity, and as a result $\overline{C1}$ is not as effective an inhibitor of the binding of protein A, as protein A is of $\overline{C1}$.

IX. Antigenic Determination of Complement Activation

The presence of certain complement components in serum can be detected antigenically by either radial immunodiffusion or nephelometric techniques (Ruddy, 1986). These procedures are the basis for quantifying C3, C4, and factor B in many clinical immunology laboratories. This approach can also be used to measure depletion or utilization of individual complement components following incubation of a serum sample with a bacterial IgG-binding protein (Balint and Jones, 1983; Nakanishi et al., 1985). These assays are generally not as quantitative as the functional assays, and caution should be employed when using these procedures with bacterial IgG-binding proteins, which are themselves capable of forming complexes with IgG, either in the serum sample used to provide the complement source or with the antibodies used in the detection assay. If antigenic assays are employed, it is essential to include a parallel series of samples incubated in the absence of Ca^{2+} or Mg^{2+}, to ensure that any change in the concentration of a complement component detected antigenically is attributable to an effect on the complement cascade and not an effect on the detection system.

X. Analysis of Complexes Formed between Bacterial Immunoglobulin-Binding Proteins and IgG

In all of the studies described thus far, the complement activation potential of bacterial immunoglobulin-binding proteins has been shown to be critically dependent on the ratio of IgG to bacterial IgG-binding protein. The interaction of bacterial IgG-binding proteins and IgG follows many of the characteristics of a classical precipitin curve. Maximal precipitation of IgG from serum occurs on addition of bacterial IgG-binding proteins when the ratio of IgG to binding protein is approximately 2:1. Analysis of the complement activating potential of isolated complexes has been achieved by isolating complexes of different compositions by sucrose gradient ultracentrifugation. In studies of the complement activating potential of rabbit IgG–protein A (PA) complexes, Langone et al. (1978b) showed that optimal complement activation occurred with an 18s complex of the composition $[(IgG)_2PA]_2$. This complex was stable for at least 96 hr at 4°C and at 37°C for at least 24 hr. The complex behaved like IgM in its ability to interact with the first component of the classical complement pathway. Other complexes displayed different ratios of IgG and protein A, including $(IgG)_2$–PA_1 and $(IgG)_3$–PA_2, which could also be detected (Langone et al., 1978b).

Analysis of complexes formed between IgG and a bacterial IgG-binding proteins is carried out most efficiently by sucrose gradient ultracentrifugation (Langone et al., 1977, 1978a,b). For comparative studies, it is convenient to use a double-labeled strategy, i.e., the IgG is labeled with one isotope, e.g., ^{125}I and the binding protein is labeled with a second, e.g., ^{131}I. If the specificity of the IgG antibody is known, it is also possible to measure functional activity of the complexes formed by binding to the appropriate immobilized antigen and testing for the ability of the complexes to bind labeled Clq, as described earlier. When this approach was carried out with IgG antibodies specific for sheep erythrocytes, it was possible to monitor the complement-fixing potential of each complex formed (Langone et al., 1978a,b). Dima et al. (1983) have extended these approaches to *in vivo* studies in mice.

XI. Summary

Complement activation by bacterial IgG-binding proteins has been shown to be dependent on a critical ratio of IgG and binding protein. In our studies, we have found that all of the complement activating potential requires the presence of IgG, and is mediated via classical pathway activation. The complement activating potential of bacterial IgG-binding proteins can be quantified by consumption of functional activity, generation of complement split products, or by reduction in the antigenic levels of individual complement components. It is difficult to determine the biological significance of a bacterial protein that can bind to the same site on IgG molecules to which the first component of complement binds, and under certain circumstances, can either inhibit or enhance the classical complement cascade.

Acknowledgment

I would like to thank Dr. Adrian Gee for reading this chapter and for his many helpful suggestions.

References

Balint, J., and Jones F. R. (1983). *Immunol. Commun* **12**, 573–579.
Boyle, M. D. P. (1990). *In* "Bacterial Immunoglobulin-Binding Proteins" (M. D. P. Boyle, ed.), Vol. 1, pp. 209–302. Academic Press, San Diego.
Boyle, M. D. P., and Borsos, T. (1980). *In* "Reticuloendothelial Society Treatise on Immunopathology" (H. Friedman, S. Reichard, and M. Escobar, eds.), Vol. 3, pp. 43–76.
Boyle, M. D. P., Faulmann, E. L., and Andres, J. M. (1988). *In* "Inflammatory Bowel Disease: Current Status and Future Approaches" (R. P. MacDermott, ed.), pp. 371–376. Excerpta Medica, Amsterdam.
Boyle, M. D. P., and Langone, J. J. (1978). *J. Natl. Cancer Inst.* **62**, 1537–1544.
Chenoweth, D. E., and Hugli, T. E. (1980). *In* "Future Perspectives in Clinical Laboratory Immunoassays" (R. M. Nakamura, ed)., pp. 443–460. Liss, New York.
Chenoweth, D. E., Cooper, S. W., Hugli, T. E., Stewart, R. W., Blackstone, E. H., and Kirklin, J. W. (1981). *New Engl. J. Med.* **304**, 497–502.
Craddock, P. R., Fehr, J., Dalmasso, A. P., Brigham, K. L., and Jacob, H. S. (1980). *J. Clin. Res.* **26**, 498A (Abstr.).
Dima, S., Medesan, C., Mots, G., Moraru, J., Sjöquist, J., and Ghetie, V. (1983). *Eur. J. Immunol.* **13**, 605–614.
Faulmann, E. L., and Boyle, M. D. P. (1987). *Mol. Immunol.* **24**, 655–660.
Fearon, D. T. (1978). *Proc. Natl. Acad. Sci. U.S.A.* **75**, 1971–1975.
Fearon, D. T., and Austen, K. F. (1975a). *J. Immunol.* **115**, 1357–1361.
Fearon, D. T., and Austen, K. F. (1975b). *Proc. Natl. Acad. Sci. U.S.A.* **72**, 3220–3225.
Frank, M. M. (1985). "Complement. Current Concepts." Upjohn, Kalamazoo, Michigan.
Gee, A. P. (1983). *In* Methods in Enzymology" (J. J. Langone and H. van Vunakis, eds.), Vol. 93, pp. 339–374. Academic Press, New York.
Gorski, J. P. (1981). *J. Immunol. Methods* **47**, 61–73.
Houle, J. J., and Hoffman, E. M. (1984). *J. Immunol.* **133**, 1444–1452.
Hugli, T. E. (1978). *Mol. Immunol.* **7**, 181–214.
Hugli, T. E. (1979). *In* "The Chemistry and Physiology of Human Plasma Proteins" (D. H. Bing, ed.), pp. 225–280. Pergamon, New York.
Hugli, T. E. (1981). *CRC Crit. Rev. Immunol.* **Feb.**, 321–366.
Hugli, T. E., and Chenoweth, D. E. (1980). *In* "Biology and Medicine" (R. M. Nakamura, W. R. Dito, E. S. and Tucker, III, eds.), pp 443–460. Liss, New York.
Hugli, T. E., and Müller-Eberhard, H. J. (1978). *Adv. Immunol.* **26**, 1–53.
Kronvall, G., and Gewurz, H. (1970). *Clin. Exp. Immunol.* **7**, 211–220.
Laky, M., Sjöquist, J., Moraru, J., and Ghetie, V. (1985). *Mol. Immunol.* **22**, 1297–1302.
Langone, J. J., Boyle, M. D. P., and Borsos T. (1977). *J. Immunol Methods* **18**, 281–293.
Langone, J. J., Boyle, M. D. P., and Borsos, T. (1978a). *J. Immunol.* **121**, 327–332.
Langone, J. J., Boyle, M. D. P., and Borsos, T. (1978b). *J. Immunol.* **121**, 333–338.
Langone, J. J., Das, C., Bennett, D., and Terman, D. S. (1984). *J. Immunol.* **133**, 1057–1063.
Mayer, M. M. (1978). *Harvey Lect. Seri.* **72**, 139–192.

Minta, J. O., and Gee, A. P. (1983). *In* "Methods in Enzymology" (J. J. Langone and H. van Vunakis, eds.), Vol. 93, pp. 375–408. Academic Press, New York.

Müller-Eberhard, H. J. (1985). *Annu. Rev. Biochem.* **44,** 697–724.

Nakanishi, K., Zbar, B., and Borsos, T. (1985). *Cancer Res.* **45,** 4122–4127.

Nardella, F. A., Schroeder, A. K., Svensson, M-L, Sjöquist, J., Barber, C., and Christensen, P. (1986). *J. Immunol.* **138,** 922–926.

Platts-Mills, T. A. E., and Ishizaka, K. (1974). *J. Immunol.* **113,** 348.

Polhill, R. B., Newman, S. L., Pruitt, K. M., and Johnston, R. B. (1978). *J. Immunol.* **121,** 371–376.

Rapp, H. J., and Borsos, T. (1970). "Molecular Basis of Complement Action." Appleton (Century-Crofts), New York.

Ruddy, S. (1986). "Manual of Clinical and Laboratory Immunology" (N. R. Rose, H. Friedman, and I. C. Fahey, eds.), pp. 175–196. American Society of Microbiology, Washington, D.C.

Ruddy, S., Gigli, I., and Austen, K. F. (1972). *New Engl. J. Med.* **287,** 489–545, 592, 642.

Satoh, P. S., Yonker, T. C., Kane, D. P., and Yeagley, V. W. (1983). *Biotechniques* **1,** 90–95.

Schröeder, A. K., Nardella, F. A., Mannik, M., Johansson, P. J. H., and Christensen, P. (1987). *J. Immunol.* **62,** 523–527.

Sjöquist, J., and Stalenheim, G. (1969). *J. Immunol.* **103,** 467–473.

Stalenheim, G., Gotze, O., Cooper, N. R., Sjöquist, J., and Müller-Eberhard, H. J. (1973). *J. Immunochem.* **10,** 501–507.

Woof, J. M., and Burton, D. R. (1990). *In* "Bacterial Immunoglobulin-Binding Proteins" (M. D. P. Boyle, ed.), Vol. 1 305–316. Academic Press, San Diego.

Wright, C., Willan, K., Sjödahl, J., Burton, D. R., and Dwek, R. (1977). *J. Biochem.* **167,** 661–668.

CHAPTER 22

Activation and differentiation of human lymphocytes by bacterial Fc-binding proteins

Douglas J. Barrett

I. Introduction

Studying the biological effects of Fc-binding proteins on human lymphocytes has been useful in dissecting the nature of T cell and B cell activation and in defining possible pathogenic roles for bacterial immunoglobulin-binding proteins. A large volume of literature has demonstrated that interaction with Fc-binding proteins can initiate both proliferation and/or differentiation of human lymphocytes (reviewed in Volume 1, Chapter 24). The biological effects are dependent on the nature of the bacterial Fc-binding protein (type I, type II, etc.), as well as the nature of the lymphocyte population. Further, the response of one cell type can be greatly influenced by the effect of the bacterial Fc-binding protein on another cell type in the same culture. For example, the insoluble form of type I Fc-binding protein induces T cell-independent B cell proliferation, whereas the soluble type I Fc-binding protein induces T cell-dependent differentiation of B cells. Thus, to properly interpret the results of studies involving activation of human lymphocytes by bacterial Fc-binding proteins, several conditions must be carefully defined, including: purification and homogeneity of lymphocyte populations, dose and purity of the Fc-binding protein, physical form in which the Fc-binding protein is presented to the lymphocyte, and the nature of the specific assays used to detect lymphocyte proliferation and lymphocyte differentiation. These considerations will be discussed in the remainder of this chapter, which describes methodology that can be used to study T and B lymphocyte activation and differentiation induced by bacterial Fc-binding proteins.

II. Lymphocyte Isolation and Purification

As reviewed in Volume 1 (Chapter 24), the purity and heterogeneity of the lymphocyte population will have a major impact on the results of studies on bacterial Fc-binding protein stimulation of human lymphocytes. In addition, accessory cells (i.e., monocytes) are generally required as antigen-presenting cells and as a source of interleukin-1 for lymphocyte activation. Thus, characterization of the phenotype and purity of the cells contained in cultures for Fc-binding protein stimulation studies are required. The following is a general guideline for the isolation and purification of human lymphocytes for such studies.

A. Peripheral Blood Lymphocyte Isolation

Lymphocytes can be isolated from whole blood by density gradient centrifugation as previously described (Maluish and Strong, 1986). Sterile, heparinized blood is diluted 1:1 in Hank's balanced salt solution (HBSS). This cell suspension is then very gently layered over cold ficoll–hypaque (specific gravity 1.078–1.082) and centrifuged at $400 \times g$ for 20 min at 4°C. Mononuclear cells are isolated from the interface between the plasma layer and the ficoll–hypaque cushion. The mononuclear cells are diluted with an equal volume of HBSS and centrifuged again at $400 \times g$ for 10 min. After one additional wash in HBSS, the cells are resuspended in RPMI 1640 medium containing 10% newborn calf serum (GIBCO; Grand Island, New York) (RPMI/NCS) at a cell concentration of $5-8 \times 10^6$ cells/ml. Monocytes are depleted by placing 10 ml of the cell suspension in 100 mm plastic tissue culture dishes (Falcon; Lincoln Park, New Jersey) and incubating for 1 hr at 37°C. While a small number of monocytes are necessary for lymphocyte activation, excessive monocyte contamination may be suppressive. The nonadherent lymphocytes are collected by decanting and they are then centrifuged at $200 \times g$ for 10 min. The pelleted lymphocytes are then resuspended in RPMI/NCS and the cell concentration is adjusted to 10×10^6 cells/ml. Monocytes that are adherent to the tissue culture dish are removed by scraping with a sterile rubber policeman, washed, and resuspended at 10×10^6 cells/ml.

B. T Cell/B Cell Separation

For some types of experiments, it may be necessary to purify T cells and B cells from the unfractionated peripheral blood lymphocytes. T cells are physically separated from B cells on the basis of their ability to form rosettes with sheep red blood cells (SRBC). SRBC are treated with 2-aminoethyl isothiouronium bromide hydrobromide (AET), as previously described (Saxon et al., 1976). These AET-SRBC are then adjusted to 5% (volume:volume) and 1 ml of this mixture is added to 3 ml of the lymphocyte suspension in a sterile 13 × 100 mm round-bottomed tube. The cell suspension is gently mixed and then centrifuged at 200 × g for 10 min at 4°C. The tube is then incubated on ice for 1 hr. Alternatively, the cells can be held at 0–4°C overnight. The majority of the clear supernatant is then removed, leaving only a small residual volume of medium (approximately 0.3 ml) over the pellet. The cell pellet is then very gently resuspended using a careful, gentle, rocking motion of the tube. When the pellet has just been freed from the bottom of the tube, the tube is held horizontally and slowly rotated to break up small clumps of cells, taking care not to dissociate the rosetted T cells. Five milliliters of cold RPMI/10% newborn calf serum is added very slowly. The cell suspension is then carefully layered over 3 ml cold ficoll–hypaque and centrifuged for 20 min at 200 × g at 4°C. Cells at the interface (non-T cells) are removed. The remainder of the ficoll–hypaque is gently aspirated without disturbing the red cell pellet, which contains the rosetted T cells. SRBC in the T cell fraction are then lysed by adding 7.0 ml of cold ammonium chloride lysing buffer, which consists of 0.155 M NH$_4$Cl, 0.1 M Na$_2$EDTA, 0.1 mM KHCO$_3$. The tube is mixed by vortexing for 2–4 min or until lysis of the SRBC is demonstrated by clarification of the solution. The T cell fraction and the non-T cell fraction are then washed twice with HBSS. To insure purity of the T cell and B cell (non-T cell) populations, the rosetting procedure just described can be repeated a second time, or alternatively, the cells may be purified utilizing the panning technique described next.

C. Panning Method for Purification of T Cell/B Cell Preparations

Panning (Sleasman et al., 1989) plates must be prepared at least 24 hr prior to utilization for cell separations. The F(ab')$_2$ fragments of goat anti-mouse immunoglobulin (Tago, Inc.; Burlingame, California) are diluted 1:500–1:1000 (approximately 5.0 µg/ml) in sterile phosphate-buffered saline, pH 7.4, containing 6.4 mg bovine serum albumin per liter (PBS/BSA). The optimal dilution of goat anti-mouse immunoglobulin to use should be determined for each lot of antibody by preliminary titration experiments. Plastic petri dishes (10 × 100 mm size; Fisher #8-757-12) are filled with 10.0 ml of diluted goat anti-mouse immunoglobulin per plate. The solution is swirled gently to cover the bottom of the plate and the plates are stored at 4°C for a minimum of 18 hr. Just prior to use, the plates are prepared by gently decanting the coating solution away and washing each plate three times with 5 ml of sterile PBS. PBS is added gently to the side of the plate, the plate is gently swirled, and the PBS is decanted. Do not allow the plate to dry between washes. To block additional binding sites on the plastic surface, 10 ml of PBS containing 2% newborn calf serum (PBS/NCS) is added to each plate and incubated at room temperature for 30 min.

For lymphocyte purification, T cells are incubated with monoclonal anti-CD20 antibodies (anti-B1; Ortho Diagnostics, Raritan, New Jersey) and B cells are incubated with anti-CD3 antibodies (OKT3; Ortho Diagnostics) to coat the residual, contaminating reciprocal population that remains after rosetting (Sleasman *et al.*, 1989). To do this, the cell suspensions are pelleted and a 1:125 dilution of monoclonal antibody in sterile PBS is added. The cell pellet is resuspended in PBS/NCS to make a final cell concentration of 15×10^6 cells/ml. The suspension is then incubated by slow rotation at 4°C for 45 min. The cell suspension is washed twice and resuspended at $5-7 \times 10^6$ cells/ml in PBS/NCS. Meanwhile, the blocking solution is decanted from the panning plates as described earlier. Three milliliters of the T cell or B cell suspension is then added to each plate. The cells are incubated on the panning plates at 4°C for 70 min with occasional gentle swirling. Nonadherent cells are then decanted from the panning plates. These are the enriched populations to be saved for further studies. The decanted cell suspension is then centrifuged and resuspended in supplemented, final tissue culture medium at a concentration of $1-2 \times 10^6$ cells/ml. The purity of the lymphocyte populations can be determined by immunofluorescence using fluorochrome-conjugated anti-CD3 and anti-B1 antibodies to enumerate T cells and B cells, respectively. The T cell and B cell fractions are finally washed twice and resuspended in a final tissue culture medium consisting of RPMI 1640 supplemented with 10% fetal bovine serum (Hyclone; Logan, Utah), 2 mM L-glutamine, N-2-N-2-hydroxyethyl-piperazine-N'-2-ethanesulfonic acid (HEPES) buffer, 100 μg/ml of streptomycin, and 100 units/ml of penicillin. Monocytes that were collected by adherence to plastic are then added to the cell suspensions at a final concentration of 5% to provide accessory cell function.

III. Assays for Lymphocyte Proliferation

Using a microculture system to assay lymphocyte proliferation, several important variables need to be standardized. The first is the geometry of the culture vessel. Flat-bottomed tissue culture plates appear to be optimal for assessing lymphocyte responses to mitogenic activation, whereas round-bottomed plates appear to be superior in optimizing lymphocyte proliferation to soluble recall antigens. In a situation where limiting cell numbers are cultured, round-bottomed plates enhance cell-to-cell contact and give optimal proliferation. The cell dose added to each microculture well is another important variable to be determined in preliminary experiments. Generally, 50,000–200,000 cells/well can be cultured in either flat-bottomed or round-bottomed plates. With some potent mitogens, as few as 10,000 cells/well can be cultured, particularly if round-bottomed plates are used. Further, the cell dose required will be determined to some degree by the extent of lymphocyte purification and the addition of monocytes back to the system. Triplicate cultures are performed for each cell dose and for each mitogen tested. Finally, the kinetics of the lymphocyte proliferative response must be examined. Generally, mitogenic responses peak at 72–96 hr, whereas proliferative responses to soluble recall antigens peak at 5–6 days (Maluish and Strong, 1986). Lymphocyte proliferation is routinely assessed by measuring triatiated thymidine incorporation into DNA during the final 6–18 hr of the culture period. The following is a prototype method for performing lymphocyte proliferation assays.

Peripheral blood mononuclear cells (PBMs) are isolated as just described (either as unfractionated PBMs or as further purified T cell or B cell populations containing 5% monocytes) and are resuspended at 1×10^6 cells/ml in supplemented, final tissue culture medium. The cell suspension is then pipetted into the wells of a 96-well microculture plate in 0.1 ml aliquots. Mitogenic, bacterial Fc-binding protein and control mitogens are diluted to twice the desired final concentration in supplemented tissue culture medium. For soluble, wild type protein A (type I Fc-binding protein) and soluble, wild type protein G (type III Fc-binding protein), we have found optimal concentrations for lymphocyte proliferation range from 5–100 μg/ml and 100–500 μg/ml, respectively (Faulmann et al., 1989). Standard mitogens are used as positive controls. For phytohemagglutinin (PHA-p; Sigma Chemical Co., St. Louis, Missouri) the optimal mitogenic concentration is between 1.0 and 5 μg/ml; for concanavalin A (Sigma) the optimal concentration is from 10–25 μg/ml; and for pokeweed mitogen (Sigma) the optimal concentration is between 1.0 and 10 μg/ml. Diluted Fc-binding protein or control mitogen is added in 0.1 ml aliquots to triplicate cultures containing the lymphocyte suspension. Control for background lymphocyte proliferation is provided by incubating cells in supplemented medium alone. Thus, the final volume in each tissue culture well is 0.2 ml. The microtiter plate is then incubated for 72 hr in an atmosphere containing 5% CO_2, with 100% humidity. On the final day of culture, 1.0 millicurie (mCi) of tritiated thymidine is added in 0.05 ml of supplemented medium and the plate is incubated for an additional 18 hr.

Tritium incorporation into the cellular DNA is then determined by harvesting the cell pellet onto glass fiber filters using a cell harvester (PHD Cell Harvester, Cambridge, Massachusetts). The filters are dried and counted in a liquid scintillation counter. Mean counts for the triplicate cultures at each dose of Fc-binding protein or control mitogen are then reported. Maximal proliferation in counts per minute (cpm) is recorded or, if desired, a stimulation index can be calculated as:

$$\text{Stimulation index} = \frac{\text{cpm in cultures stimulated by mitogen}}{\text{cpm in cultures of cells in medium alone}}$$

IV. Assays of Lymphocyte Differentiation
A. Assays of T Cell Differentiation

T cell activation *in vitro* leads to the expression of some mature T cell effector functions. Lymphokine elaboration has been used as a measure of T cell activation/differentiation in response to bacterial Fc-binding proteins. Lymphokines such as interleukin-2 (IL-2) and gamma-interferon (IFN) are secreted by activated T cells after incubation with Fc-binding proteins and can be measured by either bioassay or immunoassay.

To assess IL-2 synthesis, lymphocyte cultures are prepared as described earlier for proliferation assays. After 24–48 hr in culture, the microtiter plate is centrifuged at $100 \times g$ for 15 min to pellet the lymphocytes. The cell-free culture supernatant is carefully removed. IL-2 concentration in the supernatant can then be quantified using a bioassay and IL-2-dependent indicator cells (Palladino et al., 1983). This assay utilizes proliferation of the IL-2-dependent CTLL-2 cell line (American Type Culture Collection, Rockville, Maryland). Varying dilutions of cell culture supernatant or a reference standard IL-2 preparation (purified IL-2 [Electronucleonics, Inc., Silver Springs, Maryland], or recombinant IL-2 [Genzyme, Inc., Boston, Massachusetts]) are added to replicate cultures of 1×10^4 CTLL-2 cells in microtiter plates. Proliferation of the CTLL cell line after 18 hr in culture is assessed as described earlier, using tritiated thymidine incorporation. From a plot of counts per minute versus IL-2 concentration in the reference standard, the concentration of IL-2 can be determined for each culture supernatant. One unit of interleukin-2 activity is defined as that concentration producing half maximal proliferation of the CTLL-2 cell line.

Interferon biosynthesis by activated T cells can be assayed in culture supernatants from cells stimulated with Fc-binding proteins using a bioassay (Epstein and McManus, 1980). Cell culture supernatants are harvested 24–48 hr after stimulation by varying concentrations of the Fc-binding protein preparations, by control mitogens, and by medium alone,

Chapter 22. Lymphocyte Activation and Differentiation

as described for IL-2 generation. Human interferon activity in the supernatant is assayed in a plaque reduction assay, utilizing vesicular stomatitis virus (VSV) and the susceptible human WISH cell line (ATCC). This assay is based on the ability of T cell-derived gamma-interferon to protect WISH cells against virus-mediated destruction.

From a stock culture of WISH cells, a suspension of 5×10^5 cells/ml is made in growth medium. This medium consists of Eagles Minimal Essential Medium (EMEM), supplemented with antibiotics and 10% fetal bovine serum (FBS). A suspension of the cells is placed into the wells of flat-bottomed microtiter plates in 0.1 ml aliquots per well, containing 5×10^4 cells/well. The plates are then incubated overnight in a 5% CO_2, humidified incubator at 37°C. Before using the microtiter plates the next day, they are examined on an inverted microscope to determine if a confluent monolayer of the WISH cells has been formed. If the cells have grown to confluence, the old growth medium is removed and new maintenance medium is added. Maintenance medium consists of EMEM with 2% FBS and 0.22% sodium bicarbonate. A volume of 0.1 ml of maintenance medium is added per well. Next, 0.05 ml of experimental sample (tissue culture medium containing unknown interferon concentration) is added to duplicate wells in the top row of the microtiter plate. This results in a 1:3 dilution of the supernatant sample. This original dilution of the supernatant is then serially diluted ten-fold down the columns of the microtiter plate. The plate is then incubated for an additional 18–24 hr. At the end of this incubation period, the maintenance medium and supernatant containing interferon are removed from the wells of the microtiter plate. Next, 0.025 ml of a 1:8000 dilution of vesicular stomatitis virus is added to each well of the microtiter plate. The exact dilution of VSV should be previously determined to yield approximately 30–50 plaques per well. Controls must include wells that do not get interferon-containing samples but do receive maintenance medium alone and are subsequently challenged with the same dose of virus. This allows one to determine how well the virus has multiplied in the WISH cells. WISH cell control wells do not get supernatant sample or VSV, but do get medium alone. This allows one to determine whether plaques seen at the end of the assay are due to the effects of the virus or are due to nonspecific WISH cell death. These controls must be run on each plate. The plates are then incubated for an additional 45 min with the virus. The virus is then decanted off into a separate, biohazard disposal container. Next, 0.05 ml of methylcellulose is added to all wells including controls, and incubated for an additional 24–48 hr or until plaques in the virus control are well defined. Methylcellulose is then removed from the microtiter plate and discarded into the biohazard disposal container. The plates are stained with crystal violet to facilitate plaque enumeration.

Methylcellulose consists of 3 gm of methylcellulose in 300 ml of maintenance medium without sodium bicarbonate. This solution is then autoclaved and filter sterilized, 0.22% sodium bicarbonate in HEPES buffer is added. The crystal violet stain is made by adding 1 g of crystal violet to 100 ml of methanol to dissolve the crystal violet and then this solution is added to 400 ml of deionized water.

Specific immunoassays are currently available to quantify IL-2 (Collaborative Research) and gamma-IFN (AMGen). We have found these assays to be simple to perform and perhaps more specific, however their expense and limited sensitivity compared to the bioassays previously described limits their widespread use.

B. B Cell Differentiation to Immunoglobulin Secreting Cells

B cell responses to bacterial Fc-binding proteins can be assayed by quantifying the immunoglobulin secreted into cell culture supernatants, or alternatively, by utilizing an enzyme-linked immunospot assay (ELISPOT) that detects immunoglobulin secreting cells *in situ*. When used together, these two assays allow one to calculate immunoglobulin secretion on a per cell basis. Controls for background and mitogen activated, maximal polyclonal activation of B lymphocytes should be included with each experiment using bacterial Fc-binding proteins. Known polyclonal B cell activators, which can be used as controls to induce B cell differentiation to immunoglobulin secretion, include pokeweed mitogen (Difco or Sigma), Epstein-Barr virus (EBV) (as supernatant from the H9 cell line available from ATCC), or a combination of phorbol myristate acetate (PMA; Sigma) and ionomycin (Calbiochem, La Jolla, California). These controls are necessary to ensure the viability and functional integrity of the B cell cultures.

Unfractionated peripheral blood lymphocytes, or the purified B cell fraction (with and without added T cells) are isolated as described earlier and are cultured at a cell density of 1×10^6 cells/ml in a round-bottomed microtiter plate (0.2 ml per well) or in 1.0 ml volumes in 12×75 mm, loosely capped culture tubes. Cell cultures should be set up with varying doses of the stimulating bacterial Fc-binding proteins, as well as with a known polyclonal B cell activator such as pokeweed mitogen (or EBV), and with medium alone as controls. Assays for differentiation of B cells to immunoglobulin secreting cells are incubated for 6–10 days (average 7 days). At the end of the culture period, the cells are pelleted by centrifugation. The supernatant is removed from the cell pellet and is assayed for secreted immunoglobulin utilizing an enzyme-linked immunosorbent assay (ELISA) or a radioimmunoassay for IgG and/or IgM (Sleasman *et al.*,

1989; Barrett *et al.*, 1983). Alternatively, the cell pellet can be harvested and the number of immunoglobulin-secreting cells can be determined as spots or plaques in an ELISPOT assay on a nitrocellulose membrane utilizing a dot blot format (Barrett and Stephens, 1989). In some circumstances, the latter may be preferable to assays that quantify Ig secreted in supernatant from Fc-binding protein-stimulated cultures, since residual Fc-binding protein remaining in the supernatant may bind to Ig and interfere with solid-phase immunoassays for Ig. Both techniques are described in this section.

To detect Ig secreted into culture supernatants by ELISA (Barrett *et al.*, 1983), the cells are pelleted at the end of the culture period and the noncellular supernatant is carefully removed. The wells of flat-bottomed microtiter plates (Nunclon, NUNC, Roskilde, Denmark) are coated with 0.2 ml of a 1:1000 dilution of affinity-purified goat anti-human IgG antibody (gamma chain-specific; Cappel Laboratories, Malcerne, Pennsylvania). Anti-human IgM antibody may be substituted to alter the isotype specificity of the ELISA. The optimal working dilution of these coating antibodies must be determined in preliminary titration experiments. After washing the plate, supernatants are added to duplicate wells at 1:5 and 1:50 dilutions in PBS with 0.5% NaCl and 0.05% Tween 20 (PBS/NaCl/Tween). Reference IgG standards (Miles, Kankakee, Illinois) at concentrations between 1.0 and 1.0×10^{-4} µg/ml PBS/NaCl/Tween are added to other wells on the plate. After a 2 hr incubation and further washes, alkaline phosphatase-conjugated affinity-purified mouse anti-human IgG antibody (Cappel), diluted in PBS/NaCl/Tween is used to detect bound IgG in the ELISA. Again, a conjugated anti-human IgM may be substituted to detect secreted IgM. Optimal working dilutions of the conjugates must be determined. After an additional 2 hr incubation, the plates are washed and *p*-nitrophenyl phosphate enzyme substrate is added. After 15–30 min, the absorbance at 405 nm of converted *p*-nitrophenyl phosphate substrate is determined in a multichannel photometer (Titertek Multiskan, Helsinki, Finland). Concentrations of IgG (or IgM) in the cell culture supernatants are then calculated by comparing the absorbance of each sample with the standard curve generated by the known IgG reference standards.

As an alternative to the ELISA described, or in addition, the number of immunoglobulin-secreting cells in the culture can be quantitated in an ELISPOT assay (Barrett and Stephens, 1989). This method detects total Ig-secreting cells (IgG or IgM) as spots or plaques on a nitrocellulose membrane in a dot blot format. The assay can be made isotype-specific by using the appropriate enzyme-conjugated second antibody (anti-IgG, anti-IgM, or anti-IgA).

A nitrocellulose membrane (Bio-Rad, Richmond, California) is cut to the size of the dot blot manifold (Bio-Rad) and soaked in distilled water or buffer for 30 min. The manifold is assembled with the nitrocellulose membrane and the excess liquid is removed from wells by applying a vacuum to the manifold.

Prepare the nitrocellulose by coating with primary "capture antibody." This consists of a 1:500 dilution of affinity-purified goat anti-human Ig coating antibody (Ab) (Cappel #0201-0231) in Tris-buffered saline (TBS), which consists of 20 mM Tris in 0.5 M NaCl, pH 7.5. Add 0.1 ml of this coating solution to each of the wells of the manifold. Allow this solution to coat the nitrocellulose for 30 min at room temperature. Suction the coating antibody through the membrane by vacuum and restore the manifold to 1 atmosphere by releasing the vacuum. Block remaining reactive sites on the nitrocellulose by incubating with 0.1 ml of a blocking solution, which consists of TBS containing 1% bovine serum albumin (Sigma) for 30 min at room temperature. Suction the blocking solution through the membrane and then release the vacuum.

Adjust the harvested cell pellet to a concentration of 1×10^6 cells/ml in supplemented media and prepare serial three-fold dilutions, such that the cells can be distributed in aliquots of 0.05 ml per well. Pipette 0.05 ml of each dilution of the cells into separate wells of the manifold. Incubate the cells on the membrane at 37°C in a 5% CO_2, humidified incubator for 2 hr. Wash the cells off the membrane by adding 0.2 ml of PBS per well. Dump the wash solution out of the wells of the manifold (rather than applying suction). Repeat this washing procedure twice using TBS.

Add 0.2 ml of horseradish peroxidase conjugated, affinity-purified, anti-human Ig (Cappel #3301-0231), diluted in TBS–BSA to each well. This conjugate should be tested to determine the optimal working dilution prior to use in the assay. In general, working dilutions between 1:500 and 1:4000 are found to be optimal. Incubate the conjugate on the membrane for 30 min at room temperature. Then wash the unbound conjugate from the membrane twice with TBS, 0.2 ml/well, suctioning the wash through the manifold. Gently remove the membrane from the manifold taking care not to tear the wet nitrocellulose. Wash the membrane once more by placing it in a shallow pan with TBS and swirling or rocking gently for 30 min.

While the final wash of the membrane is occurring and immediately before use, mix the substrate reagents together. Add 60 mg of 4-chloro-1-naphthol (Sigma C-8890), 20 ml ice-cold methanol, and 0.06 ml of 30% H_2O_2 to 100 ml TBS. Drain the last TBS wash from the membrane and add the substrate to the membrane in a shallow pan. Allow the substrate to react with the conjugate, which has bound to the membrane for 15–30 min at room temperature. Drain the substrate from the nitrocellulose and wash several times with 100 ml water. Blot the nitrocellulose on filter paper and store away from light. When the membrane is dry, dark purple–blue spots can easily be seen at the sites where Ig-secreting cells rested on the membrane. Enumeration of the spots is facilitated with the aid of low power magnification (3.5 X). Count the number of spots per well and calculate the number of spot-forming cells (SFC) per 10^5 lymphocytes plated onto the nitrocellulose.

V. Conclusion

Recent studies of the mitogenic properties of recombinant protein A and protein G have demonstrated different results than those reported for the wildtype products (Faulmann *et al.*, 1989; Schrezenmeier and Fleischer, 1978). Consequently, before attributing any effect to the IgG-binding protein, care should be taken to analyze the mitogen for the presence of other bacterial products that could be responsible for the observed reactions.

References

Barrett, D. J., and Stephens, J. (1990). In preparation.
Barrett, D. J., Edwards, J. R., Pietrantuono, B. A., and Ayoub, E. M. (1983). *Cell Immunol.* **81,** 287.
Epstein, L. B., and McManus, N. H. (1980). *In* "Manual of Clinical Immunology" (N. R. Rose and H. Friedman, eds.), 2nd Ed., pp. 275–283. American Society for Microbiology, Washington, D.C.
Faulmann, E. L., Otten, R. A., Barrett, D. J., and Boyle, M. D. P. (1989). *J. Immunol. Methods,* **123,** 269–281.
Maluish, A. E., and Strong, D. M. (1986). *In* "Manual of Clinical Laboratory Immunology" (N. R. Rose, H. Friedman, and J. L. Fahey, eds.), 3rd Ed., pp. 274–281. American Society for Microbiology, Washington, D.C.
Palladino, M. A., Obata, Y., Stockert, E., and Oettgen, H. F. (1983). *Cancer Res.* **43,** 572–576.
Saxon, A., Feldhouse, J., and Robins, A. (1976). *J. Immunol. Methods,* **12,** 285.
Schrezenmeier, H., and Fleischer, B. (1978). *J. Immunol. Methods* **105,** 133–137.
Sleasman, J. W., Morimoto, C., Schlossman, S. F., and Tedder, T. F. (1990). *Eur. J. Immunol.,* in press.

CHAPTER 23

Measurement of *in vivo* leucocyte chemotaxis mediated by Fc-binding proteins

Michael J. P. Lawman
Adrian P. Gee
Patricia D. Lawman
Michael D. P. Boyle

I. Introduction

The *in vivo* measurement of vectoral, chemotactic migration has been well documented (Marasco *et al.*, 1985; Olsson and Venge, 1980; Ross, 1968; Oppenheim *et al.*, 1981; Shosham, 1981) and has been reviewed recently (Gee, 1984). These *in vitro* methods have defined, not only the existence of chemotactic compounds, but also the presence of membrane-bound receptors for these agents on responding (migrating) cells. The phenotype of these cells has also been characterized (Gee, 1984). This *in vitro* vectoral migration of cells in response to a chemical signal has been readily demonstrable using single chemotactic agents and enriched populations of cells. The measurement of chemotaxis under physiological conditions is, however, more complex. The leucocyte migrational response *in vivo* may be due to (1) the direct chemotactic response to the agent itself or (2) the generation of a physiological, chemotactic factor(s) *in vivo*. Apart from the influence of chemotactic agents, the response can also be affected by various local and systemic inhibitory or amplifying systems. The architecture at the site of inoculation may also be important. It is, therefore, difficult to prove that the accumulation of cells at any site is the direct consequence of chemotaxis and not that of random migration. With this in mind, a number of animal models have been developed to measure the role of chemotaxins in the early events of inflammation. These methods have included: (1) histopathological studies (Asherson and Allwood, 1972; Gray and Jennings, 1953), (2) radioactively labeled leucocytes (Spector *et al.*, 1967; Franco and Morley, 1976; Williams, 1979; Colditz and Movat, 1984a,b; Bamberger *et al.*, 1985), (3) Implantation–skin window (Rebuck and Crowley, 1955; Goldsmith *et al.*, 1965; Samak *et al.*, 1980; Bedard *et al.*, 1983; Goodman *et al.*, 1979; Borel and Feurer, 1978; Sveen and Hofstad, 1976; Sporn *et al.*, 1983; Feurer and Borel, 1974), and (4) air sac or pouch procedure (Selye, 1953; Lawman *et al.*, 1984, 1985; Boyle *et al.*, 1985, 1988a; Konno and Tsurufuji, 1983; Tsurufuji *et al.*, 1982).

We will emphasize the air sac technique as a method for measuring the chemotactic response to Fc-binding proteins (Lawman *et al.*, 1984; Boyle *et al.*, 1987, 1988b).

II. Air Sac Procedure

This procedure was first used in rats to study the inflammatory response (Selye, 1953). The method utilizes an air sac that is created by subdermal injection on the back of the animal. The formation of the pouch results in the disruption of the normal architecture of the skin, thereby creating an air space into which a chemotactic factor or inflammatory stimulus can be introduced. The ventral surface of the air sac is composed of a thin membrane layer, which can be removed, stained, and examined microscopically. Cells that respond to the injected compound infiltrate the air sac and attach themselves to the fascial membrane. The stained cells can then be counted and their morphology determined. This technique has been used successfully to measure the early inflammatory response in mice (Lawman *et al.*, 1984; Boyle *et al.*, 1985; Higginbotham, 1965; Clark *et al.*, 1979), rats (Selye, 1953; Konno and Tsurufuji, 1983), and rabbits.

The air sac method is simple (extensive surgical manipulation is not required), easily reproducible, and is capable of giving semiquantitative results to estimate cellular infiltrates occurring *in vivo*.

A. Air Sac Methodology
1. Materials
a. Mice. DBA-1J and DBA-2J mice were obtained from Jackson Laboratories (Bar Harbor, Maine). Other mouse strains that can be used include BALB/C and C3H/HEJ (Cumberland View Farms, Clinton, Tennessee). The mice should be about 4–8 weeks of age and of either sex.

b. Chemoattractants. The synthetic N-formylated peptide, N-formyl-L-methionyl-L-leucyl-L-phenylalanine (f-Met-Leu-Phe), was purchased from Sigma Chemical Company (St. Louis, Missouri). A stock solution of 2×10^{-2} M was made in methanol and was freshly prepared for each experiment.

c. Staphylococcal Protein A. Protein A (Pharmacia Fine Chemicals, Piscataway, New Jersey) at a 1 mg/ml stock concentration was prepared in 0.15 M phosphate-buffered saline (PBS), pH 7.2, and stored in aliquots at $-70°C$.

d. Urokinase. Urokinase was obtained from Abbot Laboratories (Chicago, Illinois) and was further purified using neutral polyacrylamide gel as previously described (Boyle *et al.*, 1987). The optimal concentration for use in migration experiments is 2×10^{-14} M.

e. Group C Streptococcus Fc-Binding Protein. A single molecular weight form of the type III Fc-binding protein (35,000 daltons) was isolated from a group C streptococcus, Strain 26 RP66 (Reis *et al.*, 1985).

B. *In Vivo* Assay Procedure

The procedure is similar to that described by Clark *et al.* (1979) and is carried out in five stages (Figure 1).

In the first stages (I and II), a connective tissue air sac is generated by injecting 0.9 ml of air subdermally on the back of the mouse. The air is injected slowly via a 25 gauge needle from a 1 ml tuberculin syringe. Once formed, 0.1 ml of the chemoattractant solution, present in the same syringe, is introduced into the sac. We have found that the ideal position for the air sac is to one side of the midline and away from the neck region. It is technically difficult to have more than one sac per mouse.

At the appropriate time after injection of the chemoattractant, the mouse is sacrificed and the air bleb and surrounding skin are surgically excised (stage III). The intact air sac is then reflected onto a microscope slide and the surrounding tissue carefully removed (stage IV). The thin membranous lining of the sac is gently stretched onto a microscope slide, fixed, and stained with Camco Quick Stain II (Baxter Scientific Products, Ocala, Florida) (stage V). The stained membrane is then examined at magnifications of 100× and 400×, and the total number of infiltrating cells scored in five randomly selected fields. The cells are classified morphologically at the higher magnification and the relative percentage of monocytes and polymorphonuclear leucocytes determined.

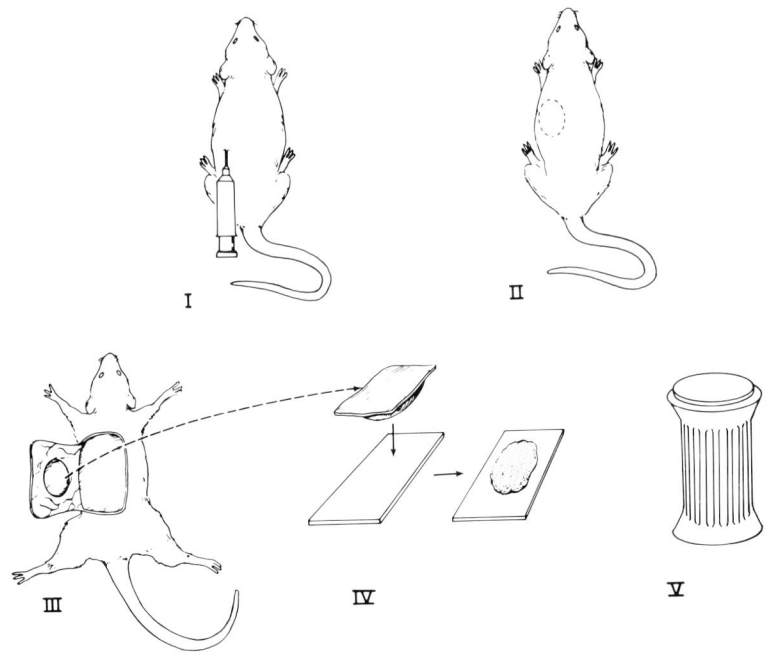

FIGURE 1
Schematic of the *in vivo* assay for chemoattractants. I–II, positioning and formation of the connective tissue air bleb. III, dissection to expose the air sac. IV, removal of the air sac and surrounding skin, and inversion onto a microscope slide. The air sac membrane is excised from the skin and gently stretched onto the slide. V, fixation and staining of the membrane. (Reproduced from Lawman *et al.*, 1985, with permission.)

By virtue of its simplicity, this method can be used to screen the effects of a variety of different chemoattractants at a range of concentrations. Kinetic studies can also be performed. Using f-Met-Leu-Phe, the chemotactic peptide, as a positive control to measure *in vivo* cell migration, both the dose response and kinetics of cell migration can be measured and the identity of the responding cells determined morphologically. Results of a typical study are shown in Figure 2. In these experiments, a stock solution of 10^{-2} M f-Met-Leu-Phe in methanol was used. Varying dilutions of the stock were made and inoculated into the air sac. The infiltrating cells were counted and the morphology determined. A 10^{-10} M concentration was found to produce optimal results. This concentration of f-Met-Leu-Phe is recommended for use as a positive chemotaxis control. The results in Figure 2 show that 10^{-10} M f-Met-Leu-Phe produced maximal infiltra-

Chapter 23. Measurement of *in Vivo* Leucocyte Chemotaxis

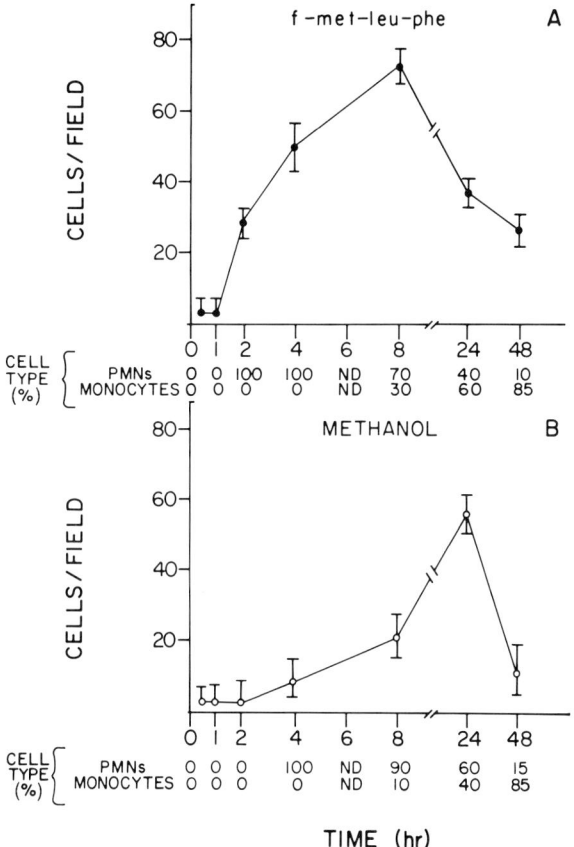

FIGURE 2
In vivo chemotactic response to f-Met-Leu-Phe as a function of time. (A) Kinetics of the response to 10^{-10} M f-Met-Leu-Phe. Differential cell counts at each time point are shown. (B) Kinetics of the response to an equivalent concentration of methanol in PBS ($10^{-6}\%$). Differential cell counts are shown for each time point. ND = not determined. (Reproduced from Lawman *et al.* (1985), with permission.)

tion of the total number of cells (granulocytes and mononuclear cells combined) and occurred in a very short time interval—approximately 5 hr after inoculation. Significant increases in cell numbers (predominantly granulocytes) can be seen at 2 hr postinjection. Since selection of the area on the membrane to be counted is subjective, the results (cell number/field) must be considered to be semiquantitative. Normally this is not a problem when the response is very strong, i.e., high numbers of migrating cells. In these cases, the pattern of infiltrating cells is uniform. When the response is low (occurring with low concentrations of chemoattractant), the infiltration tends to be localized around innovating blood vessels. This "patchy" infiltration is only observed in response to chemotactic agents and not control buffers.

Similar results have been obtained using urokinase (Boyle *et al.,* 1987). Using a range of concentrations of urokinase in a 2 hr assay, maximal numbers of granulocytes were shown to migrate into the air sac in response to the 2×10^{-14} M concentration. Interestingly, the chemotactic response was dependent upon the enzymatic activity of this serine protease. Therefore, f-Met-Leu-Phe (a nonenzymatic chemoattractant) and urokinase can both be used as positive controls in *in vivo* leucocyte migration assays.

The selection of appropriate controls for these procedures is essential. When determining the chemotactic potential of unknown agents, it is important to be able to distinguish between the response due to the selective recruitment of cells of a given phenotype and that caused by nonspecific leakage of cells, resulting from (1) the mechanical rupture of blood vessel, and/or (2) toxicity due to the buffer vehicle. In most cases, these types of nonspecific accumulations of cells contain many contaminating erythrocytes. Furthermore, an inflammatory response and a response to an irritant usually differ in their kinetics. This is illustrated in Figure 2 (lower panel), in which the maximal cell recruitment occurs at 24 hr after inoculation; this is 16 hr after the peak response to f-Met-Leu-Phe. In addition, the cell type involved is different. With the chemoattractant f-Met-Leu-Phe, at 8 hr the response is predominantly granulocytic and by 24 hr the mononuclear infiltrate dominates. In the control, however, the 24 hr peak response remains predominantly granulocytic cells. Again, this shows that chemoattractants accelerate the early events of the inflammatory response.

The air sac method has been shown to be reproducible, both in terms of animal-to-animal variation, and from experiment to experiment. Table 1 exhibits the reproducibility of experiments in response to f-Met-Leu-Phe. Consistency of results has also been shown for other chemoattractants, e.g., urokinase (Boyle *et al.,* 1987) and Fc-binding proteins (Boyle *et al.,* 1988b).

III. Use of Fc-Binding Proteins in the Air Sac Procedure

Both protein A and the type III Fc-binding protein have been shown to be chemotactic under the same conditions as the positive control, f-Met-Leu-

TABLE 1
Response of Mice to Injection of 10^{-10} M f-Met-Leu-Phe[a]

Mouse-to-Mouse Variation

Mouse	Number of cells/field[b]	
	Range	Mean ± SD[c]
A	19–31	24.6 ± 5.8
B	19–38	28.0 ± 7.6
C	20–29	25.6 ± 3.4
D	24–28	22.4 ± 4.1

Experiment-to-Experiment Variation

Experiment Number	Number of cells/field[b]	
	Range	Mean ± SD[c]
1	24–29	26.8 ± 2.2
2	19–28	24.5 ± 4.0
3	27–31	29.0 ± 1.8
4	23–27	26.3 ± 3.0

[a] Adapted from Lawman et al., 1985, with permission.
[b] The number of polymorphonuclear leukocytes in five randomly selected fields were scored 2 hr after injection with 10^{-10} M f-Met-Leu-Phe (10^{-6}% methanol). The magnification used for measurements was 400 X. Injection of 10^{-6}% methanol alone did not result in any infiltration of cells within the 2 hr time period.
[c] SD: standard deviation.

Phe (Boyle et al., 1987; 1988b). In these experiments, the procedure for generating the air sac, the inoculation of the Fc-binding proteins, and enumeration of the cell infiltrate are identical to those described earlier for f-Met-Leu-Phe. The only important difference was that these assays should be run in different inbred strains of mice. The results shown for f-Met-Leu-Phe clearly demonstrate that this method can be used to study agents that are known to be directly chemotactic *in vitro*. It would be advantageous to be able to distinguish, *in vivo*, agents that have an absolute requirement for (or can be enhanced by) the activation of complement and the generation of C5a. This can be accomplished using two strains of the same inbred mouse, namely DBA-1J and DBA-2J. DBA-1J is C5-

sufficient, whereas DBA-2J is C5-deficient. Fc-binding proteins are known to crosslink IgG molecules via the Fc region and generate complexes capable of activating complement (Langone *et al.*, 1978; Langone, 1982). The importance of complement activation in the stimulation of cell migration by Fc-binding proteins can be tested by measuring their *in vivo* chemotactic activity using these mice strains. Again, f-Met-Leu-Phe or urokinase should be used as a control, since their chemotactic activity is not dependent on the generation of C5a (Boyle *et al.*, 1987). Figure 3 illustrates the responses seen with an Fc-binding protein (type III) using the air sac model in the 1J and 2J mice. The injection of the type III Fc-binding protein produces a rapid accumulation of high numbers of granulocytes in the 1J (C5-sufficient) mouse, but a poor response in the 2J (C5-deficient) mouse. These results suggest that the ability of this Fc-binding protein to induce rapid accumulation of inflammatory cells at the site of its injection is dependent upon its ability to mediate activation of the classical complement pathway, generating the chemotactic split product,

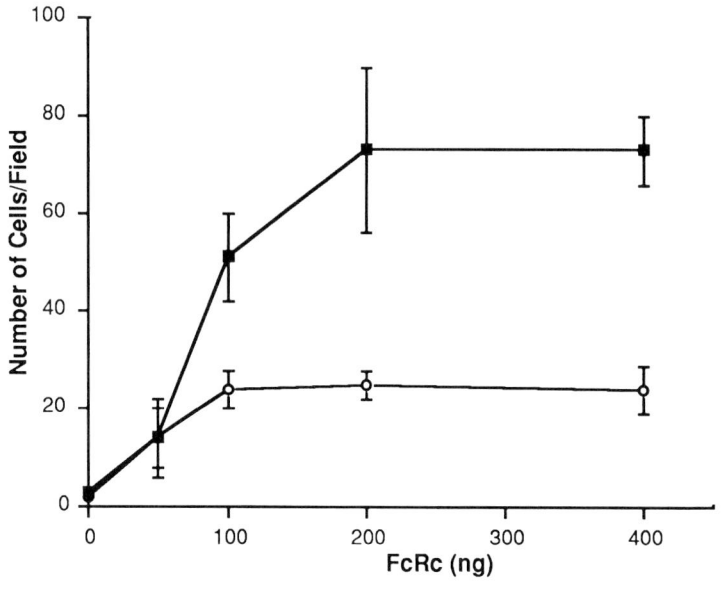

FIGURE 3
Leukocyte accumulation as a function of injection of FcRc into an air sac on the back of C5-sufficient, DBA-1J (o-o) or C5-deficient, DBA-2J (■-■) mice. Two hours after the injection of the stated concentration of FcRc into an air sac, five random, high power fields were scored for infiltrating cells using an Optomax image analyzer as described by Boyle *et al.* (1988a). (Reproduced from Boyle *et al.*, 1988b, with permission.)

C5a. Similar results have been obtained when the type I Fc-binding protein, protein A, is injected into the skin of DBA-1J or DBA-2J mice (Lawman *et al.*, 1984).

IV. Advantages and Limitations of the Air Sac Procedure

This paper describes a simple and reproducible method for studying Fc-binding proteins as potential chemoattractants *in vivo*. Both synthetic (f-Met-Leu-Phe) and physiological (urokinase) compounds can be used as controls. This method is superior to previously described *in vivo* models (Rebuck and Crowley, 1955; Southam and Levine, 1966; Snyderman *et al.*, 1971; Ogata, 1973; Lazarus and Barrett, 1974; Desai *et al.*, 1979) for the following reasons.

1. It is technically simple and easily controllable, i.e., it does not require extensive surgical manipulation or anesthesia.
2. It is remarkably reproducible from animal to animal and from day to day (Table 1).
3. It is semiquantitative, enabling both the number of infiltrating cells and their morphological type to be scored, e.g., comparison of the results obtained following injection of chemotactic agent or control buffer indicated the appearance of leukocytes that are not present in the control preparation. The localization at the site of chemoattractant administration of cells from the peripheral circulation is indicative of a chemotactic, rather than a chemokinetic response.
4. Agents that are directly chemotactic, e.g., f-Met-Leu-Phe and urokinase, can readily be distinguished from those that have an absolute requirement for, or can be enhanced by, generation of C5a, e.g., protein A or protein G (Figure 3).
5. The nature of the infiltrate and the appearance of the skin at the site of injection may be used to distinguish chemoattractant substances from irritants, e.g., injection of an irritant, such as methanol, may produce vascular disruption resulting in the presence of large numbers of erythrocytes within the infiltrate.

There are, however, two major limitations of the air sac procedure. The first is the limit to the length of the time course that can be studied. In most cases, this is around 5 days. Attempts to extend studies beyond 5 days are complicated by collapse of the air sac (reabsorption of the air), and an increase in the cellular infiltrate in control mice injected with buffer alone. Reinflating the air sac every few days does not overcome this problem. The second, and more important limitation is the subjective nature of quantitation. As stated earlier, it is impossible to be totally objective in field selection and to obtain accurate counts with "patchy" responses. Often the patchiness of the responses can be eliminated by increasing the concentration of the chemotactic stimulus (agent) in order to obtain a denser, cellular infiltrate.

In summary, the major advantages of this method are its simplicity and its accommodation of large numbers of samples. This enables multiple time points and concentrations to be studied and facilitates the use of multiple animals in each experimental protocol. This procedure is therefore of value for the rapid evaluation of the ability of bacterial Fc-binding proteins to mediate immediate or delayed hypersensitivity responses *in vivo*.

References

Asherson, G. L., and Allwood, C. G. (1972). *Immunology* **22,** 493–502.
Bamberger, D. M., Gerding, D. N., Bettin, K. M., Elson, M. K., and Forstrom, L. A. (1985). *J. Infect. Dis.* **152,** 903–912.
Bedard, P. M., Zweiman, B., and Atkins, P. C. (1983). *J. Clin. Immunol.* **3,** 84.
Borel, J. F., and Feurer, C. (1978). *J. Pathol.* **124,** 85–93.
Boyle, M. D. P., Lawman, M. J. P., Gee, A. P., and Young, M. (1985). *J. Immunol.* **134,** 564–568.
Boyle, M. D. P., Chiodo, V. A., Lawman, M. J. P., Gee, A. P., and Young, M. (1987). *J. Immunol.* **139,** 169–174.
Boyle, M. D. P., Lawman, M. J. P., Gee, A. P., and Young, M. (1988a). *In* "Methods in Enzymology" Vol. 162, pp. 101–114. Academic Press, San Diego.
Boyle, M. D. P., Faulmann, E. L., and Andres, J. M. (1988b). "Inflammatory Bowel Disease" (MacDermott, ed.), pp. 371–376. Elsevier, Amsterdam.
Clark, J. M., Menduke, H., and Wheelock, E. F. (1979). *J. Reticuloendothel. Soc.* **25,** 255–267.
Colditz, I. G., and Movat, H. Z. (1984a). *J. Immunol.* **133,** 2163–2169.
Colditz, I. G., and Movat, H. Z. (1984b). *J. Immunol.* **133,** 2163–2169.
Desai, U., Kreutzer, D. L., Showell, H., Arroyave, C. V., and Ward, P. A. (1979). *Am. J. Pathol.* **96,** 71–82.
Feurer, C., and Borel, J. F. (1974). *Antibiot. Chemother.* **19,** 161–178.
Franco, M. F., and Morley, J. (1976). *J. Immunol. Methods* **11,** 7–14.
Gee, A. P. (1984). *Mol. Cell. Biochem.* **62,** 5–11.
Goldsmith, H. S., Levin, A. G., and Southam, C. M. (1965). *Surg. Forum* **16,** 102–104.
Goodman, M. L., Way, B. A., and Irwin, J. W. (1979). *J. Pathol.* **128,** 7–14.
Gray, D. C., and Jennings, P. A. (1953). *Am. Rev. Tuberc.* **72,** 171.
Higginbotham, R. D. (1965). *J. Immunol.* **95,** 867–875.
Konno, S., and Tsurufuji, S. B. (1983). *J. Pharmacol.* **80,** 269–277.
Langone, J. J. (1982). *Adv. Immunol.* **32,** 157–252.

Chapter 23. Measurement of *in Vivo* Leucocyte Chemotaxis

Langone, J. J., Boyle, M. D. P., and Borsos, T. (1978). *J. Immunol.* **121,** 327–332.
Lawman, M. J. P., Boyle, M. D. P., Gee, A. P., and Young, M. (1984). *J. Immunol. Methods* **69,** 197–206.
Lawman, M. J. P., Boyle, M. D. P., Gee, A. P., and Young, M. (1985). *Exp. Mol. Pathol.* **43,** 274–281.
Lazarus, G. S., and Barrett, A. J. (1974). *Biochim. Biophys. Acta* **350,** 1–12.
Marasco, W. A., Becker, K. M., Feltner, D. E., Brown, C. S., Ward, P. A., and Nairn, R. (1985). *Biochemistry* **24,** 2227–2236.
Ogata, T. (1973). *Kumamoto Med.* **24,** 103–110.
Olsson, I., and Venge, P. (1980). *Allergy* **35,** 1–13.
Oppenheim, J. J., Rosenstreigh, D. L., and Potter, M. (eds). (1981). "Cellular Functions in Immunity and Inflammation." Elsevier, Amsterdam.
Rebuck, J. W., and Crowley, J. N. (1955). *Ann. N.Y. Acad. Sci.* **59,** 757–805.
Reis, K. J., Ayoub, E. M., and Boyle, M. D. P. (1985). *J. Microbiol. Methods* **4,** 45–58.
Ross, R. (1968). *Biol. Rev.* **43,** 51–96.
Samak, R., Edelstein, R., Bogucki, D., Samack, M., and Israel, L. (1980). *Biomedicine* **32,** 165–172.
Selye, N. (1953). *Proc. Soc. Exp. Biol. Med.* **82,** 328.
Shosham, S. (1981). *Int. Rev. Connect. Tissue Res.* **9,** 1–26.
Snyderman, R., Phillips, J. K., and Mergenhagen, S. E. (1971). *J. Exp. Med.* **134,** 1131–1143.
Southam, C. M., and Levine, A. G. (1966). *Blood* **27,** 734–738.
Spector, W. G., Lykke, A. W. J., and Willoughby, D. A. (1967). *J. Pathol. Bacteriol.* **93,** 101–107.
Sporn, M. B., Roberts, A. B., Shull, J. H., Smith, J. M., and Ward, J. M. (1983). *Science* **219,** 1329–1331.
Sveen, K., and Hofstad, T. (1976). *Acta Pathol. Microbiol. Scand. Sect. B* **84,** 252–258.
Tsurufuji, S., Yoshino, S., and Ohuchi, K. (1982). *Int. Arch. Allergy Appl. Immunol.* **69,** 189–198.
Williams, T. J. (1979). *Br. J. Pharmacol.* **65,** 517–524.

CHAPTER **24**

The cloning of streptococcal protein G genes

Stephen R. Fahnestock
Patrick Alexander

Genes encoding protein G, a type III Fc-binding protein, from three group G streptococcal isolates have been cloned in *Escherichia coli* and their complete DNA sequences have been determined (Fahnestock *et al.,* 1986; Filpula *et al.,* 1987; Guss *et al.,* 1986; Olsson *et al.,* 1987). The DNA sequences of the cloned genes have provided the complete amino acid sequences of the proteins they encode, facilitating the dissection of their structure and function. Comparison of the different genes has elucidated mechanisms of variation among streptococcal isolates. In addition, expression of the cloned genes and modified forms of them in *E. coli* and *Bacillus subtilis* has made available protein G and derivatives, which are of value for defining the biological properties of protein G, as well as providing immunochemical reagents with improved properties.

Here we describe the methods we have used to clone protein G genes from two group G streptococcal isolates, GX7809 and GX7805.

I. Colony Immunoassay

To facilitate screening of protein G-producing clones, we have made use of a colony immunoassay procedure (Figure 1), which is a modification of a procedure developed at Genex by James Anderson (Crop Genetics, Inc.). A circular (82 mm diameter) nitrocellulose filter (BA85, Schleicher and Schuell, Keene, New Hampshire) is placed on appropriate agar medium in a standard petri dish, and bubbles are forced out with a glass rod spreader.

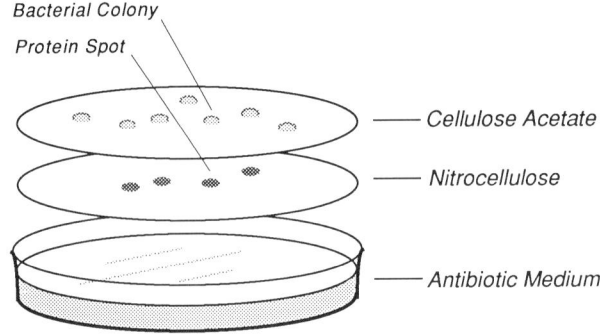

FIGURE 1
Assembly of the colony immunoassay plate.

On top of the nitrocellulose is placed a filter of cellulose acetate (OE67, Schleicher and Schuell). A glass rod spreader is used to press the cellulose acetate onto the nitrocellulose, working outward from the center. Both filters can be applied dry; however, the agar plate should be fairly fresh in order to wet both filters easily. The assembled plate can be sterilized by irradiating the open plate with a shortwave ultraviolet illuminator.

Cells are plated on top of the cellulose acetate and incubated in a normal fashion. After colonies have formed on the upper cellulose acetate filter, this filter is lifted so that the underlying nitrocellulose filter can be removed. The cellulose acetate filter, with undisturbed colonies, is replaced on the plate. The colonies need not be subjected to any cell lysis procedure, but remain intact and viable.

The principle of this procedure is that the cellulose acetate filter retains the cells, but allows any protein that is released from them (by secretion or spontaneous cell lysis) to pass through onto the nitrocellulose filter, where it is adsorbed. The adsorbed protein can then be located on the nitrocellulose with high sensitivity by any of a variety of immunochemical staining procedures. The result is an image of the overlying protein-releasing colonies, with very little distortion or loss of detail due to diffusion. When developed by the procedure described next, for example, sectoring of colonies is readily apparent when there is instability, and subtle differences can be distinguished in the intensity of the staining reaction, reflecting differences in the level of protein release.

The nitrocellulose filter is washed briefly with Tris-saline (0.01 M Tris-HCl, pH 7.4, 0.15 M NaCl), then remaining protein-binding sites are blocked with 5 ml 3% bovine serum albumin (BSA) (Sigma A-7030, St. Louis, Missouri) in Tris-saline, in a petri dish, by rocking for 30–60 min at room temperature. Protein G can be located by incubating with 1:1000 normal rabbit serum in 3% BSA-Tris-saline, washing with Tris-saline, and incubating with 1:1000 goat anti-rabbit IgG–horseradish peroxidase conjugate (Cappel 3212-0081; Accurate Chemistry and Science Corp., Westbury, New York). Alternatively, the normal rabbit serum step can be omitted. After thorough washing with Tris-saline, the filter is developed with 4-chloro-1-naphthol and hydrogen peroxide (H_2O_2). 4-Chloro-1-naphthol (18 mg) is dissolved in 6 ml methanol (ACS reagent grade), then 24 ml Tris-saline is added. Finally 30–60 microliters (μl) 30% H_2O_2 is added and the washed filter is rocked in this solution for 1–15 min, until the desired intensity is observed. The filter is then washed extensively with water and blotted dry.

By using a specific first antibody instead of the normal rabbit serum used to detect protein G (or protein A), the same procedure can be adapted to detect any protein antigen. We have used this procedure extensively to detect proteins secreted by *B. subtilis*. We have found that even proteins that accumulate intracellularly in *E. coli* can be detected readily without any cell lysis step in the procedure. Apparently there is enough spontaneous cell lysis in *E. coli* colonies to release easily detectable quantities of protein. If the pattern is to be interpreted quantitatively, however, it must be taken into account that the stain intensity will reflect both the level of protein production and the efficiency of release, whether by secretion or cell lysis.

II. Streptococcal Clinical Isolates

Group G β-hemolytic streptococci were primary isolates obtained from local hospital clinical laboratories. All eight of such isolates examined gave a positive signal on colony immunoassays for IgG-binding proteins. Three laboratory strains obtained from the American Type Culture Collection (ATCC, Rockville, Maryland) (ATCC 12394, ATCC 12395, and ATCC 9884) were negative. Six of seven clinical isolates examined gave a positive hemagglutination assay with red blood cells (RBC) coated with human IgG or with a human IgG_3 myeloma protein.

III. Preparation of Streptococcal DNA

A streptococcal isolate was grown overnight on trypticase soy agar containing 5% sheep blood. Cells eluted from such a plate were used to inoculate 250 ml Todd-Hewitt broth containing 0.02 M D,L-Thr. After 4 hr at 37°C, 83 ml 23% Gly was added, and growth was continued for 1 hr. Cells were harvested, washed with PBS (0.05 M KH_2PO_4, adjusted to pH 7.4 with NaOH, 0.15 M NaCl), and frozen in liquid nitrogen (N_2) for storage at $-70°C$.

A pellet representing half of the yield from the above 250 ml culture was thawed, washed with S7 minimal salts medium (Vasantha and Freese, 1980) containing 0.5 M sucrose, and resuspended in 10 ml of the same S7–sucrose medium. Mutanolysin (Sigma; 1 mg in 0.2 ml S7–sucrose) was added and incubated 45 min at 37°C. Protoplasts were pelleted by centrifugation in a Sorvall GLC tabletop centrifuge at 4000 rpm for 10 min at room temperature, then lysed by resuspending the pellet in 5 ml 0.1 M ethylenediaminetetraacetic acid (EDTA), pH 8.0, 0.15 M NaCl, containing 0.5 mg/ml proteinase K (Sigma). After incubation at 37°C for 55 min, 2 mM phenylmethane sulfonyl fluoride was added, and the mixture incubated at 70°C for 10 min, then cooled. The lysed, proteinase K-treated mixture was then extracted three times with chloroform-isoamyl alcohol (24:1). The aqueous phase was overlayered with an equal volume of isopropanol, and the DNA was spooled onto a pasteur pipet. The recovered DNA was washed twice with 5 ml 70% ethanol and dried under vacuum. Finally, the dried DNA was resuspended in 1 ml TEN buffer (10 mM Tris-HCl, pH 8.0, 1 mM EDTA, 50 mM NaCl).

IV. Initial Gene Cloning

The protein G gene was initially cloned from a partial restriction endonuclease *Mbo*I digest of DNA from *Streptococcus* GX7809. Approximately 5 micrograms (μg) of GX7809 DNA was digested with 4 units of endonuclease *Mbo*I in 100 μl buffer (50 mM Tris–HCl, pH 7.4, 10 mM MgSO$_4$, 100 mM NaCl), for 15 min at 37°C. Digestion was terminated by heating to 70°C for 10 min and the entire digest was applied to a 0.8% agarose gel (5 wells), which was run overnight at low voltage to fractionate the digest. The gel was stained lightly with ethidium bromide and DNA was visualized under longwave ultraviolet illumination. Material running in the size range between standards (*Hin*dIII-digested bacteriophage lambda DNA) of 4–9 kilobases (kb) was excised with a razor blade.

The gel was fragmented by forcing it through a 23 gauge needle from a 1 ml syringe and the DNA was extracted by the phenol-freeze method (Benson, 1984). Gel pieces were mixed vigorously on a Vortex mixer with an equal volume of water-saturated phenol in a 1.5 ml microfuge tube, then placed at $-70°C$. After 1 hr, the tube was allowed to thaw at room temperature, than again mixed and frozen. The frozen tube was then spun in a microfuge for 15 min at room temperature. The aqueous layer was extracted twice with phenol/chloroform/isoamyl alcohol (25:24:1), then gly-

Chapter 24. Cloning Streptococcal Protein G genes

cogen carrier (30 µg) was added and the DNA was precipitated by adding 0.1 volume 4 M LiCl, 10 mM EDTA plus 2.5 volumes ethanol. After several hours at $-20°C$, the DNA was recovered by centrifugation, washed with 70% ethanol, and dried under vacuum.

The vector for cloning in *E. coli* was the plasmid pGX1066 (Scandella *et al.*, 1985), a pBR322 derivative with a bank of restriction sites flanked by transcription terminators from phage lambda. Plasmid DNA (3 µg) was digested with endonuclease *Bam*HI, which cuts at a single site and leaves ends complementary to those generated by *Mbo*I. After digestion was complete, the DNA was treated with 1 unit calf alkaline phosphatase for 30 min at 37°C, then extracted once with phenol/chloroform/isoamyl alcohol (25:24:1), and recovered by ethanol precipitation, washed with 70% ethanol, and dried.

Digested pGX1066 vector DNA (0.5 µg) was ligated to the fractionated *Mbo*I digest of GX7809 DNA using phage T4 DNA ligase (New England Biolabs; Beverly, Massachusetts) in 20 µl of ligation buffer (25 mM Tris–HCl, pH 7.8, 10 mM MgCl$_2$, 4 mM 2-mercaptoethanol, 0.4 mM ATP). Ligation proceeded for 20 hr at 4°C. The entire ligated mixture was then used to transform 0.25 ml Ca^{2+}-shocked competent *E. coli* SK2267 (F- *gal thi* T1^r *hsd R4 recA endA sbcB15;* available from the *E. coli* Genetic Stock Center, Yale University, New Haven, Connecticut) using standard methods (Davis *et al.*, 1980). After transformation and a 30 min incubation at 37°C for expression of ampicillin resistance, the cells were pelleted, resuspended in 0.3 ml L broth, and plated on the cellulose acetate filters of three colony immunoassay plates containing 100 µg per ml ampicillin.

After overnight growth at 37°C, each plate contained about 1000 colonies. The underlying nitrocellulose filters were developed as described earlier. A single positive colony was detected. This colony was located on the corresponding cellulose acetate filter, picked, and restreaked on a colony immunoassay plate. Only three positive colonies were found among dozens of negative colonies. Each of these positive colonies was restreaked again and this time only a single positive colony was observed among many negatives. This colony was restreaked once again and this time produced about 75% positive progeny. Three of these positive colonies were restreaked again and found to produce all positive colonies.

Plasmid DNA was isolated from one of these colonies and found to consist of two species, one identical in size and restriction map to the vector pGX1066 and a second, present in barely detectable amounts, consisting of pGX1066 plus a streptococcal DNA insert of approximately 10 kb. As described previously (Fahnestock *et al.*, 1986), the smaller plasmid was found to be a cryptic derivative of pGX1066, which had lost the ampicillin resistance marker.

When this mixed plasmid DNA preparation was used to retransform *E. coli* SK2267 on colony immunoassay plates, positive colonies were observed that resembled the ones from which the plasmid was obtained. In addition, there were many intensely positive spots on the transformation plates that could not be aligned with any visible colonies. Material picked from the areas corresponding to several such spots was restreaked and in most cases produced no growth. Two such restreaked spots did produce colonies that were intensely positive. Upon examination of plasmid DNA from these strains, they were found to have lost the cryptic derivative of pGX1066 and also to have acquired a modification of the streptococcal DNA insert in the larger plasmid. In one case, there was a deletion of about 2 kb and in the other case there was an insertion of about 2 kb. Restriction mapping located the point of insertion in the larger plasmid near one end of the deletion in the smaller plasmid (Fahnestock *et al.*, 1986).

Deletion analysis located the protein G gene near one end of the streptococcal DNA insert. The distal end of the coding sequence proved to be near one end of the deletion, but not to be affected by the deletion (Fahnestock *et al.*, 1986).

The explanation for these unexpected results is probably as follows. DNA sequences adjacent to the protein G gene at its distal end are lethal to *E. coli* at high copy number. The initial positive transformant contained two plasmids, the vector pGX1066 with no insert and, at lower copy number, a plasmid with 10 kb of streptococcal DNA including the protein G gene and adjacent lethal sequences. This strain was highly unstable because the plasmid with insert was thrown off at high frequency. After several passages, a derivative was obtained in which the pGX1066 without insert had acquired a mutation that inactivated the ampicillin resistance determinant. This plasmid was now cryptic, but its presence was required in order to keep the copy number of the insert-bearing plasmid low enough to avoid lethality. The larger plasmid was required for growth on ampicillin, so the dual plasmid-containing strain was stable.

Among the retransformants, some carried plasmids in which the lethal sequences were either deleted or inactivated by insertion. These no longer required the cryptic helper plasmid, but could accommodate the altered streptococcal isolate at high copy number and were stable.

The protein G gene was found to be located entirely within a single endonuclease *Hind*III fragment of 1.9 kb. The DNA sequence of this fragment has been published in its entirety (Fahnestock *et al.*, 1986). This sequence confirms that the entire coding sequence is present, as well as an active promoter and translation initiation sequences. This fragment could be subcloned by itself into pGX1066 as well as other vectors, without adjacent sequences affected by the spontaneous deletion (Fahnestock *et al.*, 1986).

GX7809 DNA was analyzed by gel blot hybridization using the cloned 1.9 kb *Hind*III fragment (labeled by nick translation) as probe. A single *Hind*III fragment was found to hybridize to the probe, and its size was the same as the cloned *Hind*III fragment (Fahnestock *et al.*, 1986). This demonstrates that the cloned fragment was not affected by the spontaneous deletion mutation that removed adjacent lethal sequences, and that no DNA deletions or duplications occurred during cloning and subcloning. Such analysis of any cloned protein G gene is essential in view of the repetitive sequence of the gene, in order to ensure that the structure of the cloned gene accurately reflects the structure of the gene in the streptococcal chromosome.

V. Cloning of Protein G Genes from Other Isolates

With the knowledge that the unaltered 1.9 kb *Hind*III fragment containing the entire protein G gene could be subcloned directly on a high copy number plasmid, it became apparent that the gene could be separated from the adjacent lethal sequences by *Hind*III. This suggested a method for the direct cloning of protein G genes from other streptococcal isolates.

Therefore, *Hind*III digests of DNA prepared from two other isolates were analyzed by Southern blot hybridization (Fahnestock *et al.*, 1986) and probed with the GX7809 *Hind*III fragment. In each case, a single cross-hybridizing fragment was observed and in each case the fragment differed in length from the GX7809 fragment. Isolate GX7805 produced a fragment 2.4 kb in length, while the fragment from GX7817 was considerably larger at 4.5 kb.

In order to clone these fragments, areas corresponding to the appropriate molecular weights were excised from an agarose gel containing *Hind*III-digested DNA from GX7805 and GX7817 and the DNA was recovered as previously described. These fragments were then ligated to *Hind*III-digested pGX1066 and the ligated DNA was used to transform *E. coli* SK2267. Transformants were plated on colony immunoassay plates as described.

Positive colonies were obtained from the GX7805 DNA transformation. One of these proved to contain a *Hind*III fragment insert identical in size to the fragment obtained from the chromosome of GX7805. The complete DNA sequence of this fragment was determined. The difference in length between the GX7805 and GX7809 fragments was found to be due to two tandem DNA sequence duplications of 225 and 210 base pairs (bp), respectively, in the GX7805 sequence (Fahnestock, 1987; Fahnestock *et al.*, this series, Vol. 1; Filpula *et al.*, 1987). These duplications give rise to corresponding amino acid sequence duplications, resulting in a protein G product of higher molecular weight. Otherwise the DNA and protein sequences are very similar.

No positive transformants were obtained from the ligation containing the 4.5 kb GX7817 *Hind*III fragment. One possibility is that the downstream *Hind*III site is missing in this strain. If so, the 4.5 kb fragment may contain the adjacent lethal sequences that are removed by *Hind*III in the other strains.

References

Benson, S. A. (1984). *BioTechniques* **2**, 66–67.
Davis, R. W., Botstein, D., and Roth, J. R. (1980). "A Manual for Genetic Engineering, Advanced Bacterial Genetics." Cold Spring Harbor Laboratory, Cold Spring Harbor, New York.
Fahnestock, S. R. (1987). *Trends Biotechnol.* **5**, 79–84.
Fahnestock, S. R., Alexander, P., Nagle, J., and Filpula, D. (1986). *J. Bacteriol.* **167**, 870–880.
Filpula, D., Alexander, P., and Fahnestock, S. (1987). *Nucleic Acids Res.* **15**, 7210.
Guss, B., Eliasson, M., Olsson, A., Uhlèn, M., Frej, A.-K., Jornvall, H., Flock, J.-I., and Lindberg, M. (1986). *EMBO J.* **5**, 1567–1575.
Olsson, A., Eliasson, M., Guss, B., Nilsson, B., Hellman, U., Lindberg, M., and Uhlèn, M. (1987). *Eur. J. Biochem.* **168**, 319–324.
Scandella, D., Arthur, P., Mattingly, M., and Neuhold, L. (1985). *J. Cell. Biochem. Suppl. 0(9 Part B)* 203.
Vasantha, N., and Freese, E. (1980). *J. Bacteriol.* **14**, 1119–1125.

CHAPTER 25

Bacterial immunoglobulin-binding proteins—future trends

Ronald A. Otten
Michael D. P. Boyle

I. Introduction

The impact of bacterial immunoglobulin-binding proteins on immunotechnology over the past decade has been remarkable. In this volume, a variety of different applications have been described including antibody purification, antigen detection, immunoassay, immunoelectromicroscopy, and immunohistochemistry. In attempting to predict the future for this family of functionally active bacterial proteins, it is valuable to examine the ways in which the prototype molecules were identified and exploited. In Figures 1A and B, the key discoveries related to the six types of IgG-binding proteins have been detailed. These figures indicate that the type I Fc-binding protein, more frequently designated as protein A, is the most widely studied protein. The majority of the initial studies using protein A were focused on determining whether this molecule could act as a virulence factor (reviewed by Langone, 1982; Boyle, 1990a). The practical applications emerged over an extended period and this was accompanied by the recognition that protein A could bind Fab regions (Endresen, 1979; Zikán, 1980; Inganäs *et al.*, 1980) and certain isotypes of immunoglobulins other than IgG (Inganäs, 1981; Langone, 1982). By contrast, once a wild type, type III Fc-binding protein (more frequently designated as protein G) was isolated in 1984 (Reis *et al.*, 1984a; Björck and Kronvall, 1984), the major focus of the early studies was on the use of this binding protein for immunoassay and immunotechnology (Boyle, 1984; Reis *et al.*, 1984b, 1988b; Boyle *et al.*, 1985; Wallner *et al.*, 1987; Boyle and

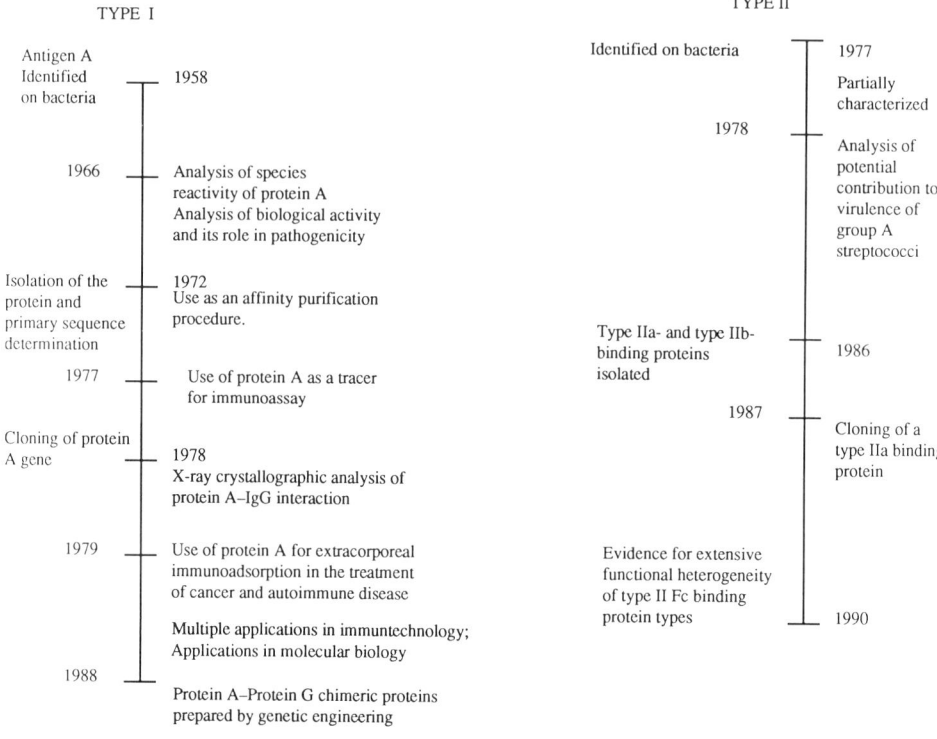

FIGURE 1A
Overview of studies of bacterial IgG-binding proteins. (For reviews Type I, see Langone, 1982; Boyle 1990a; Type II, see Faulmann and Boyle, 1990; Boyle *et al.*, 1990; Schalén and Christensen, 1990.)

Reis, 1987). The recognition that type III Fc-binding proteins had affinity for albumin (Björck *et al.*, 1987) was not immediately appreciated, since the binding of IgG to the isolated protein was not affected by the presence of a large molar excess of albumin (Myhre and Kronvall, 1980; Björck *et al.*, 1987; Faulmann *et al.*, 1989). Björck and colleagues demonstrated that the N-terminal region of the protein G molecule bound albumin and that this could be separated from the IgG-binding domains, either by chemical or enzymatic treatment of the wild type protein or by genetic engineering approaches (Åkerström *et al.*, 1987; Sjöbring *et al.*, 1988). The subsequent demonstration of F(ab')$_2$ binding and binding of α_2-macroglobulin by protein G raised intriguing questions of how this protein functions (Erntell *et al.*, 1988; Sjöbring *et al.*, 1989b).

The types IV, V, and VI Fc-binding proteins are associated with

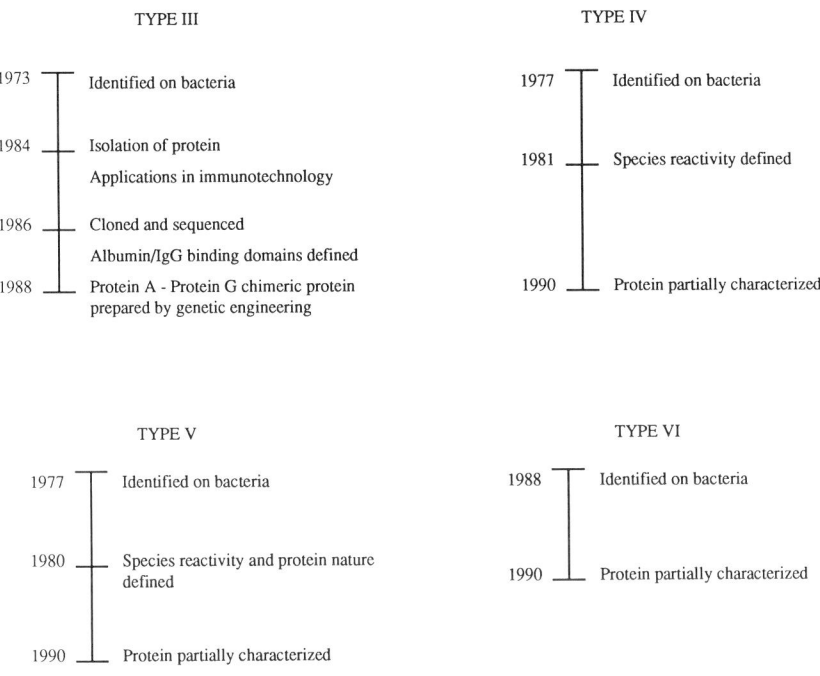

FIGURE 1B
Overview of studies of bacterial IgG-binding proteins. (For reviews, Type III, see Reis and Boyle, 1990a; Björck and Åkerström, 1990a; Type IV, see Reis et al., 1990; Type V, see Yarnall and Widders, 1990; Type VI, see Reis and Boyle, 1990b.)

animal isolates of streptococci and there have been few studies on the potential of these proteins as pathogenic factors. The type IV protein displays the most limited species reactivity of any of the binding proteins (Reis et al., 1990). Consequently, little effort has been directed toward the isolation of this binding protein.

The type V immunoglobulin-binding protein displays very similar reactivities to protein A with human IgG subclasses and the majority of other species of IgG (Myhre and Kronvall, 1981; Yarnall and Widders, 1990). However, the type V protein does not react with canine or feline IgG antibodies, which are reactive with protein A. Despite these functional similarities, there is no antigenic crossreactivity between the type I- and type V-binding proteins (Boyle and Reis, 1990). Since the type V protein does not display any unique reactivities that are not also displayed by the well characterized and readily available type I protein (protein A), there has been no major impetus to isolate the type V protein for immunotechnological applications.

The type VI immunoglobulin-binding protein is remarkable for its reactivity with rat immunoglobulin (Reis *et al.*, 1988a). This property has been used to distinguish type V-positive from type VI-positive *Streptococcus zooepidemicus* strains (Reis and Boyle, 1990b). By virtue of its high affinity for rat immunoglobulins, the type VI-binding protein is expected to be of practical value for studies involving the detection and purification of rat monoclonal antibodies.

The type II immunoglobulin-binding proteins, associated with group A streptococci, have not been studied as extensively as either the type I or type III Fc-binding proteins. Many of the earlier studies have attempted to correlate the expression of type II immunoglobulin-binding proteins by group A streptococci with pathogenicity (Burova *et al.*, 1980; Fisher *et al.*, 1986; Christensen and Schalén, 1990). The limited pattern of species reactivity has not made the type II proteins of immediate value as immunochemical reagents. However, the identification of an IgG_3-specific type IIb-binding protein may have practical value (Yarnall and Boyle, 1986b,c).

The recent discoveries of other non-IgG selective, immunoglobulin-binding proteins including protein L (Myhre and Erntell, 1985; Björck, 1988), protein P (Lindahl and Kronvall, 1988; Lindahl, 1990), and the IgA binding proteins of group A (Christensen and Oxeluis, 1975; Lindahl *et al.*, 1990) and group B (Russell-Jones *et al.*, 1984; Cleat and Timmis, 1987; Brady and Boyle, 1990) streptococci have tremendous potential for a variety of immunochemical applications. These applications are expected to follow a similar pattern of development to those described in this volume, utilizing the prototype immunoglobulin-binding proteins, protein A and protein G.

The existence of this wide range of bacterial immunoglobulin-binding proteins raises a number of theoretical and practical questions. Of particular interest to those interested in microbial pathogenesis is the question of why immunoglobulin-binding proteins are expressed by so many different bacteria? What purpose do they serve and why are they there? For the protein chemist, the structure–function relationship is of major interest. In particular, what are the structures expressed by the different bacterial-binding proteins that account for their unique profiles of species and subclass reactivities? To the immunochemist interested in practical problems in immunotechnology, the exploitation of these proteins for practical applications is the prime concern. In the remainder of this chapter, we have addressed some of these questions and outlined the future trends we perceive in these various areas of basic and applied research.

II. Role of Bacterial Immunoglobulin-Binding Proteins in Pathogenicity

The observations that certain bacteria express and secrete immunoglobulin-binding proteins that react with the same region of the Fc domain of antibody molecules to which the first component of complement also binds, suggests a possible mechanism by which these proteins could inhibit opsonophagocytosis and enhance virulence. However, animal studies have failed to provide any compelling evidence that protein A-positive *Staphylococcus aureus* strains are significantly more pathogenic than mutant strains not expressing protein A (reviewed by Langone, 1982; Boyle, 1990b). Indeed, the ability of protein A to inhibit complement activation requires conditions in which the bacterial binding protein is present in approximately a two-fold molar excess over the concentration of IgG (Langone *et al.*, 1978a,b; Boyle, 1990b). This type of ratio would be difficult to achieve for most systemic infections. However, the possibility that expression of Fc-binding proteins might provide bacteria with some selective advantage for colonizing extracellular sites cannot be excluded.

Type II immunoglobulin-binding proteins, expressed by the majority of fresh, clinical, group A streptococcal isolates have, as their major reactivity, binding to human immunoglobulins. This finding has been taken as evidence for a role for these molecules in virulence (Schalén and Christensen, 1990). Furthermore, the loss of this activity during laboratory subculture and its recovery following mouse passage have been used as arguments that these proteins play a role in the infectivity of group A streptococci. It should be noted that there is tremendous heterogeneity in type II-binding proteins (Boyle *et al.*, 1990; Faulmann and Boyle, 1990). In our mouse passage studies using two group A isolates, enhanced binding to all human IgG subclasses was only observed for one of these strains (Reis *et al.*, 1984c). The argument that immunoglobulin-binding proteins may be important for the survival of a bacteria in a given host is further compromised by the finding that the type IV-immunoglobulin binding protein, associated with certain bovine β-hemolytic streptococci, fails to bind bovine immunoglobulins (Myhre *et al.*, 1979; Reis *et al.*, 1990).

It is generally recognized that the virulence of a bacteria is the combination of a number of factors including surface and secreted molecules (Miller *et al.*, 1989). In addition, virulence factors that may be expressed in order to colonize a mucosal surface may be distinct from those molecules responsible for avoidance of opsonophagocytosis once in the blood stream or in extracellular spaces. In this regard, it is of interest that the antiphagocytic M protein of one group A streptococcal isolate (CS110) shares a common leader sequence with the type II-binding protein expressed by the same strain (Heath and Cleary, 1989; Cleary and Heath, 1990). Sequence analysis of the genes encoding the M protein and the IgG-binding protein from this strain suggest that these proteins most probably arose by some type of gene duplication event (Heath and Cleary, 1987, 1989; Cleary and Heath, 1990). The M protein is expressed on the surface of the bacteria as a coil–coil duplex (Phillips *et al.*, 1981; Fischetti *et al.*, 1988; Fischetti, 1989) and structural similarities between M proteins and the type II Fc-binding proteins have been noted (Heath and Cleary, 1987, 1989; Cleary and Heath, 1990; Boyle *et al.*, 1990). We have previously suggested that these two proteins may be capable of forming heteroduplexes on the bacterial surface (Boyle *et al.*, 1990). Such hybrid molecules might contribute to the anti-phagocytic properties of any group A strain expressing them on their surface.

The potential roles of bacterial immunoglobulin-binding proteins in virulence have been reviewed in Volume 1 of this series (see chapters by Boyle, 1990b; Widders, 1990; Brady, 1990; Christensen and Schalén, 1990). To date, there is no compelling experimental evidence that any bacterial immunoglobulin-binding protein is a virulence factor that would fulfill the requirements of Koch's postulates. Recent approaches involving the insertion of streptococcal M protein genes into nonpathogenic streptococci (Scott *et al.*, 1986; Poirier *et al.*, 1987) have enabled the effects of individual proteins in model systems to be deduced. Over the next decade, these types of approaches, coupled with determining the effects of eliminating the expression of bacterial IgG-binding protein genes by transposon mutagenesis should help to elucidate whether bacterial IgG-binding proteins play any role in the virulence of bacteria.

III. Structure–Function Relationships of Bacterial Fc-Binding Proteins

The genes encoding the type I (Duggleby and Jones, 1983; Lofdahl *et al.*, 1983; Uhlén *et al.*, 1984), type IIa (Heath and Cleary, 1987), and type III (Fahnestock *et al.*, 1986a; Guss *et al.*, 1986; Filpula *et al.*, 1987) immunoglobulin-binding proteins have been cloned and sequenced. These studies have enabled not only the primary amino acid sequences of these binding proteins to be predicted, but also have facilitated a comparison of the overall gene organization of these functionally related proteins. All of these proteins are at least bivalent in their ability to bind IgG and all contain repetitive regions in their nucleotide sequences that encode the peptides that account for their IgG-binding properties (Figure 2). Despite

Chapter 25. Future Trends 431

Type I (Protein A)

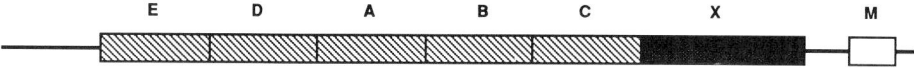

Type IIa

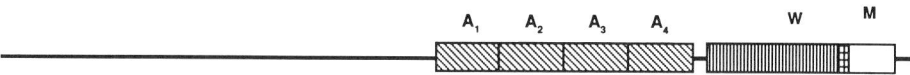

Type III (Protein G) GX7809

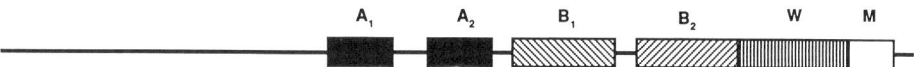

Type III (Protein G) GX7805
G148

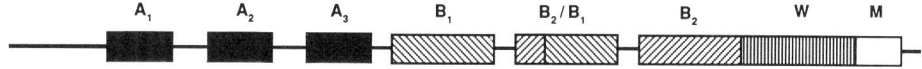

FIGURE 2
Structural profile of the genes encoding the types I, IIa, and III immunoglobulin-binding proteins. E, D, A, B, and C denote repetitive sequences that code for IgG-binding domains (58 amino acid residues/domain) within protein A (Uhlén et al., 1984; Moks et al., 1986). A_1, A_2, A_3, and A_4 designate the IgG-binding repeat region (35 amino acids/domain) of the type IIa immunoglobulin-binding protein (Heath and Cleary, 1987, 1989; Heath et al., 1990). The A domains (37 amino acids each) of the type III immunoglobulin-binding proteins represent the putative albumin-binding repeat regions located at the N-terminus (Fahnestock et al., 1990). The IgG-binding domains of protein G are designated as B_1, B_2/B_1 (hybrid), and B_2, which contain 55 amino acids each (Fahnestock et al., 1986a, 1990; Filpula et al., 1987). Variation in the number of repetitive domains contained within protein G from strain GX7809 and strain GX7805 (G148) is apparent (Fahnestock et al., 1990; Björck and Åkerström, 1990a). The cell wall-associated sequences, designated X for protein A and W for type IIa and protein G, as well as the membrane anchor regions (M) for these proteins are also illustrated (Guss et al., 1990; Heath et al., 1990; Fahnestock et al., 1986a, 1990; Filpula et al., 1987; Björck and Åkerström, 1990a). The sequences of the type III protein cloned from strain G148 by Guss et al. (1986) are identical to that obtained from strain GX7805. The type III domain designations of Fahnestock and colleagues (1990) are shown.

the functional similarities of these proteins, there is no significant homology in their primary amino acid sequences within their repetitive immunoglobulin-binding domains (Guss et al., 1990; Cleary and Heath, 1990; Björck and Åkerström, 1990a; Fahnestock et al., 1990). Protein A, the gene encoding the type I-binding protein from *Staphylococcus aureus*, has been shown to contain five adjacent nucleotide sequences encoding the IgG-binding regions (Moks et al., 1986). Each region contains approximately 58 amino acids and together these sequences account for all of the immunoglobulin-binding properties of the molecule (Uhlén et al., 1984; Moks et al., 1986). Detailed studies with the only type IIa Fc-binding protein thus far cloned and sequenced, have demonstrated that the C-terminal IgG-binding region consists of four consecutive 35 amino acid repeat regions that are responsible for the IgG-binding properties (Heath and Cleary, 1987; Heath et al., 1990). The type III-binding protein (protein G) associated with human groups C and G streptococci has been cloned from three human group G isolates (Fahnestock et al., 1986a; Guss et al., 1986; Filpula et al., 1987). The nucleotide sequences vary in the total number of IgG-binding and albumin-binding domains (Figure 2). The sequence of the gene for the type III immunoglobulin-binding protein from strain GX7809 was shown to contain two IgG-binding repeat regions (B1–B2) and two putative albumin-binding domains (A1–A2) (Fahnestock et al., 1990). The recombinant type III protein isolated from strain GX7805 contained three putative albumin-binding domains (A1–A2–A3) and three IgG-binding domains (Fahnestock et al., 1990). The additional IgG-binding domain is a hybrid of the B1 and B2 (B2/B1) that intervenes between these repeat regions (Figure 2). Each of the IgG- and albumin-binding domains in each of the strains for which sequence data are available, consist of 55 and 37 amino acids, respectively. There is a high degree of homology among the individual albumin-binding repeat regions and among the IgG-binding domains within a given protein G molecule from a single strain as well as between strains (Björck and Åkerström, 1990a; Fahnestock et al., 1990). Significant variation between individual IgG-binding repeat regions within the type I and type II Fc-binding proteins has been observed (Guss et al., 1990; Cleary and Heath, 1990). A homology gradient has been demonstrated in the amino acid composition of adjacent repeats of protein A (EDABC) (Guss et al., 1990) and in type IIa (A1A2A3A4) immunoglobulin-binding proteins (Cleary and Heath, 1990). Functional studies have indicated that the individual domains of the types I and III immunoglobulin-binding proteins are monovalent in their reactivities with nonimmune IgG and exhibit decreased affinities compared to the native protein (Moks et al., 1986; Guss et al., 1986; Fahnestock et al., 1990). Although the repetitive domains within these proteins have similar amino acid sequences, they are not identical. It is possible that changes in a single or a small number of residues might cause subtle differences in IgG-binding potential between individual domains. For instance, the E domain, which is the most divergent repeat region of protein A, was thought initially not to be an IgG-binding domain based on protein fragmentation studies (Sjödahl, 1977). However, Moks *et al.* (1986) have demonstrated that the isolated E domain expressed in *Escherichia coli* can bind human IgG. This reactivity is of a lower affinity than the isolated B repeat region of protein A, expressed in the same *E. coli* system (Moks *et al.*, 1986). Based on inhibition studies using protein A-coated cells (Hjelm *et al.*, 1975), it has been suggested that the other repeat domains (D, A, C) of protein A bind to IgG with approximately the same affinity as the isolated B region (Moks *et al.*, 1986).

Analysis of repetitive DNA sequences would suggest that some form of gene duplication event was involved in the evolution of all of the bacterial Fc-binding proteins. The presence of repetitive DNA sequences also provides the potential for intragenic recombination and the possible generation of hybrid domains. Evidence for this type of recombinational event has been provided from the analysis of type III Fc-binding proteins isolated from the different human group G isolates. Fahnestock *et al.* (1990) have demonstrated that two type III recombinant products, cloned from separate group G strains, differed by 225 and 210 base pair duplications that occurred within the albumin- and IgG-binding regions of the gene, respectively.

Recent studies on the variability of M protein types expressed by group A streptococci have been attributed to recombination among repetitive DNA regions in group A strains (Hollingshead *et al.*, 1987). This intragenic recombination can account for both differences in the size of the M protein expressed by group A strains as well as differences in antigenicity (reviewed by Fischetti, 1989). The similarity in overall gene organization of Fc-binding proteins and the M protein raises the possibility that IgG-binding protein genes could undergo a similar type of variation. This would provide a possible mechanism for the generation of the different numbers of IgG-binding domains that have been reported for type III Fc-binding proteins isolated from different human group G isolates studied (Fahnestock *et al.*, 1990) and for the apparent heterogeneity in group A Fc-binding proteins (Boyle *et al.*, 1990; Schalén and Christensen, 1990). The putative IgG binding domains of type III-binding proteins are much more homogeneous than has been observed for type I- or type II-binding proteins and thus may reflect the recombinational potential of the different bacterial species.

Protein A is the only immunoglobulin-binding protein for which detailed X-ray crystallographic data are available. The interaction of a tryptic fragment of protein A and the Fc region of a human IgG_1 myeloma has been solved by Deisenhofer and colleagues (Deisenhofer et al., 1978; Deisenhofer, 1981). In the crystal structure fragment, two contact points between the protein A–IgG_1 Fc fragment were reported (Deisenhofer, 1981). One of these regions was considered unlikely to exist in free solution and was most probably an artifact of crystallization (Deisenhofer, 1981). The second interaction occurred in the C_H2–C_H3 region of the Fc and involved hydrophobic residues in the C_H2 domain (Met 557, Ile 253, Ser 254, Leu 309, His 310, and Glu 311) and hydrophobic residues in the C_H3 domain (His 433, His 455, Tyr 436, and Asn 434) (Deisenhofer, 1981; Burton, 1985; Woof and Burton, 1990). This X-ray crystallographic analysis represents the reactivity of only one fragment of protein A with the Fc fragment of a human IgG myeloma protein of a single subclass and may not reflect the interaction of each binding domain in protein A or its mode of interaction with other reactive IgG subclasses or reactive IgG species. Different residues could be critical for reactivity with other species or subclasses of IgG. The interaction between protein A and IgG_1, described by Deisenhofer (1981), is also consistent with the limited IgG_3 reactivity of protein A. It has been found that IgG_3 antibodies of the s^+t^+ allotype will bind to protein A, while the majority of other IgG_3 allotypes are not reactive (Ito et al., 1980; Recht et al., 1981; Haake et al., 1982; van Longhem et al., 1982; Matsumato et al., 1983). The s^+t^+ allotype has a histidine residue in place of an arginine residue at position 435 of the heavy chain. Based on the X-ray crystallographic analysis, the presence of a bulky arginine side chain would be expected to disrupt the contact between protein A and IgG_3 and hence only those IgG_3 antibodies with a histidine residue (s^+t^+ allotype) in this position would be expected to bind.

A functional comparison of protein A and the type IIa-binding protein yielded interesting results. These two distinct Fc-binding proteins have very similar reactivity profiles with human IgG subclasses. Protein A reacts with human IgG_1, IgG_2, and IgG_4 (Myhre and Kronvall, 1981; Langone, 1982). The type IIa protein binds with a lower affinity to the same human IgG subclasses as protein A (Yarnall and Boyle, 1986b,c). Of particular interest is the demonstration that certain IgG_3 myelomas of the s^+t^+ allotype have been shown to react with both protein A and the type IIa protein (Yarnall and Boyle, 1986b). Due to this functional similarity, one would predict the existence of some form of structural similarity between these bacterial binding proteins. However, these proteins have completely different primary amino acid sequences and studies using monospecific, polyclonal antisera indicate that these proteins are antigenically unrelated (Yarnall and Boyle, 1986a; Boyle and Reis, 1990). Thus, a simple structure–function relationship to account for the IgG-binding properties of these molecules has yet to be established. Throughout all of these structural investigations, it has been generally assumed that all of the IgG-binding properties of a bacterial binding protein can be attributed to the same group of specific amino acids present within the IgG-binding domains. This assumption may not be valid and the observation that structurally and antigenically distinct bacterial immunoglobulin-binding proteins display a very similar profile of immunoglobulin species and subclass reactivities would suggest that many different combinations of amino acids can mediate similar reactivities.

In our studies of bacterial binding proteins, we have made a number of findings that would suggest that all of the IgG-binding properties of a given Fc-binding protein type may not be mediated by identical amino acid residues within the IgG-binding domains. This has prompted us to propose a "cassette model" to relate the IgG-binding structures of these proteins to functional activity. In this model, we postulate that a given bacterial immunoglobulin-binding protein consists of a number of unique structures or cassettes that mediate binding to a single or limited number of immunoglobulin species, classes, or subclasses. These cassettes may be composed of either unique amino acids or in some instances, one or more key residues could be a constituent of more than one cassette (overlapping cassettes). These unique and/or overlapping cassettes may be present within each repetitive immunoglobulin-binding domain or may be represented only once in the entire binding protein. The organization of functional immunoglobulin-binding cassettes within any binding protein would define its overall reactivity. This model would predict the ability to selectively modify the binding profile of any bacterial immunoglobulin-binding protein containing more than one functional cassette. For example, if reactivity with rabbit IgG was a property of a unique cassette in protein G, then amino acids within that structure could be modified, leading to loss of reactivity with rabbit IgG without loss of binding to another IgG species such as human. However, if the rabbit and human cassettes were partially overlapping, the modification of a single amino acid within the rabbit cassette could potentially change the reactivity of the binding protein with human IgG.

If the concept of functional cassettes within an immunoglobulin-binding protein is valid, a number of experimentally testable predictions can be made. (1) The loss of binding reactivity by eliminating or modifying a unique cassette should not affect the functional activity of other binding cassettes within the protein. (2) Separation of overlapping cassettes should be achievable by modification of nonoverlapping residues that are critical for the reactivity of only one cassette. Furthermore, one might speculate that specific antibodies, which abrogate the reactivity of one cassette might not interfere with the functional activity of an unrelated cassette. Serological identification of unique antigenic cassettes might be difficult however, if either the binding structures did not constitute a unique epitope or if the different cassettes were in close proximity, such that selective inhibition by direct interaction with antibody could not be distinguished from steric hindrance. Finally, a cassette model raises the possibility of "cassette shuffling" via recombination at the DNA level among regions of repetitive DNA in bacterial strains that display high recombinational frequencies. Individual strain variation in species or subclass IgG-binding potential, similar to the antigenic variation of the M protein, might be expected to occur in certain group A strains as a consequence of cassette shuffling.

At this time, there is no definitive evidence that would support a cassette model to explain the differences in IgG species reactivity among and within different types of bacterial IgG-binding proteins. However, there is considerable evidence that some of the non-IgG binding activities of these proteins can be attributed to unique, functional cassettes. Studies of the interaction of protein A with human IgG have shown reactivity not only with IgG Fc domains, but also with Fab regions of human IgM, IgG, IgA, and IgE (Inganäs *et al.*, 1980; Inganäs, 1981; Myhre, 1990). Inhibition studies, using isolated Fc and Fab fragments of human IgG have shown that these different reactivities occur within the IgG Fc-binding repeat region of the protein A molecule (Romagnani *et al.*, 1982); however, the presence of Fab fragments does not interfere with the binding of Fc fragments and vice versa, suggesting that these binding activities are mediated by independent structures within the protein A molecule. Romagnani *et al.* (1982) have demonstrated that the modification of tyrosine residues within protein A by iodination could result in a selective loss of IgG Fc-binding activity, while the alternative reactivity with Fab regions was unaffected. These findings suggest that the classic and alternative binding reactivities of protein A are mediated by two different regions, possibly unique, functional cassettes, within the IgG-binding domains of protein A.

Protein G has been shown to react with a wide variety of species and subclasses of IgG via the Fc region (Reis *et al.*, 1984b; Reis and Boyle, 1990a), the Fab region (Myhre, 1990), various species of albumin (Björck *et al.*, 1987; Faulmann *et al.*, 1989; Björck and Åkerström, 1990a), as well as the human serum proteins α_2-macroglobulin and kininogen (Sjöbring *et al.*, 1989b). DNA sequence information, as well as competitive inhibition studies and analysis of protein G fragments generated by recombinant DNA techniques, have established that the majority of these binding reactivities of protein G occur on separate regions of the molecule (Sjöbring *et al.*, 1989b; Björck and Åkerström, 1990a; Fahnestock *et al.*, 1990). As described earlier (Figure 2), the albumin-binding regions (A1, A2, etc.) and the IgG Fc-binding regions (B1, B2, etc.) have been localized to distinct, repetitive regions at the amino- and carboxy-terminal portions of protein G, respectively (Fahnestock *et al.*, 1990; Björck and Åkerström, 1990a). Recently, it has been demonstrated that α_2-macroglobulin and kininogen interact within the Fc-binding regions of the type III molecule (Sjöbring *et al.*, 1989b). In contrast, the region responsible for alternative Fab reactivity is less well defined. In competitive inhibition studies, the Fab reactivity is not affected by the presence of IgG Fc fragments, α_2-macroglobulin, or human serum albumin (Björck *et al.*, 1987; Sjöbring *et al.*, 1988; Myhre, 1990), suggesting that this reactivity may be mediated by a unique, nonoverlapping cassette.

Additional evidence for unique, functional structures within the protein G molecule has been obtained by serological approaches in our laboratory. A polyclonal anti-protein G antibody, prepared in chickens immunized with wild type protein G, was separated on a column of immobilized, recombinant protein G. The recombinant protein G that was immobilized contained only the IgG-binding domains of the binding protein. The sequences encoding the albumin binding domains had been eliminated by recombinant DNA technology. By contrast, the immunogen used to prepare the anti-protein G antibody was the native protein, containing both IgG- and albumin-binding domains. The polyclonal antiserum passed over the recombinant protein G column was recovered in two fractions. The first fraction passed directly through the column. The second fraction was eluted from the column at low pH. The ability of each fraction, following neutralization if necessary, to inhibit the binding of wild type protein G to either immobilized human serum albumin or immobilized human IgG was compared with the unfractionated antibody (Table 1). The unfractionated antibody inhibited the binding of wild type protein G to both human serum albumin and human IgG. By contrast, the serum that passed directly through the immobilized, recombinant protein G column inhibited the binding of wild type protein G to immobilized human serum albumin, but not to immobilized IgG alone. The antibody eluted from the immobilized, recombinant protein G column inhibited the binding of wild type protein G to immobilized human IgG and was without effect on its interaction with immobilized human serum albumin (Table 1). The ability to demonstrate such distinct reactivities with polyclonal antibodies raises the possibility of being able to epitope map functional domains of protein G using a panel of monoclonal antibodies. The ability of different monoclonal antibodies to selectively inhibit different species or subclass reactivities

TABLE 1
Demonstration of Antigenically and Functionally Distinct IgG- and Albumin-Binding Domains in Wild Type Protein G

Antiserum	Inhibition (%) of Wild Type Protein G Binding	
	Immobilized HuIgG[a]	Immobilized HSA[b]
Chicken anti-wild type protein G	95	95
Chicken anti-wild type protein G; Fraction I[c]	<10	95
Chicken anti-wild type protein G; Fraction II[d]	95	<10

[a] HuIgG: human IgG.
[b] HSA: human serum albumin.
[c] Fraction I contains antibodies that failed to bind to a column of immobilized recombinant protein G (devoid of albumin-binding domains).
[d] Fraction II contains antibodies that bound to and were eluted selectively from the recombinant protein G column.

might help identify unique cassettes and facilitate a more detailed structure–function analysis.

Sjöbring et al. (1989a) have provided additional support for protein G being composed of distinct binding cassettes. They have identified certain isolates of groups C and G streptococci that display IgG-binding activity in the absence of reactivity with albumin. This has been shown to be due to a deletion from the protein G gene of the sequence encoding the albumin-binding region.

While the experimental evidence we have presented would support the concept of distinct functional cassettes being involved in the different binding properties of protein A and protein G, we have presented no evidence thus far, to support the concept that the IgG species and subclass binding activities of these proteins may be dependent on more than one structure within an assigned immunoglobulin-binding domain. The most compelling evidence for the existence of distinct IgG-binding cassettes comes from comparative studies of the IgG species reactivity profiles of one form of a recombinant protein G molecule (Pharmacia Fine Chemicals, Piscataway, New Jersey), studied before and after iodination (Faulmann et al., 1989). The results of these studies, summarized in Table 2, demonstrate that this form of recombinant protein G reacted well with human, rabbit, and goat IgG. However, following radioiodination, using the mild lactoperoxidase method, the functional activity of the labeled protein is markedly different (Table 2). Once labeled, this form of protein

TABLE 2[a]
Binding Profile of One Form of a Recombinant Protein G Before and After Radioiodination

	IgG-Binding Activity		
Sample	Human	Rabbit	Goat
Pharmacia[b] recombinant protein G	+++[c]	+++	+++
^{125}I-labeled Pharmacia recombinant protein G	+++	−[d]	++[e]

[a] Adapted from Faulmann et al. (1989), with permission.
[b] Pharmacia Fine Chemicals, Piscataway, New Jersey.
[c] +++: strong binding.
[d] −: no significant binding.
[e] ++: intermediate binding.

G reacts well with human and goat IgG but displays a selective loss of reactivity with rabbit IgG (Faulmann et al., 1989). These findings would be consistent with the suggestion that within the protein G molecule, reactivity with rabbit IgG is associated with a unique cassette that is separate and distinct from the cassette that mediates reactivity with human and goat IgG.

The existence of distinct, functional IgG-binding cassettes predicts that it would be possible to select, from within a given strain, a variant or mutant that displayed different species-reactivity profiles. Previous studies from our laboratory have demonstrated the use of a colony blotting procedure to monitor expression of immunoglobulin-binding proteins by individual bacterial colonies (Yarnall et al., 1984). This approach has been used to study expression of the immunoglobulin-binding protein of a *Streptococcus zooepidemicus* isolate, S-212 (Reis et al., 1988a; Reis and Boyle, 1990b). This isolate initially displayed heterogeneity in its reactivity with goat Fc fragments (Reis and Boyle, 1990b). A single colony that expressed high levels of surface goat Fc-binding activity was selected and expanded. The resulting substrain, S-212-1, displayed a homogeneous pattern of reactivity when individual colonies were probed with goat, human, or mouse IgG (Reis and Boyle, 1990b). By contrast, colonies from within this selected substrain (S-212-1) demonstrated a high degree of heterogeneity in their reactivity with rat IgG (Reis et al., 1988a; Reis and Boyle, 1990b).

When a substrain of the original S-212 strain was selected using rat immunoglobulin as a probe (S-212-d), a colony that exhibited a high level of reactivity with rat IgG could be selected. This isolate was expanded and the colony selection procedure repeated on two further occasions. Colonies from the isolated strain (S-212-B1) obtained following this selection procedure displayed a homogeneous, high level of binding when screened in the colony blot assay with rat IgG as the probe (Reis *et al.*, 1988a; Reis and Boyle, 1990b). Furthermore, this selected strain displayed a similar, uniform colony reactivity pattern when probed with human, goat, or mouse IgG (Reis and Boyle, 1990b). Thus, depending on the method of selection, a single strain could yield distinct colonies that display different reactivity profiles. These findings suggest that the rat binding cassette was distinct from the human, mouse, and goat binding cassette(s) and that it was possible to select strains that expressed these properties independently. It is of interest that, depending on the species of IgG used to select high-expressing colonies, different functional profiles were obtained, i.e., when goat IgG was used as the probe, enhanced reactivity for mouse and human, but not rat, was observed. When rat IgG was used as the selective probe, the resulting strain displayed enhanced reactivity toward all four species. This finding would be consistent with the possibility that the rat cassette is not a unique structure but that it also contains critical elements of the cassette(s) responsible for the human, mouse, and goat reactivities of this strain, i.e., partially overlapping cassettes. It should be remembered that these studies were carried out with intact bacteria, so there are other potential explanations for these experimental findings.

The possibility that intragenic recombination among repetitive DNA sequences in immunoglobulin-binding proteins could contribute to different immunoglobulin-binding profiles would be most likely to be observed among group A streptococcal isolates. In 1986, Yarnall and Boyle demonstrated that the IgG-binding properties of one group A isolate, 64/14, were attributable to two distinct IgG-binding proteins designated type IIa and type IIb (Yarnall and Boyle, 1986c). The type IIa protein was responsible for reactivity with human IgG_1, IgG_2, IgG_4, rabbit IgG, and pig IgG. The type IIb protein bound exclusively to human IgG_3 (Yarnall and Boyle, 1986a–c; Faulmann and Boyle, 1990). The type IIa- and type IIb-binding proteins were found to be antigenically closely related and expressed independently on the cell surface (Yarnall and Boyle, 1986a). Other investigators have reported the isolation of type II Fc-binding proteins from different group A strains that display the combined immunoglobulin-binding reactivities of the type IIa and IIb proteins in a single molecule (Havlícek, 1978; Grubb *et al.*, 1982). This finding raises the possibility that a type II protein containing type IIa and type IIb functional cassettes exists in certain group A strains and that by some form of genetic rearrangement may give rise to strains expressing type IIa or type IIb activities as independent molecules.

Boyle *et al.* (1990) have described a diverse pattern of human IgG subclass reactivities among group A isolates. Some isolates have been shown to bind all four human IgG subclasses while others bind three, two, one, or zero. In addition to this variation between different strains, preliminary studies in our laboratory suggest that a single group A strain can lose certain of its subclass-binding potential during laboratory subculture. One could predict that some form of recombinational event at the DNA level could lead to the loss of a cassette and account for the differences in IgG-binding profiles observed among and within group A strains. In light of the structural similarities that exist between the DNA sequences of the type IIa Fc-binding protein and the M protein (Heath and Cleary, 1987, 1989; Cleary and Heath, 1990), it would be tempting to speculate that these variants could be due to intragenic recombination of repeating nucleotide segments, which code for the repetitive IgG-binding domains. This would provide the group A streptococcus with a mechanism for "cassette shuffling" via recombination of nucleotide segments that code for these various binding segments with a resulting variation in the ability of the protein products to interact with different human IgG subclasses.

The analysis of the structure–function relationships of bacterial immunoglobulin-binding proteins requires a great deal more experimental examination. The validity of the cassette model, which we have proposed here, can only be tested by further experimentation involving molecular genetics, chemical modification, and X-ray crystallographic analysis. The design of future studies should take into consideration the possibility that the binding interactions for reactive subclasses or species of immunoglobulins may not all be identical. Indeed the variation in DNA sequences noted between repetitive immunoglobulin-binding domains within a given bacterial binding protein may also influence the species reactivity of the resulting individual domains within the same molecule. A much more focused analysis of IgG-binding domain–IgG interaction with well defined reagents is warranted and X-ray crystallographic analysis should not be restricted to a single fragment of either the binding protein or to one species or subclass of IgG. The use of molecular genetic approaches to prepare individual binding domains combined with site-directed mutagenesis should lead to a much clearer understanding of the structure–function relationships of bacterial immunoglobulin-binding proteins.

IV. Applications Involving Immunoglobulin-Binding Proteins—Future Trends

The applications described in this volume for protein A and protein G are liable to be extended to other bacterial immunoglobulin-binding proteins like protein L (Myhre and Erntell, 1985; Björck, 1988), protein P (Lindahl and Kronvall, 1988; Lindahl, 1990), and the IgA-specific binding proteins (Christensen and Oxeluis, 1975; Russell-Jones *et al.*, 1984; Lindahl *et al.*, 1990; Brady and Boyle, 1990; Cleat and Timmis, 1990). The future directions are expected to fall into three major categories, (i) identification of new binding proteins with unique specificities and reactivities, (ii) manipulation of existing proteins to obtain more desirable reagents, and (iii) potential therapeutic applications.

A. Identification of New Bacterial Immunoglobulin-Binding Proteins

Over the past decade, a large number of new, unique, bacterial surface structures that react in a selective way with different immunoglobulin isotypes have been identified. In addition, bacterial receptors for many nonimmunoglobulin serum proteins have also been described. The ability to identify bacteria that can bind selectively to any protein of interest has been described in Chapter 2. Approaches to select high-expressing strains for isolation and characterization of these molecules have been described in Chapters 3–6. These general approaches are applicable to any bacterial binding protein and make the isolation and practical exploitation of these proteins relatively straightforward. To date, the majority of studies have been directed toward the use of IgG-binding proteins that display a wide range of species and subclass reactivities. These reagents have revolutionized immunoglobulin purification procedures and in particular, have facilitated the detection and isolation of monoclonal antibodies. The availability of proteins with nonimmune reactivity for other isotypes of immunoglobulins would have many practical applications for immunodiagnostics and for studies of humoral immunity. For example, a selective reagent for the μ heavy chain of human IgM could be used in assays for the detection of IgM antibodies as an early indicator of exposure to an infectious agent. Although many laboratories have attempted to find such a μ chain-specific binding protein, no IgM-specific bacterial binding protein has been identified to date. By contrast, a number of IgA-specific binding proteins have been described associated with certain group A (Christensen and Oxeluis, 1975; Christensen and Schalén, 1990; Lindahl *et al.*, 1990) and group B

(Russell-Jones *et al.*, 1984; Brady and Boyle, 1990; Cleat and Timmis, 1987, 1990) streptococcal isolates. These proteins are expected to be important reagents for the study of mucosal immunity. Although the use of bacterial IgA-binding proteins has not yet progressed beyond the research laboratory, we and others have demonstrated the potential for these proteins in detection of IgA (Russell-Jones *et al.*, 1984; Brady and Boyle, 1989b; Brady, 1989). Our experience has suggested that the properties of monomeric and dimeric IgA ± secretory component make it more difficult to quantify antibodies of the IgA isotype accurately using a bacterial IgA Fc-binding protein isolated from a group B streptococci than it is to quantify IgG antibodies using either protein A or protein G (Brady and Boyle, 1989a). It is, however, likely that once suitable tracer forms of bacterial IgA-binding proteins have been prepared and assay conditions for measuring IgA have been optimized, these selective bacterial binding proteins will prove to be of enormous value both in the research laboratory and in clinical immunology–microbiology laboratories. Similarly, specific proteins that would bind to human IgE would have potential value for use in radioallergosorbent assays (RAST).

At present, the major focus of research on bacterial immunoglobulin-binding proteins has been directed toward isolation and characterization of binding proteins that have been found by systematic screening of different isolates for reactivity with various species and subclasses of IgG. This approach has led to the identification of six types of IgG-binding proteins (Boyle and Reis, 1987), binding proteins for IgA (Lindahl *et al.*, 1990; Brady and Boyle, 1990; Cleat and Timmis, 1990), IgD-binding proteins (Forsgren and Grubb, 1979; Tedder, 1990), proteins binding to $F(ab')_2$ regions (Myhre, 1990; Lindahl, 1990), proteins binding to light chains (Myhre and Erntell, 1985; Björck and Åkerström, 1990b), as well as many nonimmune reactivities that have not, as yet, been completely defined (Yarnall *et al.*, 1988; Widders *et al.*, 1985; van der Merwe and Stegeman, 1985). The increasing array of organisms found to express immunoglobulin-binding proteins suggests that specific binding proteins for any species, isotype, or subclass will be identified if a large enough assortment of bacteria are screened. This possibility raises the prospect of screening bacterial isolates for a desired activity using approaches similar to those developed for screening monoclonal antibodies. Rather than selecting a bacterial isolate and determining its binding properties (i.e., screening a given hybridoma with different antigens to determine its specificity), we will start by defining the binding property desired and then screen a large selection of organisms until one that binds the ligand of interest is identified (i.e., define the antigen and screen for a hybridoma with which it will react). For this approach to be feasible, rapid screening and selection methods to identify bacteria with any desired reactivity will have to be developed.

Recent studies of bacterial immunoglobulin-binding proteins have been directed toward identifying molecules with broad species and subclass reactivities in order to obtain reagents that can be used for as many applications as possible. In the future, we expect that the trend will be toward the identification and utilization of more selective reagents. For example, the type IIb-binding protein that binds exclusively to human IgG_3 would provide the basis for development of assays to measure subclass-restricted responses or to compare the distribution of IgG_3 antibodies versus total IgG antibodies following exposure to different antigens. The availability of other human IgG subclass-selective reagents would be of value to monitor infections with certain bacteria, viruses, or parasites that are known to induce subclass-restricted responses.

The selection and/or generation of specific reagents for a given application is likely to be of major importance in determining the future directions of practical procedures involving bacterial immunoglobulin-binding proteins. The availability of bacterial binding proteins with a high affinity for constant regions of human, rat, or mouse immunoglobulin subclasses would have important practical applications for monoclonal antibody technology and for immunofluorescent procedures involving these monoclonal antibodies. The value of highly selective binding proteins, not only for immunoglobulin molecules, but also for other serum proteins is expected to continue to provide an impetus for studying the interaction of bacterial surface molecules with serum proteins.

B. Manipulation of Bacterial IgG-Binding Proteins

The use of recombinant technology has already had a major impact on immunoglobulin-binding protein technology and this trend is likely to continue. The ability to express staphylococcal and streptococcal genes in *E. coli* or *Bacillus* (Guss *et al.*, 1990; Fahnestock and Fisher, 1987; Cleary and Heath, 1990; Björck and Åkerström, 1990a; Fahnestock *et al.*, 1986a,b, 1990; Lindahl *et al.*, 1990; Cleat and Timmis, 1990) has enabled large quantities of immunoglobulin-binding proteins to be prepared without the necessity of growing large volumes of human pathogens. Furthermore, the ability to manipulate gene sequences has enabled different forms of the various binding proteins to be prepared (Moks *et al.*, 1986; Cleary and Heath, 1990; Guss *et al.*, 1986; Fahnestock *et al.*, 1990; Eliasson *et al.*, 1988). For example, the majority of recombinant forms of protein G that are available commercially have been manipulated to remove the albumin-binding domains. In addition, Eliasson and colleagues have demonstrated the feasibility of producing hybrid protein A–protein G molecules (Eliasson *et al.*, 1988, 1989). The ability to manipulate coding sequences in this way is liable to be of great importance in the future, not only for understanding the structure–function relationships of these proteins, but also for the generation of more selective immunoglobulin-binding reagents. If it is demonstrated that unique cassettes are responsible for the selective IgG-binding properties of these proteins, as we proposed earlier, then genetic engineering approaches represent the optimal strategy for generating large quantities of these selective binding structures. In addition to the applications of immunoglobulin-binding proteins to immunotechnology, Uhlén and his colleagues have demonstrated the value of plasmid vectors containing protein A sequences for many applications in molecular biology (Nilsson *et al.*, 1985; Abrahmsén *et al.*, 1986; Uhlén and Abrahmsén, 1989). DNA sequences inserted into appropriate restriction enzyme sites in these vectors result in the expression of fusion proteins that contain IgG-binding domains from protein A at the N-terminus. This property then enables the rapid affinity purification of the fusion protein on a column of immobilized IgG (Nilsson et al., 1985; Abrahmsén et al., 1986; Uhlén and Abrahmsén, 1989).

There is no question that genetic engineering technology will play a critical role in the future development and understanding of bacterial immunoglobulin-binding proteins. Indeed, the recombinant form of the IgA-binding protein associated with certain group A streptococci has been produced and isolated by Lindahl and colleagues, who were unable to isolate the wild type protein by classical protein purification procedures (Lindahl *et al.*, 1990).

C. Potential Therapeutic Applications

In this volume, the focus of applications has been toward *in vitro* techniques. Immobilized bacterial immunoglobulin-binding proteins have also been used for treatment of cancer and immune complex disease. The value of immunoglobulin-binding proteins in the treatment of disease remains controversial. For example, regression of tumors in rats or dogs treated by passage of serum over a column of immobilized protein A or with serum absorbed with *Staphylococcus aureus* Cowan I has been reported (Gordon *et al.*, 1983; Ray *et al.*, 1982; Steele *et al.*, 1974; Holohan *et al.*, 1980). However, in some studies similar findings have been observed when the serum was passed over a Sepharose column lacking any protein A (Sukumar *et al.*, 1984). Furthermore, the affinity of rat IgG for protein A is extremely low and consequently, significant removal of antibody or antibody–antigen complexes by these treatments would be most unlikely. The observation that many wild type preparations of protein A are contaminated with enterotoxins (Schrezenmeier and Fleischer, 1987) may further complicate the interpretation of these studies. Studies by Das and Langone (1989) have addressed the anti-tumor effects of protein A and staphylococcal enterotoxins and have shown, in a mouse tumor model system, that the active anti-tumor agent is protein A and that the contaminating enterotoxins present, while mitogenic, do not have anti-tumor properties.

Steele *et al.* (1974) have demonstrated the ability to detect cytotoxic anti-tumor antibodies in tumor-bearing serum following removal of blocking factors after absorption with *Staphylococcus aureus* Cowan I. Bansal *et al.* (1978) have followed up on this observation to determine the potential, therapeutic value of removing blocking factors in the treatment of patients with human colon carcinoma. Terman *et al.* (1981) treated five patients suffering from breast cancer by passage of their serum over an extracorporeal protein A column. Tumor regression was reported in three of five patients and these investigators suggest that the protein A column might be removing tumor–antigen–antibody complexes, resulting in "unblocking" the patients own immune system and releasing anti-tumor antibodies (Terman *et al.*, 1981). This study has been critically reviewed in an editorial in the same issue of the journal by Hellström and Hellström (1981), who raised a number of practical problems with the study.

In 1988, an extensive multicenter trial of the use of extracorporeal immunotherapy using columns of immobilized protein A in the treatment of patients with malignant disease was published (Messerschmidt *et al.*, 1988). Complete remission was not observed in any patient, although partial remissions were noted in some patients. Overall, there was no compelling evidence from these studies for any long term, beneficial effect of this therapeutic strategy. This study did, however, demonstrate that it was possible to carry out the extracorporeal procedure without serious adverse reactions in the patients.

The use of immobilized bacterial immunoglobulin-binding proteins in the treatment of immune complex disease is based on a more solid theoretical basis. The clinical severity of patients suffering from immune complex disease can be correlated with their level of circulating immune complexes (Dixon *et al.*, 1988; Klinman and Steinberg, 1988). The physical removal of immune complexes from the serum of patients in this population might therefore be expected to be beneficial. The results obtained in the treatment of patients with immune complex disease using extracorporeal protein A columns have recently been reviewed and demonstrate some potential benefit (Ainsworth *et al.*, 1990). This therapeutic strategy is complicated by the ability of immobilized bacterial immunoglobulin-binding proteins, in the presence of immunoglobulins, to activate the classical pathway and generate the complement anaphylatoxins, C3a and C5a (Boyle, 1990b). In addition, many inert supports to which bacterial immunoglobulin-binding proteins are immobilized have been shown to be capable of activating the alternate complement pathway in the absence of either immunoglobulins or immunoglobulin-binding proteins (Langone *et al.*, 1984; Nakanishi *et al.*, 1985). The development of better supports and methods to immobilize bacterial immunoglobulin-binding proteins, which minimize the potential problems associated with complement split product generation are expected to occur in the near future.

The potential of bacterial immunoglobulin-binding proteins for the treatment of immune complex disease will require additional, carefully controlled, double-blind clinical trials. If the therapeutic strategy of physical removal of immune complexes is shown to benefit patients with autoimmune disorders and immune complex disease, then attempts will be made to find more selective reagents. The use of protein A was initially proposed because there was a difference in affinity for IgG in complexes compared with unbound IgG (McDougal *et al.*, 1979). If this differential in binding activity between free and complexed IgG could be increased by 10–100 fold, then the ability to remove complexes in the presence of a large molar excess of monomeric IgG would be enhanced. The isolation and exploitation of more selective bacterial-binding proteins will be the focus of many laboratories in the next decade. Once again, the driving force for any practical application involving bacterial immunoglobulin-binding proteins will be directed toward identifying the problem, determining the limitations of current reagents, and modifying or finding new reagents that will achieve the desired result.

V. Summary

Bacterial immunoglobulin-binding proteins represent a family of functionally related molecules that have clearly demonstrated their versatility for use in immunotechnology. In the future, the identification and/or generation of new binding proteins with increased selectivity is liable to be the focus of the biotechnologist. Let us hope that this focus toward practicality will not dampen the enthusiasm of scientists interested in molecular pathogenesis, who will continue to ask why God gave bacteria these molecules, and that of the molecular biologists, protein chemists, and X-ray crystallographers, who will seek to unravel the nature of the selective immunoglobulin-binding properties of these bacterial binding proteins.

References

Abrahmsén, L., Moks, T., Nilsson, B., and Uhlén, M. (1986). *Nucleic Acids Res.* **14,** 7487–7500.
Ainsworth, S. K., Chen, Z., and Pilia, P. A. (1990). In "Bacterial Immunoglobulin-Binding Proteins" (M. D. P. Boyle, ed.), Vol. 1, pp. 335–346. Academic Press, San Diego.
Åkerström, B., Nielsen, E., and Björck, L. (1987). *J. Biol. Chem.* **262,** 1338–1339.
Bansal, S. C., Bansal, B. R., Thomas, H. L., Siegel, P. D., Rhoads, J. E., Cooper, D. R., Terman, D. S., and Mark, R. (1978). *Cancer* **42,** 1–18.
Björck, L. (1988). *J. Immunol.* **140,** 1194–1197.
Björck, L., and Åkerström, B. (1990a). In "Bacterial Immunoglobulin-Binding Proteins" (M. D. P. Boyle, ed.), Vol. 1, pp. 113–126. Academic Press, San Diego.
Björck, L., and Åkerström, B. (1990b). In "Bacterial Immunoglobulin-Binding Proteins" (M. D. P. Boyle, ed.), Vol. 1, pp. 267–278. Academic Press, San Diego.
Björck, L., and Kronvall, G. (1984). *J. Immunol.* **133,** 964–974.
Björck, L., Kastern, W., Lindahl, G., and Widebäck, K. (1987). *Mol. Immunol.* **24,** 1113–1122.
Boyle, M. D. P. (1984). *Biotechniques* **2,** 334–340.
Boyle, M. D. P. (1990a). In "Bacterial Immunoglobulin-Binding Proteins" (M. D. P. Boyle, ed.), Vol. 1, pp. 17–28. Academic Press, San Diego.
Boyle, M. D. P. (1990b). In "Bacterial Immunoglobulin-Binding Proteins" (M. D. P. Boyle, ed.), Vol. 1, pp. 295–304. Academic Press, San Diego.
Boyle, M. D. P., and Reis, K. J. (1987). *Biotechnology* **5,** 697–703.
Boyle, M. D. P., and Reis, K. J. (1990). In "Bacterial Immunoglobulin-Binding Proteins" (M. D. P. Boyle, ed.), Vol. 1, pp. 175–186. Academic Press, San Diego.
Boyle, M. D. P., Wallner, W. A., von Mering, G. O., and Reis, K. J. (1985). *Mol. Immunol.* **22,** 1115–1121.
Boyle, M. D. P., Faulmann, E. L., Otten, R., and Heath, D. (1990). In "Microbial Determinants of Virulence and Host Response" (E. M. Ayoub, G. H. Cassell, W. C. Branche, T. J. Henry, eds). 1990 American Society for Microbiology, Washington, DC. 19–44.
Brady, L. J. (1989). Ph.D. dissertation, University of Florida, Gainesville.
Brady, L. J. (1990). In "Bacterial Immunoglobulin-Binding Proteins" (M. D. P. Boyle, ed.), Vol. 1, pp. 365–374. Academic Press, San Diego.
Brady, L. J., and Boyle, M. D. P. (1989a). *Infect. Immun.* **57,** 1573–1581.
Brady, L. J., and Boyle, M. D. P. (1989b). *Proc. Am. Soc. Microbiol.* 146a.
Brady, L. J., and Boyle, M. D. P. (1990). In "Bacterial Immunoglobulin-Binding Proteins" (M. D. P. Boyle, ed.), Vol. 1, pp. 201–225. Academic Press, San Diego.
Burova, L. A., Christensen, P., Grubb, R., Jonsson, A., Samuelsson, G., Schalén, C., and Svensson, M. L. (1980). *Acta Pathol. Microbiol. Scand. Sect. B* **88,** 199–205.
Burton, D. R. (1985). *Mol. Immunol.* **22,** 161–206.

Chapter 25. Future Trends

Christensen, P., and Oxeluis, V.-A. (1975). *Acta Pathol. Microbiol. Scand. Sect. C* **83**, 184–188.
Christensen, P., and Schalén, C. (1990). *In* "Bacterial Immunoglobulin-Binding Proteins" (M. D. P. Boyle, ed.), Vol. 1, pp. 347–364. Academic Press, San Diego.
Cleary, P. P., and Heath, D. G. (1990). *In* "Bacterial Immunoglobulin-Binding Proteins" (M. D. P. Boyle, ed.), Vol. 1, pp. 83–100. Academic Press, San Diego.
Cleat, P. H., and Timmis, K. N. (1987). *Infect. Immun.* **55**, 11151–1155.
Cleat, P. H., and Timmis, K. N. (1990). *In* "Bacterial Immunoglobulin-Binding Proteins" (M. D. P. Boyle, ed.), Vol. 1, pp. 225–233. Academic Press, San Diego.
Das, C., and Langone, J. J. (1989). *J. Immunol.* **142**, 2943–2948.
Deisenhofer, J. (1981). *Biochemistry* **20**, 2361–2370.
Deisenhofer, J., Jones, I. A., Huber, R., Sjödahl, J., and Sjöquist, J. (1978). *Hoppe-Seyler's Z. Physiol. Chem.* **359**, 975–979.
Dixon, F. J., Cochrane, C. C., and Theofilopoulos, A. N. (1988). *In* "Immunological Diseases" (M. Samter, D. W. Talmage, M. M. Frank, K. F. Austen, and H. N. Claman, eds.), Vol. I. pp. 233–260. Little, Brown, Boston.
Duggleby, C. L., and Jones, S. A. (1983). *Nucleic Acids Res.* **11**, 3065–3076.
Eliasson, M., Olsson, A., Palmcrantz, E., Wiberg, K., Inganäs, M., Guss, B., Lindberg, M., and Uhlén, M. (1988). *J. Biol. Chem.* **263**, 4323–4327.
Eliasson, M., Andersson, R., Olsson, A., Wigzell, H., and Uhlén, M. (1989). *J. Immunol.* **142**, 575–581.
Endresen, C. (1979). *Acta Pathol. Microbiol. Scand. Sect. C* **87**, 185–189.
Erntell, M., Myhre, E. B., Sjöbring, U., and Björck, L. (1988). *Mol. Immunol.* **25**, 121–126.
Fahnestock, S. R., and Fisher, K. E. (1987). *Appl. Environ. Microbiol.* **53**, 379–384.
Fahnestock, S. R., Alexander, P., Nagle, J., and Filpula, D. (1986a). *J. Bacteriol.* **167**, 870–880.
Fahnestock, S. R., Saunders, C. W., Guyer, M. S., Löfdahl, S., Guss, B., Uhlén, M., and Lindberg, M. (1986b). *J. Bacteriol.* **165**, 1011–1014.
Fahnestock, S. R., Alexander, P., Fipula, D., and Nagle, J. (1990). *In* "Bacterial Immunoglobulin-Binding Proteins" (M. D. P. Boyle, ed.), Vol. 1, pp. 133–148. Academic Press, San Diego.
Faulmann, E. L., and Boyle, M. D. P. (1990). *In* "Bacterial Immunoglobulin-Binding Proteins" (M. D. P. Boyle, ed.), Vol. 1, pp. 69–82. Academic Press, San Diego.
Faulmann, E. L., Otten, R. A., Barrett, D. J., and Boyle, M. D. P. (1989). *J. Immunol. Methods* **123**, 269–281.
Filpula, D., Alexander, P., and Fahnestock, S. R. (1987). *Nucleic Acids Res.* **15**, 7210.
Fischetti, V. A. (1989). *Clin. Microbiol. Rev.* **2**, 285–314.
Fischetti, V. A., Parry, D. A. D., Tris, B. L., Hollingshead, S. K., Scott, J. R., and Manjula, B. N. (1988). *Proteins Struct. Funct. Genet.* **3**, 60–69.
Fisher, P. R., Daly, J. A., Lindsay, A. N., and Gooch, W. M. (1986). *Diagn. Microbiol. Infect. Dis.* **4**, 177–179.
Forsgren, A., and Grubb, A. (1979). *J. Immunol.* **122**, 1468–1472.
Gordon, B. R., Matus, R. E., Saal, S. D., MacEwen, E. G., Hurvitz, A. I., Stenzel, K. H., and Rubin, A. L. (1983). *J. Natl. Cancer Inst.* **70**, 11127–1133.
Grubb, A., Grubb, R., Christensen, P., and Schalén, C. (1982). *Int. Arch. Allergy Appl. Immunol.* **67**, 369–376.
Guss, B., Eliasson, M., Olsson, A., Uhlén, M., Frej, A. K., Jornvall, H., Flock, J. I., and Lindberg, M. (1986). *EMBO J.* **5**, 1567–1575.
Guss, B., Lindberg, M., and Uhlén, M. (1990). *In* "Bacterial Immunoglobulin-Binding Proteins" (M. D. P. Boyle, ed.), Vol. 1, pp. 29–40. Academic Press, San Diego.

Haake, D. A., Franklin, E. C., and Frangione, B. (1982). *J. Immunol.* **129,** 190–192.
Havlícek, J. (1978). *Exp. Cell Biol.* **46,** 146–151.
Heath, D. G., and Cleary, P. P. (1987). *Infect. Immun.* **55,** 1233–1238.
Heath, D. G., and Cleary, P. P. (1989). *Proc. Natl. Acad. Sci. U.S.A.* **86,** 4741–4745.
Heath, D. G., Boyle, M. D. P., and Cleary, P. P. (1990). Submitted.
Hellström, K. E., and Hellström, I. (1981). *New Engl. J. Med.* **305,** 1215–1216.
Hjelm, H., Sjödahl, J., and Sjöquist, J. (1975). *Eur. J. Biochem.* **57,** 395–403.
Hollingshead, S. K., Fischetti, V. A., and Scott, J. R. (1987). *Mol. Gen. Genet.* **207,** 196.
Holohan, T., Bowles, C., and Deisseroth, A. (1980). *Proc. Am. Assoc. Cancer Res.* **21,** 241.
Inganäs, M. (1981). *Scand. J. Immunol.* **13,** 343–352.
Inganäs, M., Johannson, S. G. O., and Bennch, H. H. (1980). *Scand. J. Immunol.* **12,** 23–31.
Ito, S., Miyazaki, T., and Matsumoto, H. (1980). *Proc. Jpn. Acad.* **56,** 226.
Klinman, D. M., and Steinberg, A. D. (1988). In "Immunological Diseases" (M. Samter, D. W. Talmage, M. M. Frank, K. F. Austen, and H. N. Claman, eds.), Vol. II, pp. 1335–1364. Little, Brown and Company, Boston.
Langone, J. J. (1982). *Adv. Immunol.* **32,** 157–252.
Langone, J. J., Boyle, M. D. P., and Borsos, T. (1978a). *J. Immunol.* **121,** 327–332.
Langone, J. J., Boyle, M. D. P., and Borsos, T. (1978b). *J. Immunol.* **121,** 333–339.
Langone, J. J., Das, C., Bennett, D., and Terman, D. S. (1984). *J. Immunol.* **133,** 1057–1063.
Lindahl, G. (1990). In "Bacterial Immunoglobulin-Binding Proteins" (M. D. P. Boyle, ed.), Vol. 1, pp. 257–266. Academic Press, San Diego.
Lindahl, G., and Kronvall, G. (1988). *J. Immunol.* **140,** 1223–1227.
Lindahl, G., Åkerström, B., Frithz, E., Hedén, L.-O., and Steinberg, L. (1990). In "Bacterial Immunoglobulin-Binding Proteins" (M. D. P. Boyle, ed.), Vol. 1, pp. 193–200. Academic Press, San Diego.
Lofdahl, S., Guss, B., Uhlén, M., Phillipson, L., and Lindberg, M. (1983). *Proc. Natl. Acad. Sci. U.S.A.* **80,** 697–701.
Matsumato, H., Ito, S., Miyakzki, T., and Ohta, T. (1983). *J. Immunol.* **131,** 1865–1870.
McDougal, J. S., Redecha, P. B., Inman, R. D., and Christian, C. L. (1979). *J. Clin. Invest.* **63,** 627–636.
Messerschmidt, G. L., Henry, D. H., Snyder, H. W., Jr., Bertram, J., Mittelman, A., Ainsworth, S., Fiore, J., Viola, M. V., Louie, J., Ambinder, E., MacKintosh, F. R., Higby, D. J., O'Brien, P., Kiprov, D., Hamburger, M., Balint, J. P., Jr., Fisher, L. D., Perkins, W., Pinsky, C. M., and Jones, F. R. (1988). *J. Clin. Oncol.* **6,** 203–212.
Miller, J. F., Mekalanos, J. J., and Falkow, S. (1989). *Science* **243,** 916–922.
Moks, T., Abrahmsen, L., Nilsson, B., Hellman, V., Sjöquist, J., and Uhlén, M. (1986). *Eur. J. Biochem.* **156,** 637–643.
Myhre, E. B. (1990). In "Bacterial Immunoglobulin-Binding Proteins" (M. D. P. Boyle, ed.), Vol. 1, pp. 243–256. Academic Press, San Diego.
Myhre, E. B., and Erntell, M. (1985). *Mol. Immunol.* **22,** 879–885.
Myhre, E. B., and Kronvall, G. (1980). *Infect. Immun.* **27,** 6–14.
Myhre, E. B., and Kronvall, G. (1981). In "Basic Concepts of *Streptococci* and Streptococcal Diseases" (S. E. Holm and P. Christensen, eds.), pp. 209–210. Reedbook, Chertsey, Surrey.
Myhre, E. B., Holmberg, O., and Kronvall, G. (1979). *Infect. Immun.* **25,** 1–10.
Nakanishi, K., Zbar, B., and Borsos, T. (1985). *Cancer Res.* **45,** 4122–4127.
Nilsson, B., Abrahamsén, L., and Uhlén, M. (1985). *EMBO J.* **4,** 1075–1080.
Phillips, G. N., Flicker, P. F., Cohen, C., Manjula, B. N., and Fischetti, V. A. (1981). *Proc. Natl. Acad. Sci. U.S.A.* **78,** 4689–4693.
Poirier, T. P., Kehoe, M. A., Whitnack, E., and Beachey, E. H. (1987). In "Streptococcal

Genetics'' (J. J. Ferretti and R. Curtis, III, eds.), pp. 117–120. American Society for Microbiology, Washington, D.C.

Ray, P. K., Raychaudhuri, S., and Allen, P. (1982). *Cancer Res.* **42**, 4970–4974.

Recht, B., Frangione, B., Frankun, E., and van Longhem, E. (1981). *J. Immunol.* **127**, 917–923.

Reis, K. J., and Boyle, M. D. P. (1990a). *In* ''Bacterial Immunoglobulin-Binding Proteins'' (M. D. P. Boyle, ed.), Vol. 1, pp. 101–112. Academic Press, San Diego.

Reis, K. J., and Boyle, M. D. P. (1990b). *In* ''Bacterial Immunoglobulin-Binding Proteins'' (M. D. P. Boyle, ed.), Vol. 1, pp. 165–174. Academic Press, San Diego.

Reis, K. J., Ayoub, E. M., and Boyle, M. D. P. (1984a). *J. Immunol.* **132**, 3091–3097.

Reis, K. J., Ayoub, E. M., and Boyle, M. D. P. (1984b). *J. Immunol.* **132**, 3098–3102.

Reis, K. J., Yarnall, M., Ayoub, E. M., and Boyle, M. D. P. (1984c). *Scand. J. Immunol.* **20**, 433–439.

Reis, K. J., Siden, E. J., and Boyle, M. D. P. (1988a). *Biotechniques* **6**, 130–136.

Reis, K. J., von Mering, G. O., Karis, M. A., Faulmann, E. L., Lottenberg, R., and Boyle, M. D. P. (1988b). *J. Immunol. Methods* **107**, 273–280.

Reis, K. J., Salpeter, J., and Boyle, M. D. P. (1990). *In* ''Bacterial Immunoglobulin-Binding Proteins'' (M. D. P. Boyle, ed.), Vol. 1, pp. 149–154. Academic Press, San Diego.

Romagnani, S., Giudizi, M. G., del Prete, G., Maggi, E., Biagiotti, R., Almerigogna, F., and Ricci, M. (1982). *J. Immunol.* **129**, 596–602.

Russell-Jones, G. J., Gotschlich, E. C., and Blake, M. S. (1984). *J. Exp. Med.* **160**, 1467–1475.

Schalén, C., and Christensen, P. (1990). *In* ''Bacterial Immunoglobulin-Binding Proteins'' (M. D. P. Boyle, ed.), Vol. 1, pp. 57–68. Academic Press, San Diego.

Schrezenmeier, H., and Fleischer, B. (1987). *J. Immunol. Methods* **105**, 133–137.

Scott, J. R., Guenther, P. C., Malone, L. M., and Fischetti, V. A. (1986). *J. Exp. Med.* **164**, 1641–1651.

Sjöbring, U., Falkenberg, C., Nielsen, E., Åkerström, B., and Björck, L. (1988). *J. Immunol.* **140**, 1595–1599.

Sjöbring, U., Björck, L., and Kastern, W. (1989a). *Mol. Microbiol.* **3**, 319–327.

Sjöbring, U., Trojnar, J., Grubb, A., Åkerström, B., and Björck, L. (1989b). *J. Immunol.* **143**, 2948–2954.

Sjödahl, J. (1977). *Eur. J. Biochem.* **73**, 343–351.

Steele, G., Jr., Ankerst, J., and Sjögren, H. O. (1974). *Int. J. Cancer* **14**, 83–92.

Sukumar, S., Zbar, B., Terata, N., and Langone, J. J. (1984). *J. Biol. Resp. Mod.* **3**, 303–315.

Tedder, T. F. (1990). *In* ''Bacterial Immunoglobulin-Binding Proteins'' (M. D. P. Boyle, ed.), Vol. 1, pp. 235–242. Academic Press, San Diego.

Terman, D. S., Young, J. B., Shearer, W. T., Ayus, C., Lehane, D., Mattioli, C., Espada, R., Howell, J. F., Yamamotot, T., Zaleski, H. I., Miller, L., Frommer, P., Feldman, L., Henry, J. F., Tillquist, R., Cook, G., and Daskal, Y. (1981). *N. Engl. J. Med.* **305**, 1195–1200.

Uhlén, M., and Abrahmsén, L. (1989). *Biochem. Soc. Trans.* **17**, 340–341.

Uhlén, M., Guss, B., Nilsson, B., Gatenbeck, S., Philipson, L., and Lindberg, M. (1984). *J. Biol. Chem.* **259**, 1695–1702.

Van der Merwe, J. P., and Stegeman, J. H. (1985). *Eur. J. Immunol.* **15**, 860–863.

Van Longhem, E. B., Frangone, B., Recht, B., and Franklin, E. C. (1982). *Scand. J. Immunol.* **15**, 275–278.

Wallner, W. A., Lawman, M. J. P., and Boyle, M. D. P. (1987). *Appl. Microbiol. Biotechnol.* **27**, 168–173.

Widders, P. R. (1990). *In* ''Bacterial Immunoglobulin-Binding Proteins'' (M. D. P. Boyle, ed.), Vol. 1, pp. 375–396. Academic Press, San Diego.

Widders, P. R., Stoke, C. R., Newby, T. J., and Bourne, F. J. (1985). *Infect. Immun.* **48,** 417–421.
Woof, J. M., and Burton, D. R. (1990). *In* "Bacterial Immunoglobulin-Binding Proteins" (M. D. P. Boyle, ed.), Vol. 1, pp. 305–316. Academic Press, San Diego.
Yarnall, M., and Boyle, M. D. P. (1986a). *Mol. Cell. Biochem.* **70,** 57–66.
Yarnall, M., and Boyle, M. D. P. (1986b). *J. Immunol.* **136,** 2670–2673.
Yarnall, M., and Boyle, M. D. P. (1986c). *Scand. J. Immunol.* **24,** 549–557.
Yarnall, M., and Widders, P. R. (1990). *In* "Bacterial Immunoglobulin-Binding Proteins" (M. D. P. Boyle, ed.), Vol. 1, pp. 155–164. Academic Press, San Diego.
Yarnall, M., Reis, K. J., Ayoub, E. M., and Boyle, M. D. P. (1984). *J. Microbiol. Methods* **3,** 83–93.
Yarnall, M., Widders, P. R., and Corbeil, L. B. (1988). *Scand. J. Immunol.* **28,** 129–137.
Zikán, J. (1980). *Folia Microbiol. (Prague)* **25,** 246–253.

Appendix

I. General Buffers
A. Phosphate Buffers

1. 10 mM Phosphate-Buffered Saline, pH 7.2
   To prepare this PBS buffer, add 8.0 g NaCl, 0.2 g KH_2PO_4, 2.9 g of Na_2HPO_4, and 0.2 g of KCl to 800 ml of distilled H_2O. Adjust the pH to 7.2 and add distilled H_2O to exactly 1000 ml. Azide (2 ml solution #31/liter) can be added to this buffer as a preservative.
2. PBS-Tween
   This 0.05% PBS-Tween buffer is prepared by adding 0.5 ml of Tween 20 to 1 liter of the PBS buffer (buffer #1). Buffers containing a higher percentage of Tween 20 can be prepared by adding proportionally greater volumes.
3. PBS–Gelatin
   PBS-gelatin (PBS–gel) is prepared by dissolving 1 g (or 5 g) of gelatin (Difco) in 100 ml PBS (buffer #1) on a stirring hot plate and then adding 900 ml of buffer #1 to yield PBS containing 0.1% gelatin or (0.5% gelatin).
4. PBS–BSA
   PBS–bovine serum albumin (BSA) is prepared by dissolving 1 g of BSA in 1 liter of the PBS buffer (buffer #1).

B. Veronal Buffers

5. Veronal-Buffered Saline Stock
   To prepare a fivefold concentrate of this VBS buffer, mix 83.0 g NaCl with 10.19 g Na_2 5-5-diethylbarbiturate (sodium barbital[1]) and dissolve in approximately 1.5 liters of distilled

---

[1] Sodium barbital is a controlled substance and cannot be ordered from a chemical supply house without an appropriate license.

H_2O. Adjust pH to 7.35 ± 0.05 with $1N$ HCl. Add distilled H_2O to exactly 2 liters.

6. Stock Trisodium Ethylenediaminetetraacetate
   To prepare this buffer (0.1 M EDTA), dissolve 37.2 g disodium ethylenediaminetetraacetate (Na_2H_2EDTA) in approximately 800 ml distilled H_2O and adust pH to 7.35 ± 0.05 with fresh 2 M NaOH. Add distilled H_2O to exactly 1 liter.

7. Veronal-Buffered Saline containing Gelatin and Divalent Cations
   This buffer (VBS-gel-metals) is prepared by mixing 200 ml of the VBS-stock solution (buffer #5) with 1 ml of the working metals solution (solution #29) and approximately 600 ml of distilled H_2O. Adjust the pH to 7.35 ± 0.05 and then add 100 ml of a 1% solution of gelatin and adjust to a final volume of exactly 1 liter. The gelatin solution is prepared by dissolving 1 g of gelatin in 100 ml of distilled H_2O on a heated stirring plate. Azide (2 ml of solution #31/liter) can be added to this buffer as a preservative. Note: This preservative should not be added to buffers used in complement assays.

8. VBS-Gel-Metals-Tween
   This buffer, containing 0.05% Tween 20, is prepared by adding 0.5 ml of Tween 20/liter of VBS-gel-metals (buffer #7).

9. EDTA-Gel Buffer
   This buffer is prepared by mixing 200 ml of the fivefold concentrate stock VBS (buffer #5) with 100 ml of stock 0.1 M EDTA (buffer #6) and adjusting the pH to 7.35 ± 0.05. Add 100 ml of a 1% gelatin solution and adjust to a final volume of exactly 1000 ml by addition of distilled H_2O. The gelatin solution is prepared by dissolving 1 g of gelatin in 100 ml of distilled H_2O on a heated stirring plate. Azide (2 ml of solution #31/liter) can be added to this buffer as a preservative.

10. EDTA-Gel-Tween
    This buffer is prepared by adding 0.5 ml of Tween 20/liter of EDTA-gel (buffer #9).

11. EGTA-Gel-Mg^{2+}
    This buffer is prepared by dissolving 3.8 g EGTA (ethyleneglycol-bis-N,N'-tetraacetic acid) in 20 ml of VBS stock (buffer #5) add 1.0 ml 2 M $MgCl_2$ (solution #27) and adjusting the pH to 7.25 ± 0.05. Then add 50 ml of a 0.2% gelatin solution and adjust to a final volume of 100 ml. The gelatin solution is prepared by dissolving 0.1 g of gelatin in 50 ml distilled H_2O on a heated stirring plate.

C. Tris Buffers

12. Tris-Buffered Saline
   A stock solution of 1 M Tris is made by dissolving 12.1 g of Tris base in 75 ml H_2O, adjusting to pH 7.4 with 1.0 M HCl, and adding H_2O to bring the final volume to 100 ml. (The pH meter used in adjusting the pH of the solution should be equipped with a calomel electrode, because frequent use of standard glass electrodes in concentrated Tris solutions will cause deterioration of the electrode performance.) The Tris-buffered saline solution (TBS) is prepared by dissolving 8.5 g of NaCl in 20 ml of the Tris stock solution and adjusting the final volume to 1000 ml with distilled H_2O. Tris solutions can be autoclaved to prevent bacterial growth during storage.

13. TBS-Tween
   This solution (0.05% TBS-Tween) is prepared by adding 0.5 ml of Tween 20/liter of TBS (buffer #12).

II. Iodination Buffers and Related Solutions

14. Radioiodination Buffer
   This phosphate buffer solution used in the protein iodination procedure is prepared as follows:

Solution A: 0.5 M KH_2PO_4: dissolve 68.04 g of anhydrous KH_2PO_4 in 1 liter of distilled H_2O.

Solution B: 0.5 M NaOH: dissolve 19.95 g of NaOH in 1 liter of distilled H_2O. To prepare 100 ml of iodination buffer, mix 8.42 ml of solution A with 5.78 ml of solution B and add approximately 80 ml of distilled H_2O. Adjust pH to 7.2 and adjust to exactly 100 ml with distilled H_2O.

15. Iodine Neutralization Solution
   The iodine neutralization solution for addition to liquid radioactive containers is prepared as follows:

Dissolve 3.99 g NaOH, 14.9 g NaI and 24.8 g $Na_2SO_3 \cdot 5 H_2O$ in 1 liter of distilled H_2O.

III. ELISA Buffers and Related Solutions

16. 0.1 M Carbonate–Bicarbonate Buffer, pH 9.6
This buffer, used for coating antigen onto microtiter plates, is prepared as follows:

Solution A: 1.0 M $NaHCO_3$: dissolve 84 g of $NaHCO_3$ in exactly 1000 ml of distilled H_2O.

Solution B: 1.0 M Na_2CO_3: dissolve 106 g of anhydrous Na_2CO_3 in exactly 1000 ml of distilled H_2O.

To prepare 1 liter of the coating buffer, mix 453 ml of solution A with 182 ml of solution B. Adjust pH to 9.6 and final volume to exactly 1000 ml. Sodium azide (2 ml solution #31/liter) may be added to each liter of coating buffer as a preservative.

IV. Electrophoresis Buffers

17. Separating Gel Buffer: 1.5 M Tris-HCl, pH 8.8
To prepare 100 ml of this buffer, dissolve 18.15 g Tris base in approximately 50 ml distilled H_2O. Adjust pH to 8.8 with 1 M HCl and dilute to exactly 100 ml with distilled H_2O. Note: When adjusting the pH, this buffer should be mixed for an extended period to ensure an accurate pH reading.

18. Stacking Gel Buffer: 0.5 M Tris–HCl, pH 6.8
To prepare 50 ml of this buffer, mix 3.0 g Tris base with 25 ml distilled H_2O. Adjust to pH 6.8 with 1 M HCl and dilute to exactly 50 ml with distilled H_2O. Note: When adjusting the pH, this buffer should be mixed for an extended period to ensure an accurate pH reading.

19. Electrode Buffer for SDS Gels, pH 8.3
To prepare 1 liter of this buffer, dissolve 3.0 g of Tris base with 14.4 g of glycine and 1.0 g of SDS in approximately 800 ml distilled H_2O. Adjust pH to 8.3 and finally dilute to exactly 1 liter with distilled H_2O.

20. SDS Sample Buffer
The sample buffer should contain the following:

Distilled H_2O	4.0 ml
0.5 M Tris-HCl, pH 6.8 (buffer #18)	1.0 ml

Glycerol	0.8 ml
10% SDS [weight/volume (w/v) in H_2O]	1.6 ml
2-Mercaptoethanol	0.4 ml
0.5% (w/v) in H_2O Bromphenol blue	0.1 ml
	8.0 ml

For unreduced samples, the mercaptoethanol should be omitted. Samples to be analyzed by SDS–PAGE should be diluted 1:2 with sample buffer and heated at 95°C for 4 min before applying to the gels. Dithiothreitol (1 ml of a 10% w/v solution in H_2O) can be used in place of mercaptoethanol as the reducing agent. The amount of water added should then be adjusted to 3.4 ml.

21. Acrylamide:BIS Stock Solution
To prepare a stock solution of 30% acrylamide and 2.67% BIS, dissolve 29.2 g acrylamide[2] and 0.8 g N,N'-methylene-bis-acrylamide (BIS) in distilled H_2O and adjust to exactly 100 ml. Filter and store at 4°C in the dark. The effective shelf-life of this solution is 30 days. Note: Acrylamide and BIS are potent neurotoxins with cumulative effects. Gloves and a mask should be worn when preparing this solution and extreme caution should be used to ensure no skin contact.

22. Separating Gel for Use in SDS–PAGE
The formulations provided are for preparing 40 ml of a 10% separating gel. If higher or lower percentage gels are required, the volume of acrylamide:BIS stock (buffer #21 and H_2O) should be adjusted accordingly.

Double distilled (dd)H_2O	16.1 ml
1.5 M Tris–HCl, pH 8.8 (buffer #17)	10.0 ml
10% SDS, weight/volume (w/v) in H_2O	0.4 ml
Acrylamide–BIS (Solution #21)	13.3 ml
10% ammonium persulfate [$(NH_4)_2S_2O_8$] (w/v in H_2O)[2]	0.2 ml
TEMED (N,N,N',N'-Tetramethylrethylenediamine)	0.02 ml
	40.0 ml

---

[2] Ammonium persulfate should be prepared immediately prior to use.

The gel should be poured immediately after preparation and covered with a layer of H_2O. Polymerization normally occurs within 60 min at ambient temperature.

23. Stacking Gel for Use in SDS–PAGE

H_2O	9.15 ml
0.5 M Tris–HCl, pH 6.8 (buffer #18)	3.75 ml
10% SDS (w/v in H_2O)	0.15 ml
Acrylamide:BIS (solution #21)	1.95 ml
10% $(NH_4)_2S_2O_8$ (w/v in H_2O)[3]	0.075 ml
TEMED	0.015 ml
	15.000 ml

V. Buffers for Use in Applications Involving Nitrocellulose

24. Wash Buffer I
This buffer is prepared as follows:

Solution A: Add 200 ml of VBS stock (buffer #5), 200 ml of distilled H_2O, and 2.5 ml Tween 20.

Solution B: Dissolve 2.5 g of gelatin in 100 ml of distilled H_2O by heating on a stir plate.

Add solution A and solution B, mix, and adjust pH to 7.35 ± 0.05 and adjust volume to exactly 1000 ml with distilled H_2O.

25. Wash Buffer II
Add 100 ml of 0.1 M EDTA (buffer #6) to 600 ml of distilled H_2O and 2.5 ml Tween 20. Dissolve 58.4 g of NaCl in this solution to make solution A. Prepare solution B by dissolving 2.5 g of gelatin in 100 ml of distilled H_2O. Mix solutions A and B, adjust pH to 7.35 ± 0.05, and finally adjust volume to exactly 1000 ml with distilled H_2O.

26. Electroblot Buffer
This buffer (25 mM Tris, 192 mM glycine, 20% methanol) is

---

[3] Ammonium persulfate should be prepared immediately prior to use.

used in procedures involving the transfer of proteins to nitrocellulose membranes. This buffer is prepared by dissolving 14.4 g glycine and 3.03 g Tris base in approximately 600 ml of distilled H_2O. Add 200 ml of methanol. Adjust to 1000 ml.

VI. General Buffers and Reagents

Metals Solution
Anhydrous magnesium chloride and calcium chloride are both very hygroscopic and will absorb large quantities of H_2O from the air. Stock solutions of these reagents should therefore be made from either fresh (previously unopened) bottles or the hydrated compounds and should be standardized gravimetrically.

27. 2 M $MgCl_2$
Dissolve 19.0 g anhydrous $MgCl_2$ in 50 ml of distilled H_2O and adjust to a final volume of 100 ml.
28. 0.3 M $CaCl_2$
Dissolve 3.33 g anhydrous $CaCl_2$ in 50 ml distilled H_2O and adjust to a final volume of 100 ml.
29. Working Metals Solution
A solution containing 1.0 M $MgCl_2$ and 0.15 M $CaCl_2$ is made by mixing equal volumes of 2 M $MgCl_2$ (solution #26) and 0.3 M $CaCl_2$ (solution #27).
30. Sterile Alsever's Solution
Alsever's solution, used for collection of erythrocytes, is prepared by dissolving 2.1 g dextrose, 0.8 g sodium citrate (dihydrate), 0.4 g NaCl, and 0.055 g citric acid in distilled H_2O to yield a final volume of 100 ml. The solution can be sterilized by passage through a 0.2 μm filter.
31. Azide Stock
A stock 10% NaN_3 solution can be made by dissolving 5.0 g NaN_3 in 50 ml H_2O. This solution should then be filtered to remove insoluble particles.
32. Glycine-HCl Buffer, pH 2.0
This buffer is used to elute bound proteins from affinity columns and is prepared as follows:
Dissolve 7.5 g of glycine in 500 ml distilled H_2O. Adjust pH to 2.0 with 1.0 M HCl and finally adjust volume to exactly 1 liter.

Index

ABC technique, and biotinylated protein A, 206–207
Acetone/detergent extraction, 55
Acid, alkaline and neutral heat, 54
Affinity chromatography, 312
Affinity chromatography using protein G-agarose, examples, 359
Affinity columns, immunoglobulin source to prepare, selection, 72–73
Affinity constant for binding between bacterial cell wall protein and its ligand procedure, determination, 100–104
Affinity purification of type III Fc-binding protein solubilized by bacteriophage lysis of group C Streptococcus 26R66, 75–77
Affinity-purified immunoglobulin-binding proteins, characterization, 77–80
  functional characterization, 80–82
  physicochemical analysis, 77–80
Agarose, precipitation, 119
Agglutination assay, 26–28
  advantages, 28
  disadvantages, 28
AIDS, 2
Air sac procedure
  advantages and limitations, 413–414
  Fc-binding proteins, use, 410–413
Albumin, reactivity of different sources of protein G with various species, 10–12
Albumin binding and background, 202
Alternate complement pathway, measurement of function, 378–379
Animal species selection, for production of polyclonal antibodies, 105–107
Anion exchange, 311
Antibody to immunoglobulin-binding proteins, detection, 110–119

Anti-immunoglobulin-binding protein antibodies, detection
  general procedure, 113–115
Anti-immunoglobulin-coated bacteria, preparation, 304–305
Antibodies for cell surface antigens, preparation, 304
Antibodies, specific, application of Fc-binding proteins for detection
  assay, development of for antibodies to a soluble agent, 183–186
  detection, 181–182
  optimization of conditions to detect anti-*Brucella* antibodies, 183–185
  rabbit IgM antibodies to sheep erythrocytes, detection, 190–194
  tumor-associated antigens, detection of antibodies, 186–190
Antibody, probing membrane, 254
Anti-*Brucella* antibodies, optimization of conditions to detect 183–185
Antigen, immobilizing, 253
Antigen, immobilizing onto microtiter plates, 153–154
Antigenic analysis of soluble immunoglobulin-binding proteins by Western blotting techniques, 120–121
Antigenic determinants on immunoglobulin-binding proteins, detection, 119–123
  assays to detect, 119–123
  agarose, precipitation, 119
  antigenic analysis of soluble immunoglobulin-binding proteins by Western blotting techniques, 120–121
  Farr assay technique, 119–120
  procedure, 121–123
Antigenic determination of complement activation, 388

461

Antigens
  colony and plaque blotting, 258–263
  detection by western blot analysis, 268
Ascites fluid or serum, 334
Assay, development of for antibodies to a soluble agent, 183–186
Assay procedure, *in vivo*, 407–410
  methodology, 406–407
Assays for detection of immunoglobulin-binding proteins, agglutination assay, 26–28
  advantages, 28
  disadvantages, 28
  microtiter agglutination test for bacterial-binding proteins, 27–28
  sensitized sheep erythrocytes, 26–27
    slide agglutination test for bacterial-binding proteins, 27
    tube agglutination test for bacterial-binding proteins, 27
Assays for lymphocyte differentiation
Assays for lymphocytic proliferation, 396–398
Autoradiographic dot blot procedure for detection of group B Streptococcal antigens, 172–173
Autoradiographic dot blot procedure to detect cell surface and secreted group B Streptococcal antigens, 173–175
Autoradiography, 255–256
Avidin, colloidal gold with, stabilization, 238–239

B cell differentiation to immunoglobulin secreting cells, 400–403
B cell/T cell differentiation, *see* T cell/B cell differentiation
Bacteria, fixation and embedding, 227
Bacteria expressing immunoglobulin-binding proteins in coagglutination assays, use, *see* Coagglutination assays
Bacterial-bound IgG-binding proteins
  for detection of specific antibodies, use, 285–286
  in place of second antibody for radioimmunoassay, use, 284–285

Bacterial cell surface immunoglobulin-binding proteins
  absorption of IgG by bacteria, 31–3
    buffers, 32
    materials, 32
    procedure, 33
    detection of residual IgG in bacterial free supernatant, 33
  assays for detection of immunoglobulin-binding proteins
    agglutination assay, 26–28
      advantages, 28
      disadvantages, 28
      microtiter agglutination test for bacterial-binding proteins, 27–28
      sensitized sheep erythrocytes, 26–27
        slide agglutination test for bacterial-binding proteins, 27
        tube agglutination test for bacterial-binding proteins, 27
  colony blot selection, 39–45
    buffers, 40
    materials, 40
    procedure, 41–45
  direct binding assay
    buffers, 31
    materials, 30–31
    procedure, 31
  direct binding of immunoglobulins to bacteria
    preparation of immunoglobulin Fc-specific probes
      absorption of immunoglobulins by bacteria, 29–30
      Fc fragments, 29–30
      iodinization of proteins, 30
      use of monoclonal antibodies or myeloma proteins, 30
  dot blot procedure, 34–37
    buffers, 34
    materials, 34
    procedure, 34–37
  methods developed, 23
  methods to enhance, 37–39
    mouse passage, 37–39
    procedure for mouse passage of bacteria, 39
  preparation, 24–25

Index

standardization, 25-26
  of number based on wet weight/volume ratio, 25
  of number based in volume/volume ratio, 25
  standardization based on measurement of turbidity, 26
storage of strains, 45-46
  blood agar plates, 46
  glycerol stocks, 45-46
  recovery of strains from glycerol stocks, 46
Bacterial immunoglobulin-binding proteins, future trends, *see* Future trends of bacterial IgG-binding proteins
Bacterial immunoglobulin proteins, isolation, *see* Isolation and functional characterization of bacterial immunoglobulin proteins
Bacterial immunoglobulin-binding proteins to analyze labeled antigens, use, 279-284
Bacterial immunoglobulins commercial source, 278
Bacterial IgG-binding proteins, detection of low affinity, 63-64
Bacterial IgG Fc-binding proteins, 3-4
Bacterial immunoglobulin-binding proteins
  distribution and function reactivity of bacterial IgG Fc-binding proteins, 3-4
  historical background, 1-2
  proteins, 4-15
    chimeric IgG-binding proteins, 15
    type I, comparisons, 4-8
    type II, 9
    type III, 9-13
    type IV, 13
    type V, 14
    type VI, 14
  second generation immunoglobulin-binding proteins, 15-17
    IgA Fc-binding proteins, 15-16
    IgD-binding proteins, 16
    protein L, 16-17
    protein P, 17
Bacterial immunosorbent reagents
  commercial source of bacterial immunoglobulins, 278
  IgG-binding capacity of bacterial immunosorbents, 276-277
  protein A-positive *Staphylococcus aureus*, 275
    fixation, 275-276
    growth, 275
  protein B-positive Streptococci, 276
  selection for use with monoclonal or polyclonal antibody, 278-279
  storage and stability, 277-278
Bacterial immunosorbents
  applications using, 279-287
  to deplete serum of IgG antibodies, 286-287
Bacterial strains, media and growth conditions, 164
Bacteriophage-associated lysin treatment, 53
Balanced salt solution (BSS), 302-303
β antigen detection
  in culture supernatants or extracts of group B streptococcus TC795, 256-257
  in extracts of group B streptococcus TC 795, 268-269
β antigen of group B Streptococci, localization of using anti-β antiserum and gold-labeled protein G, 229-231
Binding assay, for cell surface antigens, 305-306
Binding capacity of protein A, available, 323-324
Binding of first component of complement, studies, 387-388
Biotinylated IgG-binding proteins
  advantages, 205-208
  biotinylation, 208-209
    assay for percentage, 208-209
  immunohistochemical staining, 209-214
Biotinylation of proteins for use with avidin-gold, 240
Blood agar plates, 46
Blood lymphocyte isolation, peripheral, 394
Bolton-Hunter reagent, iodinating proteins, 132-133
Branhamella catarrhalis, 4
  and IgD-binding protein, 16
Brucella abortus, 4
  and protein P, 17

BSS, *see* Balanced salt solution
Buffers
  electrophoresis buffers, 456–458
  ELISA buffers and related solutions, 456
  general, 453–455
    EDTA-gel buffer, 454
    phosphate buffers, 453
    stock trisodium ethylenediaminetetraacetate, 454
    Tris-buffered saline, 455
      TBS-tween, 455
    veronal-buffered saline (VBS) stock, 453–454
  general buffers and reagents
    metals solution, 459
    iodination buffers and related solutions, 455
    iodine neutralization solution, 455
    radioiodination buffer, 455
    nitrocellulose, buffers for use in applications, 458–459
    electroblot buffer, 458–459
    wash buffer I, 458
    wash buffer II, 458

Cation exchange, 311
Cell-bound antigens, detection, 293–294
Cell surface and secreted group B Streptococcal antigens, by dot blot audioradiograph procedure, 173–175
Cell surface antigens, use of whole bacteria expressing IgG-binding proteins to detect
  bacterial strains, 301–302
  binding assay, 305–306
  preparation of anti-immunoglobulin-coated bacteria, 304–305
  preparation of antibodies, 304
  preparation of hydridoma antibody-coated bacteria, 305
  reagents and equipment, 302–307
    balanced salt solution (BSS), 302–303
    fetal bovine serum, 303
  staining and quantitation, 306–307
  variations, 307
Chemoattractants, 407

Chicken, selection of for production of polyclonal antibodies, 106–107
Chimeric IgG binding proteins, 15
Chloroform extraction, 110
Chloramine-T, iodinating proteins, 131–132
Chromatography, 200–201
  and role of protein A in multistep purification protocols, 348–352
Classical pathway complement activity, detection, 372–378
Cloning of Streptococcal protein G genes
  protein G genes from other isolates, 423–424
  colony immunoassay, 417–419
  initial gene cloning, 420–423
  preparation of Streptococcal DNA, 419–420
Clostridium perfringens, 4
  preparation, 24
  and protein P, 17
Coagglutination assays, use of bacteria expressing immunoglobulin-binding proteins
  detection of cell-bound antigens, 293–294
  detection of specific antibody, 294–296
  procedure, 291–293
  procedure for establishing to measure polyvalent soluble antigen, 296–298
Column preparation for protein A, 324–326
Column reequilibration, reuse, and storage, 329–330
Colony and plaque blotting of antigens expressed by bacteria, 258–263
Colony blot selection, 39–45
  buffers, 40
  materials, 40
  procedure, 41–45
Colloidal gold
  coupling of proteins, 221–225
  history, 217
  immunoglobulins IgA and IgG, 222
  labeling, application, 246
  particles, replica method with plasma polymerization film by glow discharge for 3-dimensional demonstration, development, 240–241

Index

Colloidal gold with avidin, stabilization, 238–239
Colloidal gold, preparation, 217–221
  glassware and solutions, 218
  15 nm gold particles, 218–219
  4.0–11.5 nm gold particles, 219
  preparative procedures, 218–221
  reducing mixture, 220
  storage of colloidal gold, 221
Competitive binding assay, 96, 115–119
Competitive binding immunoassay, developing, 135–138
Competitive binding radioimmunoassay for soluble Fc-binding proteins, 59–63
Competitive inhibition dot blot assay, 85–87
Competitive inhibition radioimmunoassay, 127–141
Complement activity, measurement, 375
Complement split products, measurement, generation, 387–388
Complement system and IgG-binding proteins
  analysis of complexes formed between bacterial IgG-binding proteins and IgG, 388–389
  antigenic determination of complement activation, 388
  complement split products generated as a consequence of complement activation mediated by bacterial IgG-binding proteins, 386–387
  detection of classical pathway complement activity, 372–378
    procedure, 373–378
      complement activity, measurement, 375
      procedure, 375–378
      sheep erythrocytes, standardization, 373–374
      sheep erythrocyte concentration, standardization, 374
      sheep erythrocytes with antibody, sensitization, 374–375
    reagents, 373
  functional activity of alternate complement pathway, measurement, 378–379
  functional complement activity, measurement, 371–372
  functional complement titration to measurement of activity of IgG-binding proteins, application, 379–380
  generation of complement split products, measurement, 387–388
    procedure, 384–386
    reagents, 382–384
    studies, 369–371
    studies of binding of first component of complement, 387–388
Complexes formed between bacterial IgG-binding proteins and IgG, analysis, 388–389
Conjugation of protein G using GMBS, 200–201
Conjugation protocol, 200
Coprococcus comes, 4
  preparation, 24

DA4-4, mouse IgG, isolation of from hybridoma tissue culture medium, 361
Direct binding assay
  buffers, 31
  materials, 30–31
  procedure, 31
Direct binding assay for detection of antibody, 147–148
Direct binding of immunoglobulins to bacteria
  preparation of immunoglobulin Fc-specific probes
    absorption of immunoglobulins by bacteria, 29–30
    Fc fragments, 29
    iodinization of proteins, 30
    use of monoclonal antibodies or myeloma proteins, 30
Dot binding, 99
Dot blot assay, 250–258
  adaption of two-stage, 172–175
  autoradiographic procedure for detection of group B Streptococcal antigens, 172–173
  competitive inhibition, 85–87

Dot blot autoradiographic procedure to detect cell surface and secreted group B Streptococcal antigens, 173–175
Dot blot procedure, 34–37
  buffers, 34
  materials, 34
  procedure, 34–37
Dot blot procedure to detect soluble bacterial immunoglobulin-binding protein, 64–66
Double-labeling techniques with different sizes of colloidal gold to localize two different antigens on thin sections, 231–234

EDTA-gel buffer, 454
Eggs, isolation of antibody from, 108–110
Electroblot buffer, 458–459
Electroblotting, for Western blot analysis, 267–268
Electrophoresis, 310
Electrophoresis buffers, 456–458
ELISA buffers and related solutions, 456
ELISA typing procedure, adaptation of two-stage RIA, 175–177
Eluting agent, selection, 74–75
Elution procedures for protein A, 328–329
Enzyme-labeled IgG-binding proteins in immunoassay, application
  development of ELISA to quantify human IgA using type III Fc-binding protein-alkaline phosphatase conjugate as tracer, 152–159
    establishing optimal concentration of each reagent, 154–156
    immobilizing antigen onto microtiter plates, 153–154
    optimization of reaction conditions for detection of human IgA, 156–159
  preparation of immunoglobulin Fc-binding protein–enzyme conjugate tracers, 149–152
    conjugation of type III Fc-binding protein to alkaline phosphatase, 151–152
      materials, 151
      procedure, 151–152
  types of assays, 147–149
    direct binding assay for detection of antibody, 147–148
    two-stage competitive binding assay for detection of soluble antigen, 149
Enzyme-labeled bacterial Fc-binding tracers, probing membrane, 257–258
Enzyme-linked immunosorbent assays (ELISA), 1
Enzymatic extraction methods, 51–55
  general comments regarding, 54
Ethanol precipitation, 310

Farr assay technique, 119–120
Fast Protein Liquid Chromatography, 151–152
Fc-binding protein antigenic characterization, comparison of functional activities, 87
Fc-binding proteins in air sac procedure, use, 410–413
Fc-binding proteins, future trends, 430–441
Fc fragments, 29
Fetal bovine serum, 303
Fluid-phase competitive inhibition assays, 84–85
Fluorescent-conjugated bacterial immunoglobulin-binding program
  comparison of recombinant protein G to wild type protein G isolated from *Streptococcus* cell membranes, 201–202
  background and albumin binding, 202
  fluorescence/protein ratios, 201–202
  functional testing, 202
  conjugation method using GMBS, 200–201
  chromatography, 200–201
  conjugation protocol, 200
  functional assay system, 201
  standard methods
    fluorescence/protein ratios, determination, 199
    linkers, commonly used, 197–199
Fluorescence/protein ratios, 201–202
  determination, 199
Functional assay system, 201, 202

Index

Functional complement titration to measurement of activity if IgG-binding proteins, application, 379–380, *see also* Complement system
Functional complement activity, measurement, 371–372
Future trends of IgG-binding proteins
 applications involving IgG-binding proteins, 442–447
  identification of new proteins, 442–444
  manipulation of proteins, 444–445
  potential therapeutic applications, 445–447
 impact, 425–428
  type II protein, 428
  type IV protein, 426–427
  type V protein, 426–427
  type VI protein, 426–427, 428
 role of in pathogenicity, 429–430
 structure–function relationships of bacterial Fc-binding proteins, 430–441

Gel filtration, 98–99
Gene cloning, initial, 420–423
Glycerol stocks, storage, 45–46
 recovery of strains from, 46
Goat serum, isolation from IgG, 359–361
Gold colloids, storage, 225
Gold labeling, procedure for on thin section, 227–231
Gold-labeling, use of for localization of immunoglobulin-binding sites and antigen-antibody complexes in bacteria, 225–231
Gold particles
 15 nm, preparing, 218–219
 4.0–11.5, preparing, 219, 220
  gold solution, 219
  reducing mixture, 220–221
Group B streptococcal-typing antisera, source, 164
Group B Streptococci, simultaneous labeling of sites of IgA binding and β antigen, 231–234
Group C Streptococcus Fc-binding protein, 407

HA, *see* Hydroxyapatite chromatography
Haemophilus somnus, 4
 preparation, 24
HIC, *see* Hydrophobic interaction chromatography
Hyaluronidase extraction, 52
Hybridoma antibody-coated bacteria, preparation, 305
Hydrophobic interaction chromatography (HIC), 311
Hydroxyapatite chromatography (HA), 311–312

IgA- and IgG-binding sites on thin sections, localizing, 227–229
IgA Fc-binding proteins, 15–16
IgA, human, optimization of reaction conditions for detection, 156–159
IgD-binding proteins, 16
IgG, absorption of by bacteria, 31–3
 buffers, 32
 materials, 32
 procedure, 33
IgG-binding capacity of bacterial immunosorbents, 276–277
IgG-binding proteins, applications involving, 442–447
IgG, human, serum or cell culture, 336–337
 equipment, 337
 materials, 336
 method, 337
IgG, mouse, *see* Mouse IgG
IgG, residual, detection of in bacterial free supernatant, 33
IgG, use of immobilized protein G to isolate determination of optimal conditions for protein G affinity chromatography, 357–358
 sample preparation, 358
 examples of affinity chromatography using protein G-agarose, 359
 comparison of purification of MOPC 21, mouse IgG_1 monoclonal antibody, loaded at pH 7.0 and at pH 5.0, 361–362
 isolation of IgG from goat serum, 359–361

isolation of DA4-4, mouse IgG, from hybridoma tissue culture medium, 361
protein G agarose, use of to make antigen-binding column, 363–365
IgG-binding protein, biotinylation, 208–209
IgG isolation from goat serum, 359–361
IgG_1 monoclonal antibodies, purification, 341–343
IgM monoclonal antibodies, purification, 343–345
Immunoassays using enzyme-labeled tracers, see Enzyme-labeled IgG-binding proteins in immunoassay
Immunoelectronmicroscopy, and use of IgG-binding proteins
  application of colloidal gold labeling, 246
  colloidal gold, coupling of proteins, 221–225
    immunoglobulins IgA and IgG, 222
    protein G from group G Streptococci and protein A from *Staphylococcus aureus*, 222–224
    storage of gold colloids, 225
    titration of amount of colloid to bind protein sample, 224–225
  colloidal gold, history, 217
  double-labeling techniques with different sizes of colloidal gold to localize two different antigens on thin sections, 231–236
    simultaneous labeling of sites of IgA binding and β antigen in group B Streptococci, 231–234
    with two different primary antibodies by silver enhancement of colloidal gold marker, 234–236
  gold-labeling, use of for localization of immunoglobulin-binding sites and antigen–antibody complexes in bacteria, 225–231
    localization of immunoglobulin-binding molecules on whole bacteria, 226–227
    procedure for gold labeling on thin section, 227–231
      fixation and embedding of bacteria, 227
      localization of IgA- and IgG-binding sites on thin sections, 227–229
      localization of β antigen of group B Streptococci using anti-β antiserum and gold-labeled protein G, 229–231
  preparation of colloidal gold, 217–221
    glassware and solutions, 218
    15 nm gold particles, 218–219
    4.0–11.5 nm gold particles, 219
    preparative procedures, 218–221
    reducing mixture, 220
    storage of colloidal gold, 221
  replica method with plasma polymerization film by glow discharge for 3-dimensional demonstration of colloidal gold particles
    development, 240–241
    technique for preparation of replicas by plasma polymerization, 241–246
  streptavidin/avidin–biotin labeling for detection of immunoglobulin-binding proteins, 236–238
    biotinylation of proteins for use with avidin–gold, 240
    for detection of immunoglobulin-binding proteins, 219–240
    stabilization of colloidal gold with avidin, 238–239
Immunogen and immunization, preparation, 107
Immunoglobulin-binding proteins, detection, 239–240
Immunoglobulin-binding proteins and polycloncal antibodies, see Polyclonal antibodies
Immunoglobulin-binding proteins in low concentrations, determination, 96–97
Immunoglobulin-binding molecules on whole bacteria, labelization, 226–227
Immunoglobulin Fc-binding protein–enzyme conjugate tracers, preparing, 149–152
  conjugation of type III Fc-binding protein to alkaline phosphatase, 151–152
  materials, 151
  procedure, 151–152

Index

Immunoglobulin source to prepare affinity columns, selection, 72–73
Immunohistochemical staining using biotinylated IgG-binding proteins, 209–214
Immunoprecipitation reactions, application of bacteria expressing immunoglobulin-binding proteins
  applications using bacterial immunosorbents, 279–287
    use of bacterial-bound IgG-binding proteins for detection of specific antibodies, 285–286
    use of bacterial-bound IgG-binding proteins in place of second antibody for radioimmunoassay, 284–285
    use of bacterial immunoglobulin-binding proteins to analyze labeled antigens, 279–284
    use of bacterial immunosorbents to deplete serum of IgG antibodies, 286–287
  general background, 274–275
  preparation of bacterial immunosorbent reagents
    commercial source of bacterial immunoglobulins, 278
    IgG-binding capacity of bacterial immunosorbents, 276–277
    protein A-positive *Staphylococcus aureus*, 275
      fixation, 275–276
      growth, 275
    protein B-positive Streptococci, 276
    selection for use with monoclonal or polyclonal antibody, 278–279
    storage and stability, 277–278
  procedures, 273–274
In vivo leucocyte chemotaxis mediated by Fc-binding proteins
  air sac procedure, advantages and limitations, 413–414
  air sac procedure
    in vivo assay procedure, 407–410
    methodology, 406–407

chemoattractants, 407
group C Streptococcus Fc-binding protein, 407
mice, 406
Staphylococcal protein A, 407
urokinase, 407
Fc-binding proteins in air sac procedure, use, 410–413
studies, 405–406
Injectable-grade monoclonal antibodies, purification
  resistance of protein A to treatment with 1 N NaOH, 346–348
  role of protein A chromatography in multistep purification protocols, 348–352
Iodine, free, separating proteins from, 133–135
Iodine neutralization solution, 455
Iodination buffers and related solutions, 455
Iodinization of protein A and protein G, 164–165
Iodinization of proteins, 30
Ion exchange, 311
Isolation and functional characterization of bacterial immunoglobulin-binding proteins
  affinity purification of type III Fc-binding protein solubilized by bacteriophage lysis of group C Streptococcus 26P66, 75–77
  characterization of affinity-purified immunoglobulin-binding proteins, 77–82
    functional characterization, 80–82
    physicochemical analysis, 77–80
  comparison of functional activities of Fc-binding proteins
    antigenic characterization, 87
    competitive inhibition dot blot assay, 85–87
    fluid-phase competitive inhibition assays, 84–85
    Western blot analysis, 82–84
  nature of sample to be purified, 73–74
  selection of eluting agent, 74–75
  selection of immunoglobulin source to prepare affinity columns, 72–73

Kinetics of antibody production, 108–110

Labeled antigens, bacterial immunoglobulin-binding proteins to analyze, 279–284
Lactoperoxidase, iodinating proteins, 132
Leucocyte chemotaxis mediated by Fc-binding proteins, in vivo, see In vivo leucocyte chemotaxis mediated by Fc-binding proteins
Ligand for protein A, choices, 320–321
Linkers, use of for labeling proteins, 197–199
Liquid chromatographic techniques, 310–311
Low affinity bacterial IgG-binding proteins, detection, 63–64
Lymphocyte differentiation and activation
  assays for lymphocyte differentiation
    B cell differentiation to immunoglobulin secreting cells, 400–403
    of T cell differentiation, 398–400
  isolation and purification, 394–398
    assays for lymphocytic proliferation, 396–398
    panning method for purification of T cell/B cell preparations, 395–396
    peripheral blood lymphocyte isolation, 394
    T cell/B cell separation, 394–395
  studies, 393–394
Lysin, treatment with bacteriophage-associated, 53
Lysostaphin extraction treatment, 53–54

Mammalian protein binding, screening procedures, 92–03
Matrix for protein A, choice, 321–322
Metals solution buffer, 459
Mice, and in vivo assay procedure, 406
Microtiter agglutination test for bacterial-binding proteins, 27–28
Monoclonal antibodies or myeloma proteins, use, 30
Monoclonal or polyclonal antibody, selection, 278–279

MOPC 21, mouse IgG_1 monoclonal antibody loaded at pH 7.0 and 5.0, 361–362
Mouse IgG, monoclonal or polyclonal, 332–336
  equipment, 332
  materials, 332
  method, 332, 334
    ascites fluid or serum, 334
    cell culture, 335–336
Mouse passage, 37–39
  procedure for mouse passage of bacteria, 39
Mutanolysin extraction, 51–52

1 N NaOH, resistance of protein A to treatment, 346–348
N-terminal sequence of type III Fc-binding proteins and fragments, 12
Neutral heat, acid and alkaline extractions, 54
Nitrocellulose, buffers for use in applications, 458–459
Nitrocellulose membranes, use of bacterial Fc-binding proteins as probes for antigen–antibody immobilized colony and plaque blotting of antigens expressed by bacteria, 258–25
  procedure, 259–261
    screening recombinant λ bacteria phage isolate for expression of streptococcal plasmin-binding protein, 261–263
  dot blot assay, 250–258
    autoradiography, 255–256
    β antigen detection in culture supernatants or extracts of group B streptococcus TC795, 256–257
    blocking membrane, 253
    immobilizing antigen, 253
    initial experiments setting up, 252
    probing membrane with antibody, 254
    probing membrane with enzyme-labeled bacterial Fc-binding tracers, 257–258
    probing membrane with radiolabeled Fc-binding tracer, 254
  techniques, 249–250
  Western blot analysis, 263–269

Index

antigens, detection, 268
β antigen detection in extracts of group B streptococcus TC 795, 268–269
electroblotting, 267–268
general considerations, 263–264
procedures, 264
sodium dodecyl sulfate polyacrylamide gel electrophoresis, 264–267
Nonenzymatic extraction procedures, 54
Normal B lymphocytes, 310

Panning method for purification of T cell/B cell preparations, 395–396
Papain digestion, 52
Pathogenicity, role of IgG-binding proteins, 429–430
PBS extraction and egg yolks, collection, 109–110
Peptococcus magnus, 4, 50
preparation, 24
Peripheral blood lymphocyte isolation, 394–395
Phosphate buffers, 453
Plasma polymerization, technique for preparation of replicas, 241–246
Polyclonal antibodies, production of to immunoglobulin-binding proteins
animal species selection, 105–107
chicken, 106–107
detection of antibody to immunoglobulin-binding proteins, 110–119
inhibition of functional activity by antibody
detection of anti-immunoglobulin-binding protein antibodies, 113–115
quantitation of specific antibodies using competitive binding assay, 115–119
whole bacteria as source of immobilized immunoglobulin-binding protein, using, 111–113
detection of antigenic determinants on immunoglobulin-binding proteins, 119–123
antigenic assays to detect, 119–123
kinetics of antibody production, 108–110
isolation of antibody from eggs, 108–110
chloroform extraction, 110
collection of yolks and PBS extraction, 109–110
preparation of immunogen and immunization, 107
Polyvalent soluble antigen, procedure for establishing a coagglutination assay to measure, 296–298
Precipitation assay and two-stage RIA typing results, summary, 168–169
Protein A
comparisons of species reactivities, 5–6, 7
commercially available derivatives, 8–9
Protein A, immobilized, use of to purify immunoglobulins
available binding capacity, 323–324
choices of ligand, 320–321
choice of matrix, 321–322
collection and detection methods, 329
column preparation, 324–326
column reequilibration, reuse, and storage, 329–330
elution procedures, 328–329
general methods using protein A-Sepharose CL-4B and protein A Sepharose 4 fast flow for mouse and human IgG purification, 332–337
human IgG, serum or cell culture, 336–337
equipment, 337
materials, 336
method, 337
mouse IgG, monoclonal or polyclonal, 332–336
equipment, 332
materials, 332
method, 332, 334
immobilized procedure, 322–323
limitations of method, 330–331
overview of purification procedure, 313–320
summary of methods for purification of immunoglobulins on protein-A Sepharose, 314–319
sample application, 327–328
sample preparation, 326–327

uses, 309–313
  affinity chromatography, 312
  anion exchange, 311
  cation exchange, 311
  electrophoresis, 310
  ethanol precipitation, 310
  hydrophobic interaction chromatography (HIC), 311
  hydroxyapatite (HA) chromatography, 311–312
  ion exchange, 311
  liquid chromatographic techniques, 310–311
  normal B lymphocytes, 310
Protein A monoclonal antibody purification
  conclusions, 352–353
  IgG_1 monoclonal antibodies, purification, 341–343
  IgM monoclonal antibodies, purification, 343–345
  injectable-grade monoclonal antibodies, purification,
    resistance of protein A to treatment with 1 N NaOH, 346–348
    role of protein A chromatography in multistep purification protocols, 348–352
  quantitation of monoclonal antibodies, 345–346
Protein A-positive *Staphylococcus aureus*, 275–276
  fixation, 275–276
  growth, 275
Protein antibodies, inhibition of functional activity by antibody detection, 113–115
Protein binding activities, determination of among bacterial cell surface proteins
Protein G-positive Streptococci, 276
Protein binding activities, determination of among bacterial cell surface proteins
  analysis of binding of Ig and others to purified bacterial surface proteins, 97–98
    binding to host proteins on solid phase, 99
    dot binding, 99
    gel filtration, 98–99
    Western blot analysis, 99–100
    competitive binding assay, 96

solid phase radioassay or enzyme-linked immunosorbent assay, 96–97
  binding of mammalian proteins, screening procedures, 92–03
  determination of affinity constant for binding between bacterial cell wall protein and its ligand
    procedure, 103–104
    theoretical considerations, 100–103
  determination of immunoglobulin-binding proteins in low concentrations
  solubilization of immunoglobulin-binding bacterial surface proteins, 93–95
Protein G
  albumin, reactivity of different sources, 10–11
  commercially available derivatives, 13
  comparisons of species reactivities, 6, 7
Protein G affinity chromatography, determination of optimal conditions, 357–358
Protein G agarose, use of to make antigen-binding column, 363–365
Protein G from group G Streptococci and protein A from *Staphylococcus aureus*, 222–224
Protein G genes from other isolates, cloning, 423–424
Protein L, 16–17
Protein P, 17
Proteins, new, identification, 442–444
Proteins, manipulation, 444–445
Proteus vulgaris, 244–246
Purified bacterial surface proteins, analysis of binding of immunoglobulins and others, 97–98
Purification of MOPC 21, mouse IgG_1 monoclonal antibody, loaded at pH 7.0 and pH 5.0, 361–362
Purification procedure, overview, 313–320
Purification of immunoglobulins on protein-A Sepharose, summary of methods, 314–319

Quantitation of antigens in two-stage competitive radioimmunoassay, 138–141

Index

Quantitation of monoclonal antibodies, 345–346
Quantitation of specific antibodies using competitive binding assay, 115–119
  materials, 116–117
  procedure, 117–119

Rabbit IgM antibodies to sheep erythrocytes, detection, 190–194
Radioimmunocytochemistry, technique using biotinylated IgG-binding proteins, 207–208
Radioimmunoassay (RIA), 1
Radioiodination buffer, 455
Radiolabeled bacterial Fc-binding proteins as tracers for soluble antigens
  competitive inhibition radioimmunoassay, 127–141
  developing competitive binding immunoassay, 135–138
  immobilizing the agent, 127–129
  quantitation of antigens in two–stage competitive radioimmunoassay, 138–141
  radiolabeling the tracer, 129–135
  studies, 125–127
Radiolabeled Fc-binding tracer, probing membrane, 254
Recombinant protein G to wild type protein G isolated from *Streptococcus* cell membranes, 201
Recombinant lambda bacteriophage isolate for expression of streptococcal plasmin-binding protein, screening, 261–263
RIA, *see* radioimmunoassay

SDS-PAGE sample buffer, 278–279
Second generation immunoglobulin-binding proteins, 15–17
  IgA Fc-binding proteins, 15–16
  IgD-binding proteins, 16
  protein L, 16–17
  protein P, 17
Secreted IgG-binding proteins, 55–68
Sheep erythrocytes
  with antibody, sensitization, 374–375
  concentration, standardization, 374
  reagents, 373
  standardization, 373–374
Sheep erythrocytes (SRBC), sensitized, 26–27
Silver enhancement of colloidal gold marker, with two different primary antibodies, 234–236
Slide agglutination test for bacterial-binding proteins, 27
Sodium dodecyl sulfate polyacrylamide gel electrophoresis, 264–267
Solid phase radioassay or enzyme-linked immunosorbent assay, 96–97
Solid phase, binding to host proteins, 99
Solubilization of immunoglobulin-binding bacterial surface proteins, 93–95
Soluble Fc-binding proteins, competitive binding radioimmunoassay, 59–63
  materials, 60
  procedure, 60–63
Soluble immunoglobulin proteins, extraction and monitoring, *see* Extraction and monitoring of soluble immunoglobulin proteins
Solubilized immunoglobulin-binding proteins, detection, 57–64
Specific antibody, detection, 294–296
SRBC, *see* Sheep erythrocytes, sensitive
Staphylococcus aureus, 4–5, 28, 39, 43–44, 56, 83, 279–284, 285
  and lysostaphin extraction treatment, 53–54
  preparation, 25
  protein A-positive, 275
    fixation, 275–276
    growth, 275
  storage and stability, 277–278
  and type VI protein, 14
Staphylococcal protein A, and *in vivo* assay procedure, 407
Stock trisodium ethylenediaminetetraacetate, 454
Streptavidin/avidin-biotin labeling for detection of immunoglobulin-binding proteins, 236–238
Streptococcal DNA, preparation, 419–420
Streptococcal protein G genes, cloning
  cloning of protein G genes from other isolates, 423–424
  colony immunoassay, 417–419

initial gene cloning, 420–423
preparation of Streptococcal DNA, 419–420
Streptococcal clinical isolates, 419
Streptococci, group B, use of Fc-binding proteins to identify cell surface and secreted antigens associated
dot blot assay, adaptation of two-stage, 172–175
dot blot autoradiographic procedure for detection of group B Streptococcal antigens, 172–173
results of dot blot autoradiographic procedure to detect cell surface and secreted group B Streptococcal antigens, 173–175
ELISA typing procedure, adaptation of two-stage RIA, 175–177
studies, 161–162
summary of precipitation assay and two-stage RIA typing results, 168–169
two-stage radioimmunoassay for detection of group B streptococcal type-specific antigens, 163–165
bacterial strains, media and growth conditions, 164
iodinization of protein A and protein G, 164–165
source of group B streptococcal-typing antisera, 164
two-stage radioimmunoassay for determination of subtypes of group B Streptococcal strains, 165
results, 165–172
typing nomenclature, 162–163
Streptococci, protein B–positive, 276
Streptococcus 26RP66, affinity purification of type III Fc-binding protein, 75–77, 80
Streptococcus dysgalactiae, 3
Streptococcus equisimilus, 3
Streptococcus mutans, 51
Streptococcus zooepidemicus, 3, 40, 44, 279, 280
and type V protein, 14
and type VI protein, 14
Streptomyces avidinii, 198
Streptomyces globisporus, 51

T cell lymphocyte differentiation, 398–400
T cell/B cell separation, 394–395
T cell/B cell preparations, panning method for purification
Taenia solium cysticeri, 213
TBS-Tween buffer, 455
Tetramethylrhodamine isothiocyanate (TRITC), 197–199
Therapeutic applications of IgG-binding proteins, potential, 445–447
Titration of amount of colloid to bind protein sample, 224–225
Tracer, radiolabeling, 129–135
important note, 130–131
iodinating proteins with Bolton-Hunter reagent, 132–133
iodinating proteins with chloramine-T, 131–132
iodinating proteins with lactoperoxidase, 132
separating proteins from free iodine, 133–135
Tris-buffered saline, 455
TRITC, *see* Tetramethylrhodamine isothiocyanate
Trypsin digestion, 52
Tube agglutination test for bacterial-binding proteins, 27
Tumor-associated antigens, detection of antibodies, 186–190
Turbidity, standardization based on measurement, 26
Two-stage competitive binding assay for detection of soluble antigen, 149
Two-stage radioimmunoassay for detection of group B streptococcal type-specific antigens, 163–165
Two-stage radioimmunoassay for determination of subtypes of group B Streptococcal strains, 165
Type I proteins, comparisons, 4–8
Type II proteins, 9
future trends, 428
Type III proteins, 9–13
Type III Fc-binding protein alkaline phosphatase conjugate, using as tracer for development of ELISA to quantify human IgA, 152–159

establishing optimal concentration of each reagent, 154–156
immobilizing antigen onto microtiter plates, 153–154
optimization of reaction conditions for detection of human IgA, 156–159
Type III Fc-binding protein, affinity purification of, 75–77
Type III Fc-binding protein to alkaline phosphatase, conjugation, 151–152
materials, 151
procedure, 151–152
Type IV proteins, 13
future trends, 426–427
Type V proteins, 14
future trends, 426–427
Type VI proteins, 14
future trends, 426–427, 428
Typing nomenclature, 162–163

Urokinase, and *in vivo* assay procedure, 407

VECSTAIN *Elite* ABC kit, 209–210, 212
Veronal-buffered saline stock, 453–454

Volume/volume ratio, standardization of bacterial cell number, 25

Wash buffer I, 458
Wash buffer II, 458
Western blot analysis, 82–84, 95, 263–269
of immunoglobulin-binding protein heterogeneity, 66–68
to study immunoglobulin-binding bacterial proteins, 99–100
Western blotting techniques, antigenic analysis of soluble immunoglobulin-binding proteins, 120–121
Wet weight/volume ratio, standardization of bacterial cell number, 25
Whole bacteria as source of immobilized immunoglobulin-binding protein, use, 111–113
materials, 112
procedure, 112–113

Yolks, egg, and PBS extraction, collection, 109–110